Kozier and Erb's
Techniques
in Clinical Nursing

Fifth Edition

AUDREY BERMAN, PhD, RN, AOCN
Professor
Associate Dean, Nursing
Coordinator Academic Computing
Samuel Merritt College
Oakland, California

SHIRLEE SNYDER, EdD, RN
Nursing Program Director
Community College of Southern Nevada
Las Vegas, Nevada

BARBARA KOZIER, RN, MN

GLENORA ERB, RN, BSN

Prentice
Hall

Upper Saddle River, New Jersey 07458

Library of Congress Cataloging-in-Publication Data

Kozier & Erb's techniques in clinical nursing / Audrey Berman
... [et al.].—5th ed.
    p. cm.
  Prev. ed. cataloged under: Techniques in clinical nursing.
  Includes bibliographical references and index.
  ISBN 0-13-028157-3
    1. Nursing. I. Title: Techniques in clinical nursing. II.
Berman, Audrey. III. Kozier, Barbara. IV. Erb, Glenora Lea,
1937-

RT41 .K723 2002
610.73—dc21

2001034047

Publisher: Julie Alexander
Executive Editor: Maura Connor
Acquisitions Editor: Nancy Anselment
Marketing Manager: Nicole Benson
Development Editor: Jeanne Allison
Editorial Assistant: Sarah Caffrey
**Director of Manufacturing
  and Production:** Bruce Johnson
Managing Editor: Patrick Walsh
Production Editor: Linda Begley, Rainbow Graphics
Production Liaison: Cathy O'Connell
Manufacturing Manager: Ilene Sanford
Design Director: Cheryl Asherman
Senior Designer: Maria Guglielmo
Cover Design: Jill Little
Cover Art: Steve Anderson
Interior Design: Jennifer Bergamini, Alamini Design
Composition: Rainbow Graphics
Printing and Binding: Banta Company, Menasha

NOTICE

Care has been taken to confirm the accuracy of information presented in this book. The authors, editors, and the publisher, however, cannot accept any responsibility for errors or omissions or for consequences from application of the information in this book and make no warranty, express or implied, with respect to its contents.

The authors and publisher have exerted every effort to ensure that drug selections and dosages set forth in this text are in accord with current recommendations and practice at time of publication. However, in view of ongoing research, changes in government regulations, and the constant flow of information relating to drug therapy and drug reactions, the reader is urged to check the package inserts of all drugs for any change in indications of dosage and for added warnings and precautions. This is particularly important when the recommended agent is a new and/or infrequently employed drug.

Pearson Education LTD.
Pearson Education Australia PTY, Limited
Pearson Education Singapore, Pte. Ltd
Pearson Education North Asia Ltd
Pearson Education Canada, Ltd.
Pearson Educación de Mexico, S.A. de C.V.
Pearson Education–Japan
Pearson Education Malaysia, Pte. Ltd

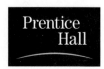
Prentice Hall

10 9 8 7 6 5 4 3 2 1
ISBN 0-13-028157-3

We dedicate this book to: Audrey's daughter, Jordanna Elise MacIntyre, who provided motivation and assistance with this book in both measurable and immeasurable ways.

Shirlee's husband, Terry J. Schnitter, whose continual love, support, and encouragement made this professional accomplishment possible and to her parents, Jean and Everett Snyder, who instilled in their daughter a love for learning.

Brief Contents

Contents

Contents *continued*

Contents *continued*

Contents *continued*

Contents *continued*

Contents *continued*

Contents *continued*

Contents *continued*

Unit VIII Wounds and Injury Care

Chapter 30 Performing Wound and Pressure Ulcer Care   619

Chapter 31 Cast Care   644

Chapter 32 Performing Perioperative Care   654

Techniques

Techniques *continued*

Techniques *continued*

Techniques *continued*

Preface

The techniques performed by nurses exemplify the integration of knowledge, skill, attitude, and critical thinking necessary for effective clinical practice in the twenty-first century. The fifth edition of *Techniques in Clinical Nursing* has been completely revised and updated to reflect the significant changes in practice that have occurred since the previous edition. It includes:

- The 166 most important techniques performed by nurses, including all common variations, organized from the simple to the more complex

- New techniques such as Standard Precautions, Implementing Seizure Precautions, Applying a Sequential Compression Device, Measuring Peak Expiratory Flow, Administering Basic Life Support to the Hospitalized Client, and Using Alginates on Wounds

- A total of 684 color illustrations and 118 new full-color photographs

Techniques in Clinical Nursing is intended as a primary textbook for nursing education programs and as a reference for practicing nurses. Content was selected based on feedback from reviewers of previous editions, a market survey by the publisher, and the extensive teaching and practice experience of the authors.

New Technique Format

Each chapter contains concise introductory material, placing the techniques in perspective to client anatomy, physiology, and pathophysiology, and provides an overview of the rationale and purpose of the techniques. The presentation of each technique follows the steps of the nursing process and contains:

- Review of the **assessment** data required before performing the technique

- As a component of the **planning** phase, when it is and is not appropriate to delegate each technique to unlicensed assistive personnel (UAP)

- **Implementation** steps, including client teaching, observation of standard infection control precautions, and client record documentation. Rationales are indicated by italic type

- Considerations in **evaluation** of the technique, focusing on steps indicated for follow-up and communication with other members of the health care team

Hallmark Features

The fifth edition builds on the successful aspects of previous editions. The strong emphasis on assisting the learner and practitioner has been maintained by including:

- Performance objectives

- Detailed step-by-step implementation

- Research and supplemental references

- Extensive use of tables, boxes, and diagrams

New Features

Age-Related Considerations

With each technique for which they are appropriate, modifications and special deliberations indicated when caring for infants, children, and elders are placed in highlighted boxes.

Modifications in Ambulatory and Community Settings

Increasingly, nurses are performing techniques in home and clinic environments that require adaptation from the steps used in hospitals. This featured content outlines client teaching regarding self-care and communication with the health care team, involvement of lay caregivers, and suggestions for altering techniques as indicated by the physical environment.

Forming Clinical Judgments

The nurse is challenged to consider appropriate responses to situations that can arise in performing the techniques in each chapter. Answers to the "Consider This" items are found in the Instructor's Manual.

Terminology

A list of key terms is found at the end of each chapter.

Acknowledgments

Special thanks to those without whom this edition would not have been possible:

- **Jeanne Allison**, Developmental Editor, who guided, facilitated, supported, and shepherded each step in the development and production of this book

- **Nancy Anselment**, Nursing Editor, without whose championing belief in the importance of this book, it would never have come to be

- **George Draper**, photographer, whose dedication to detail helped ensure the many accurate and visually clear new photographs

- **The reviewers**, who provided many helpful comments

- **The staff and patients of Summit Medical Center**, Oakland, California, for their permission and cooperation with the photographs

- **The students of Samuel Merritt College**, Oakland, California, and those of the **Community College of Southern Nevada**, Las Vegas, Nevada, for serving as models for much of the new photography

Reviewers

M. J. Basti, RN, BSN, MSN, CNAA
Cuesta Community College
San Luis Obispo, CA

Margaret W. Bellak, MN, RN
Indiana University of Pennsylvania
Indiana, PA

Janet Brown, RN, MSN, CS
Associate Professor
School of Nursing
California State University
Chico, CA

Jeanie Burt, RN, MA
Assistant Professor
School of Nursing
Harding University
Searchy, AR

Carolyn F. Duke, MSN
Assistant Professor
School of Nursing
Saint Louis University
St. Louis, MO

Toni Worthan, BSN, RN, MSN
Nursing Department
Madisonville Community College
Madisonville, KY

Techniques in Clinical Nursing

IMPLEMENTATION:
TECHNIQUE 5-1 SUPPORTING THE CLIENT'S POSITION IN BED

Equipment

The following equipment can be used when positioning clients:

- Pillows—one to six depending on client need
- Trochanter rolls
- Footboard
- Hand rolls or wrist splints, if needed
- Folded towel
- Sandbag or rolled towel

Preparation

- Check the position-change schedule for the next time and type of position change.
- Administer an analgesic, if appropriate, before changing the client's position.
- Obtain required assistance, as needed.

Performance

1. Explain to the client what you are going to do, why it is necessary, and how he or she can cooperate. Discuss how the results will be used in planning further care or treatments.

2. Wash hands and observe other appropriate infection control procedures.

3. Provide for client privacy.

Supporting a Client in Fowler's Position

1. Position the client.
   - Have the client flex the knees slightly before raising the head of the bed. *Slight knee flexion prevents the person from sliding toward the foot of the bed as the bed is raised.* Be certain the client's hips are positioned directly over the point where the bed will bend when the head is raised. *An appropriate hip position ensures that the client will be sitting upright when the head of the bed is raised.*
   - Raise the head of the bed to 45° or the angle required by or ordered for the client.

2. Provide supportive devices to align the client appropriately (see Box 5-3).
   - Place a small pillow or roll under the lumbar region of the back if you feel a space in the lumbar curvature. *The pillow supports the natural lum-*

Techniques include step-by-step instructions for each skill, as well as content regarding client teaching, observation of Standard Infection Control Precautions, and client record documentation. Rationales (*in italics*) support critical steps of each technique.

Variation: A Client Who Has Limited Strength of the Upper Extremities

- Assist the client to flex the hips and knees as in step 5 previously. Place the client's arms across the chest. *This keeps them off the bed surface and minimizes friction during movement.* Ask the client to flex the neck during the move and keep the head off the bed surface.

- Position yourself as in step 6 and place one arm under the client's back and shoulders and the other arm under the client's thighs. *This placement of the arms distributes the client's weight and supports the heaviest part of the body (the buttocks).* Shift your weight as in step 6.

Variations present alternative methods of performing certain techniques.

Delegation highlights when it is and is not appropriate to delegate a technique to unlicensed assistive personnel (UAP).

PLANNING

Delegation

Measuring and recording of oral intake and urine output is often delegated to unlicensed assistive personnel (UAP). It is important for the nurse to stress the importance of accurate measuring and recording. The UAP needs to be aware of the importance of reporting any changes in a client's intake as well as changes in color, amount, and odor of output and the presence of stool and/or urine incontinence. Certain intake such as tube feedings, parenteral fluids, intravenous medications, and catheter or tube irrigants are measured and recorded by the nurse rather than the UAP because of the need to apply professional knowledge and problem solving. Likewise, the nurse measures output from tube drainage (e.g., Hemovac, Jackson–Pratt) because of the need for cleansing the drain site to minimize the introduction of microbes into the closed system.

Urine Specimen

- Assess the client's ability and willingness to collect a timed urine specimen. If poor eyesight or hand tremors are a problem, suggest using a clean funnel to pour the urine into the container.
- Always wash hands well with warm, soapy water before and after collecting urine samples.

- Always wear gloves if handling another person's urine.

The home should have a refrigerator or other method for cooling the urine samples. Tell the client to keep the specimen container in a plastic or paper bag in the refrigerator, separate from other refrigerator contents. The client may also use a cooler with ice.

Ambulatory and Community Settings provide information related to the specific health care setting regarding client teaching about self-care, communication with the healthcare team, involvement of lay caregivers, and suggestions for altering techniques as indicated by the physical environment.

Age-Related Considerations present age-related content to alert the nurse to differences encountered with infants, children, and elders.

Urine Specimen

Infant

- The process for cleaning the perineal area and the urethral opening is similar to the process for an adult. A specimen bag, however, is used to collect the urine specimen. The specimen bag has an adhesive backing that attaches to the skin. After the infant has voided a desired amount, gently remove the bag from the skin.
- If you are having trouble obtaining a bagged urine specimen from an infant, try cutting a hole in the diaper (front for a boy and middle for a girl) and pulling part of the bag through. You can see when urine is collected without having to untape the diaper (Lindemann, 2000).

Child

- When collecting a routine urine specimen, explain the procedure in simple, nonmedical terms to the child and ask the child to void using a potty chair or a bedpan placed inside the toilet.
- Give the child a clean specimen container to play with.
- Allow a parent to assist the child, if possible. The child may feel more comfortable with a parent.

Elders

- For a clean-catch urine specimen, an older adult may have difficulty controlling the stream of urine.
- An older adult with arthritis may have difficulty holding the labia apart during the collection of a clean-catch urine specimen.

Forming Clinical Judgments

promotes critical thinking through the application of essential skills content to real-life scenarios.

FORMING CLINICAL JUDGMENTS

Consider This:

1. What should you do if I&O has been ordered for a client and the client informs you that he voided but forgot to use the urinal?
2. What if, when measuring CBG, you do not obtain enough blood to cover the indicator square on the reagent strip?
3. What should you do if the stool becomes contaminated with urine or toilet paper when collecting a stool specimen?
4. What should you do if the client or staff forgot and discarded the client's urine during the collection of a timed 24-hour urine specimen?
5. What if your assessments clearly indicate a wound infection but the culture results return indicating no growth?

Chapter 1

Foundational Techniques
Techniques

Techniques

OBJECTIVES

- Identify appropriate situations requiring handwashing.
- Correctly implement Standard Precautions, including donning and removing personal protective equipment: mask, eyewear, gown, unsterile gloves.
- Describe nursing activities that are appropriate or inappropriate to delegate to unlicensed assistive personnel.
- Describe safety measures when assisting others to perform procedures.
- Demonstrate key elements to include in the documentation of any technique or procedure.

This chapter introduces the techniques that are fundamental to all nursing care. All techniques must be performed with special attention to the use of equipment and procedures that protect the nurse and the client. In addition, techniques must be documented in the client record. Some nursing techniques are performed directly—the nurse provides the care to the client. Other nursing care is indirect—care is provided to the client by another nurse, by **unlicensed assistive personnel (UAP)**, or by family or other lay caregivers. Indirect care may only be entrusted (delegated) to others if certain conditions exist. This chapter describes the process of nurse delegation.

Safe performance of nursing care is founded on the principles of health promotion and maintenance. Therefore, the most important actions of the nurse include preventing the transmission of potentially infective organisms among the nurse, the client, and other individuals. Handwashing, standard infection precautions, and use of personal protective equipment are those fundamental techniques presented in this chapter. Further information about caring for clients who are known to have infections is found in Chapter 12.

Handwashing

Any client may harbor microorganisms that are currently harmless to the client yet potentially harmful to another person or to the same client if they find a portal of entry to a different part of the body. Handwashing is important in every setting where people are cared for, including hospitals. It is considered the most effective measure of controlling **nosocomial infections** (those that originate in the hospital) and is defined as "a vigorous, brief rubbing together of all surfaces of lathered hands" (Garner & Favero, 1998). The goal of handwashing is to remove transient microorganisms that might be transmitted to the nurse, clients, visitors, or other health care personnel. Box 1-1 lists times when nurses should wash their hands. Although handwashing is appropriate at all the listed times, washing the hands more than several times every hour damages the skin and can lead to an increase in the number of organisms transmitted from the hands. Moisturizing the skin with lotion after handwashing between clients can help protect the skin from excessive drying.

For routine client care, the Centers for Disease Control and Prevention (CDC) recommends a vigorous handwashing under a stream of water for at least 10 seconds using bar soap, granule soap, soap-filled sheets, or antimicrobial liquid soap. Liquid soaps are frequently supplied in dispensers at the sink. Antimicrobial soaps are usually provided in high-risk areas (e.g., the newborn nursery). In the following situations, the CDC recommends antimicrobial hand-

Box 1-1 *Times for Handwashing*

Unless there is an emergency,

Before
- Invasive procedures
- Caring for susceptible individuals such as newborns and immunocompromised
- Handling wounds
- Serving food

After
- Handling wounds
- Handling contaminated items such as bedpans or wet linens
- Caring for infected clients
- Removing gloves

Between
- Caring for individual clients

Note: Overwashing with soaps and detergents more than several times per hour damages the skin and can increase transmission of microorganisms (Metules 2000).

washing agents with any chemical germicides listed with the Environmental Protection Agency:

- When there are known multiple resistant bacteria
- Before invasive procedures
- In special care units, such as nurseries and intensive care units (ICUs)
- Before caring for severely immunocompromised clients

Nursing Process: Handwashing

ASSESSMENT

Determine the client's:

- Risk for acquiring an infection
- Current receipt of immunosuppressive medications
- Recent diagnostic procedures or treatments that penetrated the skin or a body cavity
- Current nutritional status
- Signs and symptoms indicating the presence of an infection:
  - Localized signs—swelling, redness, pain or tenderness with palpation or movement, palpable heat at site, loss of function of affected body part, presence of exudate
  - Systemic indications—fever, increased pulse and respiratory rates, lack of energy, anorexia, enlarged lymph nodes

Determine the location of sinks/running water and soap or soap substitutes.

Delegation

The technique of handwashing is identical for all health care providers, including unlicensed assistive personnel. Health care team members must be accountable that they and others implement appropriate handwashing procedures.

IMPLEMENTATION:

TECHNIQUE 1-1 HANDWASHING

Equipment

- Soap, foam, benzalkonium chloride–based or alcohol gel sanitizer
- Warm running water (for soap only)
- Towels (for soap and water only)

Preparation

Assess the hands.

- Nails should be kept short. *Short, natural nails are less likely to harbor microorganisms, scratch a client, or puncture gloves.*
- Remove all jewelry. *Microorganisms can lodge in the settings of jewelry and under rings. Removal facilitates proper cleaning of the hands and arms.*
- Check hands for breaks in the skin, such as hangnails or cuts. *A nurse who has open sores may require a work assignment with decreased risk for transmission of infectious organisms.*

Performance

1. If appropriate, explain to the client what you are going to do, why it is necessary, and how he or she can cooperate. Discuss how the results will be used in planning further care or treatments.

2. Turn on the water, and adjust the flow.
   - There are five common types of faucet controls:
     a. Hand-operated handles.
     b. Knee levers. Move these with the knee to regulate flow and temperature (Figure 1-1 ◆).
     c. Foot pedals. Press these with the foot to regulate flow and temperature (Figure 1-2 ◆).
     d. Elbow controls. Move these with the elbows instead of the hands.
     e. Infrared control. Motion in front of the sensor causes water to start and stop flowing automatically.
   - Adjust the flow so that the water is warm. *Warm water removes less of the protective oil of the skin than hot water.*

3. Wet the hands thoroughly by holding them under the running water, and apply soap to the hands.

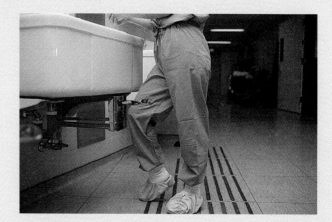

FIGURE 1-1 ◆ A knee-lever faucet control.

- Hold the hands lower than the elbows so that the water flows from the arms to the fingertips. *The water should flow from the least contaminated to the most contaminated area; the hands are generally considered more contaminated than the lower arms.*
- If the soap is liquid, apply 2 to 4 mL (1 tsp). If it is bar soap, granules, or sheets, rub them firmly between the hands.

4. Thoroughly wash and rinse the hands.
   - Use firm, rubbing, and circular movements to wash the palm, back, and wrist of each hand. Interlace the fingers and thumbs, and move the hands back and forth (Figure 1-3 ◆). Continue this motion for 10 seconds. *The circular action helps remove microorganisms mechanically.*

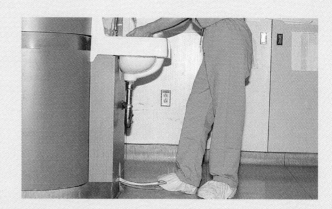

FIGURE 1-2 ◆ A foot-pedal faucet control.

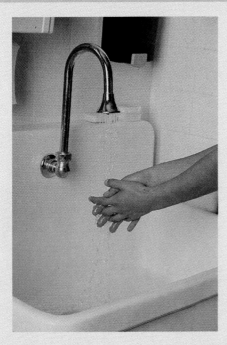

FIGURE 1-3 ◆ Interlacing the fingers during handwashing.

Interlacing the fingers and thumbs cleans the inter-digital spaces.

- Rub the fingertips against the palm of the opposite hand. *The nails and fingertips are commonly missed during handwashing* (Gould, 1997).
- Rinse the hands.

5. Thoroughly dry the hands and arms.
   - Dry hands and arms thoroughly with a paper towel. *Moist skin becomes chapped readily; chapping produces lesions.*
   - Discard the paper towel in the appropriate container.

6. Turn off the water.
   - Use a new paper towel to grasp a hand-operated control (Figure 1-4 ◆). *This prevents the nurse from picking up microorganisms from the faucet handles.*

Variation: Handwashing Before Sterile Techniques

- Apply the soap and wash as described in step 4, but hold the hands higher than the elbows during

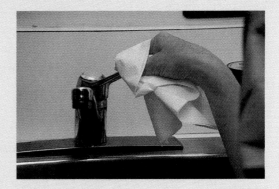

FIGURE 1-4 ◆ Using a paper towel to grasp the handle of a hand-operated faucet.

this handwash. Wet the hands and forearms under the running water, letting it run from the fingertips to the elbows so that the hands become cleaner than the elbows. (Figure 1-5 ◆). *In this way, the water runs from the area that now has the fewest microorganisms to areas with a relatively greater number.*

- After washing and rinsing, use a towel to dry one hand thoroughly in a rotating motion from the fingers to the elbow. Use a new towel to dry the other hand and arm. *A clean towel prevents the transfer of microorganisms from one elbow (least clean area) to the other hand (cleanest area).*

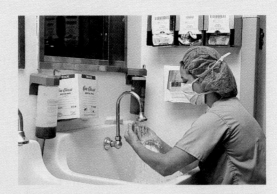

FIGURE 1-5 ◆ The hands are held higher than the elbows during a handwash before a sterile technique.

AMBULATORY AND COMMUNITY SETTINGS

Handwashing

When making a home visit:

- Keep fingernails clean, short, and well-trimmed.
- Wash hands carefully before and after any hands-on care.
- If there is no running water, use commercially

available handwashing agents that require no water.

- You may wish to bring your own bactericidal soap and paper towels for use when washing hands.
- Always turn the water off with a dry paper towel.

Standard Precautions

Microorganisms occur normally in various locations of the human body such as the surface of the skin and the gastrointestinal tract. Usually, they do not cause infection in the client. When the microorganisms enter a different part of the client's body, or the client's immune system is suppressed, infection may occur. Also, these same microorganisms could cause infection in another person. Because it is not always possible to know which clients may have infectious organisms, a set of guidelines have been established by the CDC (USDHHS, 1997) and other organizations outlining steps all health care workers must follow to reduce the chances that organisms in blood (**bloodborne pathogens**) and potentially infectious organisms from other body tissues are transmitted from the client to other persons. These are called Tier One: **Standard Precautions (SP)**. Some agencies may use an earlier term—**Universal Precautions**—reflecting their applicability in all client care situations. If the client is known to have an infection, the CDC's Tier Two: Transmission-Based Precautions are used to protect the nurse and others from acquiring the infectious organism (see Chapter 12).

Nursing Process: Standard Precautions

ASSESSMENT

- All health care providers use SP during contact with all clients.
- SP apply to:
  - Blood
  - All body fluids, excretions, and secretions except sweat and tears
  - Nonintact (broken) skin
  - Mucous membranes

PLANNING

Consider the procedures about to be performed and determine which aspects require SP. Gather all necessary equipment. Review the steps of SP as indicated.

IMPLEMENTATION:
TECHNIQUE 1-2 STANDARD PRECAUTIONS

Equipment

Depending on the specific aspects of the procedures, have available **personal protective equipment (PPE)**:

- Nonsterile (clean) gloves
- Waterproof gown
- Eye protection/goggles
- Mask

Performance

1. If PPE will be used, explain to the client why this is necessary and that SP are performed with all clients. *The client should understand that SP are used to protect clients and health care workers.*

2. Wash hands after contact with blood, body fluids, secretions, excretions, and contaminated objects (linens, dressings, instruments, or any other items that have come in contact with potentially infective material) whether or not gloves are worn. *Gloves can develop invisible holes during use. Moisture that collects on hands under gloves promotes the growth of microorganisms.*

3. Wear gloves during contact with blood, body fluids, secretions, excretions, and contaminated objects. See Technique 1-3.

4. Wear a mask, eye protection, or a face shield and a clean, waterproof gown if client care is likely to involve splashes or sprays of blood, body fluids, secretions, or excretions. See Technique 1-3.

5. Ensure that objects that have come in contact with blood, body fluids, secretions, or excretions are disposed of or cleaned properly. Check labels or procedure manuals for details regarding proper disposal or decontamination.

6. Place used needles and other "sharps" directly into puncture-resistant containers as soon as their use is completed. Do not attempt to recap needles or place sharps back in their sheaths using two hands; use the one-handed scoop technique or other safety device. *Using two hands can result in a needle-stick/puncture injury if the nurse accidentally misses the cover.*

7. Handle all soiled linen as little as possible so that the nurse's uniform or clothing is not contaminated.

8. Place all human tissue and laboratory specimens in leakproof containers. If the outside of the container becomes contaminated (soiled), place the container in a sealable plastic bag prior to transport.

Health care workers can be exposed to potentially infective materials through puncture wounds, direct contact with broken skin or wounds, or mucous membrane contact. Contact between potentially infective material and intact skin is not normally considered a risk for transmission of infection. If there is concern that the exposure has a significant risk for transmission of bloodborne pathogens such as hepatitis or human immunodeficiency virus (HIV) due to the large volume of material or percutaneous (through the skin) exposure, the nurse should follow the steps in Box 1-2.

Personal Protective Equipment

Gloves

Disposable clean gloves are worn to protect the hands when the nurse is likely to handle any potentially infective objects or materials (e.g., blood, urine, feces, sputum, mucous membranes, nonintact skin, and used equipment). Gloves also reduce the likelihood of the nurse's transmitting any potentially infectious organisms to clients. Nurses who have open sores or cuts on the hands should wear gloves for protection. Sterile gloves are used when the hands will come in contact with sterile equipment or wounds (see Chapter 12).

Gloves are to be worn when indicated, but only then. Wearing gloves when not indicated is costly and can actually increase the risk of error because working with gloves is more difficult than working with bare hands. It is not necessary to wear gloves during routine bathing (except when performing perineal care), ambulating clients, touching intact skin, handling intravenous fluid bags, taking vitals signs, or changing linens—unless, of course, body fluid spillage or contamination is present.

Many types of clean gloves contain latex rubber. Increasingly, both clients and health care workers are developing allergies to latex. In addition, latex gloves lubricated by cornstarch or powder are particularly allergenic because the latex allergen adheres to the lubricant and is aerosolized and inhaled during use. If either the client or the nurse is known to have a latex sensitivity, vinyl or other nonlatex gloves must be used.

Gowns

Clean (cloth) or disposable (paper) gowns or plastic aprons are worn when the nurse's uniform is likely to become soiled. Generally, disposable gowns are used in hospitals. The gown must have a waterproof layer, making it impermeable to liquids and body fluids.

Face Masks/Face Shields/Eyewear

In Standard Precautions, masks are worn to prevent potentially infective material from entering the

---

Box 1-2 *Steps to Follow After Exposure to Bloodborne Pathogens*

- Report the incident immediately to appropriate personnel within the agency.
- Complete an injury report.
- Seek appropriate evaluation and follow-up. This includes:
  - Identification and documentation of the source individual when feasible and legal
  - Testing of the source individual's blood when feasible and consent is given
  - Making results of the test available to the source individual's health care provider
  - Testing of blood of exposed nurse (with consent)
  - Postexposure prophylaxis if medically indicated with hepatitis vaccine or antiviral agents
  - Medical and psychological counseling regarding personal risk of infection or risk of infecting others
- For a puncture/laceration:
  - Encourage bleeding
  - Wash/clean the area with soap and water
  - Initiate first-aid and seek treatment if indicated

- For a mucous membrane exposure (eyes, nose, mouth), saline or water flush for 5 to 10 minutes

HIV Postexposure Protocol (PEP)

- For "high-risk" exposure (high blood volume *and* source with a high HIV titer): three-drug treatment is encouraged. Must be started within 1 hour.
- For "increased-risk" exposure (high blood volume *or* source with a high HIV titer): three-drug treatment is encouraged. Must be started within 1 hour.
- For "low-risk" exposure (neither high blood volume nor source with a high HIV titer): two-drug treatment is offered. Must be started within 1 hour.
- Drug prophylaxis is for 4 weeks.
- Drug regimens vary. Drugs commonly used are zidovudine, lamivudine, and indinavir.
- HIV antibody tests done shortly after exposure (baseline), and 6 weeks, 3 months, and 6 months afterward.

nurse's mouth, nose, or eyes during procedures in which blood or other body fluids may splash near the nurse's face. A one-piece unit consisting of a paper mask with a clear plastic shield rising from the mask to protect the eyes is commonly used (see Figure 1-6 ◆). If the nurse wears prescription eyeglasses, goggles may be worn over the glasses.

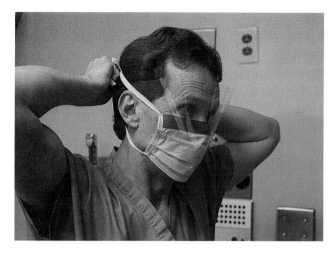

FIGURE 1-6 ◆ A face mask and eye protection covering the nose, mouth, and eyes.

Performance

1. Explain to the client what you are going to do, why it is necessary, and how he or she can cooperate.

2. Wash your hands.

3. Don a clean gown.
   - Pick up a clean gown and allow it to unfold in front of you without allowing it to touch any area soiled with body substances.
   - Slide the arms and the hands through the sleeves.
   - Fasten the ties at the neck to keep the gown in place.
   - Overlap the gown at the back as much as possible, and fasten the waist ties or belt (Figure 1-7 ◆). *Overlapping securely covers the uniform at the back. Waist ties keep the gown from falling away from the body and prevent inadvertent soiling of the uniform.*

4. Don the face mask.
   - Locate the top edge of the mask. The mask usually has a narrow metal strip along the edge.
   - Hold the mask by the top two strings or loops.
   - Place the upper edge of the mask over the bridge of the nose, and tie the upper ties at the back of the head or secure the loops around the ears. If glasses are worn, fit the upper edge of the mask under the glasses. *With the edge of the mask under the glasses, clouding of the glasses is less likely to occur.*
   - Secure the lower edge of the mask under the chin, and tie the lower ties at the nape of the

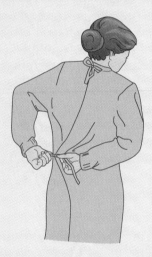

FIGURE 1-7 ◆ Overlapping the gown at the back to cover the nurse's uniform.

neck. *To be effective, a mask must cover both the nose and the mouth, because air moves in and out of both.*
   - If the mask has a metal strip, adjust this firmly over the bridge of the nose. *A secure fit prevents both the escape and the inhalation of microorganisms around the edges of the mask and the fogging of eyeglasses.*
   - Wear the mask only once, and do not wear any mask longer than the manufacturer recommends or once it becomes wet. *A mask should be used only once because it becomes ineffective when moist.*
   - Do not leave a used face mask hanging around the neck.

5. Don clean disposable gloves.

- No special technique is required.
- If you are wearing a gown, pull the gloves up to cover the cuffs of the gown. If you are not wearing a gown, pull the gloves up to cover the wrists.

6. To remove soiled personal protective equipment, remove the gloves first because they are the most soiled.

   - If wearing a gown that is tied at the waist in front, undo the ties before removing gloves.
   - Remove the first glove by grasping it on its palmar surface just below the cuff, taking care to touch only glove to glove (Figure 1-8 ◆). *This keeps the soiled parts of the used gloves from touching the skin of the wrist or hand.*
   - Pull the first glove completely off by inverting or rolling the glove inside out.
   - Continue to hold the inverted removed glove by the fingers of the remaining gloved hand. Place the first two fingers of the bare hand inside the cuff of the second glove (Figure 1-9 ◆). *Touching the outside of the second soiled glove with the bare hand is avoided.*
   - Pull the second glove off the fingers by turning it inside out. This pulls the first glove inside the second glove. *The soiled part of the glove is folded to the inside to reduce the chance of transferring any microorganisms by direct contact.*
   - Using the bare hand, continue to remove the gloves, which are now inside out, and dispose of them in the waste container (Figure 1-10 ◆).

7. Wash your hands.

8. Remove the mask.

   - If using a mask with strings, first untie the *lower* strings of the mask. *This prevents the top part of the mask from falling onto the chest.*
   - Untie the top strings, and while holding the ties securely, remove the mask from the face. *This prevents hand contact with the moistened, contaminated portion of the mask.*

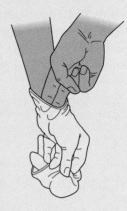

FIGURE 1-9 ◆ Inserting fingers to remove the second contaminated glove.

or

If side loops are present, lift the side loops up and away from the ears and face.

- Discard a disposable mask in the waste container.
- Wash the hands again if they have become contaminated by accidentally touching the soiled part of the mask.

9. Remove the gown when preparing to leave the room. Unless a gown is grossly soiled with body substances, no special precautions are needed to remove it. If a gown is grossly soiled:

   - Avoid touching soiled parts on the outside of the gown, if possible. *The top part of the gown may be soiled, for example, if you have been holding an infant with a respiratory infection.*
   - Grasp the gown along the inside of the neck and pull down over the shoulders.
   - Roll up the gown with the soiled part inside, and discard it in the appropriate container.

10. Remove protective eyewear and dispose of properly or place in the appropriate receptacle for cleaning.

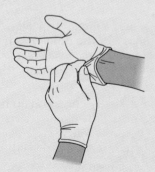

FIGURE 1-8 ◆ Plucking the palmar surface below the cuff of a contaminated glove.

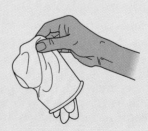

FIGURE 1-10 ◆ Holding the contaminated gloves, which are inside out.

Standard Precautions/Personal Protective Equipment

- All aspects of Standard Precautions apply equally in the clinic, home, or long-term care setting.
- Ensure that there is an adequate supply of gloves, gowns, masks, and eyewear.
- Ensure that procedures are in place for removal and disposal of used materials.
- Teach the client and family appropriate aspects of Standard Precautions.

EVALUATION

Conduct any follow-up indicated during your care of the client. Ensure that an adequate supply of equipment is available for the next health care provider.

Delegation

Since approximately the mid-1990s, increasing numbers of UAP have been used in health care settings to increase the work that can be performed by nurses. These "nurse extenders" may be persons identified as certified nursing aides/assistants, home health aides, patient care technicians, orderlies, surgical technicians, or a variety of other titles. They have had diverse degrees of training and experience. They are employees and do not include family members or friends who provide some client care. Each state or province nurse practice act specifies which actions constitute the legal practice of nursing, which actions are the purview only of nurses, and which may be del-egated to others. **Delegation** refers to indirect care—the intended outcome is achieved through the work of someone supervised by a nurse.

It is not possible to generate an exhaustive list of exactly which actions may or may not be delegated to UAP. Examples of tasks that may and may not be delegated are in Box 1-3. A statement regarding delegation is included with the steps for each technique in this book. The unlicensed person may not delegate tasks to another person. Principles guiding the nurse's decision to delegate ensure the safety and quality of outcomes. These principles are listed in Box 1-4. Once the decision has been made to delegate, the nurse must communicate clearly to the UAP and verify that the UAP understands:

- The specific tasks to be done for each client
- When each task is to be done
- The expected outcomes for each task, including parameters outside of which the unlicensed person must immediately report to the nurse (and any action that must urgently be taken)

Box 1-3 *Examples of Tasks That May and May Not Be Delegated to Unlicensed Assistive Personnel*

Tasks That **May** Be Delegated to Unlicensed Assistive Personnel	Tasks That **May Not** Be Delegated to Unlicensed Assistive Personnel
• Vital signs	• Assessment
• Intake and output	• Interpretation of data
• Patient transfers and ambulation	• Nursing diagnosis
• Postmortem care	• Creation of a nursing care plan
• Bathing	• Evaluation of care effectiveness
• Feeding	• Care of invasive lines
• Clean catheterization	• Parenteral medications
• Gastrostomy feedings in established systems	• Venipuncture
• Safety	• Insertion of nasogastric tubes
• Weighing	• Client education
• Simple dressing changes	• Triage
• Suction of chronic tracheostomies	• Telephone advice
• Basic life support (cardiopulmonary resuscitation [CPR])	• Sterile procedures

- Who is available to serve as a resource if needed
- When and in what format (written or verbal) a report on the tasks is expected

A specific task that can be delegated to one UAP may not be appropriate for a different UAP, depending on the UAP's experience and individual skill sets. Also, a task that is appropriate for the UAP to perform with one client may not be appropriate with a different client or the same client under altered circumstances. For example, routine vital signs may be delegated to the UAP for a client in stable condition but would not be delegated for the same client who has become unstable.

It is important to note that the nurse is not held legally responsible for the acts of the unlicensed person but is accountable for the quality of the act of delegation. Delegation can be an extremely useful strategy in providing thorough and effective nursing care. Skill in delegation, however, must be learned and developed over time. The nurse should not hesitate to consult with others regarding the appropriateness of delegation.

Assisting with Procedures

When procedures are performed by the physician or other health care provider, the nurse may be asked to participate in a number of different ways: preparing the client and/or the support persons, monitoring and assisting the client during the procedure, caring for the client after the procedure, and documenting the client's response to the procedure. The procedure may be performed at the bedside, in an examining room, or sometimes in the emergency or special procedures department of a hospital. Many procedures are invasive, involving insertion of an instrument, often a needle, through the skin and withdrawing some fluid or tissue (see Table 1-1 for examples). The fluid or tissue is usually placed in a special container and sent to the hospital laboratory for examination. Although the techniques for taking specimens are considered safe, complications can occur with each of them. The knowledge and skill of the assisting nurse can help minimize complications and maximize the therapeutic value of the procedure.

Nursing Process: Assisting with Procedures

ASSESSMENT

1. Review the physician's order for the procedure, if available. Note carefully the time and place of the planned procedure, any medications or techniques to be performed prior to the procedure (e.g., giving enemas, starting an IV, administering eyedrops), and any documents that must be available.

2. Determine if the client has had this procedure performed previously. If so, obtain the client's knowledge of the procedure and ability to cooperate, how it was performed, and the client's reactions to the procedure. *This information helps the nurse determine what teaching or precautions are needed.*

3. Assess for pertinent health factors, for example, the presence of dyspnea or any drug allergies, particularly allergies to drugs contained in local anes-

TABLE 1-1	COMMON STUDIES INVOLVING REMOVAL OF BODY FLUID OR TISSUES		
Name	**Type of Specimen**	**Source**	**Common Tests**
Lumbar puncture	Spinal fluid	Subarachnoid space of the spinal canal	Pressure, appearance, sugar, protein, cell count, bacteria
Abdominal paracentesis	Ascitic fluid	Peritoneal cavity	Cell count, cells, specific gravity, protein
Thoracentesis	Pleural fluid	Pleural cavity	Cell count, protein
Bone marrow biopsy	Bone marrow	Iliac crest, posterior superior iliac spine, or sternum	Cells, iron
Liver biopsy	Liver tissue	Liver	Carcinoma, cells
Amniocentesis	Amniotic fluid	Amniotic sac	Fetal maturity, genetic abnormalities
Vaginal examination	Cells, secretions	Cervical os or vaginal floor	Papanicolaou test, culture

thetics and skin antiseptics, which could present a problem during the study.

4. Measure vital signs before the procedure.

PLANNING

Carefully review the procedure that will be performed. Reflect on the sequence of events, how long it will take, and what may be required of the client and the nurse at each step. Determine if more than one nurse or assistant will be needed. Arrange for someone to care for other clients if necessary.

Delegation

Unlicensed personnel may be delegated the task of assisting the nurse or other health care provider with some techniques. However, if these activities require the assistant to perform techniques not generally expected of unlicensed personnel, such as sterile technique, they may not be delegated to the UAP. As always, the nurse must verify the UAP's abilities and experience, plus be knowledgeable about agency and regulatory policies and procedures.

IMPLEMENTATION:
TECHNIQUE 1-4 ASSISTING WITH INVASIVE PROCEDURES

Equipment

- Varies according to the procedure.
- Always have extra sterile gloves and other common supplies available.

Preparation

- Ensure that the results of relevant laboratory tests are available
- Determine if a consent form has been signed. Some agencies require a signed consent from the client for special procedures.
- Coordinate the services of personnel from other departments who are involved in the procedure.

Performance

1. Explain to the client what you and any other health care providers are going to do, why it is necessary, and how he or she can cooperate. Discuss how the results will be used in planning further care or treatments.

2. Observe appropriate infection control procedures.

3. Provide for client privacy.

4. Prepare the client.
   - Have the client empty the bladder and bowels prior to the procedure. *This prevents unnecessary discomfort.*
   - Position the client as required for the procedure.
   - Drape the client to expose only the necessary area.

5. Open any sterile trays or equipment that is needed. Fill in labels and laboratory slips with the client's identification data.

- Check with the person performing the procedure to determine the best time for opening supplies.

6. Prepare and provide equipment and medications needed during the procedure.
   - Maintain sterility of dressings, needles, syringes, specimen containers, and other equipment (see Chapter 12).
   - Draw up or pour medications/solutions as needed. If the practitioner is wearing sterile gloves and will be drawing the medication from a vial that you are holding (nonsterile outside), show the practitioner the label and say the name and concentration of the fluid before it is aspirated. For example, show the label while you say "epinephrine one to ten thousand" or "xylocaine one percent without epinephrine" and then tilt the vial top so the practitioner can access it with a needle (Figure 1-11 ◆).

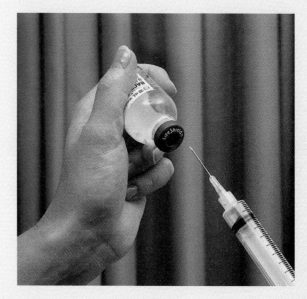

FIGURE 1-11 ◆ Holding a vial.

7. Support the client during the procedure.

- If you are not needed to handle equipment or supplies for the practitioner, position yourself where you can observe and reassure the client.

- Observe the client closely for signs of distress, for example, abnormal pulse, respirations, skin color, or blood pressure; altered level of consciousness.

8. Label any specimens and arrange for them to be sent immediately to the laboratory. *Incorrect identification of specimens can lead to subsequent error of diagnosis or therapy for the client.*

9. Provide required nursing care after the procedure.

- Assist the client to a comfortable position.

- Measure vital signs.

- Wash off any antiseptic or other product applied to the skin.

- Observe the insertion site for swelling or bleeding.

 10. **Document** the procedure and findings in the client record using forms or checklists supplemented by narrative notes when appropriate.

EVALUATION

- Perform follow-up care based on findings that deviated from expected or normal for the client. Relate findings to previous assessment data if available.

- Report significant deviations from normal to the physician.

Documenting Procedures

There are several reasons why it is critically important that all patient care activities are documented in the client record. These include facilitating continuity of care through ongoing communication among health care providers, promoting effective care through the ability to examine results of previous care and care plans, meeting legal and accreditation requirements, and providing data for research and reimbursement. A variety of **documentation** formats, such as the problem-oriented medical record and source-orientated record, are used in different agencies. Records may be written or electronic. In most cases, care is documented through a combination of checklists, forms, and narrative notes. No matter what format is used, key requirements of documenting procedures are the same. See Box 1-5.

BOX 1-5 *Documentation*

As with all documentation, write legibly, in ink, objectively; use approved abbreviations only; and sign with your name and title. For each procedure, include:

- Date and time it was performed, using the agency preference for 12- or 24-hour clock times

- Name of the physician or other practitioner who performed the procedure

- The exact procedure performed (e.g., right subclavian IV inserted; bone marrow biopsy, left iliac crest)

- Number, color, character, and amount of any specimens, fluid, or tissue obtained

- Any pressure, measurements, or other readings (including vital signs) taken

- Client teaching done prior to, during, and following the procedure

- Client's reaction and tolerance of the procedure

- Nurse's interventions and care following the procedure

SAMPLE RECORDING: Lumbar Puncture

Date	Time	Notes
5/24/01	1500	Lumbar puncture performed by Dr Guido. Four 2-mL specimens of cloudy serous CSF sent to lab. Initial pressure 130 mm. Closing pressure 100 mm. No apparent discomfort. Resting. _____ SNicols, NS

BOX 1-5 *Documentation (continued)*

SAMPLE RECORDING: Soap Suds Enema

Date	Time	Notes
10/02/02	0830	600-cc soap suds enema delivered and retained by patient for 15 minutes. Client assisted to commode. Returned large amount dark brown, soft stool. C/o mild abdominal cramping during procedure, relieved after passing stool. Returned to bed with rails up, call light in reach. Client verbalizes awareness of need to increase fluid and fiber intake to promote bowel regularity. _____ JMacIntyre, RN

Chapter Summary

TERMINOLOGY

bloodborne pathogens
delegation
documentation

nosocomial infections
personal protective equipment (PPE)
Standard Precautions (SP)

Universal Precautions
unlicensed assistive personnel
  (UAP)

FORMING CLINICAL JUDGMENTS

Consider This:

1. You are preparing to perform vital signs on a client who has been experiencing explosive vomiting and diarrhea. What specific precautions (gown, gloves, mask, eyewear) would you take?

2. After caring for a client with hepatitis, upon removing your gown you notice that you have blood on your arm. What would you do?

3. Although you have assisted physicians with several invasive procedures such as a thoracentesis, this will be the first time you assist with a liver biopsy. How will you prepare and what will you tell the physician about your abilities?

4. You observe a nursing assistant bathing and changing the linens on a client who has been incontinent of stool. The assistant is not wearing gloves or any other personal protective equipment. How would you respond?

5. You are considering asking the orderly to assist with a recent new admission. The client has been admitted with a fractured hip. Which tasks of the admission may you delegate to the orderly? Explain how you reached that conclusion.

RELATED RESEARCH

Paulson, D. S., Fendler, E. J., Dolan, M. J., & Williams, R. A. (1999). A close look at alcohol gel as an antimicrobial sanitizing agent. *American Journal of Infection Control, 27*(4), 332–338.

References

Borton, D. (1997). Isolation precautions: Clearing up the confusion. *Nursing, 27*(1), 49–51.

Crow, S. (1997). Your guide to gloves: Learn when to use—not abuse—a good thing. *Nursing, 27*(3), 26.

Friedman, M. M., & Rhinehart, E. (1999). Putting infection control principles into practice in home care. *Nursing Clinics of North America, 34*, 463–482.

Garner, J. S., & Favero, M. S. (1998). Guideline for handwashing and hospital environmental control, 1985, Updated. *Morbidity and Mortality Weekly Report, 37*(24). [Available online at www.cdc.gov].

Global Consensus Conference: Final recommendations. (1999). *American Journal of Infection Control, 27*, 503–513.

Gritter, M. (1998). The latex threat. *American Journal of Nursing, 98*(9), 26–33.

Gould, D. (1997). Practical procedures for nurses: Handwashing. *Nursing Times, 93*(37), 2.

Habel, M. (2000). *Delegating nursing care to unlicensed assistive personnel.* Available from CME Resource #118. Sacramento, CA.

Hanchett, M. (1998). Implementing standard precautions in home care. *Home Care Manager, 2*(2), 16–20.

Hansten, R., & Washburn, R. (1998). *Clinical delegation skills: A handbook for professional practice,* 2nd ed. Gaithersburg, MD: Aspen.

Kiernan, M. (1999). Handwashing in infection control. *Community Nurse, 5*(7), 19–20.

Kingston, J. (1999). Infection control: Is everybody doing it? *Nursing Times, 95*(44), 60–62.

Mayone-Ziomek, J. M. (1998). Handwashing in health care. *Medsurg Nursing, 6*, 364–369.

McConnell, E. A. (1999). Proper handwashing technique. *Nursing, 29*(4), 26.

Metules, T. J. (2000). Tips for nurses who wash too much. *RN, 63*(3), 34–37.

Parker, L. J. (1999). Importance of handwashing in the prevention of cross-infection. *British Journal of Nursing, 8*, 716, 718–720.

Parkman, C. A. (1996). Delegation: Are you doing it right. *American Journal of Nursing, 96*(9), 42–48.

Perry, C., & Barnett, J. (1998). Principles of universal precautions. *Emergency Nurse, 6*(6), 25–28.

Schick, R. (1999). Product focus: Handwashing techniques. *Nursing Homes, 48*(6), 63–67.

Shulmeister, L. (1999). I know handwashing is important, but . . . *Clinical Journal of Oncology Nursing, 3*, 139–140.

Sommer, B. (1999). Protecting our patients and ourselves. *Home Care Provider, 4*(1), 30–35.

U. S. Department of Health and Human Services, Centers for Disease Control and Prevention. (1997, September 8). Draft guidelines for infection control in healthcare personnel, 1997. *Federal Register, 62*, 173.

Zimmerman, P. G. (1997). Delegating to unlicensed assistive personnel. *Nursing, 27*(5), 71.

Chapter 2

Vital Signs

Techniques

OBJECTIVES

- Describe factors that affect the vital signs and accurate measurement of them.
- Identify the normal range for each vital sign measured in adults.
- Identify the variations in normal body temperature, pulse, respirations, and blood pressure that occur from infancy to old age.
- Compare oral, rectal, axillary, and tympanic methods of measuring body temperature.
- Identify indications and contraindications for using oral, rectal, axillary, and tympanic body temperature sites.
- Identify nine pulse sites commonly used to assess the pulse and state the reasons for their use.
- List the characteristics that should be included when assessing pulses.
- Explain how to measure both the apical pulse and the apical–radial pulse.
- Describe assessment of the rate, depth, rhythm, and characteristics of respirations.
- Differentiate systolic from diastolic blood pressure.
- Describe five phases of Korotkoff's sounds.
- Describe various methods and sites used to measure blood pressure.
- Identify when it is appropriate to delegate measurement of vital signs to unlicensed assistive personnel.

Vital Signs

The four **vital signs,** or **cardinal signs,** are body temperature, pulse, respirations, and blood pressure. Recently, many agencies such as the Veterans Administration have designated pain as a fifth vital sign, to be assessed at the same time as each of the other four. Pain assessment is covered in Chapter 14. These signs, which should be looked at both individually and collectively, enable nurses to monitor the functions of the body. The signs reflect changes that otherwise might not be observed. Monitoring a client's vital signs should not be an automatic or routine procedure; it should be a thoughtful, scientific assessment. Vital signs should be evaluated with reference to the client's present and prior health status and compared to accepted normal standards. If findings appear inconsistent with those anticipated, they should immediately be rechecked. Vital signs vary with the client's age. See Table 2-1 for a summary of the normal values of the vital signs at various ages.

When and how often to assess a specific client's vital signs are chiefly nursing judgments, depending on the client's health status. Some agencies have policies about taking clients' vital signs, and physicians may specifically order assessment of a vital sign (e.g., "Blood pressure q2h"). Ordered assessments, however, should be considered the minimum; nurses should measure clients' vital signs more often if their health status requires it. Examples of times to assess vital signs are listed in Box 2-1.

Body Temperature

Body temperature is the balance between the heat produced by the body and the heat lost from the body. There are two kinds of body temperature: core temperature and surface temperature. **Core temperature** is the temperature of the deep tissues of the body (e.g., abdominal cavity and pelvic cavity). The normal core body temperature is not an exact point on a scale but a range of temperatures. When measured orally, the average body temperature of an adult is between 36.7°C (98°F) and 37°C (98.6°F) (see Figure 2-1 ◆). The surface temperature is the temperature of the skin, the subcutaneous tissue, and fat. Surface temperature, by contrast, rises and falls in response to the environment.

Factors Affecting Body Temperature

Nurses should be aware of factors that can affect a client's body temperature so that they can recognize normal temperature variations and understand the significance of body temperature measurements that deviate from normal. Normally, a person's temperature can vary as much as 1.0°C (1.8°F) from early morning to late afternoon. Exercise and stress increase body temperature temporarily (see Figure 2-1). As seen in Table 2-1, older adults' temperatures are often lower than those of middle age adults.

BOX 2-1 *Times to Assess Vital Signs*

- On the client's admission to a health care agency, to obtain baseline data
- When a client has a change in health status or reports symptoms such as chest pain or feeling hot or faint
- According to a nursing or medical order
- Before and after surgery or an invasive diagnostic procedure
- Before and after the administration of a medication that could affect the respiratory or cardiovascular systems (e.g., before giving a digitalis preparation)
- Before and after any nursing intervention that could affect the vital signs (e.g., ambulating a client who has been on bed rest)

TABLE 2-1	**VARIATIONS ON NORMAL VITAL SIGNS BY AGE**				
	Average Value				
Age	**Oral Temperature**	**Pulse**	**Respirations**	**Blood Pressure**	
Newborn	36.8°C (98.2°F) (axillary)	130	35	73/55	
1 year	36.8°C (98.2°F) (axillary)	120	30	90/55	
5–8 years	37.0°C (98.6°F)	100	20	95/57	
10 years	37.0°C (98.6°F)	70	20	102/62	
Teen	37.0°C (98.6°F)	75	18	120/80	
Adult	37.0°C (98.6°F)	80	16	120/80	
Older adult (> 70 years)	36.0°C (96.8°F)	70	16	Increased diastolic	

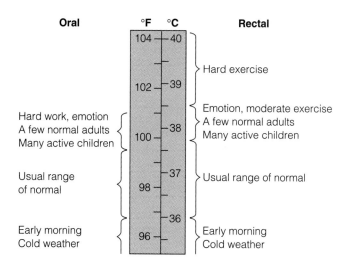

Oral | °F | °C | Rectal

FIGURE 2-1 ◆ Estimated ranges of body temperature in normal persons. Courtesy Charles C Thomas, publisher, Springfield, IL, 1948.

Alterations in Body Temperature

Pyrexia

A body temperature above the usual range is called **pyrexia, hyperthermia,** or (in lay terms) **fever.** A very high fever (e.g., 41°C [105.8°F]) is called **hyperpyrexia.** Signs of fever the nurse may assess are shown in Box 2-2. A client with a fever is said to be **febrile.**

Hypothermia

Hypothermia is a core body temperature below the lower limit of normal. Death usually occurs when the temperature falls below 34°C (93.2°F). With severe hypothermia, sleepiness and even coma are likely to develop, which depress the activity of heat control mechanisms further and prevent shivering. Clinical signs of hypothermia are shown in Box 2-3.

Body Temperature Assessment Sites

There are a number of body sites for measuring body temperature. The most common are oral, rectal, tympanic, and axillary. Each of the sites has advantages and disadvantages. When possible, the body tempera-

---

Box 2-2 *Clinical Signs of Fever*

- Increased heart rate
- Increased respiratory rate and depth
- Shivering
- Pallid, cold skin (during chill stage)
- Flushed, warm skin
- Complaints of feeling cold (during chill stage)
- "Gooseflesh" appearance of the skin (during chill stage)

Box 2-3 *Clinical Signs of Hypothermia*

- Severe shivering (initially)
- Feelings of cold and chills
- Pale, cool, waxy skin
- Hypotension
- Decreased urinary output
- Lack of muscle coordination
- Disorientation
- Drowsiness progressing to coma

---

ture is usually measured orally (by mouth). Traditionally, the oral method was not used for clients receiving oxygen, because the accuracy of the measurement was considered questionable. However, evidence suggests that oral readings are accurate in clients receiving oxygen by nasal cannula, aerosol mask, Venturi mask, and nasal prongs.

Rectal temperature readings are considered the most accurate. In some agencies, taking temperatures rectally is contraindicated for clients with myocardial infarctions. It is believed that inserting a rectal thermometer can stimulate the vagus nerve, which in turn can cause myocardial damage.

Measurements of temperature in the axilla (armpit) are about 0.65°C (1°F) less than the rectal temperature. Clients for whom the axillary method of temperature assessment is appropriate include clients with oral inflammation or wired jaws, clients recovering from oral surgery, clients who can breathe only through their mouths (e.g., following nasal surgery), irrational clients, and clients for whom oral, tympanic, and rectal temperatures are contraindicated.

The tympanic membrane, or nearby tissue in the ear canal, is another core body temperature site. Tympanic membrane temperature readings average 1.1 to 1.5°F higher than oral temperature readings. Because temperature sensors applied directly to the tympanic membrane can be uncomfortable and involve risk of membrane injury or perforation, non-invasive infrared thermometers are used. Electronic tympanic thermometers are used extensively in both inpatient and ambulatory care settings.

Measuring Body Temperature

Nursing Process: Body Temperature

ASSESSMENT

1. Based on the purpose of taking the temperature and the client's age, determine the most appropriate method of measuring the client's temperature.
   - The oral route is most common. Do not take an

oral temperature if the client has had oral surgery or has any lesions in the mouth.

- Rectal temperatures are very accurate and may be used for clients who cannot tolerate an oral thermometer or who may have a seizure, are confused, or are comatose. Do not take a rectal temperature on anyone who has had rectal surgery, has lower gastrointestinal disorders, is immunosuppressed, has a clotting disorder, or has significant hemorrhoids.
- Axillary temperatures are the least accurate but the most safe.
- Tympanic (ear) thermometers are noninvasive and quick (2 to 3 seconds). They may not always return consistent temperatures.

2. Consider the client's overall condition. Is the temperature being taken as part of a routine examination or assessment of a current illness?

- If fever or hypothermia is suspected, the most accurate measurement possible should be obtained.
- If fever or hypothermia is suspected, know what the last temperature reading was. In this way, you can estimate if the temperature reading you obtain is likely to be accurate.

PLANNING

Delegation

Measurement of the client's temperature can be delegated to unlicensed assistive personnel (UAP) or family members/caregivers. The interpretation of an abnormal temperature and determination of appropriate responses are done by the nurse.

Types of Thermometers

Traditionally, body temperatures have been measured using *mercury-in-glass thermometers*. Glass thermometers can be hazardous, however, due to exposure to mercury (toxic to humans) and broken glass should the thermometer crack or break. In 1998, the United States Environmental Protection Agency and the American Hospital Association agreed to the goal of eliminating mercury from health care environments. Some hospitals no longer use mercury thermometers, and several cities have banned the sale and manufacture of them. However, the nurse may still encounter mercury thermometers and must be well versed in their safe use. Oral glass thermometers may have long, slender tips; short, rounded tips; or pear-shaped tips (Figure 2-2 ◆). The rounded thermometer can be used at the rectal as well as other sites. In some agencies, thermometers may be color-coded. For example, red-colored thermometers may be used for rectal temperatures and blue-colored ones for oral and axillary temperatures.

Electronic thermometers offer another method of assessing body temperatures. They can provide a reading in only 2 to 60 seconds, depending on the model.

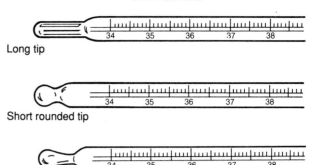

CENTIGRADE

Long tip

Short rounded tip

Pear-shaped tip

Three types of thermometer tips (Centigrade scale).

FIGURE 2-2 ◆ Three types of thermometer tips (Centigrade scale).

The equipment consists of a battery-operated portable electronic unit, a probe that the nurse attaches to the unit, and a probe cover, which is usually disposable (Figure 2-3 ◆). Some models have a different circuit for each method of measurement, and the nurse needs to make sure that the correct circuit is switched on before taking the temperature.

Chemical disposable thermometers come in individual cases and are discarded after use. Disposable thermometers may be particularly useful if the client has a communicable disease. One type has small chemical dots at one end that respond to body heat by changing color, thereby providing a reading of the body temperature (Figure 2-4 ◆).

Temperature-sensitive tape may also be used to obtain a general indication of body surface temperature. When applied to the skin, usually of the forehead or abdomen, the tape responds by changing color (Figure

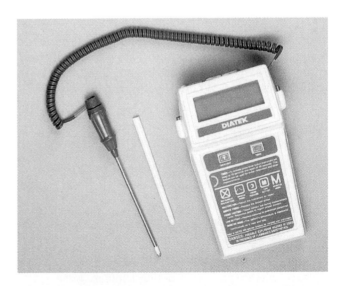

FIGURE 2-3 ◆ An electronic thermometer. Note the probe and probe cover.

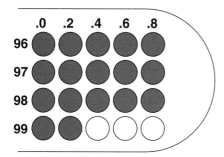

FIGURE 2-4 ◆ Chemical dot thermometer showing a reading of 99.2°F.

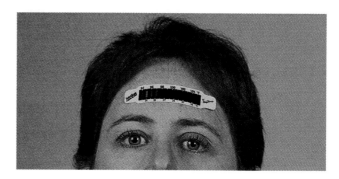

FIGURE 2-5 ◆ Temperature-sensitive tape.

2-5 ◆). After the length of time specified by the manufacturer (e.g., 15 seconds), a color appears on the tape. The nurse compares the color with the legend on the package and then removes and discards the tape. This method is particularly useful at home and for infants whose temperatures are to be monitored for any reason. Skin strips may, however, register falsely elevated readings, so high readings should be validated with another temperature measurement device.

Infrared thermometers sense body heat in the form of infrared energy given off by a heat source, which in the ear canal is primarily the tympanic membrane. Because the infrared thermometer makes no contact with the tympanic membrane or moist mucous membrane, the risk of spreading infection is reduced.

IMPLEMENTATION:
TECHNIQUE 2-1 ASSESSING BODY TEMPERATURE

Equipment

- Thermometer
- Thermometer sheath or cover
- Lubricant for a rectal temperature
- Disposable gloves
- Towel for axillary temperature
- Tissues/wipes

Preparation

- Check that all equipment is functioning normally. If necessary, shake a glass thermometer down to below 35°C (95°F). *Mercury will not fall below the starting level if the client's temperature is less than that. Beginning with the thermometer on a very low temperature allows the nurse to note that the mercury has risen to the client's actual temperature.*

Performance

1. Explain to the client what you are going to do, why it is necessary, and how he or she can cooperate. Discuss how the results will be used in planning further care or treatments.

2. Wash hands and observe appropriate infection control procedures. Don gloves if performing a rectal temperature.

3. Provide for client privacy.

4. Place the client in the appropriate position (e.g., lateral or Sim's position for inserting a rectal thermometer).

5. Place the thermometer (see Box 2-4).
   - Apply a protective sheath or probe cover if appropriate.
   - Lubricate a rectal thermometer.

6. Wait the appropriate amount of time: 2 to 3 minutes for an oral or rectal temperature using a mercury thermometer, 6 to 9 minutes for an axillary temperature with a mercury thermometer. Electronic and tympanic thermometers will indicate that the reading is complete through a light or tone. Check package instructions for length of time to wait prior to reading chemical dot or tape thermometers.

7. Remove the thermometer and discard the cover or wipe with a tissue if necessary.

8. Read the temperature and record it on your worksheet. If the temperature is obviously too high, too low, or inconsistent with the client's condition, recheck it with a thermometer known to be functioning properly.

Variation

Be sure to record the temperature from an electronic thermometer before replacing the probe into the

BOX 2-4 *Thermometer Placement*

Oral	Place the bulb on either side of the frenulum (Figure 2-6 ◆).

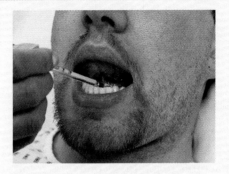

FIGURE 2-6 ◆ Oral thermometer placement.

Rectal	Apply disposable gloves (Figure 2-7 ◆).
	Instruct the client to take a slow deep breath during insertion.
	Never force the thermometer if resistance is felt.
	Insert 1½ inches (3.5 cm) in adults.

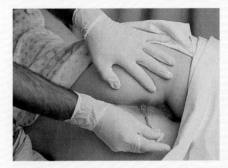

FIGURE 2-7 ◆ Inserting a rectal thermometer.

Axillary	Pat the axilla dry if very moist (Figure 2-8 ◆).
	The bulb is placed in the center of the axilla.

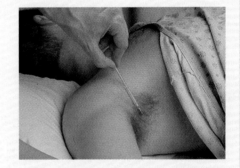

FIGURE 2-8 ◆ Axillary thermometer placement.

Tympanic	Pull the pinna slightly upward and backward (Figure 2-9 ◆).
	Point the probe slightly anteriorly, toward the eardrum.
	Insert the probe slowly using a circular motion until snug.

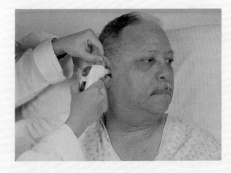

FIGURE 2-9 ◆ Pull the pinna of the ear up and back while inserting the tympanic thermometer.

charging unit. With many models, replacing the probe erases the temperature from the display.

9. Wash the thermometer if necessary and return it to the storage location.

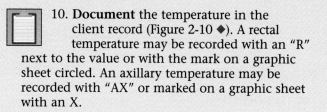

10. **Document** the temperature in the client record (Figure 2-10 ◆). A rectal temperature may be recorded with an "R" next to the value or with the mark on a graphic sheet circled. An axillary temperature may be recorded with "AX" or marked on a graphic sheet with an X.

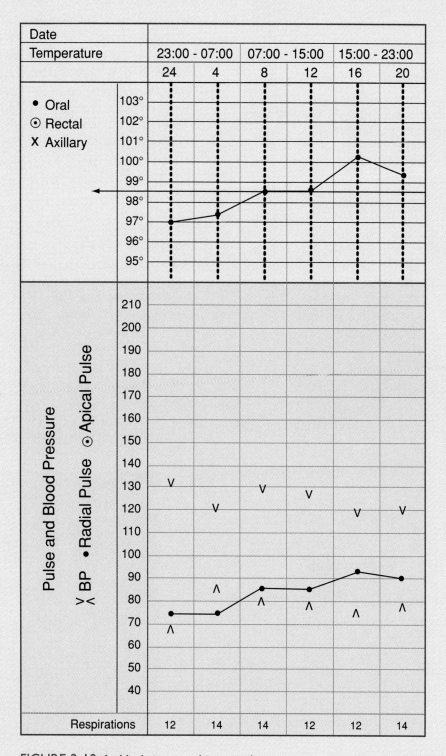

FIGURE 2-10 ◆ Vital signs graphic record.

AMBULATORY AND COMMUNITY SETTINGS

Temperature

- When making a home visit, take a thermometer with you in case the client does not have a functional thermometer of his or her own.
- Examine the thermometer used by the client in the home for safety and proper functioning.
- Observe the client/caregiver taking and reading a temperature. Provide reinforcement and teaching as indicated, including the importance of reporting the site and type of thermometer used and the preference to use one consistently.

- Check that the client knows how to record the temperature. Provide a recording chart/table if indicated.
- Discuss means of keeping the thermometer clean and avoiding cross-contamination.
- Ensure that the client has water-soluble lubricant available if using a rectal thermometer.
- Discuss environmental control modifications that should be taken during illness or extreme climate conditions (e.g., heating, air conditioning, appropriate clothing and bedding).

AGE-RELATED CONSIDERATIONS

Temperature
Infant

- Using the axillary site, you may need to hold the infant's arm against the chest (Figure 2-11 ◆).

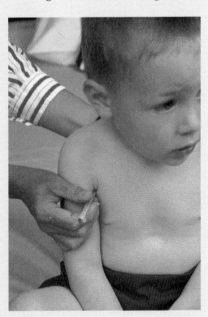

FIGURE 2-11 ◆ Axillary thermometer placement—child.

- Axillary route may not be as accurate as other routes for detecting fevers in children (Bindler & Ball, 1999).
- The tympanic route is fast and convenient. Place infant supine and stabilize the head. Pull the pinna straight back and slightly downward. Direct the probe tip anteriorly and insert far enough to seal the canal.
- Avoid the tympanic route in a child with active ear infections or tympanic membrane drainage tubes.
- The rectal route is least desirable in infants.

Child

- Tympanic or axillary sites are commonly preferred.
- For the tympanic route, have the child held on an adult's lap with the child's head held gently against the adult for support. Pull the pinna straight back and upward for children over age 3 (Figure 2-12 ◆).
- Avoid the tympanic route in a child with active ear infections or tympanic membrane drainage tubes.
- The oral route may be used for children over age 3, but nonbreakable, electronic thermometers are recommended.
- For a rectal temperature, place the child prone across your lap or in a side-lying position with the

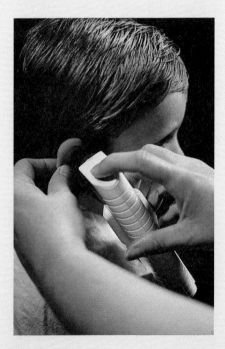

FIGURE 2-12 ◆ Pull the pinna of the ear back and up for placement of a tympanic thermometer in a child over 3 years of age, back and down for children under age 3.

Temperature (*continued*)

knees flexed. Insert the thermometer 1 inch into the rectum.

Elders

- Elders' temperatures tend to be lower than those of middle-aged adults.
- Elders' temperatures are strongly influenced by

both environmental and internal temperature changes.

- Elders can develop significant buildup of ear cerumen that may interfere with tympanic thermometer readings.
- Elders are more likely to have hemorrhoids. Inspect the anus before taking a rectal temperature.

EVALUATION

- Compare the results with the client's previous temperatures.
- Conduct appropriate follow-up such as notifying the physician, giving a medication, or altering the client's environment. This includes teaching the client how to lower an elevated temperature through actions such as increasing fluid intake, coughing and deep breathing, or removing heavy coverings.

Pulse

Pulse is the term used to describe the rate, rhythm, and volume of the heartbeat as it is assessed at either central or peripheral locations. The pulse is a wave of blood created by contraction of the left ventricle of the heart. Generally, the pulse wave represents the volume output by each cardiac contraction and the compliance of the arteries. Compliance of the arteries is the distensibility of the arteries (i.e., their ability to contract and expand). The rate of the pulse is expressed in beats per minute (BPM).

In a healthy person, the pulse reflects the heartbeat; that is, the pulse rate is the same as the rate of the ventricular contractions of the heart. However, in some types of cardiovascular disease, the heartbeat and pulse rates can differ. For example, a client's heart may produce very weak or small pulse waves that are not detectable in a peripheral pulse. In these instances, the nurse should assess the heartbeat (apical pulse) and the peripheral pulse. (See the section on assessing the apical pulse later in this chapter.) A **peripheral pulse** is a pulse located in the periphery of the body (e.g., in the foot, hand, or neck). The **apical pulse** is a central pulse located at the apex of the heart.

Factors Affecting Pulse Rate

- *Age.* As age increases, the pulse rate gradually decreases. See Table 2-1 for specific variations in pulse rates from birth to adulthood.
- *Sex.* After puberty, the average male's pulse rate is slightly lower than the female's.

- *Exercise.* The pulse rate normally increases with activity. Both the resting pulse and rate of increase in exercising athletes may be less than the average person because of greater cardiac size, strength, and efficiency.
- *Fever.* The pulse rate increases (a) in response to the lowered blood pressure that results from peripheral vasodilatation associated with elevated body temperature and also (b) because of the increased metabolic rate.
- *Medications.* Some medications decrease the pulse rate, and others increase it. For example, cardiotonics (e.g., digitalis preparations) will decrease the heart rate, whereas epinephrine will increase it.
- *Hypovolemia/dehydration.* Loss of fluid from the vascular system increases pulse rate.
- *Stress.* Stress, emotions such as fear and anxiety, and the perception of severe pain increase the rate as well as the force of the heartbeat.
- *Position.* When a person is sitting or standing, blood pools in dependent vessels of the venous system. Pooling results in a transient decrease in the venous blood return to the heart and a subsequent reduction in blood pressure, increasing cardiac rate, force of the ventricular contractions, and tone of the veins and arteries.

Pulse Assessment Sites

The pulse is commonly taken in nine sites (Figure 2-13 ◆):

1. *Temporal,* where the temporal artery passes over the temporal bone of the head. The site is superior (above) and lateral to (away from the midline of) the eye.
2. *Carotid,* at the side of the neck below the lobe of the ear, where the carotid artery runs between the trachea and the sternocleidomastoid muscle.
3. *Apical,* at the apex of the heart. In an adult this is located in the left chest, about 8 cm (3 in.) left of the sternum (breastbone) at the fifth intercostal space.
4. *Brachial,* at the inner aspect of the biceps muscle of the arm or medially in the antecubital space.

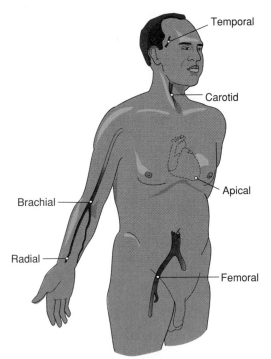

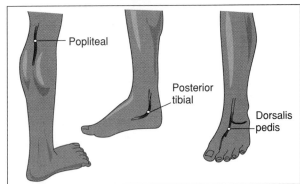

FIGURE 2-13 ◆ Nine sites for assessing pulse.

TABLE 2-2	REASONS FOR USING SPECIFIC PULSE SITES

Pulse Site	Reasons for Use
Radial	Readily accessible
Temporal	Used when radial pulse is not accessible
Carotid	Used for infants Used in cases of cardiac arrest Used to determine circulation to the brain
Apical	Routinely used for infants and children up to 3 years of age Used to determine discrepancies with radial pulse Used in conjunction with some medications
Brachial	Used to measure blood pressure Used during cardiac arrest for infants
Femoral	Used in cases of cardiac arrest Used for infants and children Used to determine circulation to a leg
Popliteal	Used to determine circulation to the lower leg
Posterior tibial	Used to determine circulation to the foot
Pedal	Used to determine circulation to the foot

Nursing Process: Assessing the Peripheral Pulses

ASSESSMENT

1. Peripheral pulses may be assessed as either an indicator either of cardiac function or of vascular integrity. As an indicator of cardiac function, the peripheral pulse is used to:
   - Provide baseline data for subsequent evaluation
   - Identify whether the pulse rate is within normal range
   - Determine whether the pulse rhythm is regular
   - Monitor and assess changes in the client's health status
   - Monitor clients at risk for pulse alterations (e.g., those with a history of heart disease or experiencing cardiac **arrhythmias**, hemorrhage, acute pain, infusion of large volumes of fluids, fever).

   As an indicator of vascular integrity, the peripheral pulse is used to:
   - Determine whether the pulse volume is normal
   - Compare the equality of corresponding peripheral pulses on each side of the body
   - Determine the adequacy of blood flow to a particular part of the body

2. In order to provide a complete picture of the client's cardiovascular health, also assess for other clinical signs of cardiovascular alterations (e.g.,

5. *Radial,* where the radial artery runs along the radial bone, on the thumb side of the inner aspect of the wrist.

6. *Femoral,* where the femoral artery passes alongside the inguinal ligament.

7. *Popliteal,* where the popliteal artery passes behind the knee.

8. *Posterior tibial,* on the medial surface of the ankle where the posterior tibial artery passes behind the medial malleolus.

9. *Pedal* (dorsalis pedis), where the dorsalis pedis artery passes over the bones of the foot. This artery can be palpated by feeling the dorsum of the foot on an imaginary line from the middle of the ankle to the space between the big toe and second toe.

Some reasons for use of each site are given in Table 2-2.

dyspnea, fatigue, pallor, cyanosis, palpitations, syncope, impaired peripheral tissue perfusion as evidenced by skin discoloration and cool temperature) and factors that may alter pulse rate (e.g., emotional status and activity level).

PLANNING

Delegation

Measurement of the client's radial pulse can be delegated to UAP or family members/caregivers. Reports of abnormal pulse rates or rhythms require reassessment by the nurse, who also determines appropriate action if the abnormality is confirmed. Due to the skill required in locating and interpreting peripheral pulses other than the radial artery and in using Doppler ultrasound devices, UAP are generally not delegated these techniques.

IMPLEMENTATION:
TECHNIQUE 2-2 ASSESSING PERIPHERAL PULSES

Equipment

- Watch with a second hand or indicator
- If using Doppler ultrasound stethoscope (DUS), the transducer probe, the stethoscope headset, transmission gel, and tissues/wipes

Preparation

If using the DUS, check that the equipment is functioning normally.

Performance

1. Explain to the client what you are going to do, why it is necessary, and how he or she can cooperate. Discuss how the results will be used in planning further care or treatments.

2. Wash hands and observe appropriate infection control procedures.

3. Provide for client privacy.

4. Select the pulse point. Normally, the radial pulse is taken, unless it cannot be exposed or circulation to another body area is to be assessed.

5. Assist the client to a comfortable resting position. When the radial pulse is assessed, with the palm facing downward, the client's arm can rest alongside the body or the forearm can rest at a 90-degree angle across the chest. For the client who can sit, the forearm can rest across the thigh, with the palm of the hand facing downward or inward.

6. Palpate and count the pulse. Place two or three middle fingertips lightly and squarely over the pulse point (Figure 2-14 ◆). *Using the thumb is contraindicated because the thumb has a pulse that the nurse could mistake for the client's pulse.*
   - Count for 15 seconds and multiply by 4. Record the pulse in beats per minute on your worksheet. If taking a client's pulse for the first time, when obtaining baseline data, or if the pulse is irregu-

lar, count for a full minute. An irregular pulse also requires taking the apical pulse.

7. Assess the pulse rhythm and volume.
   - Assess the pulse rhythm by noting the pattern of the intervals between the beats. A normal pulse has equal time periods between beats. If this is an initial assessment, assess for 1 minute.
   - Assess the pulse volume. A normal pulse can be felt with moderate pressure, and the pressure is equal with each beat. A forceful pulse volume is full; an easily obliterated pulse is weak. Record the rhythm and volume on your worksheet.

8. **Document** the pulse rate, rhythm, and volume and your actions in the client record (Figure 2-10). Also record pertinent related data such as variation in pulse rate compared to normal for the client and abnormal skin color and skin temperature in the nurse's notes.

Variation: Using a DUS

- Plug the stethoscope headset into one of the two output jacks located next to the volume control. DUS units may have two jacks so that a second person can listen to the signals. See Figure 2-15 ◆.
- Apply transmission gel either to the probe at the narrow end of the plastic case housing the transducer, or to the client's skin. *Ultrasound beams do not travel well through air. The gel makes an airtight seal, which then promotes optimal ultrasound wave transmission.*
- Press the "on" button.
- Hold the probe against the skin over the pulse site. Use a light pressure, and keep the probe in contact with the skin (Figure 2-16 ◆). *Too much pressure can stop the blood flow and obliterate the signal.*
- Adjust the volume if necessary. Distinguish artery sounds from vein sounds. The artery sound (signal) is distinctively pulsating and has a pumping quality. The venous sound is intermittent and varies

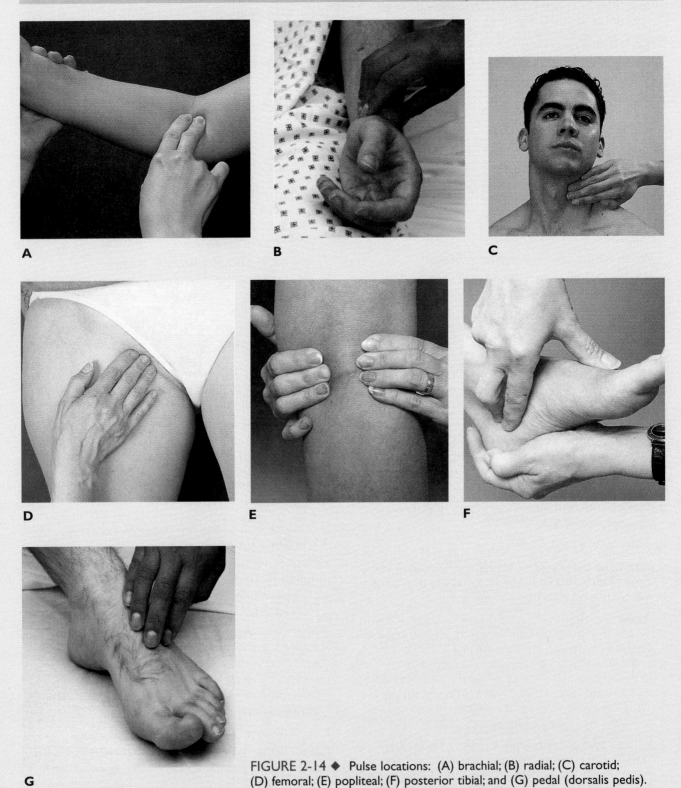

A

B

C

D

E

F

G

FIGURE 2-14 ◆ Pulse locations: (A) brachial; (B) radial; (C) carotid; (D) femoral; (E) popliteal; (F) posterior tibial; and (G) pedal (dorsalis pedis).

with respirations. Both artery and vein sounds are heard simultaneously through the DUS because major arteries and veins are situated close together throughout the body. If arterial sounds cannot be easily heard, then reposition the probe.

• After assessing the pulse, remove all the gel from the probe to prevent damage to its surface. Clean the transducer with aqueous solutions. *Alcohol or other disinfectants may damage the face of the transducer.* Remove all gel from the client.

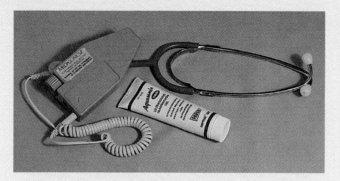

FIGURE 2-15 ◆ An ultrasound (Doppler) stethoscope.

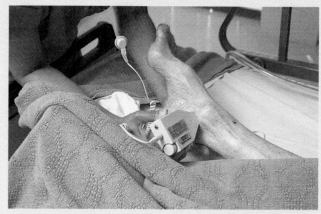

FIGURE 2-16 ◆ Using an ultrasound (Doppler) stethoscope to assess the posterior tibial pulse.

EVALUATION

- Compare the pulse rate to baseline data or normal range for age of client.
- Relate pulse rate and volume to other vital signs; pulse rhythm and volume to baseline data and health status.
- If assessing peripheral pulses, evaluate equality, rate, and volume in corresponding extremities.
- Conduct appropriate follow-up such as notifying the physician or giving medication.

Nursing Process: Assessing an Apical Pulse

ASSESSMENT

1. Assess the apical pulse of an adult with an irregular peripheral pulse, clients with cardiac disease, and clients receiving medications to improve heart action.

2. In order to provide a complete picture of the client's cardiovascular health, also assess for other clinical signs of cardiovascular alterations (e.g., dyspnea, fatigue, pallor, cyanosis, syncope) and factors that may alter pulse rate (e.g., emotional status or activity level).

PLANNING

Delegation

Unlicensed assistive personnel are generally not responsible for assessing apical pulses.

IMPLEMENTATION:
TECHNIQUE 2-3 ASSESSING AN APICAL PULSE

Equipment

- Watch with a second hand or indicator
- Stethoscope
- Antiseptic wipes
- If using DUS, the transducer probe, the stethoscope headset, transmission gel, and tissues/wipes

Preparation

If using the DUS, check that the equipment is functioning normally.

Performance

1. Explain to the client what you are going to do, why it is necessary, and how he or she can cooper-ate. Discuss how the results will be used in planning further care or treatments.

2. Wash hands and observe appropriate infection control procedures.

3. Provide for client privacy.

4. Position the client appropriately in a comfortable supine position or to a sitting position. Expose the area of the chest over the apex of the heart.

5. Locate the apical impulse. This is the point over the apex of the heart where the apical pulse can be most clearly heard. It is also referred to as the **point of maximal impulse (PMI)**.

   - Palpate the angle of Louis (the angle between the manubrium, the top of the sternum, and the body of the sternum). It is palpated just below the suprasternal notch and is felt as a prominence (Figure 2-17 ◆).

• Slide your index finger just to the left of the client's sternum, and palpate the second intercostal space.

• Place your middle or next finger in the third intercostal space, and continue palpating downward until you locate the apical impulse, usually at about the fifth intercostal space if the client is an adult.

• Palpate the apical impulse. Move your index finger laterally along the fifth intercostal space to the midclavicular line (MCL). Normally, the apical impulse is palpable at or just medial to the MCL (Figure 2-17).

6. Auscultate and count heartbeats.

• Use antiseptic wipes to clean the earpieces and diaphragm of the stethoscope if their cleanliness is in doubt. *The diaphragm must be cleaned and disinfected if soiled with body substances.*

• Warm the diaphragm of the stethoscope by holding it in the palm of the hand for a moment. *The metal of the diaphragm is usually cold and can startle the client when placed immediately on the chest.*

• Insert the earpieces of the stethoscope into your ears in the direction of the ear canals, or slightly forward, to facilitate hearing.

• Tap your finger lightly on the diaphragm to be sure it is the active side of the head. If necessary, rotate the head to select the diaphragm side (see Figure 2-18 ◆).

• Place the diaphragm of the stethoscope over the apical impulse and listen for the normal S_1 and S_2 heart sounds, which are heard as "lub-dub" (Figure 2-19 ◆). *The heartbeat is normally loudest over the apex of the heart.* Each lub-dub is counted as one heartbeat. *The two heart sounds are produced by closure of the valves of the heart. The S_1*

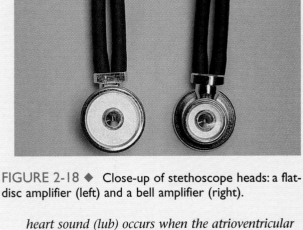

FIGURE 2-18 ◆ Close-up of stethoscope heads: a flat-disc amplifier (left) and a bell amplifier (right).

heart sound (lub) occurs when the atrioventricular valves close after the ventricles have been sufficiently filled. The S_2 heart sound (dub) occurs when the semilunar valves close after the ventricles empty.

• If the rhythm is regular, count the heartbeats for 30 seconds and multiply by 2. If the rhythm is irregular, count the beats for 60 seconds. *A 60-second count provides a more accurate assessment of an irregular pulse than a 30-second count.*

7. Assess the rhythm and the strength of the heartbeat.

• Assess the rhythm of the heartbeat by noting the pattern of intervals between the beats. A normal pulse has equal time periods between beats.

• Assess the strengths (volume) of the heartbeat. Normally, the heartbeats are equal in strength and can be described as strong or weak.

8. **Document** the pulse site, rate, rhythm, and volume and your actions in the client record. Also record pertinent related data such as variation in pulse rate compared to normal for the client and abnormal skin color and skin temperature.

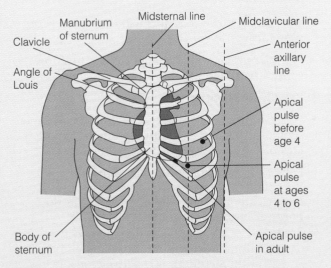

FIGURE 2-17 ◆ Location of the apical pulse—adult and child.

Labels: Manubrium of sternum; Midsternal line; Midclavicular line; Clavicle; Angle of Louis; Anterior axillary line; Apical pulse before age 4; Apical pulse at ages 4 to 6; Body of sternum; Apical pulse in adult

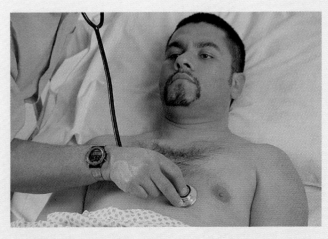

FIGURE 2-19 ◆ Taking an apical pulse using the flat-disc amplifier.

EVALUATION

- Relate pulse rate to other vital signs; pulse rhythm to baseline data and health status.
- Report to the physician any abnormal findings such as irregular rhythm, reduced ability to hear the heartbeat, pallor, cyanosis, dyspnea, tachycardia, or bradycardia.
- Conduct appropriate follow-up such as administering medication ordered based on apical heart rate.

Nursing Process: Assessing an Apical–Radial Pulse

ASSESSMENT

Measurement of the apical and radial pulse simultaneously is done to determine adequacy of peripheral circulation or presence of **pulse deficit.**

PLANNING

Delegation

Unlicensed assistive personnel are generally not responsible for assessing **apical–radial pulses** using the one-nurse technique. UAP may perform the radial pulse count for the two-nurse technique.

IMPLEMENTATION:
TECHNIQUE 2-4 ASSESSING AN APICAL–RADIAL PULSE

Equipment

- Watch with a second hand or indicator
- Stethoscope
- Antiseptic wipes

Preparation

If using the two-nurse technique, ensure that the other nurse is available at this time.

Performance

1. Explain to the client what you are going to do, why it is necessary, and how he or she can cooperate. Discuss how the results will be used in planning further care or treatments.

2. Wash hands and observe appropriate infection control procedures.

3. Provide for client privacy.

4. Position the client appropriately. Assist the client to assume the position described for taking the apical pulse. See Technique 2-3, Step 4. If previous measurements were taken, determine what position the client assumed, and use the same position. *This ensures an accurate comparative measurement.*

5. Locate the apical and radial pulse sites. In the two-nurse technique, one nurse locates the apical impulse by palpation or with the stethoscope while the other nurse palpates the radial pulse site. See Techniques 2-2 and 2-3.

6. Count the apical and radial pulse rates.

Two-Nurse Technique

- Place the watch where both nurses can see it. The nurse who is taking the radial pulse may hold the watch.

- Decide on a time to begin counting. A time when the second hand or indicator is on 12, 3, 6, or 9 is usually selected. The nurse taking the radial pulse says "Start" at the same time. *This ensures that simultaneous counts are taken.*

- Each nurse counts the pulse rate for 60 seconds. Both nurses end the count when the nurse taking the radial pulse says, "Stop." *A full 60-second count is necessary for accurate assessment of any discrepancies between the two pulse sites.*

- The nurse who assesses the apical rate also assesses the apical pulse rhythm and volume (i.e., whether the heartbeat is strong or weak). If the pulse is irregular, note whether the irregular beats come at random or at predictable times.

- The nurse assessing the radial pulse rate also assesses the radial pulse rhythm and volume.

One-Nurse Technique

- Assess the apical pulse for 60 seconds.
- Assess the radial pulse for 60 seconds.

7. **Document** the apical and radial (AR) pulse rates, rhythm, volume, and any pulse deficit in the client record. Also record related data such as variation in pulse rate compared to normal for the client and other pertinent observations, such as pallor, cyanosis, or dyspnea.

AMBULATORY AND COMMUNITY SETTINGS

Pulse

- Be sure the client is resting in a comfortable position.

- If the client is taking medications that affect heart rate, teach the client or family member to measure the client's pulse.

AGE-RELATED CONSIDERATIONS

Pulse

Infant

- Use the apical pulse for the heart rate of newborns, infants, and children 2 to 3 years old to establish baseline data for subsequent evaluation; to determine whether the cardiac rate is within normal range; and to determine if the rhythm is regular.

- Place a baby in the supine position, and offer a pacifier if the baby is crying or restless. Crying and physical activity will increase the pulse rate. For this reason, take the apical pulse rate of infants and small children before assessing body temperatures.

- Locate the apical pulse one or two spaces above the adult apex during infancy.

- Brachial, popliteal, and femoral pulses may be palpated. Due to a normally low blood pressure and rapid heart rate, infants' other distal pulses may be hard to feel.

Child

- To take a peripheral pulse, position the child comfortably in the adult's arms, or have the adult

remain close by. This may decrease anxiety and yield more accurate results.

- To assess the apical pulse, assist a young child to a comfortable supine or sitting position.

- Demonstrate the procedure to the child using a stuffed animal or doll, and allow the child to handle the stethoscope before beginning the procedure. This will decrease anxiety and promote cooperation.

- The apex of the heart is normally located in the fourth intercostal space in young children, and the fifth intercostal space in children 7 years of age and over.

- Locate the apical impulse along the fourth intercostal space, between the MCL and the anterior axillary line (see Figure 2-16).

Elders

- If the client has severe hand or arm tremors, the radial pulse may be difficult to count.

EVALUATION

- Relate pulse rate and rhythm to other vital signs, to baseline data, and to general health status.

- Report to the physician any changes from previous measurements or any discrepancy between the two pulses.

- Conduct appropriate follow-up such as administering medication or other actions to be taken for a discrepancy in the AR pulse rates.

Respirations

Respiration is the act of breathing. It includes the intake of oxygen and the output of carbon dioxide. The term **inhalation** or **inspiration** refers to the intake of air into the lungs. **Exhalation** or **expiration** refers to breathing out or the movement of gases from the lungs to the atmosphere. **Ventilation** is another word that is used to refer to the movement of air in and out of the lungs. **Hyperventilation** refers to very

deep, rapid respirations. **Hypoventilation** refers to very shallow respirations.

There are two types of breathing that nurses observe: costal breathing (thoracic breathing) and diaphragmatic breathing (abdominal breathing). **Costal breathing** can be observed by the movement of the chest upward and outward. **Diaphragmatic breathing** is observed by the movement of the abdomen, which occurs as a result of the diaphragm's contraction and downward movement.

Factors Affecting Respirations

- *Age.* As age increases, the respiratory rate gradually decreases. (See Table 2-1.)

- *Exercise.* Respirations increase in rate and depth with exercise.

- *Fever.* The respiratory rate will be faster in clients with an elevated temperature.

- *Medications.* Narcotics and other central nervous system depressants often slow the respiratory rate.

• *Stress.* Anxiety is likely to increase respiratory rate and depth.

Assessing Respirations

The rate, depth, rhythm, and special characteristics of respirations should be assessed. *Respiratory rate* is described in breaths per minute. A healthy adult normally takes between 15 and 20 breaths per minute.

The *depth* of a person's respirations can be established by watching the movement of the chest. Respiratory depth is generally described as normal, deep, or shallow. *Deep respirations* are those in which a large volume of air is inhaled and exhaled, inflating most of the lungs. *Shallow respirations* involve the exchange of a small volume of air and often the minimal use of lung tissue. During a normal inspiration and expiration, an adult takes in about 500 mL of air.

Respiratory rhythm or pattern refers to the regularity of the expirations and the inspirations. Normally, respirations are evenly spaced. Respiratory rhythm can be described as *regular* or *irregular*. An infant's respiratory rhythm may be less regular than an adult's.

Respiratory quality or character refers to those aspects of breathing that are different from normal, effortless breathing. Normal breathing is silent, but a number of abnormal sounds such as a wheeze are obvious to the nurse's ear. Many sounds occur as a result of the presence of fluid in the lungs and are most clearly heard with a stethoscope. See Chapter 3, pages 49–50, for auscultation and percussion methods used to assess lung sounds. Additional terms used to describe respirations are in Box 2-5.

Nursing Process: Respirations

ASSESSMENT

1. Measurement of the rate, rhythm, and character of respirations is used to:
   • Acquire baseline data against which future measurements can be compared
   • Monitor abnormal respirations and respiratory patterns and identify changes
   • Assess respirations before the administration of a medication that can depress respirations (an abnormally slow respiratory rate may warrant withholding the medication)
   • Monitor respirations following the administration of a general anesthetic or any medication that influences respirations
   • Monitor clients at risk for respiratory alterations

BOX 2-5 *Breathing Patterns and Sounds*

Breathing Patterns

Rate
• **Eupnea**—normal respiration that is quiet, rhythmic, and effortless
• **Tachypnea**—rapid respiration marked by quick, shallow breaths
• **Bradypnea**—abnormally slow breathing
• **Apnea**—cessation of breathing

Volume
• *Hyperventilation*—prolonged and deep breaths
• *Hypoventilation*—shallow respirations

Rhythm
• **Cheyne–Stokes breathing**—rhythmic waxing and waning of respirations, from very deep to very shallow breathing and temporary apnea

Ease or Effort
• **Dyspnea**—difficult and labored breathing during which the individual has a persistent, unsatisfied need for air and feels distressed
• **Orthopnea**—ability to breathe only in upright sitting or standing positions

Breath Sounds

Audible Without Amplification
• **Stridor**—shrill, harsh sound heard during inspiration
• **Wheeze**—continuous, high-pitched musical squeak or whistling sound on expiration and sometimes on inspiration
• *Bubbling*—gurgling sounds heard as air passes through secretions

Chest Movements
• *Intercostal **retraction***—indrawing between the ribs
• *Substernal retraction*—indrawing beneath the sternum
• *Suprasternal retraction*—indrawing above the sternum
• **Flail chest**—ballooning out of the chest wall through injured rib spaces; results in **paradoxical breathing,** during which the chest wall balloons on expiration but is depressed or sucked inward on inspiration

Secretions and Coughing
• **Hemoptysis**—the presence of blood in the sputum
• *Productive cough*—a cough accompanied by expectorated secretions
• *Nonproductive cough*—a dry, harsh cough without secretions

(e.g., those with fever, pain, acute anxiety, chronic obstructive pulmonary disease, respiratory infection, pulmonary edema or emboli, chest trauma or constriction, brain stem injury)

2. In order to assess the client's general pulmonary health, examine skin and mucous membrane color (e.g., cyanosis or pallor); position assumed for breathing (e.g., use of orthopneic position); signs of cerebral anoxia (e.g., irritability, restlessness, drowsiness, or loss of consciousness); chest movements (e.g., retractions between the ribs or above or below the sternum); activity tolerance; chest pain; dyspnea; and medications affecting respiratory rate.

PLANNING

Delegation

Counting and observing respirations may be delegated to UAP. The follow-up assessment, interpretation of abnormal respirations, and determination of appropriate responses are done by the nurse.

IMPLEMENTATION:
TECHNIQUE 2-5 ASSESSING RESPIRATIONS

Equipment

• Watch with a second hand or indicator

Preparation

For a routine assessment of respirations, determine the client's activity schedule and choose a suitable time to monitor the respirations. A client who has been exercising will need to rest for a few minutes to permit the accelerated respiratory rate to return to normal.

Performance

1. Explain to the client what you are going to do, why it is necessary, and how he or she can cooperate. Discuss how the results will be used in planning further care or treatments.

2. Wash hands and observe appropriate infection control procedures.

3. Provide for client privacy.

4. Observe or palpate and count the respiratory rate.
   • The client's awareness that you are counting the respiratory rate could cause the client voluntarily to alter the respiratory pattern. If you anticipate this, place a hand against the client's chest to feel the chest movements with breathing, or place the client's arm across the chest and observe the chest movements while supposedly taking the radial pulse.
   • Count the respiratory rate for 30 seconds if the respirations are regular. Count for 60 seconds if they are irregular. An inhalation and an exhalation count as one respiration.

5. Observe the depth, rhythm, and character of respirations.
   • Observe the respirations for depth by watching the movement of the chest. *During deep respirations, a large volume of air is exchanged; during shallow respirations, a small volume is exchanged.*
   • Observe the respirations for regular or irregular rhythm. *Normally, respirations are evenly spaced.*
   • Observe the character of respirations—the sound they produce and the effort they require. *Normally, respirations are silent and effortless.*

 6. **Document** the respiratory rate, depth, rhythm, and character on the appropriate record (Figure 2-10).

AMBULATORY AND COMMUNITY SETTINGS

Respirations

• Assess the home setting for factors that could interfere with breathing, such as exhaust, gas, or paint fumes or persons who smoke.

• If the client has just come in from another room, allow the client to rest a minute or two before counting respirations.

• Have an adult hold a child gently to reduce movement while counting respirations.

AGE-RELATED CONSIDERATIONS

Respirations
Infant

• An infant or child who is crying will have an abnormal respiratory rate and will need quieting before respirations can be accurately assessed.

• If necessary, place your hand gently on the infant's abdomen to feel the rapid rise and fall during respirations.

Respirations (*continued*)
Child

- Because young children are diaphragmatic breathers, observe the rise and fall of the abdomen. If necessary, place your hand gently on the abdomen to feel the rapid rise and fall during respirations.

Elders

- Ask the client to remain quiet or count respirations after taking the pulse.

EVALUATION

- Relate respiratory rate to other vital signs, in particular pulse rate, respiratory rhythm, and depth to baseline data and health status.
- Report to the physician respiratory rate significantly above or below the normal range and any notable change in respirations from previous assessments; irregular respiratory rhythm; inadequate respiratory depth; abnormal character of breathing—orthopnea, wheezing, stridor, or bubbling; and any complaints of dyspnea.
- Conduct appropriate follow-up such as administering appropriate medications or treatments, positioning the client to ease breathing, and requesting involvement of other members of the health care team such as the respiratory therapist.

Blood Pressure

Arterial blood pressure is a measure of the pressure exerted by blood as it pulsates through the arteries. Because blood moves in waves, there are two blood pressure measures: the **systolic** pressure, the pressure of the blood as a result of contraction of the ventricles (i.e., the pressure of the height of the blood wave); and the **diastolic** pressure, the pressure when the ventricles are at rest. Diastolic pressure, then, is the lower pressure, present at all times within the arteries. The difference between the diastolic and systolic pressures is called the **pulse pressure**.

Factors Affecting Blood Pressure

- *Age.* Newborns have a mean systolic pressure of 73 mm Hg. Systolic and diastolic pressures rise gradually with age until adulthood. In elders, the arteries are more rigid and less yielding to the pressure of the blood. This produces an elevated systolic pressure. Because the walls no longer retract as flexibly with decreased pressure, the diastolic pressure is also higher. (See Table 2-1.)
- *Sex.* Women usually have lower blood pressures than men of the same age, most likely due to hormonal variations. After menopause, women generally have higher blood pressures than before.
- *Exercise.* Physical activity increases blood pressure.

For reliable assessment of resting blood pressure, wait 20 to 30 minutes following exercise.

- *Medications.* Many medications may increase or decrease the blood pressure.
- *Stress.* Stimulation of the sympathetic nervous system increases cardiac output and vasoconstriction of the arterioles, thus increasing the blood pressure reading. However, severe pain can produce vasodilation and decrease blood pressure greatly.
- *Race.* African American males over 35 years have higher blood pressures than European American males of the same age.
- *Obesity.* Both childhood and adult obesity predispose persons to hypertension.
- *Diurnal variations.* Blood pressure is usually lowest early in the morning, when the metabolic rate is lowest, then rises throughout the day and peaks in the late afternoon or early evening.
- *Fever/Heat/Cold.* Because of increased metabolic rate, fever can increase blood pressure. However, external heat causes vasodilation and decreased blood pressure. Cold causes vasoconstriction and elevates blood pressure.

Blood Pressure Assessment Sites

Blood pressure is usually assessed in the client's arm using the brachial artery and a standard stethoscope. Assessing the blood pressure on a client's thigh using the popliteal artery is usually indicated in these situations:

- The blood pressure cannot be measured on either arm (e.g., because of burns, trauma, or bilateral mastectomy).
- The blood pressure in one thigh is to be compared with the blood pressure in the other thigh.
- The blood pressure cuff is too large for the upper extremities.

Blood pressure is *not* measured on a client's arm or thigh in the following situations:

- The client has had breast or axilla (or hip) surgery on that side.
- The client has an intravenous infusion or a blood transfusion in that limb.
- The client has an arteriovenous fistula (e.g., for renal dialysis) in that limb.

Measuring Blood Pressure

There are two common *noninvasive indirect methods* of measuring blood pressure: the auscultatory and palpatory methods. The *auscultatory method* is commonly used in hospitals, clinics, and homes. External pressure is applied to a superficial artery and the nurse reads the pressure from the sphygmomanometer while listening through a stethoscope for the five phases of sounds called Korotkoff's sounds (Figure 2-20 ◆).

The systolic pressure is the point where the first tapping sound is heard (phase 1). In adults, the diastolic pressure is the point where the sounds become inaudible (phase 5). The phase 5 reading may be zero; that is, the muffled sounds are heard even when there is no air pressure in the blood pressure cuff. For complete accuracy, the phase 4 and 5 readings should be recorded.

The *palpatory method* is sometimes used when Korotkoff's sounds cannot be heard and electronic equipment to amplify the sounds is not available. The nurse palpates the pulsations of the artery as the pressure in the cuff is released. The systolic pressure is read from the sphygmomanometer when the first pulsation is felt. A single whiplike vibration, felt in addition to the pulsations, identifies the point at which the pressure in the cuff nears the diastolic pressure. This vibration is no longer felt when the cuff pressure is below the diastolic pressure. To palpate the diastolic pressure, the nurse applies light to moderate pressure over the pulse point.

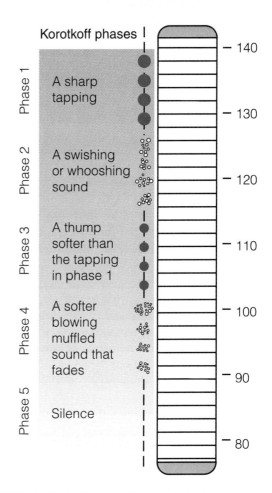

FIGURE 2-20 ◆ Korotkoff's sounds. In the illustration, the blood pressure is 138/90 or 138/102/90.

Nursing Process: Blood Pressure

ASSESSMENT

1. Blood pressure readings are used to:
   - Provide a baseline measure of arterial blood pressure for subsequent evaluation
   - Determine the client's hemodynamic status (e.g., stroke volume of the heart and blood vessel resistance)
   - Identify and monitor changes in blood pressure resulting from a disease process and medical therapy (e.g., presence or history of cardiovascular disease, renal disease, circulatory shock, or acute pain; rapid infusion of fluids or blood products)
   - Determine client's safety in performing activity such as arising after extended bed rest or recovery from anesthesia

2. In order to assess the client's general pulmonary health, examine for signs and symptoms of **hypertension** (e.g., headache, ringing in the ears, flushing of face, nosebleeds, fatigue); signs and symptoms of **hypotension** (e.g., tachycardia, dizziness, mental confusion, restlessness, cool and clammy skin, pale or cyanotic skin); factors affecting blood pressure (e.g., activity, emotional stress, pain, and time the client last smoked or ingested caffeine).

PLANNING

Delegation

Blood pressure measurement may be delegated to UAP. The interpretation of abnormal blood pressure readings and determination of appropriate responses are done by the nurse.

IMPLEMENTATION:
TECHNIQUE 2-6 ASSESSING BLOOD PRESSURE

Equipment
- Stethoscope or DUS

- Blood pressure cuff of the appropriate size (newborn, infant, child, small adult, adult, large adult, thigh). The blood pressure cuff consists of a rubber

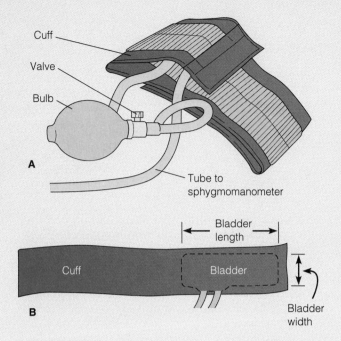

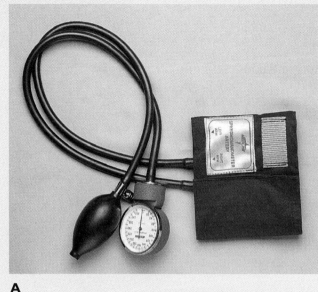

FIGURE 2-21 ◆ (A) Blood pressure cuff and bulb, (B) bladder.

bag that can be inflated with air, called the *bladder* (Figure 2-21 ◆). It is usually covered with cloth and has two tubes attached to it. One tube connects to a rubber bulb that inflates the bladder. When turned counterclockwise, a small valve on the side of this bulb releases the air in the bladder. When the valve is tightened (turned clockwise), air pumped into the bladder remains there. The other tube is attached to a sphygmomanometer (Figure 2-22 ◆).

Blood pressure cuffs come in various sizes. The width should be 40 percent of the circumference, or 20 percent wider than the diameter of the midpoint of the limb on which it is used (Figure 2-23 ◆). The length of the bladder also affects the accuracy of measurement. The bladder should be sufficiently long almost to encircle the limb and to cover at least two-thirds of its circumference. If the cuff is too small, a false high systolic reading will occur.

• Sphygmomanometer. The **sphygmomanometer** indicates the pressure of the air within the bladder. There are two types of sphygmomanometers: *aneroid* and *mercury* (Figure 2-22). The aneroid sphygmomanometer is a calibrated dial with a needle that points to the calibrations. The mercury sphygmomanometer is a calibrated cylinder filled with mercury. The pressure is indicated at the point to which the meniscus of the mercury (the crescent-shaped top surface of the column) rises. It is important to view the meniscus at eye level to avoid distortions in the reading.

Some agencies use electronic sphygmomanometers, which eliminate the need to listen to the sounds of the client's systolic and diastolic blood

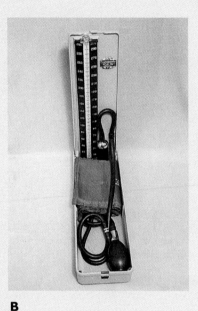

FIGURE 2-22 ◆ Blood pressure equipment: (A) an aneroid manometer and cuff and (B) a mercury manometer and cuff.

pressures through a stethoscope. With some electronic sphygmomanometers, as the pressure in the cuff is lowered, a light flashes to indicate the systolic and diastolic pressures.

Preparation

1. Ensure that the equipment is intact and functioning properly. Check for leaks in the rubber tubing of the sphygmomanometer.

2. Make sure that the client has not smoked or ingested caffeine within 30 minutes prior to measurement.

Performance

1. Explain to the client what you are going to do,

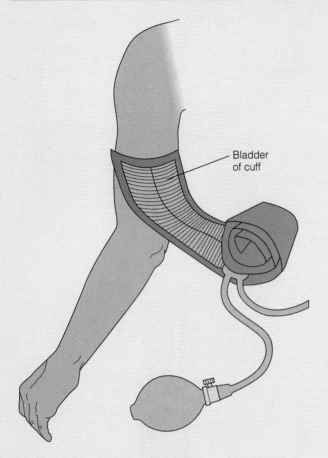

FIGURE 2-23 ◆ Determining the bladder of a blood pressure cuff is 40 percent of the arm circumference or 20 percent wider than the diameter of the midpoint of the limb.

Bladder of cuff

why it is necessary, and how he or she can cooperate. Discuss how the results will be used in planning further care or treatments.

2. Wash hands and observe appropriate infection control procedures.

3. Provide for client privacy.

4. Position the client appropriately.

- The adult client should be sitting unless otherwise specified. Both feet should be flat on the floor because *legs crossed at the knee result in elevated systolic and diastolic blood pressures* (Foster-Fitzpatrick, Oritz, Sibilano, Marcentonio, & Braun, 1999).

- The elbow should be slightly flexed with the palm of the hand facing up and the forearm supported at heart level. Readings in any other position should be specified. The blood pressure is normally similar in sitting, standing, and lying positions, but it can vary significantly by position in certain persons. *The blood pressure increases when the arm is below heart level and decreases when the arm is above heart level.*

- Expose the upper arm.

5. Wrap the deflated cuff evenly around the upper arm. Locate the brachial artery (see Figure 2-13). Apply the center of the bladder directly over the artery. *The bladder inside the cuff must be directly over the artery to be compressed if the reading is to be accurate.*

- For an adult, place the lower border of the cuff approximately 2.5 cm (1 in) above the antecubital space.

6. If this is the client's initial examination, perform a preliminary palpatory determination of systolic pressure. *The initial estimate tells the nurse the maximal pressure to which the manometer needs to be elevated in subsequent determinations. It also prevents underestimation of the systolic pressure or overestimation of the diastolic pressure should an* **auscultatory gap** *occur.*

- Palpate the brachial artery with the fingertips.

- Close the valve on the pump by turning the knob clockwise.

- Pump up the cuff until you no longer feel the brachial pulse. At that pressure, the blood cannot flow through the artery. Note the pressure on the sphygmomanometer at which the pulse is no longer felt. *This gives an estimate of the maximum pressure required to measure the systolic pressure.*

- Release the pressure completely in the cuff, and wait 1 to 2 minutes before making further measurements. *A waiting period gives the blood trapped in the veins time to be released. Otherwise, false high systolic readings will occur.*

7. Position the stethoscope appropriately.

- Cleanse the earpieces with alcohol or recommended disinfectant.

- Insert the ear attachments of the stethoscope in your ears so that they tilt slightly forward. *Sounds are heard more clearly when the ear attachments follow the direction of the ear canal.*

- Ensure that the stethoscope hangs freely from the ears to the diaphragm. *Rubbing the stethoscope against an object can obliterate the sounds of the blood within an artery.*

- Place the bell side of the amplifier of the stethoscope over the brachial pulse. *Because the blood pressure is a low-frequency sound, it is best heard with the bell-shaped diaphragm.* Hold the diaphragm with the thumb and index finger.

8. Auscultate the client's blood pressure.

- Pump up the cuff until the sphygmomanometer is 30 mm Hg above the point where the brachial pulse disappeared.

- Release the valve on the cuff carefully so that the pressure decreases at the rate of 2 to 3 mm Hg per second. *If the rate is faster or slower, an error in measurement may occur.*

- As the pressure falls, identify the manometer reading at each of the five phases.
- Deflate the cuff rapidly and completely.
- Wait 1 to 2 minutes before making further determinations. *This permits blood trapped in the veins to be released.*
- Repeat the above steps once or twice as necessary to confirm the accuracy of the reading.

9. If this is the client's initial examination, repeat the procedure on the client's other arm. There should be a difference of no more than 10 mm Hg between the arms. The arm found to have the higher pressure should be used for subsequent examinations.

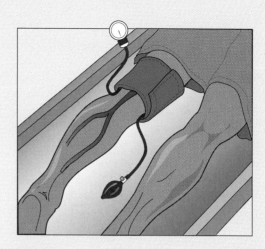

FIGURE 2-24 ◆ Measuring blood pressure in the client's thigh.

Variation: Obtaining a Blood Pressure by the Palpation Method

If it is not possible to use a stethoscope to obtain the blood pressure or if Korotkoff's sounds cannot be heard, palpate the radial or brachial pulse site as the cuff pressure is released. The manometer reading at the point where the pulse reappears is a mean pressure between systolic and diastolic.

10. Remove the cuff from the client's arm.

11. Wipe the cuff with an approved disinfectant. *Cuffs can become significantly contaminated.*

12. **Document** and report pertinent assessment data according to agency policy. Record two pressures in the form "130/80" where "130" is the systolic (phase 1) and "80" is the diastolic (phase 5) pressure. Record three pressures in the form "130/110/90," where "130" is the systolic, "110" is the first diastolic (phase 4), and "90" is the second diastolic (phase 5) pressure. Use the abbreviations RA for right arm and LA for left arm. Record a difference of greater than 10 mm Hg in the arms.

Variation: Taking a Thigh Blood Pressure

- Help the client to assume the prone position. If the client cannot assume this position, measure the blood pressure while the client is in the supine position with the knee slightly flexed. Slight flexing of the knee will facilitate placing the stethoscope on the popliteal space (Figure 2-24 ◆).

- Expose the thigh, taking care not to expose the client unduly.
- Locate the popliteal artery (see Figure 2-13).
- Wrap the cuff evenly around the midthigh with the compression bladder over the posterior aspect of the thigh and the bottom edge above the knee. *The bladder must be directly over the posterior popliteal artery if the reading is to be accurate.*
- If this is the client's initial examination, perform a preliminary palpatory determination of systolic pressure by palpating the popliteal artery.
- In adults, the systolic pressure in the popliteal artery is usually 20 to 30 mm Hg higher than that in the brachial artery because of use of a larger bladder; the diastolic pressure is usually the same.

Variation: Using an Electronic Indirect Blood Pressure Monitoring Device

- Place the blood pressure cuff on the extremity according to the manufacturer's guidelines.
- Turn on the blood pressure switch.
- If appropriate, set the device for the desired number of minutes between blood pressure determinations (Figure 2-25 ◆).
- When the device has determined the blood pressure reading, note the digital results.

AMBULATORY AND COMMUNITY SETTINGS

Blood Pressure

- If the client takes blood pressure readings at home, use the same equipment or calibrate it against a system known to be accurate.
- Observe the client or family member taking the blood pressure and provide feedback if further instruction is needed.

- If the client is in a chair or low bed, position yourself so that you maintain the client's arm at heart level and you can read the sphygmomanometer at eye level.

AGE-RELATED CONSIDERATIONS

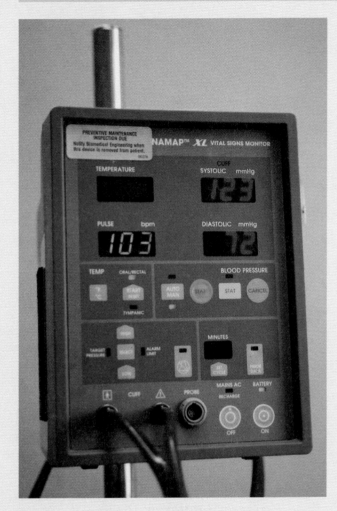

FIGURE 2-25 ◆ Electronic BP (adult).

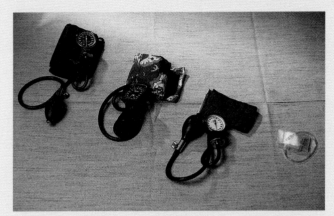

FIGURE 2-26 ◆ Pediatric blood pressure cuffs (with manometers).

Child

• Explain each step of the process and what it will feel like. Demonstrate on a doll.

• Use the palpation technique for children under 3 years old.

• Cuff bladder width should be 40 percent and length should be 80 to 100 percent of the arm circumference (Figure 2-26 ◆).

• Take the blood pressure prior to other uncomfortable procedures so that the blood pressure is not artificially elevated by the discomfort.

• In children, the diastolic pressure is considered to be the onset of phase 4, where the sounds become muffled.

• In children, the thigh pressure is about 10 mm Hg higher than the arm.

Elders

• Skin may be very fragile. Do not allow cuff pressure to remain high any longer than necessary.

• Determine if the client is taking antihypertensives and, if so, when the last dose was taken.

• If the client has arm contractures, assess the blood pressure by palpation, with the arm in a relaxed position. If this is not possible, take a thigh blood pressure.

Blood Pressure

Infant

• Use a pediatric stethoscope with small diaphragm.

• The lower edge of the blood pressure cuff can be closer to the antecubital space of an infant.

• Use the palpation method if auscultation with a stethoscope or Doppler is unsuccessful.

• Arm and thigh pressures are equivalent in children under 1 year of age.

EVALUATION

• Relate blood pressure to other vital signs, to baseline data, and health status.

• Report any significant change in the client's blood pressure. Also report these findings:

• Systolic blood pressure of an adult above 140 mm Hg

• Diastolic blood pressure of an adult above 90 mm Hg

• Systolic blood pressure of an adult below 100 mm Hg

- Conduct appropriate follow-up such as administration of medication. If the blood pressure is significantly higher or lower than usual, implement appropriate safety precautions.

Oxygen Saturation

A pulse **oximeter** is a noninvasive device that measures a client's arterial blood **oxygen saturation** (SaO$_2$) by means of a sensor attached to the client's finger (Figure 2-27 ◆), toe, nose, earlobe, or forehead (or around the hand or foot of a neonate). The pulse oximeter can detect hypoxemia before clinical signs and symptoms, such as dusky skin or nailbed color.

The pulse oximeter's *sensor* has two parts: (a) two light-emitting diodes (LEDs)—one red, the other infrared—that transmit light through nails, tissue, venous blood, and arterial blood; and (b) a photodetector placed directly opposite the LEDs (e.g., the other side of the finger, toe, or nose). The photodetector measures the amount of red and infrared light absorbed by oxygenated and deoxygenated hemoglobin in arterial blood and reports it as SaO$_2$. Normal SaO$_2$ is 95 to 100 percent, and an SaO$_2$ below 70 percent is life threatening.

Factors Affecting Oxygen Saturation Readings

- *Hemoglobin.* If the hemoglobin is fully saturated with oxygen, the SaO$_2$ will appear normal even if the total hemoglobin level is low. Thus, the client could be severely anemic and have inadequate oxygen to supply the tissues but the pulse oximeter would return a normal value.

- *Circulation.* The oximeter will not return an accurate reading if the area under the sensor has impaired circulation.

- *Activity.* Shivering or excessive movement of the sensor site may interfere with accurate readings.

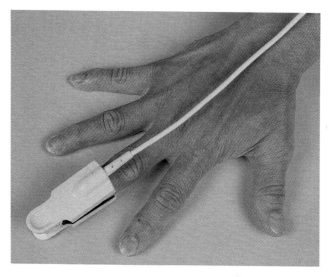

FIGURE 2-27 ◆ Fingertip oximeter sensor (adult).

Nursing Process: Measuring Oxygen Saturation

ASSESSMENT

1. Based on the client's age and physical condition, determine the best location for a pulse oximeter sensor.

2. Consider the client's overall condition including risk factors for development of hypoxemia (e.g., respiratory or cardiac disease) and hemoglobin level.

3. Determine vital signs, skin and nailbed color, and tissue perfusion of extremities as baseline data.

4. Assess for allergy to adhesive.

PLANNING

Delegation

Application of the pulse oximeter sensor and recording of the SaO$_2$ value may be delegated to UAP. The interpretation of the oxygen saturation value and determination of appropriate responses are done by the nurse.

IMPLEMENTATION:
TECHNIQUE 2-7 ASSESSING OXYGEN SATURATION (PULSE OXIMETER)

Equipment

- Nail polish remover as needed
- Alcohol wipe
- Sheet or towel
- Pulse oximeter

Pulse oximeters with various types of sensors are available from several manufacturers. The *oximeter unit* consists of an inlet connection for the sensor cable, a faceplate that indicates (a) the oxygen saturation measurement (expressed as a percentage) and (b) the pulse rate. Cordless units are also available (Figure 2-28 ◆). A preset alarm system signals high and low SaO$_2$ measurements and a high and low pulse rate. The high and low SaO$_2$ levels are generally preset at 100 percent and 85 percent, respectively, for adults. The high and low pulse rate alarms are usually preset at 140 and 50 beats per minute for adults. These alarm

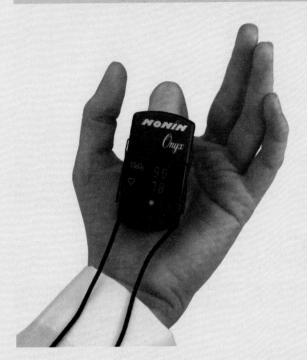

FIGURE 2-28 ◆ Fingertip oximeter sensor (cordless).
Courtesy Nonin Medical Inc.

limits can, however, be changed according to the manufacturer's directions.

Preparation

Check that the oximeter equipment is functioning normally.

Performance

1. Explain to the client what you are going to do, why it is necessary, and how he or she can cooperate. Discuss how the results will be used in planning further care or treatments.

2. Wash hands and observe appropriate infection control procedures.

3. Provide for client privacy.

4. Choose a sensor appropriate for the client's weight, size, and desired location. Because weight limits of sensors overlap, a pediatric sensor could be used for a small adult.
   • If the client is allergic to adhesive, use a clip or sensor without adhesive. If using an extremity, assess the proximal pulse and capillary refill at the point closest to the site.
   • If the client has low tissue perfusion due to peripheral vascular disease or therapy using vasoconstrictive medications, use a nasal sensor or a reflectance sensor on the forehead. Avoid using lower extremities that have a compromised circu-

lation and extremities that are used for infusions or other invasive monitoring.

5. Prepare the site.
   • Clean the site with an alcohol wipe before applying the sensor.
   • It may be necessary to remove a female client's nail polish or acrylic nails because *they can interfere with accurate measurements.*

6. Apply the sensor, and connect it to the pulse oximeter.
   • Make sure the LED and photodetector are accurately aligned (i.e., opposite each other on either side of the finger, toe, nose, or earlobe). Many sensors have markings to facilitate correct alignment of the LEDs and photodetector.
   • Attach the sensor cable to the connection outlet on the oximeter. Turn on the machine according to the manufacturer's directions. Appropriate connection will be confirmed by an audible beep indicating each arterial pulsation. Some devices have a wheel that can be turned clockwise to increase the pulse volume and counterclockwise to decrease it.
   • Ensure that the bar of light or waveform on the face of the oximeter fluctuates with each pulsation and reflects the pulse volume or strength.

7. Set and turn on the alarm.
   • Check the preset alarm limits for high and low oxygen saturation and high and low pulse rates. Change these alarm limits according to the manufacturer's directions as indicated. Ensure that the audio and visual alarms are on before you leave the client. A tone will be heard and a number will blink on the faceplate.

8. Ensure client safety.
   • Inspect and/or move or change the location of an adhesive toe or finger sensor every 4 hours and a spring-tension sensor every 2 hours.
   • Inspect the sensor site tissues for irritation from adhesive sensors.

9. Ensure the accuracy of measurement.
   • Minimize motion artifacts by using an adhesive sensor, or immobilize the client's monitoring site. *Movement of the client's finger or toe may be misinterpreted by the oximeter as arterial pulsations.*
   • If indicated, cover the sensor with a sheet or towel to block large amounts of light from external sources (e.g., sunlight, procedure lamps, or bilirubin lights in the nursery). *Large amounts of outside light may be sensed by the photodetector and alter the SaO$_2$ value.*

 10. **Document** the oxygen saturation on the appropriate record at designated intervals.

Pulse Oximetry

- Pulse oximetry is a quick, inexpensive, noninvasive method of assessing oxygenation. Like an automatic blood pressure cuff, it also provides a pulse rate reading. Use in the ambulatory or home setting whenever indicated.

- If the client requires frequent or continuous home monitoring, teach the client and family how to apply and maintain the equipment. Remind them to rotate the site periodically and assess for skin trauma.

AGE-RELATED CONSIDERATIONS

Pulse Oximetry

Infant

- If an appropriate-sized finger or toe sensor (Figure 2-29 ◆) is not available, consider using an earlobe or forehead sensor.
- The high and low SaO_2 levels are generally preset at 95 percent and 80 percent for neonates.
- The high and low pulse rate alarms are usually preset at 200 and 100 for neonates.

Child

- Instruct the child that the sensor does not hurt. Disconnect the probe whenever possible to allow for movement.

Elders

- Use of vasoconstrictive medications, poor circulation, or thickened nails may make finger or toe sensors inaccurate.

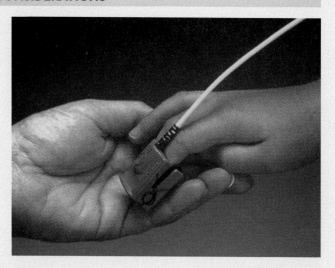

FIGURE 2-29 ◆ Finger tip oximeter sensor (child).
Courtesy Nonin Medical Inc.

EVALUATION

- Compare the oxygen saturation to the client's previous oxygen saturation level. Relate to pulse rate and other vital signs.

- Conduct appropriate follow-up such as notifying the physician, adjusting oxygen therapy, or providing breathing treatments.

Chapter Summary

TERMINOLOGY

apical pulse
apical–radial pulse
apnea
arrhythmia
auscultatory gap
bradypnea
cardinal signs
Cheyne–Stokes breathing
core temperature
costal breathing
diaphragmatic breathing
diastolic
dyspnea
eupnea
exhalation
expiration

febrile
fever
flail chest
hemoptysis
hyperpyrexia
hypertension
hyperthermia
hyperventilation
hypotension
hypothermia
hypoventilation
inhalation
inspiration
orthopnea
oximeter
oxygen saturation

paradoxical breathing
peripheral pulse
point of maximal impulse (PMI)
pulse deficit
pulse pressure
pyrexia
respiration
retraction
sphygmomanometer
stridor
systolic
tachypnea
ventilation
vital signs
wheeze

FORMING CLINICAL JUDGMENTS

Consider This:

1. What should you do if the client has been eating or smoking within the past 30 minutes and you wish to take the temperature?

2. How should you proceed if the client is not cooperative and able to understand your instructions regarding the use of an oral glass thermometer?

3. What are several reasons why is it important to know by what route the last temperature reading was taken, when, and what the resultant temperature reading was?

4. In an emergency, the radial pulse may not be accessible or palpable. What other two sites are useful in such situations?

5. When assessing pulses in the foot, what is the next action to take if neither the posterior tibial nor dorsalis pedis pulse can be felt?

6. While you are counting respirations following counting the client's pulse, the client asks why it is taking so long. What would be an appropriate response?

7. If using a mercury manometer for blood pressure reading in the home, at what height should you place the mercury column?

8. While releasing the cuff and auscultating the blood pressure, the client coughs loudly and jerks the arm, resulting in your inability to accurately hear the Korotkoff's sounds. In detail, how should you proceed?

9. The pulse oximeter on the client's finger reads 85 percent. The client's skin is warm and has normal color; the client is awake and oriented, temperature is 98.8°F, apical pulse 78, BP 136/84. What would be your next actions?

RELATED RESEARCH

Beckstrand, R. L., Wilshaw, R., Moran, S., & Schaalje, G. B. (1996). Practice applications of research: Supralingual temperatures compared to tympanic and rectal temperatures. *Pediatric Nursing, 22*, 436–438.

Foster-Fitzpatrick, L., Ortiz, A., Sibilano, H., Marcantonio, R., & Braun, L. T. (1999). The effects of crossed leg on blood pressure measurement. *Nursing Research, 48*, 105–108.

Lanham, D. M., Walker, B., Klocke, E., and Jennings, M. (1999). Accuracy of tympanic temperature readings in children under 6 years of age. *Pediatric Nursing, 25*(1), 39–42.

Manian, F. A., & Griesenauer, S. (1998). Lack of agreement between tympanic and oral temperature measurements in adult hospitalized patients. *American Journal of Infection Control, 26*, 428–430.

Moniaci, V., & Kraus, M. (1997). Determining the relationship between invasive and noninvasive blood pressure values. *Neonatal Network, 16*(1), 51–56.

REFERENCES

_____. (1997). Consult stat. Guidelines for monitoring BP at home. *RN, 60*(1), 57.

_____. (2000). Consult stat. Tips for getting more reliable O$_2$ saturation reading. *RN, 63*(2), 73.

Ball, J., & Bindler, R. (1999). *Pediatric nursing: Caring for children*. Stamford, CT: Appleton & Lange.

Bayne, C. G. (1997). Technology assessment: Vital signs: Are we monitoring the right parameters? *Nursing Management, 28*(5), 74–76.

Bindler, R., & Ball, J. (1999). *Quick reference to pediatric clinical skills*. Stamford, CT: Appleton & Lange.

Braun, S. K., Preston, P., & Smith, R. N. (1998). Getting a better read on thermometry. *RN, 61*(3), 57–60.

Bushey, P., Chulay, M., & Holland, S. (1997). Correlation of indirect blood pressure measurements and systemic blood pressure. *Critical Care Nurse, 17*, 12.

Cowan, T. (1997). Product review: Ambulatory blood pressure monitors. *Professional Nurse, 12*, 373–376.

Faria, S. H. (1999). Assessment of vital signs in the child. *Home Care Provider, 4*, 222–223.

Faria, S. H. (1999). Patient assessment: Assessment of peripheral arterial pulses. *Home Care Provider, 4*, 140–141.

Foster-Fitzpatrick, L., Ortiz, A., Sibilano, H., Marcantonio, R., & Braun, L. T. (1999). The effects of crossed leg on blood pressure measurement. *Nursing Research, 48*, 105–108.

Graves, J. W. (1999). The clinical utility of out-of-office self-measurement of blood pressure. *Home Healthcare Consultant, 6*(11), 26–29.

Karch, A. M., & Karch, F. E. (2000). Practice errors: When a blood pressure isn't routine. *American Journal of Nursing, 100*(3), 23.

McConnell, E. A. (1999). Do's and don'ts: Performing pulse oximetry. *Nursing, 29*(11), 17.

National Institutes of Health, National Heart, Lung, and Blood Institute. (1997). *The sixth report of the Joint National Committee on Prevention, Detection, Evaluation, and Treatment of High Blood Pressure*. NIH Publication #98-4080.

Nicholls, P. H. (1997). Consult stat. Wrist and finger BP monitors offer accurate alternatives. *RN, 60*(4), 64.

O'Toole, S. (1998). Temperature measurement devices. *Professional Nurse, 13*, 779–782.

Roper, M. (1996). Back to basics: Assessing orthostatic vital signs. *American Journal of Nursing, 96*(8), 43–46.

Schiff, L. (2000). Pulse oximeters. *RN 63*(8), 65–66, 68.

Torrance, C., & Semple, M. (1997). Practical procedures for nurses: Assessing pulse—1. *Nursing Times, 93*(41), insert 2.

Torrance, C., & Elley, K. (1997). Practical procedures for nurses: Assessing pulse—2. *Nursing Times, 93*(42), insert 2.

Weiss, M. E., Sitzer, V., Clarke, M., Haley, K., Richards, M., Sanchez, A., & Gocka, I. (1998). A comparison of temperature measurements using three ear thermometers. *Applied Nursing Research, 11*, 158–166.

Woo, E. K. (1998). Device errors: Infant skin temperature probes: Follow these safety tips for use. *Nursing, 28*(7), 31.

Chapter 3

Assessing Adult Health

Techniques

OBJECTIVES

- Define terms associated with health assessment.
- Describe 10 components of a nursing health history.
- Identify purposes of the physical health examination.
- Explain the four methods of examining.
- Explain the significance of selected physical findings.
- Identify expected outcomes of health assessment.
- Identify the various steps in selected assessment procedures.
- Describe suggested sequencing to conduct a physical health assessment in an orderly fashion.
- Discuss variations in assessment techniques appropriate for clients of different ages.

Nursing Health History

The nursing health history interview is the first part of the assessment of the client's health status and is usually carried out before the physical examination. This is a structured interview designed to collect specific health data and to obtain a detailed health record of the client. Its purposes are:

- To elicit information about all the variables that may affect the client's health status
- To obtain data that help the nurse understand and appreciate the client's life experiences
- To initiate a nonjudgmental, trusting interpersonal relationship with the client

The nurse uses the data obtained in collaboration with the client to develop individualized care. Components of the nursing history include (1) biographic data, (2) chief complaint or reason for visit, (3) history of present illness (current health status), (4) past history, (5) family history of illness, (6) lifestyle, (7) social data, (8) psychological data, and (9) patterns of health care. Content of each of these components is described in Box 3-1. In addition, a review of systems (also called a screening interview) may be done. This involves a brief review of the essential functioning of each body part or physiologic system. In collecting history data, the nurse applies knowledge of the variations in verbal and nonverbal communication styles among persons of different cultures. See Table 3-1.

Physical Health Examination

A complete health assessment is generally conducted moving from the head to the toes. However, the procedure can vary in many ways according to the age of the individual, the severity of the illness, the preferences of the nurse, and the agency's priorities and procedures. Regardless of what procedure is used, the assessment is conducted in a systematic and efficient manner that conserves energy and time and requires the fewest position changes for the client.

Prepare the client by explaining what will be done, the reasons for the examination, and what the client can expect. Prepare the environment by obtaining all necessary equipment, including adequate lighting, drapes for privacy, and adjusting the room temperature. Equipment commonly used in performing an examination is shown in Table 3-2.

Methods of Examining

Four primary techniques are used in the physical examination: inspection, palpation, percussion, and auscultation.

Box 3-1 *Components of a Nursing Health History*

Biographic Data

Client's name, address, age, sex, marital status, occupation, religious preference, health care financing, and usual source of medical care.

Chief Complaint or Reason for Visit

The answer given to the question "What is troubling you?" or "What brought you to the hospital or clinic?" The chief complaint should be recorded in the client's own words.

History of Present Illness

- When the symptoms started
- Whether the onset of symptoms was sudden or gradual
- How often the problem occurs
- Exact location of the distress
- Character of the complaint (e.g., intensity of pain or quality of sputum, emesis, or discharge)
- Activity in which the client was involved when the problem occurred
- Phenomena or symptoms associated with the chief complaint
- Factors that aggravate or alleviate the problem

Past History

- *Childhood illnesses,* such as chickenpox, mumps, measles, rubella (German measles), rubeola (red measles), streptococcal infections, scarlet fever, rheumatic fever, and other significant illnesses
- *Childhood immunizations* and the date of the last tetanus shot
- *Allergies* to drugs, animals, insects, or other environmental agents and the type of reaction that occurs
- *Accidents and injuries:* how, when, and where the incident occurred, type of injury, treatment received, and any complications
- *Hospitalization* for serious illnesses: reasons for the hospitalization, dates, surgery performed, course of recovery, and any complications
- *Medications:* all currently used prescription and over-the-counter medications, such as aspirin, nasal spray, vitamins, or laxatives

Family History of Illness

To ascertain risk factors for certain diseases, the ages of siblings, parents, and grandparents and their current state of health or (if they are deceased) the cause of death are obtained. Particular attention should be given to disorders such as heart disease, cancer, diabetes, hypertension, obesity, allergies, arthritis, tuberculosis, bleeding, alcoholism, and any mental health disorders.

Lifestyle

- *Personal habits:* the amount, frequency, and duration of substance use (tobacco, alcohol, coffee, cola, tea, and illicit or recreational drugs)
- *Diet:* description of a typical diet on a normal day or any special diet, number of meals and snacks per day, who cooks and shops for food, ethnically distinct food patterns, and allergies
- *Sleep/rest patterns:* usual daily sleep/wake times, difficulties sleeping, and remedies used for difficulties
- *Activities of daily living (ADLs):* any difficulties experienced in the basic activities of eating, grooming, dressing, elimination, and locomotion
- *Recreation/hobbies:* exercise activity and tolerance, hobbies and other interests, and vacations

Social Data

- *Family relationships/friendships:* The client's support system in times of stress (who helps in time of need?); what effect the client's illness has on the family; and whether any family problems are affecting the client. See also the discussion of family assessment in Chapter 12.
- *Ethnic affiliation:* Health customs and beliefs; cultural practices that may affect health care and recovery. See also detailed ethnic/cultural assessment guide in Chapter 13.
- *Educational history:* Data about the client's highest level of education attained and any past difficulties with learning.
- *Occupational history:* Current employment status, the number of days missed from work because of illness, any history of accidents on the job, any occupational hazards with a potential for future disease or accident, the client's need to change jobs because of past illness, the employment status of both spouses or partners and the way child care is handled, and the client's overall satisfaction with the work.
- *Economic status:* Information about how the client is paying for medical care (including what kind of medical and hospitalization coverage the client has), and whether the client's illness presents financial concerns.
- *Home and neighborhood conditions:* Home safety measures and adjustments in physical facilities that may be required to help the client manage a physical disability, activity intolerance, and activities of daily living; the availability of neighborhood and community services to meet the client's needs.

- *Major stressors* experienced in the past year and the client's perception of them.
- *Usual coping pattern* with a serious problem or a high level of stress.
- *Communication style.* Ability to verbalize appropriate emotion; nonverbal communication—such as eye movements, gestures, use of touch, and posture; interactions with support persons; and the congruence of nonverbal behavior and verbal expression.

All health care resources the client is currently using and has used in the past. These include the family physician, specialists (e.g., ophthalmologist or gynecologist), dentist, folk practitioners (e.g., herbalist or curandero), health clinic, or health center; whether the client considers the care being provided adequate; and whether access to health care is a problem.

Inspection

Inspection is visual examination, that is, assessing by using the sense of sight. The nurse inspects with the naked eye and with a lighted instrument such as an **otoscope** (used to view the ear). Use of the senses of hearing and smell may also be considered part of inspection. Inspection should be systematic, so that nothing is missed.

Palpation

Palpation is the examination of the body using the sense of touch. The pads of the fingers are used because their concentration of nerve endings makes them highly sensitive to tactile discrimination. Palpation is used to determine (1) texture (e.g., of the hair); (2) temperature (e.g., of a skin area); (3) vibration (e.g., of a joint); (4) position, size, consistency,

---

TABLE 3-1	CULTURAL NORMS RELEVANT TO HEALTH ASSESSMENT

Here are a few examples of different cultural norms in nonverbal communication. Cultural norms will vary within a culture, and from generation to generation. Therefore, it is extremely important to make few assumptions, observe carefully, and ask your client about preferences. Your assessment and care will benefit greatly from this awareness of differences.

Eye Contact

Keep in Mind—Eye contact and the handshake hold different shades of meaning for different cultures. For example, some Native American communities consider direct eye contact an invasion of privacy and a firm handshake aggressive. Many Asian cultures avoid eye contact as a sign of respect for the other individual. The nurse of Western European descent might believe that a client who avoids direct eye contact is somewhat suspicious, and that a weak handshake signifies disinterest.

Touch and Personal Space

Keep in Mind—European Americans tend to keep a certain amount of personal space between themselves and others, typically three feet, and use touch sparingly. French people typically feel comfortable standing very close to others, and are more comfortable touching. Cultural groups such as Orthodox Jews and Chinese Americans may consider excessive touching, especially from the opposite sex, offensive.

Use of Body Language

Keep in Mind—Body language can easily be misinterpreted during the assessment, so pay careful attention to the assumptions you are making based on your own cultural norms. For example, European Americans typically nod to indicate agreement or approval. Asian Americans may nod to be polite, but this may not actually indicate agreement.

Nursing Implications—Be careful not to assume things about your client based on the norms for your own cultural group. For example, if you value eye contact as a sign of interest, you may incorrectly assume your client is disinterested if he or she does not maintain eye contact. In fact, the client may be trying to show respect for you. Observing your client with family and other individuals is a helpful way to learn about his or her usual pattern of eye contact.

Nursing Implications—Note patterns of touch between family members, or individuals of the same culture. Just as with eye contact, it may be difficult for you to change your habits of touch and personal space. However, if you sense unease in your clients, reevaluate your actions to be more sensitive to their comfort level. When in doubt, ask your client if he or she feels comfortable in the situation.

Nursing Implications—Make sure that you are not relying solely on nonverbal clues to determine if your client understands or agrees with you. Instead of asking, "Did you understand how we will test your blood?" and relying on a nod as the affirmation, you might ask, "Can you explain how we will test your blood?" Also try to follow up your questions so that you actually hear a verbal "yes" or a "no" response.

TABLE 3-2 **EQUIPMENT AND SUPPLIES**

Supplies	Purpose
Flashlight or penlight	To assist viewing of the pharynx and cervix or to determine the reactions of the pupils of the eye
Laryngeal or dental mirror	To observe the pharynx and oral cavity
Nasal speculum	To permit visualization of the lower and middle turbinates; usually, a penlight is used for illumination
Ophthalmoscope	A lighted instrument to visualize the interior of the eye
Otoscope	A lighted instrument to visualize the eardrum and external auditory canal (a nasal speculum may be attached to the otoscope to inspect the nasal cavities)
Percussion (reflex) hammer	An instrument with a rubber head to test reflexes
Tuning fork	A two-pronged metal instrument used to test hearing acuity and vibratory sense
Vaginal speculum (various sizes)	To assess the cervix and the vagina
Assorted containers and slides	For specimens
Cotton applicators	To obtain specimens
Disposable pads	To absorb liquid
Drapes	To cover the client
Gloves (sterile and unsterile)	To protect the nurse
Lubricant	To ease insertion of instruments (e.g., vaginal speculum)
Sterile safety pins	To test sensory function
Tongue blades (depressors)	To depress the tongue during assessment of the mouth and pharynx

From *Fundamentals of nursing: Concepts, process, and practice,* 6th ed., by B. Kozier, G. Erb, A. Berman, & K. Burke, 2000, Upper Saddle River, NJ: Prentice Hall Health.

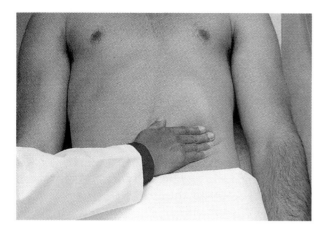

FIGURE 3-1 ◆ The position of the hand for light palpation.

and mobility of organs or masses; (5) distention (e.g., of the urinary bladder); (6) presence and rate of peripheral pulses; and (7) tenderness or pain.

There are two types of palpation: light and deep. Light (superficial) palpation should always precede deep palpation, because heavy pressure on the fingertips can dull the sense of touch. For *light palpation,* the nurse extends dominant hand fingers parallel to the skin surface and presses gently downward while moving the hand in a circular fashion (Figure 3-1 ◆).

Deep palpation is done with two hands (bimanually) or one hand. In deep bimanual palpation, the nurse extends the dominant hand as for light palpation, then places the finger pads of the nondominant hand on the dorsal surfaces of the distal interphalangeal joint of the middle three fingers of the dominant hand (Figure 3-2 ◆). The top hand applies pressure while the lower hand remains relaxed to perceive the tactile sensations. For deep palpation using one hand, the finger pads of the dominant hand press over the area to be

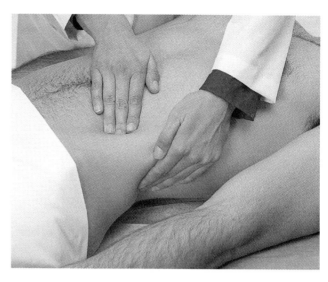

FIGURE 3-3 ◆ Deep palpation using the lower hand to support the body while the upper hand palpates the organ.

palpated. Often, the other hand is used to support a mass or organ from below (Figure 3-3 ◆).

Percussion

In **percussion,** the body surface is struck to elicit sounds that can be heard or vibrations that can be felt. There are two types of percussion: direct and indirect. In *direct percussion,* the nurse strikes the area to be percussed directly with the pads of two, three, or four fingers or with the pad of the middle finger. The strikes are rapid, and the movement is from the wrist. This technique is useful in percussing an adult's sinuses (Figure 3-4 ◆). The second type, *indirect percussion,* is the striking of an object (e.g., a finger) held against the body area to be examined. In this technique, the middle finger of the nondominant hand, referred to as the

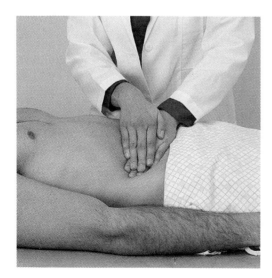

FIGURE 3-2 ◆ The position of the hand for deep bimanual palpation.

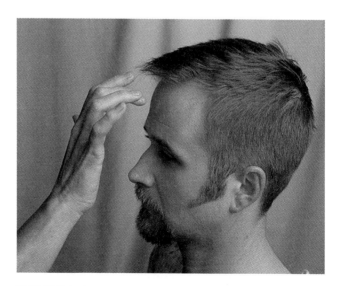

FIGURE 3-4 ◆ Direct percussion. Using one hand to strike the surface of the body.

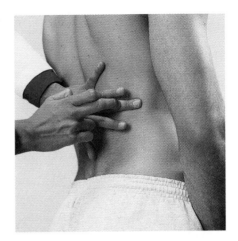

FIGURE 3-5 ◆ Indirect percussion. Using the finger of one hand to strike the finger of the other hand.

pleximeter, is placed firmly on the client's skin. Only the distal phalanx and joint of this finger should be in contact with the skin. Using the tip of the flexed middle finger of the other hand, called the **plexor**, the nurse strikes the pleximeter, usually at the distal interphalangeal joint or a point between the distal and proximal joints (Figure 3-5 ◆). The striking motion comes from the wrist; the forearm remains stationary. The angle between the plexor and the pleximeter should be 90 degrees, and the blows must be firm, rapid, and short to obtain a clear sound. Percussion is used to determine the size and shape of internal organs by establishing their borders. It indicates whether tissue is fluid-filled, air-filled, or solid. Percussion elicits five types of sound: **flatness, dullness, resonance, hyperresonance,** and **tympany.** See Table 3-3 for characteristics of the sounds and examples of where they may be heard.

Auscultation

Auscultation is the process of listening to sounds produced within the body, such as with the use of a stethoscope that amplifies the sounds and conveys them to the nurse's ears. The stethoscope should be 30 to 25 cm (12 to 14 in) long, with both a flat-disc and a bell-shaped diaphragm. (See Figure 2-18 on page 28.) The flat-disc diaphragm best transmits high-pitched sounds (e.g., bronchial sounds), and the bell-shaped diaphragm best transmits low-pitched sounds, such as some heart sounds.

Auscultated sounds are described according to their pitch, intensity, duration, and quality. The **pitch** is the frequency of the vibrations (the number of vibrations per second). Low-pitched sounds (e.g., some heart sounds) have fewer vibrations per second than high-pitched sounds (e.g., bronchial sounds). The intensity (amplitude) refers to the loudness or softness of a sound. Some body sounds are loud (e.g., bronchial sounds heard over the trachea), whereas others are soft (e.g., normal breath sounds heard in the lungs). The duration of a sound is its length (long or short). The quality of sound is a subjective description of a sound (e.g., whistling, gurgling, or snapping).

General Survey

Health assessment begins with a general survey that includes observation of the client's general appearance, mental status, vital signs, height, and weight. Many of the components of the general survey, such as body build, posture, hygiene, and mental status, are observed while taking the client's health history.

General Appearance and Mental Status

The general appearance and behavior of an individual must be assessed in terms of culture, educational level, socioeconomic status, and current circumstances. For example, an individual who has recently experienced a personal loss may appropriately appear depressed. Also, the client's age, sex, and race are useful factors in interpreting findings that suggest increased risk for known conditions.

PLANNING

Delegation

Due to the substantial knowledge and skill required, assessment of general appearance and mental status is

TABLE 3-3	PERCUSSION SOUNDS				
Sound	**Intensity**	**Pitch**	**Duration**	**Quality**	**Example of Location**
Flatness	Soft	High	Short	Extremely dull	Muscle, bone
Dullness	Medium	Medium	Moderate	Thudlike	Liver, heart
Resonance	Loud	Low	Long	Hollow	Normal lung
Hyperresonance	Very loud	Very low	Very long	Booming	Emphysematous lung
Tympany	Loud	High (distinguished mainly by musical timbre)	Moderate	Musical	Stomach filled with gas (air)

From *Fundamentals of nursing: Concepts, process, and practice,* 6th ed., by B. Kozier, G. Erb, A. Berman, & K. Burke, 2000, Upper Saddle River, NJ: Prentice Hall Health.

not delegated to unlicensed assistive personnel (UAP). However, many aspects are observed during usual care and may be recorded by persons other than the nurse.

Abnormal findings must be validated and interpreted by the nurse.

Equipment

• None.

Performance

1. Explain to the client what you are going to do, why it is necessary, and how he or she can cooper-ate. Discuss how the results will be used in planning further care or treatments.

2. Wash hands and observe appropriate infection control procedures.

3. Provide for client privacy.

ASSESSMENT	NORMAL FINDINGS	DEVIATIONS FROM NORMAL
4. Observe body build, height, and weight in relation to the client's age, lifestyle, and health.	Proportionate, varies with lifestyle	Excessively thin or obese
5. Observe the client's posture and gait, standing, sitting, and walking.	Relaxed, erect posture; coordinated movement	Tense, slouched, bent posture; uncoordinated movement; tremors
6. Observe the client's overall hygiene and grooming. Relate these to the person's activities prior to the assessment.	Clean, neat	Dirty, unkempt
7. Note body and breath odor in relation to activity level.	No body odor or minor body odor relative to work or exercise; no breath odor	Foul body odor; ammonia odor; acetone breath odor; foul breath
8. Observe for signs of distress in posture or facial expression.	No distress noted	Bending over because of abdominal pain, wincing, or labored breathing
9. Note obvious signs of health or illness (e.g., in skin color or breathing).	Healthy appearance	Pallor; weakness; obvious illness
10. Assess the client's attitude.	Cooperative	Negative, hostile, withdrawn
11. Note the client's affect/mood; assess the appropriateness of the client's responses.	Appropriate to situation	Inappropriate to situation
12. Listen for quantity of speech (amount and pace), quality (loudness, clarity, inflection), and organization (coherence of thought, overgeneralization, vagueness).	Understandable, moderate pace Exhibits thought association	Rapid or slow pace. Uses generalizations; lacks association; exhibits confabulation
13. Listen for relevance and organization of thoughts.	Logical sequence: makes sense; has sense of reality	Illogical sequence: flight of ideas; confusion

14. **Document** findings in the client record using forms or checklists supplemented by narrative notes when appropriate. See Figure 3-6 ♦.

ADMISSION DATA

Date 4-16-01 Time 3:15p.m. Primary Language English

Arrived Via: ☐ Wheelchair ☐ Stretcher ☑ Ambulatory

From: ☐ Admitting ☐ ER ☑ Home ☐ Nursing Home ☐ Other

Admitting M.D. R. Katz   Time Notified 5 p.m.

ORIENTATION TO UNIT

	YES NO		YES NO
Arm Band Correct	☒ ☐	Visiting Hours	☒ ☐
Allergy Band	☒ ☐	Smoking Policy	☒ ☐
Telephone	☒ ☐	TV, Lights, Bed Controls,	
Electrical Policy	☒ ☐	Call Lights, Side Rails	☒ ☐
Educational Mat'l	☒ ☐	Nurses Station	☒ ☐
(TV Brochure)	☒ ☐		

Family M.D. R. Katz

Weight 125 lb. Height 5ft. 2in. BP:R — L 122/80

Temp. 103F Pulse 92, weak Resp 28, shallow

Source Providing Information ☑ Patient ☐ Other

Unable to Obtain History ☐

Reason for Admission (Onset, Duration, Pt.'s Perception) "Chest cold" X 2 weeks S.O.B on exertion. "Lung pain, fever," "Dr. says I have pneumonia."

ALLERGIES & REACTIONS

Drugs Penicillin

Food/Other

Signs & Symptoms rash, nausea

Blood Reaction ☐ Yes ☑ No Dyes/Shellfish ☐ Yes ☑ No

MEDICATIONS

Current Meds	Dose/Freq.	Last Dose
Synthroid	0.1 mg. daily	4-16, 8 a.m.

Disposition of Meds: ☒ Home ☐ Pharmacy ☐ Safe *At Bedside

MEDICAL HISTORY

☑ No Major Problems   ☐ Gastro

☐ Cardiac   ☐ Arthritis

☐ Hyper/Hypotension   ☐ Stroke

☐ Diabetes   ☐ Seizures

☐ Cancer   ☐ Glaucoma

☐ Respiratory   ☑ Other Childbirth-1998

Surgery/Procedures	Date
Appendectomy	1978
Partial thyroidectomy	1991

SPECIAL ASSISTIVE DEVICES

☐ Wheelchair ☐ Contacts ☐ Venous ☐ Dentures

☐ Braces ☐ Hearing Aid Access ☐ Partial

☐ Cane/Crutches ☐ Prosthesis Device ☐ Upper

☐ Walker ☐ Glasses ☐ Epidural Catheter ☐ Lower

☐ Other None

VALUABLES

Patient informed Hospital not responsible for personal belongings.

Valuables Disposition: ☐ Patient ☐ Safe ☐ Given to

Patient/SO Signature None

PSYCHOSOCIAL HISTORY

Recent Stress None

Coping Mechanism Not assessed because of fatigue

Support System Husband, coworkers, friends

Calm: ☑ Yes ☐ No

Anxious: ☐ Yes ☑ No Facial muscles tense; trembling

Religion Catholic. Would want Last Rites

Tobacco Use: ☐ Yes ☑ No

Alcohol Use: ☐ Yes ☑ No

Drug Use: ☐ Yes ☑ No

NEUROLOGICAL

Oriented: ☑ Person ☑ Place ☑ Time ☐ Confused ☐ Sedated
☐ Alert ☐ Restless ☑ Lethargic ☐ Comatose

Pupils: ☑ Equal ☐ Unequal ☑ Reactive ☐ Sluggish
☐ Other 3mm.

Extremity Strength: ☑ Equal ☐ Unequal

Speech: ☑ Clear ☐ Slurred ☐ Other

MUSCULO-SKELETAL

Normal ROM of Extremities ☑ Yes ☐ No

☑ Weakness ☐ Paralysis ☐ Contractures ☐ Joint Swelling ☑ Pain
☐ Other ↓ related to fatigue   when coughing

RESPIRATORY

Pattern: ☐ Even ☐ Uneven ☑ Shallow ☑ Dyspnea
☑ Other diminished breath sounds

Breathing Sounds: ☐ Clear ☑ Other inspiratory crackles

Secretions: ☐ None ☑ Other pink, thick sputum

Cough: ☐ None ☑ Productive ☐ Nonproductive

CARDIOVASCULAR

Pulses: Apical Rate 92-W ☑ Reg. ☐ Irregular ☐ Pacemaker
S = Strong W = Weak A = Absent D = Doppler

Radial R 92 L ___ Pedal R — L —

Edema: ☑ Absent ☐ Present Site

Perfusion: ☐ Warm ☐ Dry ☑ Diaphoretic ☐ Cool (Hot)

GASTROINTESTINAL

Oral Mucosa ☐ Normal ☑ Other pale and dry

Bowel Sounds: ☑ Normal ☐ Other Abd. soft

Wt. Change: ☐ ☑ N/V Stool Frequency/Character 1/day; soft

Last B/M 4-15-01 ☐ Ostomy (type)

Equip.

GENITOURINARY

Urine: Last Voided This morning

☐ Normal ☐ Anuria ☐ Hematuria ☐ Dysuri ☐ Incontinent

☒ Other ↓ amount & frequency since ill

☐ Catheter (type) ___ Other

LMP 4-1-01 ☐ Vaginal/Penile Discharge

Other

SELF CARE

Need Assist with: ☐ Ambulating ☐ Elimination
☐ Meals ☒ Hygiene ☐ Dressing
While fatigued

Amanda Aquilini [F. age 28]
#4637651

**NORTH BROWARD HOSPITAL DISTRICT
NURSING ADMINISTRATION ASSESSMENT**

FIGURE 3-6 ◆ Nursing assessment form.

NUTRITION

General Appearance: ☑ Well Nourished ☐ Emaciated
☐ Other _____
Appetite: ☐ Good ☐ Fair ☑ Poor -x2 days
Diet _Liquid_ Meal Pattern _3/day_
☐ Feeds Self ☐ Assist ☐ Total Feed

SKIN ASSESSMENT

Color: ☐ Normal ☐ Flushed ☑ Pale ☐ Dusky ☐ Cyanotic
☐ Jaundiced ☑ Other _Cheeks flushed, hot_
General Description _Surgical scars:_
RLQ abdomen; anterior neck
_____
_____
_____
_____

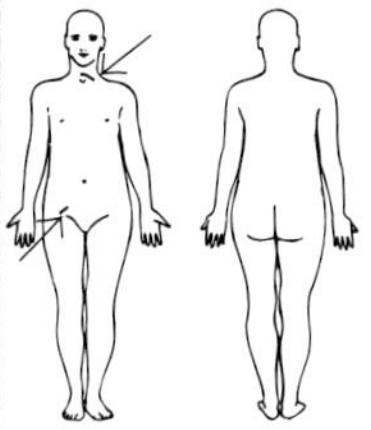

Note Cultures Obtained _____
_____
_____

PRESSURE SORE ™AT RISKʃ SCREENING CRITERIA

OVERALL SKIN CONDITION Grade			BOWEL AND BLADDER CONTROL Grade			REHABILITATIVE STATE Grade		
	0	Turgor (elasticity adequate, skin warm and moist)	✓	0	Always able to ask for bedpan		0	Fully ambulatory
✓	1	Poor turgor, skin cold & dry		1	Incontinence of urine	✓	1	Ambulated with assistance
	2	Areas mottled, red or denuded		2	Incontinence of feces		2	Chair to bed ambulation only
	3	Existing skin ulcer/lesions		3	Totally incontinent Confined to bed		3	Confined to bed
							4	Immobile in bed

NUTRITIONAL STATE Grade			MENTAL STATE Grade		
	0	Eats all	✓	0	Alert and clear
✓	1	Eats very little		1	Confused
	2	Refuses food often		2	Disoriented/senile
	3	Tube feeding		3	Stuporous
	4	Intravenous feeding		4	Unconcious

CHRONIC DISEASE STATUS
(i.e. COPD, ASCVD. Peripheral Vascular Disease, Diabetes, or Renal Disease, Cancer, Motor or Sensory Deficits, Elderly, Other)

Grade		
✓	0	Absent
	1	One Present
	2	Two Present
	3	Three or more Present

TOTAL _____ Refer to Skin Care Protocol

FALLS SCREENING

If one or more of the following are checked institute fall precautions/plan of care
☐ History of Falls ☐ Unsteady Gait ☐ Confusion/Disorientation ☐ Dizziness

If two or more of the following are checked institute fall precautions/plan of care
☐ Age over 80 ☐ Utilizes cane, walker, w/c ☐ Sleeplessness
☐ Impaired vision ☐ Urgency/frequency in elimination
☐ Multiple Diagnoses ☐ Impaired hearing
☐ Inability to understand or follow directions ☐ Medication/Sedative /Diuretic etc.

NURSE SIGNATURE/TITLE	DATE	TIME
Mary Medina, RN	4-16-01	3:30pm
NURSE SIGNATURE/TITLE	DATE	TIME

EDUCATION/DISCHARGE PLANNING

1. What do you know about your present illness? _"Dr. says I have pneumonia." "I will have an I.V."_
2. What information do you want or need about your illness? _____
3. Would you like family/SO involved in your care? _Husband, Michael_
4. How long do you expect to be in the hospital? _"1-2 days"_
5. What concerns do you have about leaving the hospital? _____

CHECK APPROPRIATE BOX

Will patient need post discharge assistance with ADLs/physical functioning? ☐ Yes ☑ No ☐ Unknown

Does patient have family capable of and willing to provide assistance post discharge?
☑ Yes ☐ No ☐ Unknown ☐ No family

Is assistance needed beyond that which family can provide?
☐ Yes ☑ No ☐ Unknown

Previous admission in the last six months?
☐ Yes ☑ No ☐ Unknown

Patient lives with _Husband and 1 child_
Planned discharge to _Home_
Comments: _Fatigue and anxiety may have interfered with learning. Re-teach anything covered at admission, later._

Social Services Notified ☐ Yes ☑ No

NARRATIVE NOTES

S--c/o sharp chest pain when coughing and dyspnea on exertion. States unable to carry out regular daily exercise for past week. Coughing relieved "if I sit up and sit still." Nausea associated with coughing. Having occasional "chills." Occasionally becomes frightened, stating, "I can't breathe." Well groomed but "too tired to put on make-up."

O--Chest expansion < 3cm, no nasal flaring or use of accessory muscles. Breath sounds and insp. crackles in Ⓡ upper and lower chest.

Assesses own supports as "good" (eg, relationship c̄ husband). Is "worried" about daughter. States husband will be out of town until tomorrow. Left 3-year-old daughter with neighbor. Concerned too about her work (is attorney). "I'll never get caught up." Had water at noon—no food today. Informed of need to save urine for 24 hr. specimen. IV D₅W LR 1000 mL started in Ⓡ arm, 100 mL/hr. Slow capillary refill. Keeping head of bed ↑ to facilitate breathing.

✱✱ **NORTH BROWARD HOSPITAL DISTRICT**
NURSING ADMINISTRATION ASSESSMENT

FIGURE 3-6 ◆ (continued)

TECHNIQUE 3-1 ASSESSING APPEARANCE AND MENTAL STATUS (*continued*)

AMBULATORY AND COMMUNITY SETTINGS

General Survey

- Assess the client in private whenever possible. If a family member is needed to assist with recall of events or translation, obtain the client's permission.

- Use your own equipment when possible in measuring vital signs. Bring a tape measure for measuring height. Recognize that the client's home scale for measuring weight may not be accurate.

AGE-RELATED CONSIDERATIONS

General Survey

Infant

- Measure height of children under age 2 in the supine position with knees fully extended.
- Weigh without clothing.
- Include measurement of head circumference until age 2.

Child

- Weigh in underwear only.

Elders

- Allow extra time for clients to answer questions.
- Adapt questioning techniques as appropriate for clients with hearing or visual limitations.

EVALUATION

- Perform a detailed follow-up examination of individual systems based on findings that deviated from expected or normal for the client. Relate findings to previous assessment data if available.

- Report significant deviations from normal to the physician.

Vital Signs

Vital signs are measured (1) to establish baseline data against which to compare future measurements and (2) to detect actual and future health problems. See Chapter 2 for measurements of temperature, pulse, respirations, and blood pressure.

Height and Weight

In adults, the ratio of weight to height provides a general measure of health. By asking clients about their height and weight before actually measuring them, the nurse obtains some idea of the person's self-image. Excessive discrepancies between the client's responses and the measurements may provide clues to actual or potential problems in self-concept. It is also important that the nurse and client be aware of any weight gains or losses over a specific time period.

The nurse measures height with a measuring stick attached to weight scales or to a wall. The client removes the shoes and stands erect, with heels together, buttocks and head against the measuring stick, and eyes looking straight ahead. The nurse raises the L-shaped sliding arm on the weight scale until it rests on top of the client's head, or places a small flat object, such as a ruler or book, on the client's head. The edge of the ruler should abut the measuring guide. More accurate results can be obtained with a right-angled instrument.

Weight is usually measured when a client is admitted and often regularly (e.g., each morning before breakfast). When accuracy is essential, the nurse should use the same scale each time (since every scale weighs differently), take the measurements at the same time each day, and make sure the client wears the same kind of clothing. The client stands on a platform, and the weight is read from a digital display panel or a balancing arm. Clients who cannot stand are weighed on bed and chair scales (Figures 3-7 ◆ and 3-8 ◆). The bed scales have canvas straps or a stretcherlike apparatus. A machine lifts the client above the bed, and the weight is reflected either on a digital display panel or on a balance arm like that of a standing scale.

Integument

The integument includes the skin, hair, and nails. The examination begins with a generalized inspection using a good source of lighting, preferably indirect natural daylight.

Skin

Assessment of the skin involves inspection and palpation. Using the olfactory sense, the nurse may detect unusual skin odors, usually most evident in the skin folds or in the axillae. Pungent body odor is frequently related to poor hygiene, hyperhidrosis (excessive per-

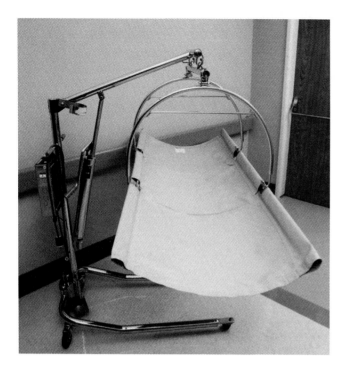

FIGURE 3-7 ◆ Bed scale.

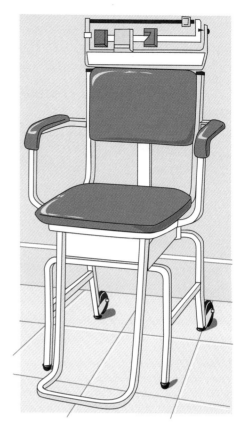

FIGURE 3-8 ◆ Chair scale.

spiration), or **bromhidrosis** (foul-smelling perspiration).

Dark-skinned clients normally have areas of lighter pigmentation, such as the palms, lips, and nailbeds. **Hyperpigmentation** (increased pigmentation) and **hypopigmentation** (decreased pigmentation) may also result from changes in the distribution of melanin (the dark pigment) in the epidermis. **Vitiligo** is seen as patches of hypopigmented skin, while albinism is the complete or partial lack of melanin in the skin, hair, and eyes. Other localized color changes may indicate a problem. **Edema**, the presence of excess interstitial fluid, appears swollen, shiny, and taut and tends to blanch skin color. Color variations may appear differently in clients depending on their underlying skin color (see Table 3-4).

PLANNING

Review characteristics of primary and secondary skin lesions if necessary (see Figure 3-9 ◆). Ensure that adequate lighting is available.

Delegation

Due to the substantial knowledge and skill required, assessment of the skin is not delegated to UAP. However, the skin is observed during usual care and these persons should record their findings. Abnormal findings must be validated and interpreted by the nurse.

TABLE 3-4	VARIATIONS IN SKIN COLOR	
Color	**Common Location**	**Cultural Variation**
Pallor (pale)	Buccal mucosa In people with light skin may also be evident in the face, the conjuctiva of the eyes, and the nails	Absence of underlying red tones in very dark-skinned persons In black-skinned clients, may appear ashen gray In brown-skinned clients, may appear as a yellowish brown tinge
Cyanosis (a bluish tinge)	Nailbeds, lips, and buccal mucosa	In dark-skinned clients, palpebral conjunctiva and palms and soles may also show cyanosis
Jaundice (a yellowish tinge)	Sclera of the eyes; mucous membranes; skin	Do not confuse jaundice with the normal yellow pigmentation in the sclera of a dark-skinned or black client; if jaundice is suspected, the posterior part of the hard palate should also be inspected for a yellowish color tone
Erythema (redness)	Skin	May not be visible in very dark skin

Macule, Patch   Flat, unelevated change in color. *Macules* are 1 mm to 1 cm in size and circumscribed. Examples: freckles, measles, petechiae, flat moles. *Patches* are larger than 1 cm and may have an irregular shape. Examples: port wine birthmark, vitiligo (white patches), rubella.

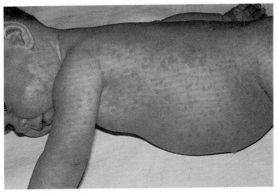

Diffuse, discrete erythematous macules (rubella)

Nodule, Tumor   Elevated, solid, hard mass that extends deeper into the dermis than a papule. *Nodules* have a circumscribed border and are 0.5 to 2 cm. Examples: squamous cell carcinoma, fibroma. *Tumors* are larger than 2 cm and may have an irregular border. Examples: malignant melanoma, hemangioma.

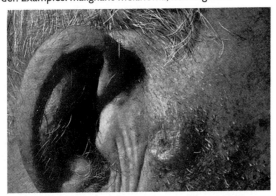

Solitary, shiny brown, ½-inch nodule (squamous cell carcinoma)

Cyst   A 1-cm or larger, elevated, encapsulated, fluid-filled or semisolid mass arising from the subcutaneous tissue or dermis. Examples: sebaceous and epidermoid cysts, chalazion of the eyelid

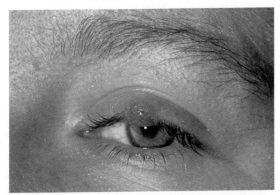

Reddened, circumscribed swelling on upper eyelid (chalazion)

Papule, Plaque   Circumscribed, solid elevation of skin. *Papules* are less than 1 cm. Examples: warts, acne, pimples, elevated moles. *Plaques* are larger than 1 cm. Examples: psoriasis, rubeola.

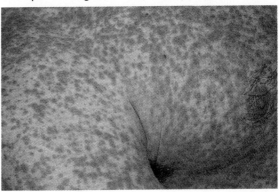

Diffuse, varying-sized, confluent maculo-papular lesions (rubeola)

Vesicle, Bulla   A circumscribed, round or oval, thin translucent mass filled with serous fluid or blood. Vesicles are less than 0.5 cm. Examples: herpes simplex, early chicken pox, small burn blister. *Bullae* are larger than 0.5 cm. Examples: large blister, second-degree burn, herpes simplex.

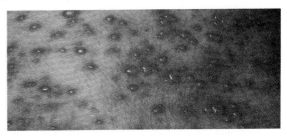

Clustered vesicles on an erythematous base (chickenpox)

Wheal   A reddened, localized collection of edema fluid; irregular in shape. Size varies. Examples: hives, mosquito bites.

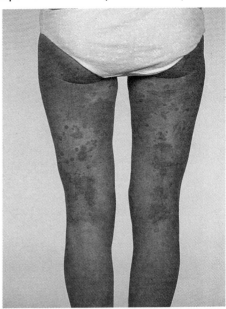

Diffuse, elevated, reddened lesions of varying size on backs of legs (hives)

FIGURE 3-9 ◆ Selected skin lesions (primary and secondary).

Pustule Vesicle or bulla filled with pus. Examples: acne vulgaris, impetigo.

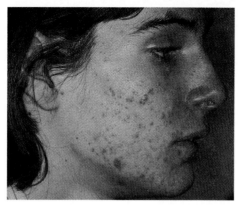

Diffuse, varying-sized, erythematous pustules on the cheeks (acne vulgaris)

Secondary Skin Lesions

Atrophy

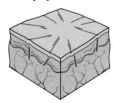

A translucent, dry, paperlike, sometimes wrinkled skin surface resulting from thinning or wasting of the skin due to loss of collagen and elastin.

Examples Striae, aged skin.

Erosion

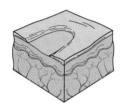

Wearing away of the superficial epidermis causing a moist, shallow depression. Because erosions do not extend into the dermis, they heal without scarring.

Examples Scratch marks, ruptured vesicles.

Lichenification

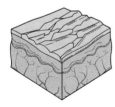

Rough, thickened, hardened area of epidermis resulting from chronic irritation such as scratching or rubbing.

Example Chronic dermatitis.

Scales

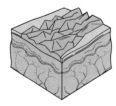

Shedding flakes of greasy, keratinized skin tissue. Color may be white, gray, or silver. Texture may vary from fine to thick.

Examples Dry skin, dandruff, psoriasis, and eczema.

Crust

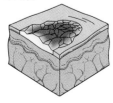

Dry blood, serum, or pus left on the skin surface when vesicles or pustules burst. Can be red-brown, orange, or yellow. Large crusts that adhere to the skin surface are called scabs.

Examples Eczema, impetigo, herpes, or scabs following abrasion.

Ulcer

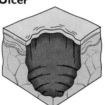

Deep, irregularly shaped area of skin loss extending into the dermis or subcutaneous tissue. May bleed. May leave scar.

Examples Pressure ulcers, stasis ulcers, chancres.

Fissure

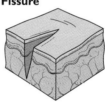

Linear crack with sharp edges, extending into the dermis.

Examples Cracks at the corners of the mouth or in the hands, athlete's foot.

Scar

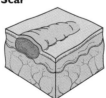

Flat, irregular area of connective tissue left after a lesion or wound has healed. New scars may be red or purple; older scars may be silvery or white.

Examples Healed surgical wound or injury, healed acne.

Keloid

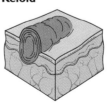

Elevated, irregular, darkened area of excess scar tissue caused by excessive collagen formation during healing. Extends beyond the site of the original injury. Higher incidence in people of African descent.

Examples Keloid from ear piercing or surgery.

Equipment

- Millimeter ruler
- Examination gloves
- Magnifying glass

Performance

1. Explain to the client what you are going to do, why it is necessary, and how he or she can cooperate. Discuss how the results will be used in planning further care or treatments.

2. Wash hands and observe appropriate infection control procedures.

3. Provide for client privacy.

4. Inquire if the client has any history of the following: pain or itching; presence and spread of any lesions, bruises, abrasions, or pigmented spots; previous experience with skin problems; associated clinical signs; family history; presence of problems in other family members; related systemic conditions; use of medications, lotions, or home remedies; excessively dry or moist feel to the skin; tendency to bruise easily; any association of the problem to season of year, stress, occupation, medications, recent travel, housing, personal contact, and so on; any recent contact with allergens (e.g., metal paint).

ASSESSMENT	NORMAL FINDINGS	DEVIATIONS FROM NORMAL
5. Inspect skin color (best assessed under natural light and on areas not exposed to the sun).	Varies from light to deep brown; from ruddy pink to light pink; from yellow overtones to olive	Pallor, cyanosis, jaundice, erythema
6. Inspect uniformity of skin color.	Generally uniform except in areas exposed to the sun; areas of lighter pigmentation (palms, lips, nailbeds) in dark-skinned people	Areas of either hyperpigmentation or hypopigmentation
7. Assess edema, if present (i.e., location, color, temperature, shape, and the degree to which the skin remains indented or pitted when pressed by a finger). See Box 3-2.		
8. Inspect, palpate, and describe skin lesions (see Figure 3-9). Apply gloves if lesions are open or draining. Palpate lesions to determine shape and texture. Describe lesions according to type or structure, color, distribution, and configuration. See Box 3-3.	Freckles, some birthmarks, some flat and raised nevi; no abrasions or other lesions	Various interruptions in skin integrity
9. Observe and palpate skin moisture.	Moisture in skin folds and the axillae (varies with environmental temperature and humidity, body temperature, and activity)	Excessive moisture (e.g., in hyperthermia); excessive dryness (e.g., in dehydration)
10. Palpate skin temperature. Compare the two feet and the two hands, using the backs of your fingers.	Uniform; within normal range	Generalized hyperthermia (e.g., in fever); generalized hypothermia (e.g., in shock); localized hyperthermia (e.g., in infection); localized hypothermia (e.g., in arteriosclerosis)
11. Note skin turgor (fullness or elasticity) by lifting and pinching the skin on an extremity.	When pinched, skin springs back to previous state	Skins stays pinched or tented or moves back slowly (e.g., in dehydration)

12. **Document** findings in the client record using forms or checklists supplemented by narrative notes when appropriate. Draw location of skin lesions on body surface diagrams (see Figure 3-10 ◆).

<table>
<tr><td>

BOX 3-2 *Scale for Describing Edema*

- 1+ Barely detectable (2 mm)
- 2+ Indentation of 2–4 mm
- 3+ Indentation of 5–7 mm
- 4+ Indentation of more than 7 mm

</td><td>

BOX 3-3 *Describing Skin Lesions*

- *Type or structure.* Skin lesions are classified as *primary* (those that appear initially in response to some change in the external or internal environment of the skin) and *secondary* (those that do not appear initially but result from modifications such as chronicity, trauma, or infection of the primary lesion). For example, a vesicle (primary lesion) may rupture and cause an erosion (secondary lesion).
- *Size, shape, and texture.* Note size in millimeters and whether the lesion is circumscribed or irregular; round or oval-shaped; flat, elevated, or depressed; solid, soft, or hard; rough or thickened; fluid-filled or has flakes.
- *Color.* There may be no discoloration, one discrete color (e.g., red, brown, or black), several colors, as with *ecchymosis* (a bruise), in which an initial dark red or blue color fades to a yellow color. When color changes are limited to the edges of a lesion, they are described as *circumscribed;* when spread over a large area, they are described as *diffuse.*
- *Distribution.* Distribution is described according to the location of the lesions on the body and symmetry or asymmetry of findings in comparable body areas.
- *Configuration.* Configuration refers to the arrangement of lesions in relation to each other. Configurations of lesions may be annular (arranged in a circle); clustered together or grouped; linear (arranged in a line); arc- or bow-shaped; merged together or indiscrete; follow the course of cutaneous nerves; or meshed in the form of a network.

</td></tr>
</table>

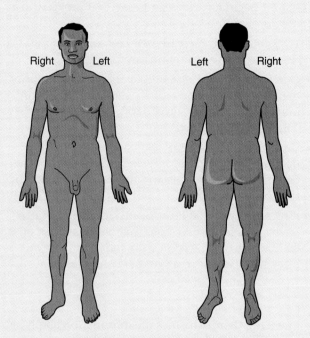

Right   Left   Left   Right

FIGURE 3-10 ◆ Diagram for charting skin lesions.

AMBULATORY AND COMMUNITY SETTINGS

Assessing the Skin

- When making a home visit, take a penlight or examination lamp with you in case there is inadequate lighting.
- If skin lesions are suggestive of physical abuse, follow state regulations for follow-up and reporting.

Signs of abuse may include a pattern of bruises, unusual location of burns, or lesions not easily explainable. If lesions are present in adults or verbal-age children, conduct the interview and assessment in private.

AGE-RELATED CONSIDERATIONS

Assessing the Skin

Infant

- Newborns may be jaundiced for several weeks after birth.
- Newborns may have milia (whiteheads), small white nodules over the nose and face, and vernix caseosa (white, cheesy, greasy material on the skin).
- In dark-skinned races, areas of hyperpigmentation may be found in the sacral area.

- If a rash is present, inquire in detail about immunization history.
- Assess skin turgor by pinching the skin on the abdomen.

Child

- In dark-skinned races, areas of hyperpigmentation may be found in the sacral area.
- As puberty approaches, skin may change in oiliness and acne may appear.

Assessing the Skin (continued)

- If a rash is present, inquire in detail about immunization history.

Elders

- Changes in white skin occur at an earlier age than in black skin.
- The skin loses its elasticity and wrinkles. Wrinkles first appear on the skin of the face and neck, which are abundant in collagen and elastic fibers.
- The skin appears thin and translucent because of loss of dermis and subcutaneous fat.
- The skin is dry and flaky because sebaceous and sweat glands are less active. Dry skin is more prominent over the extremities.
- The skin takes longer to return to its natural shape after being tented between the thumb and finger.
- Flat tan to brown-colored macules, referred to as *senile lentigines* or *melanotic freckles,* are normally apparent on the back of the hand and other skin areas that are exposed to the sun. These macules may be as large as 1 to 2 cm.
- Warty lesions *(seborrheic keratoses)* with irregularly shaped borders and a scaly surface often occur on the face, shoulders, and trunk. These benign lesions begin as yellowish to tan and progress to a dark brown or black.
- *Vitiligo* tends to increase with age and is thought to result from an autoimmune response.
- Cutaneous tags *(acrochordons)* are most commonly seen in the neck and axillary regions. These skin lesions vary in size and are soft, often flesh-colored, and pedicled.
- Visible, bright red, fine dilated blood vessels *(telangiectasias)* commonly occur as a result of the thinning of the dermis and the loss of support for the blood vessel walls.
- Pink to slightly red lesions with indistinct borders *(actinic keratoses)* may appear at about age 50, often on the face, ears, backs of the hands, and arms. They may become malignant if untreated.

EVALUATION

- Compare findings to previous skin assessment data if available to determine if lesions or abnormalities are changing.
- Report significant deviations from normal to the physician.

Hair

Assessing a client's hair includes inspecting the hair, considering developmental changes, and determining the individual's hair care practices and the factors influencing them. Much of the information about hair can be obtained by questioning the client.

Normal hair is resilient and evenly distributed. In people with severe protein deficiency (kwashiorkor), the hair color is faded and appears reddish or bleached, and the texture is coarse and dry. Some therapies for cancer cause **alopecia** (hair loss), and some disease conditions cause the hair to be more coarse or thinner.

PLANNING

Delegation

Due to the substantial knowledge required, assessment of the hair is not delegated to UAP. However, many

Equipment

- Examination gloves

Performance

1. Explain to the client what you are going to do, why it is necessary, and how he or she can cooperate. Discuss how the results will be used in planning further care or treatments.

2. Wash hands, apply gloves, and observe other appropriate infection control procedures.

3. Provide for client privacy.

4. Inquire if the client has any history of the following: recent use of hair dyes, rinses, or curling or straightening preparations; recent chemotherapy (if alopecia is present); presence of disease, such as hypothyroidism, which can be associated with dry, brittle hair.

ASSESSMENT	NORMAL FINDINGS	DEVIATIONS FROM NORMAL
5. Inspect the evenness of growth over the scalp.	Evenly distributed hair	Patches of hair loss (i.e., alopecia)
6. Inspect hair thickness or thinness.	Thick hair	Very thin hair (e.g., in hypothyroidism)
7. Inspect hair texture and oiliness.	Silky, resilient hair	Brittle hair (e.g., hypothyroidism); excessively oily or dry hair
8. Note presence of infections or infestations by parting the hair in several areas.	No infection or infestation	Flaking, sores, lice, nits (louse eggs), and ringworm
9. Inspect amount of body hair.	Variable	Hirsutism (abnormal hairiness) in women.

 10. **Document** findings in the client record using forms or checklists supplemented by narrative notes when appropriate.

AMBULATORY AND COMMUNITY SETTINGS

Assessing the Hair

- When making a home visit, ask to see the products the client usually uses on the hair. Assist the client to determine if the products are appropriate for the client's type of hair and scalp (e.g., for dry or oily hair). Provide education regarding hygiene of the hair and scalp.

- When making a home visit, examine the equipment that the client uses on the hair. Provide client teaching regarding appropriate combs and brushes, and safety in using electric hairstyling appliances such as hair dryers.

AGE-RELATED CONSIDERATIONS

Assessing the Hair

Infant

- It is normal for infants to have either very little or a great deal of body and scalp hair.

Child

- As puberty approaches, axillary and pubic hair will appear.

Elders

- There may be loss of scalp, pubic, and axillary hair.
- In women, the hair of the eyebrows and some facial hair become coarse.
- Hairs of the eyebrows, ears, and nostrils become bristle-like and coarse.

---

aspects are observed during usual care and may be recorded by persons other than the nurse. Abnormal findings must be validated and interpreted by the nurse.

EVALUATION

Report significant deviations from normal to the physician.

Nails

Parts of the nail are shown in Figure 3-11 ◆. Nails are inspected for nail plate shape, angle between the nail

and the nailbed, nail texture, nailbed color, and the intactness of the tissues around the nails.

PLANNING

Delegation

Due to the substantial knowledge required, assessment of the nails is not delegated to UAP. However, many aspects are observed during usual care and may be recorded by persons other than the nurse. Abnormal findings must be validated and interpreted by the nurse.

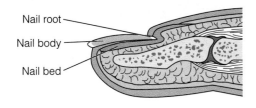
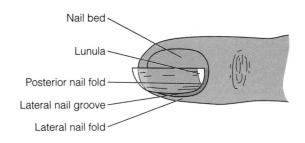

FIGURE 3-11 ◆ The parts of the nail.

IMPLEMENTATION:
TECHNIQUE 3-4 ASSESSING THE NAILS

Equipment

• None.

Performance

1. Explain to the client what you are going to do, why it is necessary, and how he or she can cooperate. Discuss how the results will be used in planning further care or treatments.

2. Wash hands and observe appropriate infection control procedures.

3. Provide for client privacy.

4. Inquire if the client has any history of the following: presence of diabetes mellitus, peripheral circulatory disease, previous injury, or severe illness.

ASSESSMENT	NORMAL FINDINGS	DEVIATIONS FROM NORMAL
5. Inspect fingernail plate shape to determine its curvature and angle.	Convex curvature; angle between nail and nailbed of about 160 degrees (Figure 3-12A ◆).	Spoon nail (Figure 3-12B); **clubbing** (180 degrees or greater) (Figure 3-12C and D)
6. Inspect fingernail and toenail texture.	Smooth texture	Excessive thickness (e.g., result of poor circulation, iron-deficiency anemia); excessive thinness or presence of grooves or furrows (e.g., in iron-deficiency anemia); Beau's lines (transverse white lines or grooves; Figure 3-12E)
7. Inspect fingernail and toenail bed color.	Highly vascular and pink in light-skinned clients; dark-skinned clients may have brown or black pigmentation in longitudinal streaks	Bluish or purplish tint (may reflect cyanosis); pallor (may reflect poor arterial circulation)
8. Inspect tissues surrounding nails.	Intact epidermis	Hangnails; paronychia (inflammation)
9. Perform **blanch test** of capillary refill. Press two or more nails between your thumb and index finger; look for blanching and return of pink color to nailbed.	Prompt return of pink or usual color	Delayed return of pink or usual color (may indicate circulatory impairment)

10. **Document** findings in the client record using forms or checklists supplemented by narrative notes when appropriate.

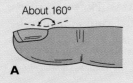
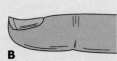
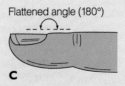
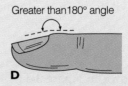
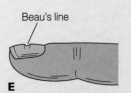

FIGURE 3-12 ◆ (A) A normal nail, showing the convex shape and the nail plate angle of about 160 degrees; (B) a spoon-shaped nail; (C) early clubbing; (D) late clubbing; (E) Beau's lines.

Assessing the Nails

- If indicated, teach the client or family member about proper nail care, including how to trim and shape the nails to avoid paronychia.

Assessing the Nails

Infant

- Newborns' nails grow very quickly, are extremely thin, and tear easily.

Child

- Bent, bruised, or ingrown toenails may indicate shoes that are too tight.
- Nail biting should be discussed with the family member.

Elders

- The nails grow more slowly and thicken.
- Longitudinal bands commonly develop, and the nails tend to split.
- Bands across the nails may indicate protein deficiency; white spots, zinc deficiency; and spoon-shaped nails, iron deficiency.

EVALUATION

- Perform a detailed follow-up examination of other individual systems based on findings that deviated from expected or normal for the client. Relate findings to previous assessment data if available.
- Report significant deviations from normal to the physician.

Head

During an examination of the head, the nurse often inspects and palpates simultaneously, as well as auscultating. The nurse examines the skull, face, eyes, ears, nose, sinuses, mouth, and pharynx.

Skull and Face

There is a large range of normal shapes of skulls. A normal head size is referred to as **normocephalic.** Names of areas of the head are derived from names of the underlying bones: frontal, parietal, occipital, mastoid process, mandible, maxilla, and zygomatic (Figure 3-13 ◆).

Many disorders cause a change in facial shape or condition. Kidney or cardiac disease can cause edema of the eyelids. Hyperthyroidism can cause **exophthalmos,** a protrusion of the eyeballs with elevation of the upper eyelids, resulting in a startled or staring expression. Hypothyroidism, or myxedema, can cause a dry, puffy face with dry skin and coarse features and thinning of scalp hair and eyebrows. Increased adrenal hormone production or administration can cause a round face with reddened cheeks, referred to as *moon face,* and excessive hair growth on the upper lips, chin, and sideburn areas. Prolonged illness, starvation, and dehydration can result in sunken eyes, cheeks, and temples.

PLANNING

Delegation

Due to the substantial knowledge and skill required, assessment of the skull and face is not delegated to UAP. However, many aspects are observed during usual care and may be recorded by persons other than the nurse. Abnormal findings must be validated and interpreted by the nurse.

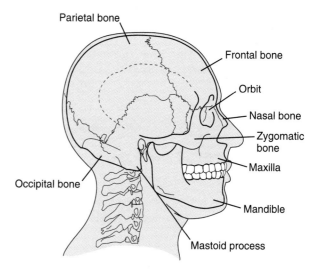

FIGURE 3-13 ◆ Bones of the head.

Equipment

• None.

Performance

1. Explain to the client what you are going to do, why it is necessary, and how he or she can cooperate. Discuss how the results will be used in planning further care or treatments.

2. Wash hands and observe appropriate infection control procedures.

3. Provide for client privacy.

4. Inquire if the client has any history of the following: any past problems with lumps or bumps, itching, scaling, or dandruff; any history of loss of consciousness, dizziness, seizures, headache, facial pain, or injury; when and how any lumps occurred; length of time any other problem existed; any known cause of problem; associated symptoms, treatment, and recurrences.

ASSESSMENT	NORMAL FINDINGS	DEVIATIONS FROM NORMAL
5. Inspect the skull for size, shape, and symmetry.	Rounded (normocephalic and symmetrical, with frontal, parietal, and occipital prominences); smooth skull contour	Lack of symmetry; increased skull size with more prominent nose and forehead; longer mandible (may indicate excessive growth hormone or increased bone thickness)
6. Palpate the skull for nodules or masses and depressions. Use a gentle, rotating motion with the fingertips. Begin at the front and palpate down the midline, then palpate each side of the head.	Smooth, uniform consistency; absence of nodules or masses	Sebaceous cysts; local deformities from trauma
7. Inspect the facial features (e.g., symmetry of structures and of the distribution of hair).	Symmetric or slightly asymmetric facial features; palpebral fissures equal in size; symmetric nasolabial folds	Increased facial hair; thinning of eyebrows; asymmetric features; exophthalmos; myxedema facies; moon face
8. Inspect the eyes for edema and hollowness.		Periorbital edema; sunken eyes
9. Note symmetry of facial movements. Ask the client to elevate the eyebrows, frown, or lower the eyebrows, close the eyes tightly, puff the cheeks, and smile and show the teeth. (See Technique 3-19, Assessing the Cranial Nerves, on page 123.)	Symmetric facial movements	Asymmetric facial movements (e.g., eye on affected side cannot close completely); drooping of lower eyelid and mouth; involuntary facial movements (i.e., tics or tremors)

 10. **Document** findings in the client record using forms or checklists supplemented by narrative notes when appropriate.

AGE-RELATED CONSIDERATIONS

Assessing the Skull and Face

Infant

• Most newborns' heads are shaped according to the method of delivery for the first week.

• The posterior fontanel (soft spot) usually closes by 8 weeks, but the anterior fontanel may remain up to 18 months.

• Voluntary head control should be present by about 6 months of age.

Perform a detailed follow-up examination of other systems based on findings that deviated from expected or normal for the client. Relate findings to previous assessment data if available. Report significant deviations from normal to the physician.

Eyes and Vision

It is recommended that people under age 40 have their eyes tested every 3 to 5 years, or more frequently if there is a family history of diabetes, hypertension, blood dyscrasia, or eye disease (e.g., glaucoma). After age 40, an eye examination is recommended every 2 years to rule out the possibility of glaucoma. Examination of the eyes commonly includes assessment of visual acuity (the degree of detail the eye can discern in an image), ocular movement, visual fields (the area an individual can see when looking straight ahead), and external structures. For the anatomic structures of the eye, see Figures 3-14 ◆ and 3-15 ◆.

Many people wear eyeglasses or contact lenses to correct common refractive errors of the lens of the eye: **myopia** (nearsightedness), **hyperopia** (farsightedness), and **presbyopia** (loss of elasticity of the lens and thus loss of ability to see close objects). **Astigmatism**, an uneven curvature of the cornea that prevents horizontal and vertical rays from focusing on the retina, is a common problem that may occur in conjunction with myopia and hyperopia.

Common inflammatory visual problems that nurses may encounter in clients include conjunctivitis, dacryocystitis, hordeolum, iritis, and contusions or hematomas of the eyelids and surrounding structures. **Conjunctivitis** (inflammation of the bulbar and palpebral conjunctiva) may result from foreign bodies, chemicals, allergenic agents, bacteria, or viruses.

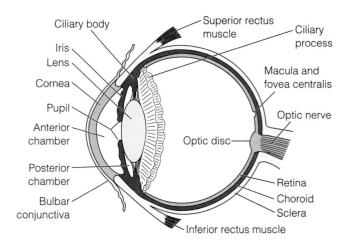

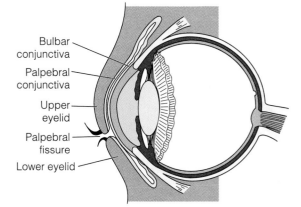

FIGURE 3-15 ◆ Anatomic structures of the eye.

Redness, itching, tearing, and mucopurulent discharge occur. During sleep, the eyelids may become encrusted and matted together. **Dacryocystitis** (inflammation of the lacrimal sac) is manifested by tearing and a discharge from the nasolacrimal duct. **Hordeolum (sty)** is a redness, swelling, and tenderness of the hair follicle and glands that empty at the edge of the eyelids. **Iritis** (inflammation of the iris) may be caused by local or systemic infections and results in pain, tearing, and photophobia (sensitivity to light). Contusions or **hematomas** are "black eyes" resulting from injury.

Cataracts tend to occur in those over 65 years old. This opacity of the lens or its capsule, which blocks light rays, in frequently corrected by surgery. Cataracts may also occur in infants due to a malformation of the lens if the mother contracted rubella in the first trimester of pregnancy. **Glaucoma** (a disturbance in the circulation of aqueous fluid, which causes an increase in intraocular pressure) is the most frequent cause of blindness in people over 40. It can be controlled if diagnosed early. Danger signs of glaucoma include blurred or foggy vision, loss of peripheral vision, difficulty focusing on close objects, difficulty adjusting to dark rooms, and seeing rainbow-colored rings around lights.

Eyelids that lie at or below the pupil margin are referred to as *ptosis* and are usually associated with

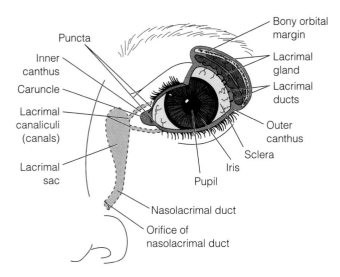

FIGURE 3-14 ◆ The external structures and lacrimal apparatus of the eye.

aging, edema from drug allergy or systemic disease (e.g., kidney disease), congenital lid muscle dysfunction, neuromuscular disease (e.g., myasthenia gravis), and third cranial nerve impairment. Eversion, an out-turning of the eyelid, is called *ectropion;* inversion, an inturning of the lid, is called *entropion*. These abnormalities are often associated with scarring injuries or the aging process.

Pupils are normally black, equal in size (about 3 to 7 mm in diameter), and have round, smooth borders. Cloudy pupils are often indicative of cataracts. Enlarged pupils (**mydriasis**) may indicate injury or glaucoma, or result from certain drugs (e.g., atropine). Constricted pupils (**miosis**) may indicate an inflammation of the iris or result from such drugs as morphine or pilocarpine. Unequal pupils (**anisocoria**) may result from a central nervous system disorder;

however, slight variations may be normal. The iris is normally flat and round. A bulging toward the cornea can indicate increased intraocular pressure.

PLANNING

Place the client in an appropriate room for assessing the eyes and vision. The nurse must be able to control natural and overhead lighting during some portions of the examination.

Delegation

Due to the substantial knowledge and skill required, assessment of the eyes and vision are not delegated to UAP. However, many aspects are observed during usual care and may be recorded by persons other than the nurse. Abnormal findings must be validated and interpreted by the nurse.

IMPLEMENTATION:
TECHNIQUE 3-6 ASSESSING THE EYES AND VISION

Equipment

- Cotton-tipped applicator
- Gauze square
- Examination gloves
- Millimeter ruler
- Penlight
- Snellen's or E chart
- Opaque card

Performance

1. Explain to the client what you are going to do, why it is necessary, and how he or she can cooper-

ate. Discuss how the results will be used in planning further care or treatments.

2. Wash hands, apply gloves, and observe appropriate infection control procedures.

3. Provide for client privacy.

4. Inquire if the client has any history of the following: family history of diabetes, hypertension, blood dyscrasia, eye disease, injury, or surgery; client's last visit to an ophthalmologist; current use of eye medications; use of contact lenses or eyeglasses; hygienic practices for corrective lenses; current symptoms of eye problems (e.g., changes in **visual acuity**, blurring of vision, tearing, spots, photophobia, itching, or pain).

ASSESSMENT	NORMAL FINDINGS	DEVIATIONS FROM NORMAL
External Eye Structures		
5. Inspect the eyebrows for hair distribution and alignment and skin quality and movement (ask client to raise and lower the eyebrows).	Hair evenly distributed; skin intact Eyebrows symmetrically aligned; equal movement	Loss of hair; scaling and flakiness of skin Unequal alignment and movement of eyebrows
6. Inspect the eyelashes for evenness of distribution and direction of curl.	Equally distributed; curled slightly outward	Turned inward (see inversion of eyelid, below)
7. Inspect the eyelids for surface characteristics (e.g., skin quality and texture), position in relation to the cornea, ability to blink, and frequency of blinking. For proper visual examination of the upper eyelids, elevate the eyebrows with your thumb and index fingers, and have the client close the eyes (Figure 3-16 ◆). Inspect the lower eyelids while the client's eyes are closed.	Skin intact; no discharge; no discoloration Lids close symmetrically Approximately 15 to 20 involuntary blinks per minute; bilateral blinking When lids open, no visible sclera above corneas, and upper and lower borders of cornea are slightly covered	Redness, swelling, flaking, crusting, plaques, discharge, nodules, lesions Lids close asymmetrically, incompletely, or painfully Rapid, monocular, absent, or infrequent blinking Ptosis, ectropion, or entropion; rim of sclera visible between lid and iris

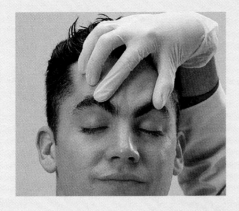

FIGURE 3-16 ◆ Inspecting the upper eyelids.

ASSESSMENT	NORMAL FINDINGS	DEVIATIONS FROM NORMAL
8. Inspect the bulbar conjunctiva (that lying over the sclera) for color, texture, and the presence of lesions. Retract the eyelids with your thumb and index finger, exerting pressure over the upper and lower bony orbits, and ask the client to look up, down, and from side to side.	Transparent; capillaries sometimes evident; sclera appears white (yellowish in dark-skinned clients)	Jaundiced sclera (e.g., in liver disease); excessively pale sclera (e.g., in anemia); reddened sclera; lesions or nodules (may indicate damage by mechanical, chemical, allergenic, or bacterial agents)
9. Inspect the palpebral conjunctiva (that lining the eyelids) by everting the lids. Note color, texture, and the presence of lesions. Evert both lower lids, and ask the client to look up. Then gently retract the lower lids with the index fingers.	Shiny, smooth, and pink or red	Extremely pale (possible anemia); extremely red (inflammation); nodules or other lesions
10. Evert the upper lids if a problem is suspected (see Box 3-4).		

Box 3-4 *Everting the Upper Eyelid*

- Ask the client to look down while keeping the eyes slightly open. *Closing the eyelids contracts the orbicular muscle, which prevents lid eversion.*

- Gently grasp the client's eyelashes with the thumb and index finger. Pull the lashes gently downward. *Upward or outward pulling on the eyelashes causes muscle contraction.*

- Place a cotton-tipped applicator stick about 1 cm above the lid margin, and push it gently downward while holding the eyelashes (Figure 3-17 ◆). These

actions evert the lid (i.e., flip the lower part of the lid over on top of itself).

- Hold the margin of the everted lid or the eyelashes against the ridge of the upper bony orbit with the applicator stick or the thumb (Figure 3-18 ◆).

- Inspect the conjunctiva for color, texture, lesions, and foreign bodies.

- To return the lid to its normal position, gently pull the lashes forward, and ask the client to look up and blink.

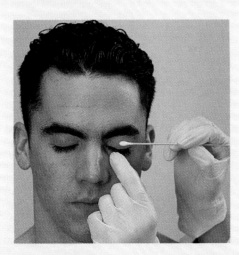

FIGURE 3-17 ◆ Placing the applicator stick.

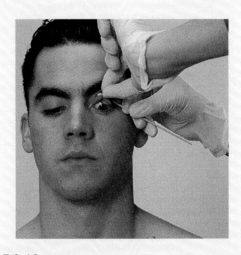

FIGURE 3-18 ◆ Holding the margin of the everted eyelid.

ASSESSMENT	NORMAL FINDINGS	DEVIATIONS FROM NORMAL
External Eye Structures *continued*		
11. Inspect and palpate the lacrimal gland (see Box 3-5).	No edema or tenderness over lacrimal gland	Swelling or tenderness over lacrimal gland
12. Inspect and palpate the lacrimal sac and nasolacrimal duct (see Box 3-5).	No edema or tearing	Evidence of increased tearing; regurgitation of fluid on palpation of lacrimal sac
13. Inspect the cornea for clarity and texture. Ask the client to look straight ahead. Hold a penlight at an oblique angle to the eye, and move the light slowly across the corneal surface.	Transparent, shiny, and smooth; details of the iris are visible In older people, a thin, grayish white ring around the margin, called *arcus senilis*, may be evident	Opaque; surface not smooth (may be the result of trauma or abrasion) Arcus senilis in clients under age 40 is abnormal
14. Perform the corneal sensitivity (reflex) test to determine the function of the fifth (trigeminal) cranial nerve. Ask the client to keep both eyes open and look straight ahead. Approach from behind and beside the client, and lightly touch the cornea with a corner of the gauze.	Client blinks when the cornea is touched, indicating that the trigeminal nerve is intact	One or both eyelids fail to respond
15. Inspect the anterior chamber for transparency and depth. Use the same oblique lighting as used to test the cornea.	Transparent No shadows of light on iris Depth of about 3 mm	Cloudy Crescent-shaped shadows on far side of iris Shallow chamber (possible glaucoma)
16. Inspect the pupils for color, shape, and symmetry of size. Pupil charts are available in some agencies. See Figure 3-21 ◆ for variations in pupil diameters.	Black in color; equal in size; normally 3 to 7 mm in diameter; round, smooth border, iris flat and round	Cloudiness, mydriasis, miosis, anisocoria; bulging of iris toward cornea
17. Assess each pupil's direct and consensual reaction to light to determine the function of the third (oculomotor) and fourth (trochlear) cranial nerves (see Box 3-6).	Illuminated pupil constricts (direct response) Nonilluminated pupil constricts (consensual response)	Neither pupil constricts Unequal responses Absent responses

---

Box 3-5 *Palpating the Lacrimal Gland, Lacrimal Sac, and Nasolacrimal Duct*

Lacrimal Gland

- Using the tip of your index finger, palpate the lacrimal gland (Figure 3-19 ◆).
- Observe for edema between the lower lid and the nose.

Lacrimal Sac and Nasolacrimal Duct

- Observe for evidence of increased tearing.
- Using the tip of your index finger, palpate inside the lower orbital rim near the inner canthus (Figure 3-20 ◆).

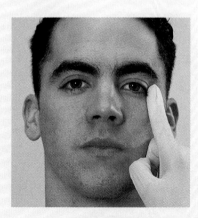

FIGURE 3-19 ◆ Palpating the lacrimal gland.

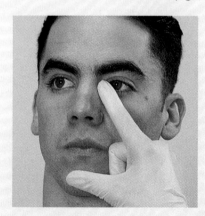

FIGURE 3-20 ◆ Palpating the lacrimal sac and nasolacrimal duct.

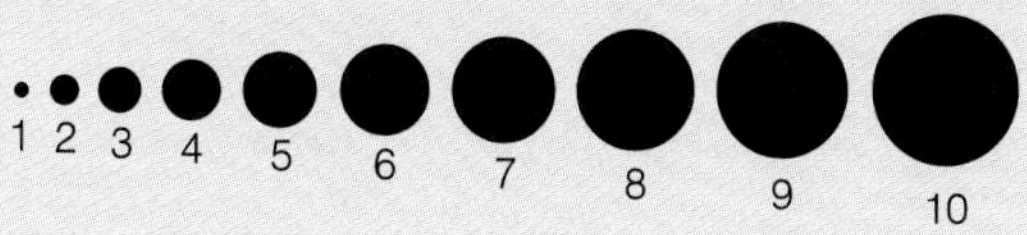

1 2 3 4 5 6 7 8 9 10

FIGURE 3-21 ◆ Variations in pupil diameters in millimeters.

Box 3-6 *Assessing Pupil Reactions*

Direct and Consensual Reaction to Light

- Partially darken the room.
- Ask the client to look straight ahead.
- Using a penlight or flashlight and approaching from the side, shine a light on the pupil.
- Observe the response of the illuminated pupil. It should constrict (direct response).
- Shine the light on the pupil again, and observe the response of the other pupil. It should also constrict (consensual response).

Reaction to Accommodation

- Hold an object (a penlight or pencil) about 10 cm (4 in) from the bridge of the client's nose.
- Ask the client to look first at the top of the object and then at a distant object (e.g., the far wall) behind the penlight. Alternate the gaze from the near to the far object.
- Observe the pupil response. The pupils should constrict when looking at the near object and dilate when looking at the far object.
- Next, move the penlight or pencil toward the client's nose. The pupils should converge. To record normal assessment of the pupils, use the abbreviation PERRLA (pupils equally round and react to light and accommodation).

ASSESSMENT	NORMAL FINDINGS	DEVIATIONS FROM NORMAL
18. Assess each pupil's reaction to accommodation. See Box 3-6.	Pupils constrict when looking at near object; pupils dilate when looking at far object; pupils converge when near object is moved toward nose	One or both pupils fail to constrict, dilate, or converge
Visual Fields		
19. Assess peripheral **visual fields** to determine function of the retina and neuronal visual pathways to the brain and second (optic) cranial nerve (see Box 3-7).	When looking straight ahead, client can see objects in the periphery	Visual field smaller than normal (possible glaucoma); one-half vision in one or both eyes (indicates nerve damage)
Extraocular Muscle Tests		
20. Assess six ocular movements to determine eye alignment and coordination. These can be performed on clients over 6 months of age (see Box 3-8).	Both eyes coordinated, move in unison, with parallel alignment End-point nystagmus (rapid involuntary movement of the eyeball on the extreme lateral gaze)	Eye movements not coordinated or parallel; one or both eyes fail to follow a penlight in specific directions (e.g., strabismus [cross-eye or squint]) Nystagmus other than end-point (may indicate neurologic impairment)
Visual Acuity		
21. Assess near vision by providing adequate lighting and asking the client to read from a magazine or newspaper held at a distance of 36 cm (14 in). If the client normally wears corrective lenses, the glasses or lenses should be worn during the test.	Able to read newsprint	Difficulty reading newsprint unless due to aging process
22. Assess distance vision, asking the client to wear corrective lenses, unless they are used for reading only, that is, for distances of only 36 cm (12 to 14 in) (see Box 3-9).	20/20 vision on Snellen chart from age 6 onward	Denominator of 40 or more on Snellen chart with corrective lenses
23. Perform functional vision tests if the client is unable to see the top line (20/200) of the Snellen chart (see Box 3-10).		Functional vision only (e.g., light perception, hand movements, counting fingers at 1 ft)

BOX 3-7 *Assessing Peripheral Visual Fields*

• Have the client sit directly facing you at a distance of 60 to 90 cm (2 to 3 ft).

• Ask the client to cover the right eye with a card and look directly at your nose.

• Cover or close your eye directly opposite the client's covered eye (i.e., your left eye), and look directly at the client's nose.

• Hold an object (e.g., a penlight or pencil) in your fingers, extend your arm, and move the object into the visual field from various points in the periphery. The object should be at an equal distance from the client and yourself. Ask the client to tell you when the moving object is first spotted.

  a. To test the *temporal field* of the left eye, extend and move your right arm in from the client's right periphery. Temporally, peripheral objects can be seen at right angles (90 degrees) to the central point of vision.

  b. To test the *upward field* of the left eye, extend and move the right arm down from the upward periphery. The upward field of vision is normally 50 degrees because the orbital ridge is in the way.

  c. To test the *downward field* of the left eye, extend and move the right arm up from the lower periphery. The downward field of vision is normally 70 degrees because the cheekbone is in the way.

  d. To test the *nasal field* of the left eye, extend and move your left arm in from the periphery (Figure

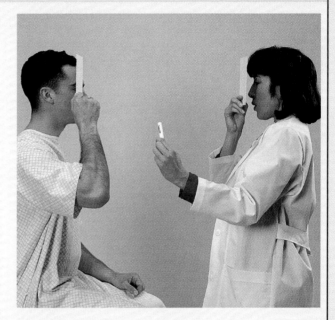

FIGURE 3-22 ◆ Assessing the client's left peripheral vision.

3-22 ◆). The nasal field of vision is normally 50 degrees away from the central point of vision because the nose is in the way.

• Repeat the above steps for the right eye, reversing the process.

BOX 3-8 *Assessing the Six Ocular Movements*

• Stand directly in front of the client, and hold the penlight at a comfortable distance (e.g., 30 cm [1 ft]) in front of the client's eyes.

• Ask the client to hold the head in a fixed position facing you and to follow the movements of the penlight with the eyes *only*.

• Move the penlight in a slow, orderly manner through the six cardinal fields of gaze, that is, from the center of the eye along the lines of the arrows in Figure 3-23 ◆ and back to the center.

• Stop the movement of the penlight periodically so that nystagmus can be detected.

    These six positions are used because six muscles guide the movements of each eye. Four *rectus* muscles (superior, inferior, lateral, and medial) move the eye in the direction indicated. Two *oblique* muscles (superior and inferior) rotate the eyeball on its axis. Cranial nerves III (oculomotor), IV (trochlear), and VI (abducens) innervate these muscles. Moving the object through the six positions can identify a nonfunctioning muscle or associated cranial nerve.

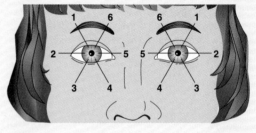

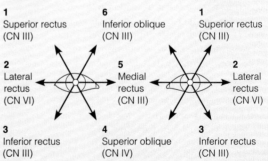

1 Superior rectus (CN III)	6 Inferior oblique (CN III)	1 Superior rectus (CN III)
2 Lateral rectus (CN VI)	5 Medial rectus (CN III)	2 Lateral rectus (CN VI)
3 Inferior rectus (CN III)	4 Superior oblique (CN IV)	3 Inferior rectus (CN III)

FIGURE 3-23 ◆ The six muscles that govern eye movement.

Box 3-9 *Assessing Distance Vision*

- Ask the client to stand or sit 6 m (20 ft) from a Snellen or character chart (Figure 3-24 ◆), cover the eye not being tested, and identify the letters or characters on the chart.
- Take three readings: right eye, left eye, both eyes.
- Record the readings of each eye and both eyes, that is, the smallest line from which the person is able to read one-half or more of the letters.

At the end of each line of the Snellen chart are standardized numbers (fractions). The top line is 20/200. The numerator (top number) is always 20, the distance the person stands from the chart. The denominator (bottom number) is the distance from which the normal eye can read the chart. Therefore, a person who has 20/40 vision, can see at 20 feet from the chart what a normal-sighted person can see at 40 feet from the chart. Visual acuity is recorded as "s̄c" (without correction), or "c̄c" (with correction). You can also indicate how many letters were misread in the line; for example, "visual acuity 20/40—2c̄c" indicates that two letters were misread in the 20/40 line by a client wearing corrective lenses.

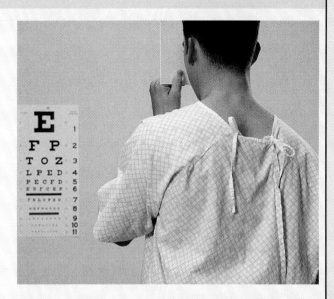

FIGURE 3-24 ◆ Testing distance vision.

Box 3-10 *Performing Functional Vision Tests*

Light Perception

Shine a penlight into the client's eye from a lateral position, and then turn the light off. Ask the client to tell you when the light is on or off. If the client knows when the light is on or off, the client has light perception, and the vision is recorded as "LP."

Hand Movements (H/M)

Hold your hand 30 cm (1 ft) from the client's face, and move it slowly back and forth, stopping it periodically.

Ask the client to tell you when your hand stops moving. If the client knows when your hand stops moving, record the vision as "H/M 1 ft."

Counting Fingers (C/F)

Hold up some of your fingers 30 cm (1 ft) from the client's face, and ask the client to count your fingers. If the client can do so, note on the vision record "C/F 1 ft."

24. **Document** findings in the client record using forms or checklists supplemented by narrative notes when appropriate.

AMBULATORY AND COMMUNITY SETTINGS

Assessing the Eyes and Vision

- When making a home visit, take your equipment and charts with you. Also include a tape measure to lay out the 20 feet for distance vision testing.

- Use the assessment as an opportunity to reinforce proper eye care and need for regular vision testing.

AGE-RELATED CONSIDERATIONS

Assessing the Eyes and Vision

Infant

- Infants 4 weeks of age should gaze at and follow objects.
- Ability to focus with both eyes should be present by 6 months of age.

Child

- Epicanthal folds, common in Asian cultures, may cover the medial canthus and cause eyes to appear misaligned.
- Dark-skinned children's sclerae may be darker and have small brown macules.
- Preschool children's acuity can be checked with picture cards or the E chart. Acuity should approach 20/20 by 6 years of age.

Elders

Visual Acuity

- Visual acuity decreases as the lens of the eye ages and becomes more opaque and loses elasticity.
- The ability of the iris to accommodate to darkness and dim light diminishes.
- Peripheral vision diminishes.
- The adaptation to light (glare) and dark decreases.
- Accommodation to far objects often improves, but accommodation to near objects decreases.
- Color vision declines; older people are less able to perceive purple colors and to discriminate pastel colors.

- Many older people wear corrective lenses; they are most likely to have hyperopia. Visual changes are due to loss of elasticity (presbyopia) and transparency of the lens.

External Eye Structures

- The skin around the orbit of the eye may darken.
- The eyeball may appear sunken because of the decrease in orbital fat.
- Skin folds of the upper lids may seem more prominent, and the lower lids may sag.
- The eyes may appear dry and lusterless because of the decrease in tear production from the lacrimal glands.
- A thin, grayish white arc or ring (*arcus senilis*) appears around part or all of the cornea. It results from an accumulation of a lipid substance on the cornea. The cornea tends to cloud with age.
- The iris may appear pale with brown discolorations as a result of pigment degeneration.
- The conjunctiva of the eye may appear paler than that of younger adults and may take on a slightly yellow appearance because of the deposition of fat.
- Pupil reaction to light and accommodation is normally symmetrically equal but may be less brisk.
- The pupils can appear smaller in size, unequal, and irregular in shape because of sclerotic changes in the iris.

EVALUATION

- Perform a detailed follow-up examination of other systems based on findings that deviated from expected or normal for the client. Relate findings to previous assessment data if available.
- Report significant deviations from normal to the physician. Persons with denominators of 40 or more on the Snellen or character chart, with or without corrective lenses, need to be referred to an ophthalmologist.

Ears and Hearing

Nursing assessment of the ear includes direct inspection and palpation of the external ear, inspection of the remaining parts of the ear by an otoscope, and determination of auditory acuity. Audiometric evalua-

tions, conducted by an audiometrist, measure hearing at various decibels and are recommended for the elderly or other persons with suspected hearing loss.

To inspect the external ear canal and tympanic membrane, the nurse inserts an otoscope into the external auditory canal. In some practice settings, the generalist nurse does not perform otoscopic examinations.

PLANNING

It is important to conduct the ear and hearing examination in an area that is quiet. In addition, the location should allow the client to be positioned sitting or standing at the same level as the nurse.

Delegation

Due to the substantial knowledge and skill required, assessment of the ears and hearing is not delegated to UAP. However, many aspects are observed during

Equipment

• Otoscope with several sizes of ear specula

Performance

1. Explain to the client what you are going to do, why it is necessary, and how he or she can cooperate. Discuss how the results will be used in planning further care or treatments.

2. Wash hands and observe appropriate infection control procedures.

3. Provide for client privacy.

4. Inquire if the client has any history of the following: family history of hearing problems or loss; presence of any ear problems; medication history, especially if there are complaints of ringing in ears; any hearing difficulty: its onset, factors contributing to it, and how it interferes with activities of daily living; use of a corrective hearing device: when and from whom it was obtained.

5. Position the client comfortably, seated if possible.

ASSESSMENT	NORMAL FINDINGS	DEVIATIONS FROM NORMAL
Auricles		
6. Inspect the auricles for color, symmetry of size, and position. To inspect position, note the level at which the superior aspect of the auricle attaches to the head in relation to the eye.	Color same as facial skin Symmetrical Auricle aligned with outer canthus of eye, about 10 degrees from vertical (Figure 3-25 ◆).	Bluish color of earlobes (e.g., cyanosis); pallor (e.g., frostbite); excessive redness (inflammation or fever) Asymmetry Low-set ears (associated with a congenital abnormality, such as Down syndrome)
7. Palpate the auricles for texture, elasticity, and areas of tenderness. • Gently pull the auricle upward, downward, and backward. • Fold the pinna forward (it should recoil). • Push in on the tragus. • Apply pressure to the mastoid process.	Mobile, firm, and not tender; pinna recoils after it is folded	Lesions (e.g., cysts); flaky, scaly skin (e.g., seborrhea); tenderness when moved or pressed (may indicate inflammation or infection of external ear)
External Ear Canal and Tympanic Membrane		
8. Using an otoscope, inspect the external ear canal for **cerumen,** skin lesions, pus, and blood (see Box 3-11).	Distal third contains hair follicles and glands Dry cerumen, grayish-tan color; or sticky, wet cerumen in various shades of brown	Redness and discharge Scaling Excessive cerumen obstructing canal
9. Inspect the tympanic membrane for color and gloss.	Pearly gray color, semitransparent (Figure 3-28 ◆)	Pink to red, some opacity Yellow-amber White Blue or deep red Dull surface

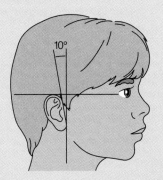

Normal alignment

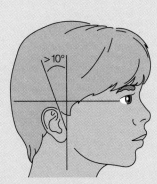

Low-set ears and deviation in alignment

FIGURE 3-25 ◆ Normal alignment of ears.

BOX 3-11 *Inspecting the Ears with an Otoscope*

- Attach a speculum to the otoscope. Use the largest diameter that will fit the ear canal without causing discomfort. This achieves maximum vision of the entire ear canal and tympanic membrane.
- Tip the client's head away from you, and straighten the ear canal. For an adult, straighten the ear canal by pulling the pinna up and back (Figure 3-26 ◆). Straightening the ear canal facilitates vision of the ear canal and the tympanic membrane.

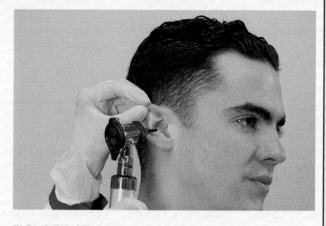

FIGURE 3-27 ◆ Inserting an otoscope.

- Hold the otoscope either (a) right side up, with your fingers between the otoscope handle and the client's head or (b) upside down, with your fingers and the ulnar surface of your hand against the client's head (Figure 3-27 ◆). This stabilizes the head and protects the eardrum and canal from injury if a quick head movement occurs.
- Gently insert the tip of the otoscope into the ear canal, avoiding pressure by the speculum against either side of the ear canal. The inner two-thirds of the ear canal is bony; if the speculum is pressed against either side, the client will experience discomfort.

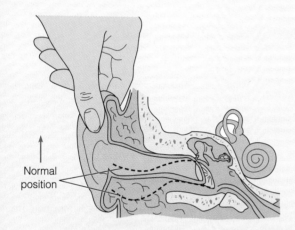

Normal position

FIGURE 3-26 ◆ Straightening the ear canal of an adult.

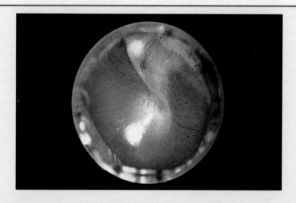

FIGURE 3-28 ◆ Normal tympanic membrane.

ASSESSMENT	NORMAL FINDINGS	DEVIATIONS FROM NORMAL
Gross Hearing Acuity Tests		
10. Assess client's response to normal voice tones. If client has difficulty hearing the normal voice, proceed with the following tests.	Normal voice tones audible	Normal voice tones not audible (e.g., requests nurse to repeat words or statements, leans toward the speaker, turns the head, cups the ears, or speaks in loud tone of voice)
10A. Perform the watch tick test. The ticking of a watch has a higher pitch than the human voice.	Able to hear ticking in both ears	Unable to hear ticking in one or both ears
• Have the client occlude one ear. Out of the client's sight, place a ticking watch 2 to 3 cm (1 to 2 in) from the unoccluded ear. • Ask what the client can hear. Repeat with the other ear.		

Gross Hearing Acuity Tests *continued*

ASSESSMENT	NORMAL FINDINGS	DEVIATIONS FROM NORMAL
10B. Tuning Fork Tests Perform Weber's test to assess bone conduction (see Box 3-12).	Sound is heard in both ears or is localized at the center of the head (Weber negative)	Sound is heard better in impaired ear, indicating a bone-conductive hearing loss or sound is heard better in ear without a problem, indicating a sensorineural disturbance (Weber positive)
Conduct the Rinne test to compare air conduction to bone conduction (see Box 3-12).	Air-conducted (AC) hearing is greater than bone-conducted (BC) hearing (i.e., AC > BC [positive Rinne])	Bone conduction time is equal to or longer than the air conduction time (i.e., BC > AC or BC = AC [negative Rinne; indicates a conductive hearing loss])

Box 3-12 *Performing Tuning Fork Tests*

Weber's Test

This test assesses bone conduction by testing the lateralization (sideward transmission) of sounds.

- Hold the tuning fork at its base. Activate it by tapping the fork gently against the back of your hand near the knuckles or by stroking the fork between your thumb and index fingers. It should be made to ring softly.
- Place the base of the vibrating fork on top of the client's head (Figure 3-29 ◆) and ask where the client hears the noise.

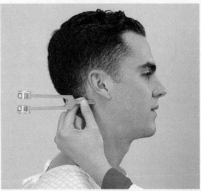

A

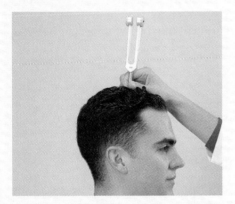

FIGURE 3-29 ◆ Weber's test tuning fork placement.

Rinne Test

This test compares air conduction to bone conduction.

- Ask the client to block the hearing in one ear intermittently by moving a fingertip in and out of the ear canal.
- Hold the handle of the activated tuning fork on the mastoid process of one ear (Figure 3-30A ◆) until the client states that the vibration can no longer be heard.
- Immediately hold the still vibrating fork prongs in

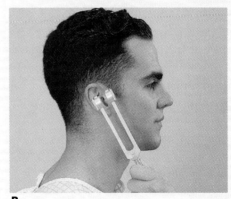

B

FIGURE 3-30 ◆ Rinne's test tuning fork placement.
(A) Base of the tuning fork on the mastoid process;
(B) tuning fork prongs placed in front of the client's ear.

front of the client's ear canal (Figure 3-30B ◆). Push aside the client's hair if necessary. Ask whether the client now hears the sound. Sound conducted by air is heard more readily than sound conducted by bone. The tuning fork vibrations conducted by air are normally heard longer.

---

11. **Document** findings in the client record using forms or checklists supplemented by narrative notes when appropriate.

AMBULATORY AND COMMUNITY SETTINGS

Assessing the Ears and Hearing

- Ensure that the examination is conducted in a quiet place. In particular, elders will have difficulty accurately reporting results of hearing tests if there is excessive outside noise.

- If necessary, ask the adult present with an infant or child to assist in holding the child still during the examination.

AGE-RELATED CONSIDERATIONS

Assessing the Ears and Hearing

Infant

- To assess gross hearing, ring a bell from behind the infant or have the parent call the child's name to check for a response. At 3 to 4 months of age, the child will turn the head and eyes toward the sound.

Child

- To inspect the external canal and tympanic membrane in children less than 3 years old, pull the pinna down and back. Insert the speculum only one-fourth to one-half inch.

Elders

- The skin of the ear may appear dry and be less resilient because of the loss of connective tissue.

- Increased coarse and wirelike hair growth occurs along the helix, antihelix, and tragus.
- The pinna increases in both width and length, and the earlobe elongates.
- Earwax is drier.
- The tympanic membrane is more translucent and less flexible. The intensity of the light reflex may diminish slightly.
- Sensorineural hearing loss occurs.
- Generalized hearing loss (**presbycusis**) occurs in all frequencies, although the first symptom is the loss of high-frequency sounds: the *f, s, sh,* and *ph* sounds. To such persons, conversation can be distorted and result in what appears to be inappropriate or confused behavior.

---

usual care and may be recorded by persons other than the nurse. Abnormal findings must be validated and interpreted by the nurse.

EVALUATION

- Perform a detailed follow-up examination of the neurologic system based on findings that deviated from expected or normal for the client. Relate findings to previous assessment data if available.

- Report significant deviations from normal to the physician.

Nose and Sinuses

A nurse can inspect the nasal passages very simply with a flashlight. However, a nasal speculum, which is a lighted instrument, facilitates examination of the nasal chambers. Assessment of the nose includes inspection and palpation of the external nose (the upper third of

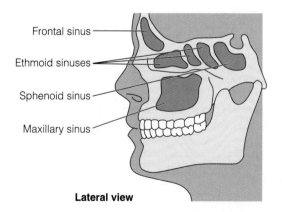

Frontal sinus

Ethmoid sinuses

Sphenoid sinus

Maxillary sinus

Lateral view

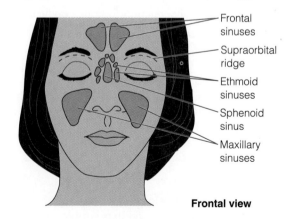

Frontal sinuses

Supraorbital ridge

Ethmoid sinuses

Sphenoid sinus

Maxillary sinuses

Frontal view

FIGURE 3-31 ◆ The facial sinuses.

the nose is bone; the remainder is cartilage); patency of the nasal cavities; and inspection of the nasal cavities. The nurse also inspects and palpates the facial sinuses (Figure 3-31 ◆). Advanced practitioners may perform transillumination of the sinuses. If the client reports difficulty or abnormality in smell, the nurse may test the client's olfactory sense by asking the client to identify common odors such as coffee or mint. Ask the client to close the eyes, and place vials containing the scent under the client's nose to do this.

PLANNING

Delegation

Due to the substantial knowledge and skill required, assessment of the nose and sinuses is not delegated to UAP. However, many aspects are observed during usual care and may be recorded by persons other than the nurse. Abnormal findings must be validated and interpreted by the nurse.

IMPLEMENTATION:
TECHNIQUE 3-8 ASSESSING THE NOSE AND SINUSES

Equipment

- Examination gloves
- Nasal speculum
- Flashlight/penlight

Performance

1. Explain to the client what you are going to do, why it is necessary, and how he or she can cooperate. Discuss how the results will be used in planning further care or treatments.

2. Wash hands, apply gloves, and observe appropriate infection control procedures.

3. Provide for client privacy.

4. Inquire if the client has any history of the following: allergies, difficulty breathing through the nose, sinus infections, injuries to nose or face, nosebleeds; any medications taken; any changes in sense of smell.

5. Position the client comfortably, seated if possible.

ASSESSMENT	NORMAL FINDINGS	DEVIATIONS FROM NORMAL
Nose		
6. Inspect the external nose for any deviations in shape, size, or color and flaring or discharge from the nares.	Symmetric and straight No discharge or flaring Uniform color	Asymmetric Discharge from nares Localized areas of redness or presence of skin lesions
7. Lightly palpate the external nose to determine any areas of tenderness, masses, and displacements of bone and cartilage.	Not tender; no lesions	Tenderness on palpation; presence of lesions
8. Determine patency of both nasal cavities. Ask the client to close the mouth, exert pressure on one naris, and breathe through the opposite naris. Repeat the procedure to assess patency of the opposite naris.	Air moves freely as the client breathes through the nares	Air movement is restricted in one or both nares
9. Inspect the nasal cavities using a flashlight or a nasal speculum (see Box 3-13).		
10. Observe for the presence of redness, swelling, growths, and discharge.	Mucosa pink Clear, watery discharge No lesions	Mucosa red, edematous Abnormal discharge (e.g., purulent) Presence of lesions (e.g., polyps)
11. Inspect the nasal septum between the nasal chambers.	Nasal septum intact and in midline	Septum deviated to the right or to the left.
Facial Sinuses		
12. Palpate the maxillary and frontal sinuses for tenderness.	Not tender	Tenderness in one or more sinuses

BOX 3-13 *Using a Nasal Speculum*

- Hold the speculum in your right hand to inspect the client's left nostril and your left hand to inspect the client's right nostril.
- Tip the client's head back.
- Facing the client, insert the tip of the closed speculum (blades together) about 1 cm or up to the point at which the blade widens. Care must be taken to avoid pressure on the sensitive nasal septum (Figure 3-32 ◆).
- Stabilize the speculum with your index finger against

the side of the nose. Use the other hand to position the head and then to hold the light.
- Open the speculum as much as possible and inspect the floor of the nose (vestibule), the anterior portion of the septum, the middle meatus, and the middle turbinates. The posterior turbinate is rarely visualized because of its position (Figure 3-33 ◆).
- Inspect the lining of the nares and the integrity and position of the nasal septum.

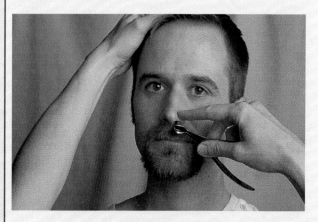

FIGURE 3-32 ◆ Using a nasal speculum.

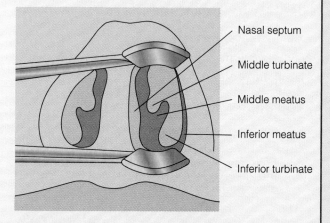

Nasal septum

Middle turbinate

Middle meatus

Inferior meatus

Inferior turbinate

FIGURE 3-33 ◆ The nasal turbinates.

---

 13. **Document** findings in the client record using forms or checklists supplemented by narrative notes when appropriate.

AGE-RELATED CONSIDERATIONS

Assessing the Nose and Sinuses

Infant

- A speculum is usually not necessary to examine the septum, turbinates, and vestibule. Instead, push the tip of the nose upward with the thumb and shine a light into the nares.

Child

- A speculum is usually not necessary to examine the septum, turbinates, and vestibule. It might cause the child to be apprehensive. Instead, push the tip

of the nose upward with the thumb and shine a light into the nares.
- Ethmoid sinuses develop by age 6. Sinus problems in children under this age are rare.

Elders

- The sense of smell markedly diminishes because of a decrease in the number of olfactory nerve fibers and atrophy of the remaining fibers. Older persons are less able to identify and discriminate odors.
- Nosebleeds may result from hypertensive disease or other arterial vessel changes.

EVALUATION

- Perform a detailed follow-up examination of other systems based on findings that deviated from

expected or normal for the client. Relate findings to previous assessment data if available.
- Report significant deviations from normal to the physician.

Mouth and Oropharynx

Assessment of the mouth and pharynx includes a number of structures: lips, inner and buccal mucosa, the tongue and floor of the mouth, teeth and gums, hard and soft palates, uvula, salivary glands, tonsillar pillars, and tonsils (Figure 3-34 ◆).

Dental caries (cavities) and periodontal disease (pyorrhea) are two problems that most frequently affect the teeth. Both are commonly associated with plaque and tartar deposits. **Plaque** is an invisible soft film that adheres to the enamel surface of teeth; it consists of bacteria, molecules of saliva, and remnants of epithelial cells and leukocytes. When plaque is unchecked, tartar (dental calculus) forms. **Tartar** is a visible, hard deposit of plaque and dead bacteria that forms at the gum lines. Tartar buildup can alter the fibers that attach the teeth to the gum and eventually disrupt bone tissue. Periodontal disease is characterized by **gingivitis** (red, swollen *gingiva*, i.e., gum), bleeding, receding gum lines, and the formation of pockets between the teeth and gums. In advanced periodontal disease, the teeth are loose, and pus is evident when the gums are pressed.

Other problems nurses may see are **glossitis** (inflammation of the tongue), **stomatitis** (inflammation of the oral mucosa), and **parotitis** (inflammation of the parotid salivary gland). The accumulation of foul matter (food, microorganisms, and epithelial elements) on the teeth and gums is referred to as **sordes**.

PLANNING

If possible, arrange for the client to sit with the head against a firm surface such as a headrest or examina-

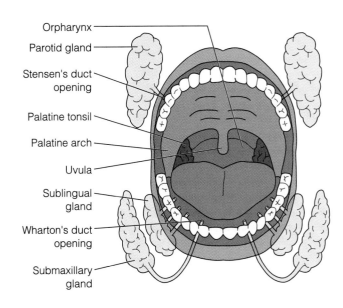

FIGURE 3-34 ◆ Anatomic structures of the mouth.

Labels: Orpharynx, Parotid gland, Stensen's duct opening, Palatine tonsil, Palatine arch, Uvula, Sublingual gland, Wharton's duct opening, Submaxillary gland

tion table. This makes it easier for the client to hold the head still during the examination.

Delegation

Due to the substantial knowledge and skill required, assessment of the mouth and oropharynx is not delegated to UAP. However, many aspects are observed during usual care and may be recorded by persons other than the nurse. Abnormal findings must be validated and interpreted by the nurse.

IMPLEMENTATION:
TECHNIQUE 3-9 ASSESSING THE MOUTH AND OROPHARYNX

Equipment

- Examination gloves
- Tongue depressor
- 2" × 2" gauze pads
- Flashlight or penlight

Performance

1. Explain to the client what you are going to do, why it is necessary, and how he or she can cooper-

ate. Discuss how the results will be used in planning further care or treatments.

2. Wash hands, apply gloves, and observe appropriate infection control procedures.

3. Provide for client privacy.

4. Inquire if the client has any history of the following: routine pattern of dental care, last visit to dentist; length of time ulcers or other lesions have been present; any denture discomfort; any medications client is receiving.

5. Position the client comfortably, seated if possible.

ASSESSMENT	NORMAL FINDINGS	DEVIATIONS FROM NORMAL
Lips and Buccal Mucosa		
6. Inspect the outer lips for symmetry of contour, color, and texture. Ask the client to purse the lips as if to whistle.	Uniform pink color (darker, e.g., bluish hue, in Mediterranean groups and dark-skinned clients)	Pallor; cyanosis Blisters; generalized or localized swelling; fissures, crusts, or scales (may result from

ASSESSMENT	NORMAL FINDINGS	DEVIATIONS FROM NORMAL
Lips and Buccal Mucosa *continued*		
6. (*continued*)	Soft, moist, smooth texture Symmetry of contour Ability to purse lips	excessive moisture, nutritional deficiency, or fluid deficit) Inability to purse lips (indicative of facial nerve damage)
7. Inspect and palpate the inner lips and buccal mucosa for color, moisture, texture, and the presence of lesions (see Box 3-14).	Uniform pink color (freckled brown pigmentation in dark-skinned clients) Moist, smooth, soft, glistening, and elastic texture (drier oral mucosa in elderly due to decreased salivation)	Pallor; white patches (leukoplakia) Excessive dryness Mucosal cysts; irritations from dentures; abrasions, ulcerations; nodules
Teeth and Gums		
8. Inspect the teeth and gums while examining the inner lips and buccal mucosa (see Box 3-14).	32 adult teeth Smooth, white, shiny tooth enamel Pink gums (bluish or dark patches in dark-skinned clients) Moist, firm texture to gums No retraction of gums (pulling away from the teeth)	Missing teeth; ill-fitting dentures Brown or black discoloration of the enamel (may indicate staining or the presence of caries) Excessively red gums Spongy texture; bleeding; tenderness (may indicate periodontal disease) Receding, atrophied gums; swelling that partially covers the teeth
9. Inspect the dentures. Ask the client to remove complete or partial dentures. Inspect their condition, noting in particular broken or worn areas.	Smooth, intact dentures	Ill-fitting dentures; irritated and excoriated area under dentures
Tongue/Floor of the Mouth		
10. Inspect the surface of the tongue for position, color, and texture. Ask the client to protrude the tongue.	Central position Pink color (some brown pigmentation on tongue borders in dark-skinned clients); moist; slightly rough; thin whitish coating Smooth, lateral margins; no lesions	Deviated from center (may indicate damage to hypoglossal [twelfth cranial] nerve) Smooth red tongue (may indicate iron, vitamin B_{12}, or vitamin B_3 deficiency) Dry, furry tongue (associated with fluid deficit) Nodes, ulcerations, discolorations (white or red areas); areas of tenderness
11. Inspect tongue movement. Ask the client to roll the tongue upward and move it from side to side.	Moves freely; no tenderness	Restricted mobility
12. Inspect the base of the tongue, the mouth floor, and the frenulum. Ask the client to place the tip of the tongue against the roof of the mouth.	Smooth tongue base with prominent veins	Swelling, ulceration
13. Palpate the tongue and floor of the mouth for any nodules, lumps, or excoriated areas. To palpate the tongue, use a piece of gauze to grasp its tip (stabilize it), and with the index finger of your other hand, palpate the back of the tongue, its borders, and its base (Figure 3-38 ◆). To assess function of the glossopharyngeal and hypoglossal nerves, see the neurologic assessment, later in this chapter.	Smooth with no palpable nodules	Swelling, nodules
Salivary Glands		
14. Inspect salivary duct openings for any swelling or redness (see Figure 3-34).	Same as color of buccal mucosa and floor of mouth	Inflammation (redness and swelling)

Box 3-14 *Inspecting and Palpating the Lip, Mucosa, Teeth, Gums*

Inner Lip and Front Teeth

- Apply examination gloves.
- Ask the client to relax the mouth, and, for better visualization, pull the lip outward away from the teeth.
- Grasp the lip on each side between the thumb and index finger (Figure 3-35 ◆).
- Palpate any lesions for size, tenderness, and consistency.
- Inspect the front teeth and gums.

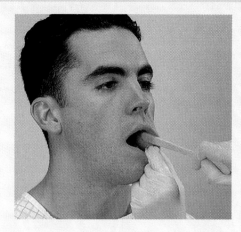

FIGURE 3-36 ◆ Inspecting the buccal mucosa.

fillings and caries. Observe the number of teeth, tooth color, the state of fillings, dental caries, and tartar along the base of the teeth. Note the presence and fit of partial or complete dentures.

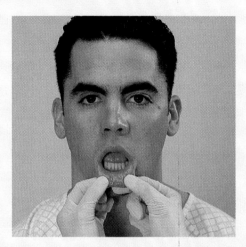

FIGURE 3-35 ◆ Inspecting the mucosa of the lower lip.

Buccal Mucosa and Back Teeth

- Ask the client to open the mouth. Using a tongue depressor, retract the cheek (Figure 3-36 ◆). View the surface buccal mucosa from top to bottom and back to front. A flashlight or penlight will help illuminate the surface. Repeat the procedure for the other side.
- Ask the client to open the mouth again. Using penlight to assist visualization, move a finger along the inside cheek. Another finger may be moved outside the cheek.
- Examine the back teeth. For proper vision of the molars, use the index fingers of both hands to retract the cheek (Figure 3-37 ◆). Ask the client to relax the lips and first close, then open, the jaw. Closing the jaw assists in observation of tooth alignment and loss of teeth; opening the jaw assists in observation of dental

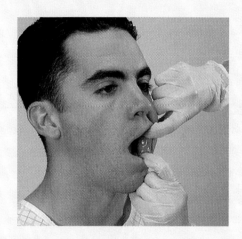

FIGURE 3-37 ◆ Inspecting the back teeth.

Gums

- Inspect the gums around the molars. Observe for bleeding, color, retraction (pulling away from the teeth), edema, and lesions.
- Assess the texture of the gums by gently pressing the gum tissue with a tongue depressor.

ASSESSMENT	NORMAL FINDINGS	DEVIATIONS FROM NORMAL
Palates and Uvula		
15. Inspect the hard and soft palates for color, shape, texture, and the presence of bony prominences. Ask the client to open the mouth wide and tilt the head backward.	Light pink, smooth, soft palate Lighter pink hard palate, more irregular texture	Discoloration (e.g., jaundice or pallor) Palates the same color Irritations

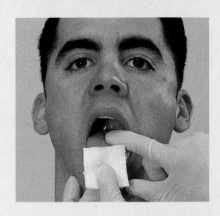

FIGURE 3-38 ◆ Palpating the tongue.

ASSESSMENT	NORMAL FINDINGS	DEVIATIONS FROM NORMAL
Palates and Uvula *continued*		
15. (*Continued*) Then, press tongue with a tongue depressor as necessary, and use a penlight for appropriate visualization.		Bony growths (exostoses) growing from the hard palate
16. Inspect the uvula for position and mobility while examining the palates. To observe the uvula, ask the client to say "ah" so that the soft palate rises.	Positioned in midline of soft palate	Deviation to one side from tumor or trauma; immobility (may indicate damage to trigeminal [fifth cranial] nerve or vagus [tenth cranial] nerve)
Oropharynx and Tonsils		
17. Inspect the oropharynx for color and texture. Inspect one side at a time to avoid eliciting the gag reflex. To expose one side of the oropharynx, press a tongue blade against the tongue on the same side about halfway back while the client tilts the head back and opens the mouth wide. Use a penlight for illumination, if needed.	Pink and smooth posterior wall	Reddened or edematous; presence of lesions, plaques, or drainage
18. Inspect the tonsils (behind the fauces) for color, discharge, and size.	Pink and smooth No discharge Of normal size (see Box 3-15 for a grading system to describe the size of tonsils)	Inflamed Presence of discharge Swollen
19. Elicit the gag reflex by pressing the posterior tongue with a tongue depressor.	Present	Absent (may indicate problems with glossopharyngeal or vagus nerves)

 20. **Document** findings in the client record using forms or checklists supplemented by narrative notes when appropriate.

> ### Box 3-15 *Grading System to Describe Size of Tonsils*
>
> - *Grade 1 (normal):* The tonsils are behind the tonsillar pillars (i.e., the soft structures supporting the soft palate).
> - *Grade 2:* The tonsils are between the pillars and the uvula.
> - *Grade 3:* The tonsils touch the uvula.
> - *Grade 4:* One or both tonsils extend to the midline of the oropharynx.

Assessing the Mouth and Oropharynx

• Although clients may be sensitive to discussion of their personal hygiene practices, use the assessment as an opportunity to provide teaching regarding appropriate oral and dental care for the entire family. Refer clients to a dentist if indicated.

Assessing the Mouth

Infant

• Inspect the palate for a cleft.

Child

• Tooth development should be appropriate for age.
• White spots on the teeth may indicate excessive fluoride ingestion.
• Drooling is common up to 2 years of age.
• The tonsils are normally larger in children than in adults and commonly extend beyond the palatine arch until the age of 11 or 12 years.

Elders

• The oral mucosa may be drier than that of younger persons because of decreased salivary gland activity. Decreased salivation occurs only in elderly people taking prescribed medications such as antidepressants, antihistamines, decongestants, diuretics, antihypertensives, tranquilizers, antispasmodics, and antineoplastics. Extreme dryness is associated with dehydration.
• Some receding of the gums occurs, giving an appearance of increased toothiness.
• There may be a brownish pigmentation to the gums, especially in black persons.
• Taste sensations diminish. Sweet and salty tastes are lost first. Elderly persons may add more salt and sugar to food than they did when they were younger. Diminished taste sensation is due to atrophy of the taste buds and a decreased sense of smell. It indicates diminished function of the fifth and seventh cranial nerves.
• Tiny purple or bluish black swollen areas (varicosities) under the tongue, known as *caviar spots*, are not uncommon.
• The teeth may show signs of staining, erosion, chipping, and abrasions due to loss of dentin. Tooth loss occurs as a result of dental disease but is preventable with good dental hygiene.
• The gag reflex may be slightly sluggish.

EVALUATION

• Perform a detailed follow-up examination of neurological and other systems based on findings that deviated from expected or normal for the client. Relate findings to previous assessment data if available.
• Report significant deviations from normal to the physician.

Neck

Examination of the neck includes the muscles, lymph nodes, trachea, thyroid gland, carotid arteries, and jugular veins. Areas of the neck are defined by the sternocleidomastoid muscles, which divide each side of the neck into two triangles: the anterior and posterior (Figure 3-39 ◆). The trachea, thyroid gland, anterior cervical nodes, and carotid artery lie within the anterior triangle (the carotid artery runs parallel and anterior to the sternocleidomastoid muscle) (Figure 3-40 ◆). The supraclavicular and posterior lymph nodes lie within the posterior triangle (Figure 3-41 ◆ and Table 3-5).

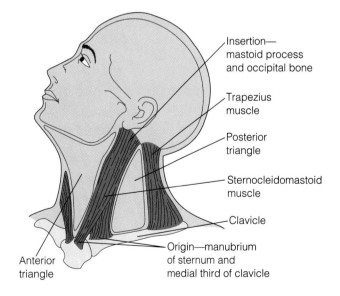

Insertion— mastoid process and occipital bone

Trapezius muscle

Posterior triangle

Sternocleidomastoid muscle

Clavicle

Origin—manubrium of sternum and medial third of clavicle

Anterior triangle

FIGURE 3-39 ◆ Major muscles of the neck.

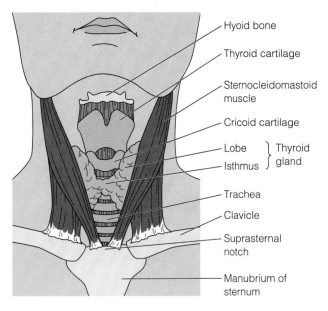

FIGURE 3-40 ◆ Structures of the neck.

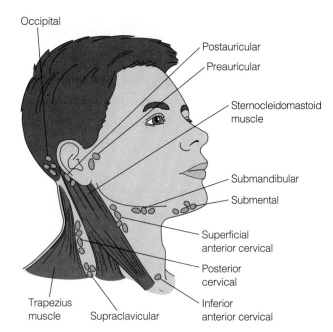

FIGURE 3-41 ◆ Lymph nodes of the neck.

PLANNING

Delegation

Due to the substantial knowledge and skill required, assessment of the neck is not delegated to UAP.

However, many aspects are observed during usual care and may be recorded by persons other than the nurse. Abnormal findings must be validated and interpreted by the nurse.

TABLE 3-5	LYMPH NODES OF THE HEAD AND NECK	
Node Center	**Location**	**Area Drained**
Head		
Occipital	At the posterior base of the skull	The occipital region of the scalp and the deep structures of the back of the neck
Postauricular (mastoid)	Behind the auricle of the ear or in front of the mastoid process	The parietal region of the head and part of the ear
Preauricular	In front of the tragus of the ear	The forehead and upper face
Floor of Mouth		
Submandibular (submaxillary)	Along the medial border of the lower jaw, halfway between the angle of the jaw and the chin	The chin, upper lip, cheek, nose, teeth, eyelids, part of the tongue and of the floor of the mouth
Submental	Behind the tip of the mandible, in the midline, under the chin	The anterior third of the tongue, gums, and floor of the mouth
Neck		
Superficial (anterior) cervical chain	Along the anterior to the sternocleidomastoid muscle	The skin and neck
Posterior cervical chain	Along the anterior aspect of the trapezius muscle	The posterior and lateral regions of the neck, occiput, and mastoid
Deep cervical chain	Under the sternocleidomastoid muscle	The larynx, thyroid gland, trachea, and upper part of the esophagus
Supraclavicular	Above the clavicle, in the angle between the clavicle and the sternocleidomastoid muscle	The lateral regions of the neck and lungs

From *Fundamentals of nursing: Concepts, process, and practice*, 6th ed., by B. Kozier, G. Erb, A. Berman, & K. Burke, 2000, Upper Saddle River, NJ: Prentice Hall Health.

Equipment

• None.

Performance

1. Explain to the client what you are going to do, why it is necessary, and how he or she can cooperate. Discuss how the results will be used in planning further care or treatments.

2. Wash hands and observe appropriate infection control procedures.

3. Provide for client privacy.

4. Inquire if the client has any history of the following: Any problems with neck lumps; neck pain or stiffness; when and how any lumps occurred; any previous diagnoses of thyroid problems; and any other treatments provided (e.g., surgery, radiation).

ASSESSMENT	NORMAL FINDINGS	DEVIATIONS FROM NORMAL
Neck Muscles		
5. Inspect the neck muscles (sternocleidomastoid and trapezius) for abnormal swellings or masses. Ask the client to hold the head erect.	Muscles equal in size; head centered	Unilateral neck swelling; head tilted to one side (indicates presence of masses, injury, muscle weakness, shortening of sternocleidomastoid muscle, scars)
6. Observe head movement. Ask client to:	Coordinated, smooth movements with no discomfort	Muscle tremor, spasm, or stiffness
• Move the chin to the chest (determines function of the sternocleidomastoid muscle).	Head flexes 45 degrees	Limited range of motion; painful movements; involuntary movements (e.g., up-and-down nodding movements associated with Parkinson's disease)
• Move the head back so that the chin points upward (determines function of the trapezius muscle).	Head hyperextends 60 degrees	Head hyperextends less than 60 degrees
• Move the head so that the ear is moved toward the shoulder on each side (determines function of the sternocleidomastoid muscle).	Head laterally flexes 40 degrees	Head laterally flexes less than 40 degrees
• Turn the head to the right and to the left (determines function of the sternocleidomastoid muscle).	Head laterally rotates 70 degrees	Head laterally rotates less than 70 degrees
7. Assess muscle strength.		
• Ask the client to turn the head to one side against the resistance of your hand. Repeat with the other side (determines the strength of the sternocleidomastoid muscle).	Equal strength	Unequal strength
• Shrug the shoulders against the resistance of your hands (determines the strength of the trapezius muscles).	Equal strength	Unequal strength
Lymph Nodes		
8. Palpate the entire neck for enlarged lymph nodes, using the guidelines shown in Box 3-16.	Not palpable	Enlarged, palpable, possibly tender (associated with infection and tumors)
Trachea		
9. Palpate the trachea for lateral deviation. Place your fingertip or thumb on the trachea in the suprasternal notch (see Figure 3-40), and then move your finger laterally to the left and the right in spaces bordered by the clavicle, the anterior aspect of the sternocleidomastoid muscle, and the trachea.	Central placement in midline of neck; spaces are equal on both sides	Deviation to one side, indicating possible neck tumor; thyroid enlargement; enlarged lymph nodes

Box 3-16 *Palpating Neck Lymph Nodes*

- Face the client, and bend the client's head forward slightly or toward the side being examined to relax the soft tissue and muscles.
- Palpate the nodes using the pads of the fingers. Move the fingertips in a gentle, rotating motion.
- When examining the submental and submandibular nodes, place the fingertips under the mandible on the side nearest the palpating hand, and pull the skin and subcutaneous tissue laterally over the mandibular surface so that the tissue rolls over the nodes.
- When palpating the supraclavicular nodes, have the client bend the head forward to relax the tissues of the anterior neck and to relax the shoulders so that the clavicles drop. Use your hand nearest the side to be examined when facing the client (i.e., your left hand for the client's right nodes). Use your free hand to flex the client's head forward if necessary. Hook your index and third fingers over the clavicle lateral to the sternocleidomastoid muscle (Figure 3-42 ◆).
- When palpating the anterior cervical nodes and posterior cervical nodes, move your fingertips slowly in a forward circular motion against the sternocleidomastoid and trapezius muscles, respectively.

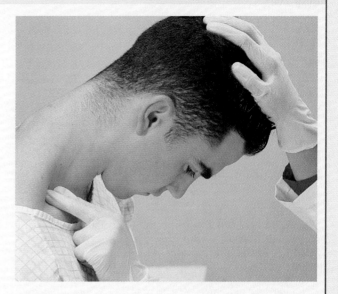

FIGURE 3-42 ◆ Palpating the supraclavicular lymph nodes.

- To palpate the deep cervical nodes, bend or hook your fingers around the sternocleidomastoid muscle.

ASSESSMENT	NORMAL FINDINGS	DEVIATIONS FROM NORMAL
Thyroid Gland		
10. Inspect the thyroid gland.		
• Stand in front of the client.		
• Observe the lower half of the neck overlying the thyroid gland for symmetry and visible masses.	Not visible on inspection	Visible diffuseness or local enlargement
• Ask the client to hyperextend the head and swallow. If necessary, offer a glass of water to make it easier for the client to swallow. This action determines how the thyroid and cricoid cartilages move and whether swallowing causes a bulging of the gland.	Gland ascends during swallowing but is not visible	Gland is not fully movable with swallowing
11. Palpate the thyroid gland for smoothness. Note any areas enlargement, masses, or nodules. See Box 3-17 for palpation methods.	Lobes may not be palpated If palpated, lobes are small, smooth, centrally located, painless, and rise freely with swallowing.	Solitary nodules
12. If enlargement of the gland is suspected, auscultate over the thyroid area for a bruit (a soft rushing sound created by turbulent blood flow). Use the bell-shaped diaphragm of the stethoscope.	Absence of bruit	Presence of bruit

 13. **Document** findings in the client record using forms or checklists supplemented by narrative notes when appropriate.

Box 3-17 *Palpating the Thyroid Gland*

Stand in front of or behind the client, and ask the client to lower the chin slightly. Lowering the chin relaxes the neck muscles, facilitating palpation.

Posterior Approach

- Place your hands around the client's neck, with your fingertips on the lower half of the neck over the trachea (Figure 3-43 ◆).
- Ask the client to swallow (taking a sip of water, if necessary), and feel for any enlargement of the thyroid isthmus as it rises. The isthmus lies across the trachea, below the cricoid cartilage (see Figure 3-40).
- To examine the right thyroid lobe, have the client lower the chin slightly and turn the head slightly to the right (the side being examined). With your left fingers, displace the trachea slightly to the right. With your right fingers, palpate the right thyroid lobe. Have the client swallow while you are palpating.

- Repeat the last step, in reverse, to examine the left thyroid lobe.

Anterior Approach

- Place the tips of your index and middle fingers over the trachea, and palpate the thyroid isthmus as the client swallows.
- To examine the right thyroid lobe, have the client lower the chin slightly and turn the head slightly to the right. With your right fingers, displace the trachea slightly to the client's right (your left). With your left fingers, palpate the right thyroid lobe (Figure 3-44 ◆).
- To examine the left thyroid lobe, repeat the above step in reverse.

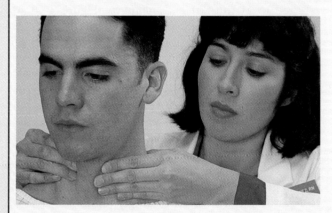

FIGURE 3-43 ◆ Palpating the thyroid (posterior approach).

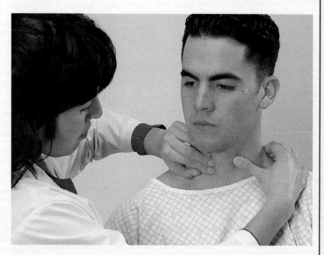

FIGURE 3-44 ◆ Palpating the thyroid (anterior approach).

AGE-RELATED CONSIDERATIONS

Assessing the Neck

Infant

- Examine the neck while the child is lying supine. Neck mobility is determined by lifting the head and turning it from side to side.
- An infant's neck is normally short, lengthening by about age 3 to 4. This makes palpation of the trachea difficult.

Child

- An infant's neck is normally short, lengthening by about age 3 to 4. This makes palpation of the trachea difficult.

EVALUATION

- Perform a detailed follow-up examination of other systems based on findings that deviated from

expected or normal for the client. Relate findings to previous assessment data if available.

- Report significant deviations from normal to the physician.

Thorax and Lungs

Assessing the thorax and lungs is frequently critical to assessing the client's aeration status. The client's posture is important to note. Some people with chronic respiratory problems tend to bend forward or even prop their arms on a support to elevate their clavicles. This posture is an attempt to expand the chest fully and thus breathe with less effort.

Chest Wall Landmarks

The nurse must be familiar with a series of imaginary lines on the chest wall and be able to locate the position of each rib and some spinous processes. These landmarks help the nurse to identify the position of underlying organs (e.g., lobes of the lung). Figure 3-45 ◆ shows the anterior, lateral, and posterior series of lines. Locating the position of each rib and certain spinous processes is essential for identifying underlying lobes of the lung. Figure 3-46 ◆ shows anterior, right and left lateral views, and posterior view of the chest and underlying lungs. Each lung is first divided into the upper and lower lobes by an oblique fissure that runs from the level of the spinous process of the third thoracic vertebra (T3) to the level of the sixth rib at the midclavicular line. The right upper lobe is abbreviated RUL; the right lower lobe, RLL. Similarly, the left upper lobe is abbreviated LUL; the left lower lobe, LLL. The right lung is further divided by a minor fissure into the right upper lobe and right middle lobe (RML). This fissure runs anteriorly from the right midaxillary line at the level of the fifth rib to the level of the fourth rib.

These specific landmarks (i.e., T3 and the fourth, fifth, and sixth ribs) are located as follows: The starting point for locating the ribs anteriorly is the angle of Louis, the junction between the body of the sternum and the manubrium (the handlelike superior part of the sternum that joins with the clavicles). The superior border of the second rib attaches to the sternum at this manubriosternal junction (Figure 3-47 ◆). The nurse can identify the manubrium by first palpating the clavicle and following its course to its attachment at the manubrium. The nurse then palpates and counts distal ribs and intercostal spaces (ICSs) from the second rib. It is important to note that an ICS is numbered according to the number of the rib immediately *above* the space. When palpating for rib identification, the nurse should palpate along the midclavicular line rather than the sternal border, because the rib cartilages are very close at the sternum. Only the first seven ribs attach directly to the sternum.

The counting of ribs is more difficult on the posterior than on the anterior thorax. For identifying underlying lung lobes, the pertinent landmark is T3. The starting point for locating T3 is the spinous process of the seventh cervical vertebra (C7), also referred to as the *vertebra prominens* (Figure 3-48 ◆). When the client flexes the neck anteriorly, a prominent process can be observed and palpated. This is the spinous process of the seventh cervical vertebra. If two spinous processes are observed, the superior one is C7, and the inferior one is the spinous process of the first thoracic vertebra (T1). The nurse then palpates and counts the spinous processes from C7 to T3. Each spinous process up to T4 is adjacent to the corresponding rib number (e.g., T3 is adjacent to the third rib). After T4, however, the spinous processes project obliquely, causing the spinous process of the vertebra to lie, not over its correspondingly numbered rib, but over the rib below. Thus, the spinous process of T5 lies over the body of T6 and is adjacent to the sixth rib.

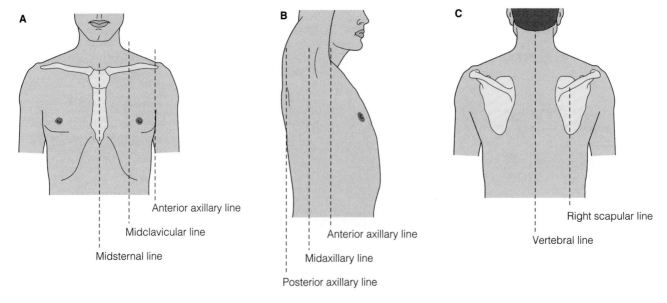

A

Anterior axillary line

Midclavicular line

Midsternal line

B

Anterior axillary line

Midaxillary line

Posterior axillary line

C

Right scapular line

Vertebral line

FIGURE 3-45 ◆ Chest wall landmarks (A) anterior; (B) lateral; (C) posterior.

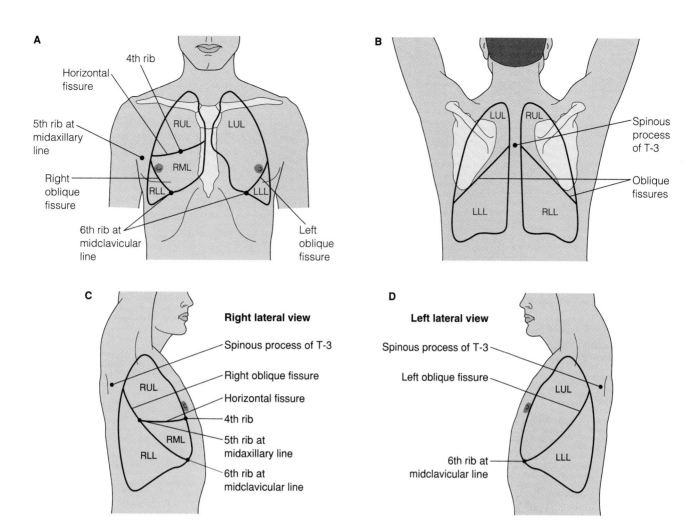

A

4th rib

Horizontal fissure

5th rib at midaxillary line

Right oblique fissure

RUL

LUL

RML

RLL

LLL

6th rib at midclavicular line

Left oblique fissure

B

LUL

RUL

Spinous process of T-3

Oblique fissures

LLL

RLL

C

Right lateral view

Spinous process of T-3

Right oblique fissure

Horizontal fissure

4th rib

5th rib at midaxillary line

6th rib at midclavicular line

RUL

RML

RLL

D

Left lateral view

Spinous process of T-3

Left oblique fissure

LUL

6th rib at midclavicular line

LLL

FIGURE 3-46 ◆ Chest wall landmarks with underlying lungs.

Chest Shape and Size

In adults, the thorax is oval. Its diameter measured in the anteroposterior direction is smaller than its transverse diameter (Figure 3-49 ◆). In addition, the diameter of the thorax is smaller at the top than at the base.

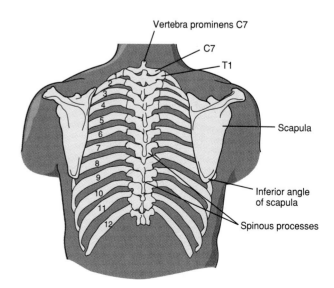

Manubrium of sternum

Manubriosternal junction (angle of Louis)

Clavicle

First intercostal space

Second intercostal space

Body of sternum

Xiphoid

Costal angle

Costal margin

1 2 3 4 5 6 7 8 9 10

Vertebra prominens C7

C7

T1

Scapula

Inferior angle of scapula

Spinous processes

FIGURE 3-47 ◆ Location of the anterior ribs, angle of Louis, and sternum.

FIGURE 3-48 ◆ Location of the posterior ribs in relation to the spinous processes.

Clinical appearance

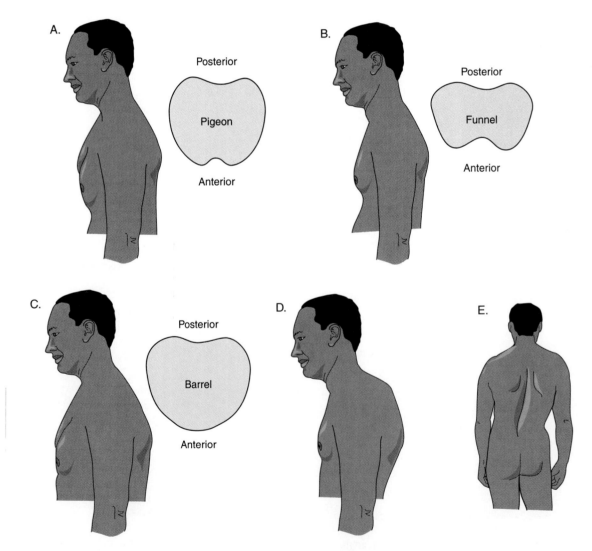

Cross section of thorax

Posterior

Transverse diameter

Anterior

FIGURE 3-49 ◆ Configuration of the thorax showing oval shape, anteroposterior diameter, and transverse diameter.

There are several deformities of the chest (Figure 3-50 ◆). Pigeon chest (pectus carinatum), a permanent deformity, may be caused by rickets. A narrow transverse diameter, an increased anteroposterior diameter, and a protruding sternum characterize pigeon chest. A funnel chest (pectus excavatum), a congenital defect, is the opposite of pigeon chest in that the sternum is depressed, narrowing the anteroposterior diameter. Because the sternum points posteriorly in clients with a funnel chest, abnormal pressure on the heart may result in altered function. A barrel chest, in which the ratio of the anteroposterior to transverse diameter is 1 to 1, is seen in clients with thoracic kyphosis (excessive convex curvature of the thoracic spine) and emphysema (chronic pulmonary condition in which the air sacs, or alveoli, are dilated and distended). Scoliosis is a lateral deviation of the spine.

Breath Sounds

Assessment of the lungs and thorax includes all methods of examination: inspection, palpation, percussion,

A.

Posterior

Pigeon

Anterior

B.

Posterior

Funnel

Anterior

C.

Posterior

Barrel

Anterior

D.

E.

FIGURE 3-50 ◆ Chest deformities. (A) pigeon chest; (B) funnel chest; (C) barrel chest; (D) kyphosis; (E) scoliosis.

TABLE 3-6	NORMAL BREATH SOUNDS		
Type	**Description**	**Location**	**Characteristics**
Vesicular	Soft-intensity, low-pitched, "gentle sighing" sounds created by air moving through smaller airways (bronchioles and alveoli)	Over peripheral lung; best heard at base of lungs	Best heard on inspiration, which is about 2.5 times longer than the expiratory phase (5:2 ratio)
Bronchovesicular	Moderate-intensity and moderate-pitched "blowing" sounds created by air moving through larger airways (bronchi)	Between the scapulae and lateral to the sternum at the first and second intercostal spaces	Equal inspiratory and expiratory phases (1:1 ratio)
Bronchial (tubular)	High-pitched, loud, "harsh" sounds created by air moving through the trachea	Anteriorly over the trachea; not normally heard over lung tissue	Louder than vesicular sounds; have a short inspiratory phase and long expiratory phase (1:2 ratio)

From *Fundamentals of nursing: Concepts, process, and practice*, 6th ed., by B. Kozier, G. Erb, A. Berman, & K. Burke, 2000, Upper Saddle River, NJ: Prentice Hall Health.

and auscultation. Abnormal or **adventitious breath sounds** occur when air passes through narrowed airways or airways filled with fluid or mucus, or when pleural linings are inflamed. See Table 3-6 for normal breath sounds. Adventitious sounds are often superimposed over normal sounds (Table 3-7).

PLANNING

For efficiency, the nurse usually examines the posterior chest first, then the anterior chest. For posterior and lateral chest examinations, the client is uncovered to the waist and in a sitting position. A sitting or lying position may be used for anterior chest examination. The sitting position is preferred because it maximizes chest expansion.

Delegation

Due to the substantial knowledge and skill required, assessment of the thorax and lungs is not delegated to UAP. However, many aspects of breathing are observed during usual care and may be recorded by persons other than the nurse. Abnormal findings must be validated and interpreted by the nurse.

TABLE 3-7	ADVENTITIOUS BREATH SOUNDS		
Name	**Description**	**Cause**	**Location**
Crackles (rales)	Fine, short, interrupted crackling sounds; alveolar rales are high-pitched. Sound can be simulated by rolling a lock of hair near the ear. Best heard on inspiration but can be heard on both inspiration and expiration. May not be cleared by coughing.	Air passing through fluid or mucus in any air passage	Most commonly heard in the bases of the lower lung lobes
Gurgles (rhonchi)	Continuous, low-pitched, coarse, gurgling, harsh, louder sounds with a moaning or snoring quality. Best heard on expiration but can be heard on both inspiration and expiration. May be altered by coughing.	Air passing through narrowed air passages as a result of secretions, swelling, tumors	Loud sounds can be heard over most lung areas but predominate over the trachea and bronchi
Friction rub	Superficial grating or creaking sounds heard during inspiration and expiration. Not relieved by coughing.	Rubbing together of inflamed pleural surfaces	Heard most often in areas of greatest thoracic expansion (e.g., lower anterior and lateral chest)
Wheeze	Continuous, high-pitched, squeaky musical sounds. Best heard on expiration. Not usually altered by coughing.	Air passing through a constricted bronchus as a result of secretions, swelling, tumors	Heard over all lung fields

From *Fundamentals of nursing: Concepts, process, and practice*, 6th ed., by B. Kozier, G. Erb, A. Berman, & K. Burke, 2000, Upper Saddle River, NJ: Prentice Hall Health.

Equipment

- Stethoscope
- Skin marker/pencil
- Centimeter ruler

Performance

1. Explain to the client what you are going to do, why it is necessary, and how he or she can cooperate. Discuss how the results will be used in planning further care or treatments.

2. Wash hands and observe appropriate infection control procedures.

3. Provide for client privacy. In women, drape the anterior chest when it is not being examined.

4. Inquire if the client has any history of the following: family history of illness, including cancer, allergies, tuberculosis; lifestyle, including smoking and occupational hazards (e.g., inhaling fumes); any medications being taken; current problems (e.g., swellings, coughs, wheezing, pain).

ASSESSMENT	NORMAL FINDINGS	DEVIATIONS FROM NORMAL
Posterior Thorax		
5. Inspect the shape and symmetry of the thorax from posterior and lateral views. Compare the anteroposterior diameter to the transverse diameter.	Anteroposterior to transverse diameter in ratio of 1:2 Chest symmetric	Barrel chest; increased anteroposterior to transverse diameter Chest asymmetric
6. Inspect the spinal alignment for deformities. Have the client stand. From a lateral position, observe the three normal curvatures (cervical, thoracic, and lumbar).	Spine vertically aligned	Exaggerated spinal curvatures (kyphosis, lordosis); lateral deviation of spine (scoliosis)
7. Palpate the posterior thorax.		
• For clients who have no respiratory complaints, rapidly assess the temperature and integrity of all chest skin.	Skin intact; uniform temperature	Skin lesions; areas of hyperthermia
• For clients who do have respiratory complaints, palpate all chest areas for bulges, tenderness, or abnormal movements. Avoid deep palpation for painful areas, especially if a fractured rib is suspected. In such a case, deep palpation could lead to displacement of the bone fragment against the lungs.	Chest wall intact; no tenderness; no masses	Lumps, bulges; depressions; areas of tenderness; movable structures (e.g., rib)
8. Palpate the posterior chest for respiratory excursion (thoracic expansion). Place the palms of both your hands over the lower thorax with your thumbs adjacent to the spine and your fingers stretched laterally (Figure 3-51 ◆). Ask the client to take a deep breath while you observe the movement of your hands and any lag in movement.	Full and symmetric chest expansion (i.e., when the client takes a deep breath, your thumbs should move apart an equal distance and at the same time; normally the thumbs separate 3 to 5 cm [1.5 to 2 in] during deep inspiration)	Asymmetric and/or decreased chest expansion
9. Palpate the chest for vocal (tactile) fremitus, the faintly perceptible vibration felt through the chest wall when the client speaks.	Bilateral symmetry of vocal femitus Fremitus is heard most clearly at the apex of the lungs Low-pitched voices of males are more readily palpated than higher pitched voices of females	Decreased or absent fremitus (associated with pneumothorax) Increased fremitus (associated with consolidated lung tissue, as in pneumonia)
• Place the palmar surfaces of your fingertips or the ulnar aspect of your hand or closed fist on the posterior		

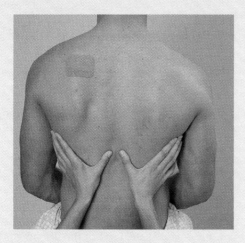

FIGURE 3-51 ◆ Position of the hands for measuring posterior respiratory excursion.

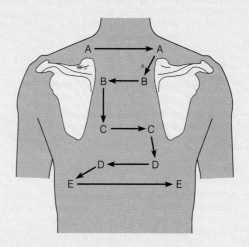

FIGURE 3-52 ◆ Areas and sequence for palpating tactile fremitus—posterior chest.

ASSESSMENT	NORMAL FINDINGS	DEVIATIONS FROM NORMAL
Posterior Thorax *continued*		
chest, starting near the apex of the lungs (Figure 3-52 ◆, position A). • Ask the client to repeat such words as "blue moon" or "one, two, three." • Repeat the two steps, moving your hands sequentially to the base of the lungs, through positions B–E in Figure 3-52. • Compare the fremitus on both lungs and between the apex and the base of each lung, using either one hand and moving it from one side of the client to the corresponding area on the other side *or* two hands that are placed simultaneously on the corresponding areas of each side of the chest.		
10. Percuss the thorax (see Box 3-18).	Percussion notes resonate, except over scapula Lowest point of resonance is at the diaphragm (i.e., at the level of the eighth to tenth rib posteriorly) *Note:* Percussion on a rib normally elicits dullness	Asymmetry in percussion Areas of dullness or flatness over lung tissue (associated with consolidation of lung tissue or a mass)
11. Percuss for diaphragmatic excursion (movement of the diaphragm during maximal inspiration and expiration) (see Box 3-18).	Excursion is 3 to 5 cm (1 to 2 in) bilaterally in females and 5 to 6 cm (2 to 3 in) in males Diaphragm is usually slightly higher on the right side	Restricted excursion (associated with lung disorder)
12. Auscultate the chest using the flat-disc diaphragm of the stethoscope (best for transmitting the high-pitched breath sounds). • Use the systematic zigzag procedure used in percussion (Figure 3-53 ◆) • Ask the client to take slow, deep breaths through the mouth. Listen at each point to the breath sounds during a complete inspiration and expiration. • Compare findings at each point with the corresponding point on the opposite side of the chest.	Vesicular and bronchovesicular breath sounds (see Table 3-6)	Adventitious breath sounds (e.g., crackles, rhonchi, wheeze, friction rub; see Table 3-7) Absence of breath sounds (associated with collapsed and surgically removed lung lobes

BOX 3-18 *Percussing the Thorax*

Percussing for Normal Thorax Sounds

Percussion of the thorax is performed to determine whether underlying lung tissue is filled with air or liquid, or solid material and to determine the positions and boundaries of certain organs. Because percussion penetrates to a depth of 5 to 7 cm (2 to 3 in), it detects superficial rather than deep lesions. Percussion sounds and tones are described in Table 3-3.

• Ask the client to bend the head and fold the arms forward across the chest. This separates the scapula and exposes more lung tissue to percussion.

• Percuss in the intercostal spaces at about 5-cm (2-in) intervals in a systematic sequence (Figure 3-53). Figure 3-54 ◆ shows normal percussion sounds in the posterior chest.

• Compare one side of the lung with the other.

• Percuss the lateral thorax every few inches, starting at the axilla and working down to the eighth rib.

Percussing for Diaphragmatic Excursion

• Ask the client to take a deep breath and hold it while you percuss downward along the scapular line until dullness is produced at the level of the diaphragm. Mark this point with a marking pencil, and repeat the procedure on the other side of the chest.

• Ask the client to take a few normal breaths and then expel the last breath completely and hold it while you percuss upward from the marked point to assess and mark the diaphragmatic excursion during deep expiration on each side.

• Measure the distance between the two marks.

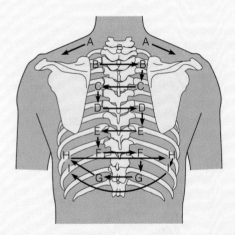

FIGURE 3-53 ◆ Sequence for posterior chest percussion.

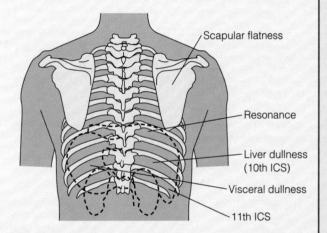

FIGURE 3-54 ◆ Normal percussion sounds on the posterior chest.

ASSESSMENT	NORMAL FINDINGS	DEVIATIONS FROM NORMAL
Anterior Thorax		
13. Inspect breathing patterns (e.g., respiratory rate and rhythm).	See Chapter 2, pages 31–32	See Chapter 2, Box 2-5, for abnormal breathing patterns and sounds
14. Inspect the costal angle (angle formed by the intersection of the costal margins) and the angle at which the ribs enter the spine.	Costal angle is less than 90 degrees, and the ribs insert into the spine at approximately a 45-degree angle (see Figure 3-47)	Costal angle is widened (associated with chronic obstructive pulmonary disease)
15. Palpate the anterior chest (see posterior chest palpation).		
16. Palpate the anterior chest for respiratory excursion. • Place the palms of both your hands on the lower thorax, with your fingers laterally along the lower rib cage	Full symmetric excursion; thumbs normally separate 3 to 5 cm (1.5 to 2 in)	Asymmetric and/or decreased respiratory excursion

Anterior Thorax *continued*

and your thumbs along the costal margins (Figure 3-55 ◆).
- Ask the client to take a deep breath while you observe the movement of your hands.

17. Palpate tactile fremitus in the same manner as for the posterior chest and using the sequence shown in Figure 3-56 ◆. If the breasts are large and cannot be retracted adequately for palpation, this part of the examination is usually omitted.	Same as posterior vocal fremitus. Fremitus is normally decreased over heart and breast tissue.	Same as posterior fremitus
18. Percuss the anterior chest systematically. • Begin above the clavicles in the supraclavicular space, and proceed downward to the diaphragm (Figure 3-57 ◆). • Compare one side of the lung to the other. • Displace female breasts for proper examination.	Percussion notes resonate down to the sixth rib at the level of the diaphragm but are flat over areas of heavy muscle and bone, dull on areas over the heart and the liver, and tympanic over the underlying stomach (Figure 3-58 ◆).	Asymmetry in percussion notes Areas of dullness or flatness over lung tissue
19. Auscultate the trachea.	Bronchial and tubular breath sounds (see Table 3-6)	Adventitious breath sounds (see Table 3-7)
20. Auscultate the anterior chest. Use the sequence used in percussion (see Figure 3-57), beginning over the bronchi between the sternum and the clavicles.	Bronchovesicular and vesicular breath sounds (see Table 3-6)	Adventitious breath sounds (see Table 3-7)

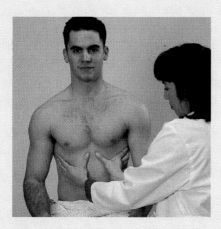

FIGURE 3-55 ◆ Position of the hands for measuring anterior respiratory excursion.

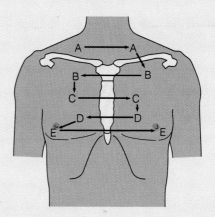

FIGURE 3-56 ◆ Areas and sequence for palpating tactile fremitus—anterior chest.

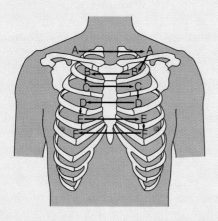

FIGURE 3-57 ◆ Sequence for anterior chest percussion.

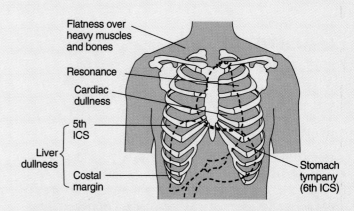

FIGURE 3-58 ◆ Normal percussion sounds on the anterior chest.

21. **Document** findings in the client record using forms or checklists supplemented by narrative notes when appropriate.

AGE-RELATED CONSIDERATIONS

Assessing the Thorax and Lungs

Infant

- The thorax is rounded; that is, the diameter from the front to the back (anteroposterior) is equal to the transverse diameter. It is also cylindrical, having a nearly equal diameter at the top and the base.
- To assess tactile fremitus, place the hand over the crying infant's chest.
- Auscultated sounds will be louder and harsher.
- Infants tend to breathe more abdominally than thoracically.

Child

- By 6 years of age, the anteroposterior diameter has decreased in proportion to the transverse one.
- Children tend to breathe more abdominally than thoracically up to age 6.

Elders

- The thoracic curvature may be accentuated (kyphosis) because of osteoporosis and changes in cartilage, resulting in collapse of the vertebrae.
- Kyphosis and osteoporosis alter the size of the chest cavity as the ribs move downward and forward.

- The anteroposterior diameter of the chest widens, giving the person a barrel-chested appearance. This is due to loss of skeletal muscle strength in the thorax and diaphragm and constant lung inflation from excessive expiratory pressure on the alveoli.
- Breathing rate and rhythm are unchanged at rest; the rate normally increases with exercise but may take longer to return to the preexercise rate.
- Inspiratory muscles become less powerful, and the inspiration reserve volume decreases. A decrease in depth of respiration is therefore apparent.
- Expiration may require the use of accessory muscles. The expiratory reserve volume significantly increases because of the increased amount of air remaining in the lungs at the end of a normal breath.
- Deflation of the lung is incomplete.
- Small airways lose their cartilaginous support and elastic recoil; as a result, they tend to close, particularly in basal or dependent portions of the lung.
- Elastic tissue of the alveoli loses its stretchability and changes to fibrous tissue. Exertional capacity decreases.
- Cilia in the airways decrease in number and are less effective in removing mucus; elderly clients are therefore at greater risk for pulmonary infections.

EVALUATION

Relate findings to previous assessment data if available. Report significant deviations from normal to the physician.

Cardiovascular and Peripheral Vascular Systems

Heart

Heart function can be assessed to a large degree by findings in the history, by symptoms such as shortness of breath, by the client's general appearance (e.g., cyanosis and edema of the legs suggest impaired func-

tion), and by pulse rate, rhythm, and quality. Direct examination of the heart, however, offers more specific information, including the heart sounds, the heart size, and such findings as **lifts, heaves,** or murmurs (more prolonged sounds during systole and diastole). Nurses assess heart functions through observations (inspection), palpation, and auscultation, in that sequence. Auscultation is more meaningful when other data are obtained first.

The nurse must determine the heart's exact location. In the average adult, most of the heart lies behind and to the left of the sternum. A small portion (the right atrium) extends to the right of the sternum. The upper portion of the heart (both atria), referred to as its base, lies toward the back. The lower portion (the ventricles), referred to as its apex, points forward. The apex of the left ventricle actually touches the anterior chest wall at or medial to the left midclavicular line

(MCL) and at or near the fifth left intercostal space (LICS), which is slightly below the left nipple (see Figure 2-17 on page 28). This point where the apex touches the anterior chest wall is known as the **point of maximal impulse (PMI).**

The precordium, the area of the chest overlying the heart, is inspected and palpated simultaneously for the presence of abnormal pulsations. Several heart sounds can be heard by auscultation. The first heart sound, S_1, occurs when the atrioventricular (AV) valves close. Although the right and left AV valves do not close simultaneously, the closures occur closely enough to be heard as one sound (S_1), a dull, low-pitched sound described as "lub." After this, the semilunar valves close, producing the second heart sound, S_2, described as "dub." S_2 has a higher pitch than S_1 and is also shorter. These two sounds, S_1 and S_2 ("lub-dub"), occur within 1 second or less, depending on the heart rate.

The two heart sounds are best heard over the aortic, pulmonic, tricuspid, and apical areas associated with the closure of the respective valves (Figure 3-59 ◆). Associated with these sounds are systole and diastole. Systole is the period in which the ventricles contract. It begins with the first heart sound and ends at the second heart sound. Systole is normally shorter than diastole. Diastole is the period in which the ventricles relax. It starts with the second sound and ends at the subsequent first sound. Normally, no sounds are audible during these periods (Figure 3-60 ◆). The experienced nurse, however, may perceive extra heart sounds (S_3 and S_4) during diastole. Both sounds are low in pitch and heard best at the apical site, with the bell of the stethoscope, and with the client lying on the left side. S_3 occurs early in diastole right after S_2 and sounds like "lub-dub-ee" (S_1, S_2, S_3) or "Kentuc-ky." It often disappears when the client sits up. S_3 is normal in children and young adults. In older adults, it may indicate heart failure. S_4 is rarely heard in healthy clients. It occurs near the very end of diastole just before S_1 and creates the sound of "*dee*-lub-dub"

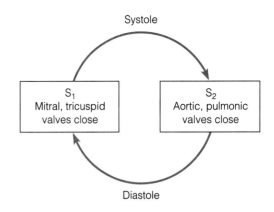

FIGURE 3-60 ◆ Relationship of heart sounds to systole/diastole.

(S_4, S_1, S_2) or "*Ten*-nessee." S_4 may be heard in many elderly clients and can be a sign of hypertension. Normal heart sounds are summarized in Table 3-8.

Central Vessels

The carotid arteries supply oxygenated blood to the head and neck (Figure 3-61 ◆). Because they are the only source of blood to the brain, prolonged occlusion of one of these arteries can result in serious brain damage. When cardiac output is diminished, the peripheral pulses may be difficult or impossible to feel, but the carotid pulse should be felt easily.

The carotid is auscultated for a bruit, and if a bruit is found, the carotid artery is then palpated for a thrill. A bruit (a blowing or swishing sound) is created by turbulence of blood flow due either to a narrowed arterial channel (common in older people) or to a condition, such as anemia or hyperthyroidism, which increases cardiac output. A thrill, which frequently accompanies

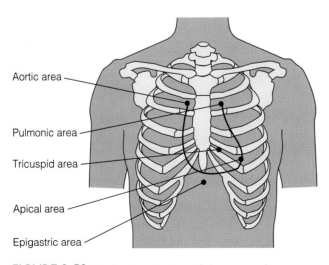

FIGURE 3-59 ◆ Anatomic sites of the precordium.

Aortic area
Pulmonic area
Tricuspid area
Apical area
Epigastric area

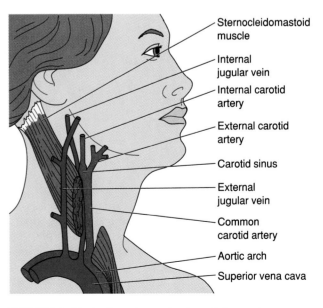

FIGURE 3-61 ◆ Arteries and veins of the neck.

Sternocleidomastoid muscle
Internal jugular vein
Internal carotid artery
External carotid artery
Carotid sinus
External jugular vein
Common carotid artery
Aortic arch
Superior vena cava

| TABLE 3-8 | NORMAL HEART SOUNDS | | | | |

Sound or Phase	Description	Aortic	Pulmonic	Tricuspid	Apical
		Area			
S_1	Dull, low-pitched, and longer than S_2; sounds like "lub"	Less intensity than S_2	Less intensity than S_2	Louder than or equal to S_2	Louder than or equal to S_2
Systole	Normally silent interval between S_1 and S_2				
S_2		Louder than S_1	Louder than S_1; abnormal if louder than the aortic S_2 in adults over 40 years of age	Less intensity than or equal to S_1	Less intensity than or equal to S_1
Diastole	Normally silent interval between S_2 and next S_1				

From *Fundamentals of nursing: Concepts, process, and practice*, 6th ed., by B. Kozier, G. Erb, A. Berman, & K. Burke, 2000, Upper Saddle River, NJ: Prentice Hall Health.

a bruit, is a vibrating sensation like the purring of a cat or water running through a hose. It, too, indicates turbulent blood flow due to arterial obstruction.

The jugular veins drain blood from the head and neck directly into the superior vena cava and right side of the heart (Figure 3-61). The external jugular veins are superficial and may be visible above the clavicle. The internal jugular veins lie deeper along the carotid artery and may transmit pulsations onto the skin of the neck. Normally, external neck veins are distended and visible when a person lies down; they are flat and not as visible when a person stands up, because gravity encourages venous drainage. Bilateral jugular vein distention (JVD) may indicate right-sided heart failure.

PLANNING

Heart examinations are usually performed while the client is in a semireclined position. The practitioner stands at the client's right side, where palpation of the cardiac area is facilitated and optimal inspection allowed.

Delegation

Due to the substantial knowledge and skill required, assessment of the heart and central vessels is not delegated to UAP. However, many aspects of cardiac function are observed during usual care and may be recorded by persons other than the nurse. Abnormal findings must be validated and interpreted by the nurse.

IMPLEMENTATION:
TECHNIQUE 3-12 ASSESSING THE HEART AND CENTRAL VESSELS

Equipment

- Stethoscope
- Centimeter ruler

Performance

1. Explain to the client what you are going to do, why it is necessary, and how he or she can cooperate. Discuss how the results will be used in planning further care or treatments.

2. Wash hands and observe appropriate infection control procedures.

3. Provide for client privacy.

4. Inquire if the client has any history of the following: family history of incidence and age of heart disease, high cholesterol levels, high blood pressure, stroke, obesity, congenital heart disease, arterial disease, hypertension, and rheumatic fever; client's past history of rheumatic fever, heart murmur, heart attack, varicosities, or heart failure; present symptoms indicative of heart disease (e.g., fatigue, dyspnea, orthopnea, edema, cough, chest pain, palpitations, syncope, hypertension, wheezing, hemoptysis); presence of diseases that affect the heart (e.g., obesity, diabetes, lung disease, endocrine disorders); lifestyle habits that are risk factors for cardiac disease (e.g., smoking, alcohol intake, eating and exercise patterns, areas and degree of stress perceived).

ASSESSMENT	NORMAL FINDINGS	DEVIATIONS FROM NORMAL
5. Simultaneously inspect and palpate the precordium for the presence of abnormal pulsations, lifts, or heaves. To locate the valve areas of the heart, see Box 3-19.		
• Inspect and palpate the aortic and pulmonic areas, observing them at an angle and to the side, to note the presence or absence of pulsations. Observing these areas at an angle increases the likelihood of seeing pulsations.		
• Inspect and palpate the tricuspid area for pulsations and heaves or lifts.	No pulsations No lift or heave	Pulsations Diffuse lift or heave, indicating enlarged or overactive right ventricle
• Inspect and palpate the apical area for pulsation, noting its specific location (it may be displaced laterally or lower) and diameter. If displaced laterally, record the distance between the apex and the MCL in centimeters.	Pulsations visible in 50 percent of adults and palpable in most PMI in fifth LICS at or medial to MCL Diameter of 1 to 2 cm ($\frac{1}{3}$ to $\frac{1}{2}$ in) No lift or heave	PMI displaced laterally or lower (indicates enlarged heart) Diameter over 2 cm (indicates enlarged heart or aneurysm) Diffuse lift or heave lateral to apex (indicates enlargement or overactivity of left ventricle)
• Inspect and palpate the epigastric area at the base of the sternum for abdominal aortic pulsations.	Aortic pulsations	Bounding abdominal pulsations (e.g., aortic aneurysm)
6. Auscultate the heart in all four anatomic sites: aortic, pulmonic, tricuspid, and apical (mitral). Auscultation need not be limited to these areas; however, the nurse may need to move the stethoscope to find the most audible sounds for each client. Box 3-20 describes the steps involved in auscultating the heart.	S_1: Usually heard at all sites Usually louder at apical area S_2: Usually heard at all sites Usually louder at base of heart Systole: Silent interval. Slightly shorter duration than diastole at normal heart rate (60 to 90 beats/min) Diastole: silent interval. Slightly longer duration than systole at normal heart rates S_3 in children and young adults S_4 in many older adults	Increased or decreased intensity Varying intensity with different beats Increased intensity at aortic area Increased intensity at pulmonic area Sharp-sounding ejection clicks S_3 in older adults S_4 may be a sign of hypertension

Carotid Arteries

ASSESSMENT	NORMAL FINDINGS	DEVIATIONS FROM NORMAL
7. Palpate the carotid artery, using extreme caution (see Box 3-21).	Symmetric pulse volumes Full pulsations, thrusting quality Quality remains same when client breathes, turns head, and changes from sitting to supine position Elastic arterial wall	Asymmetric volumes (possible stenosis or thrombosis) Decreased pulsations (may indicate impaired left cardiac output) Increased pulsations Thickening, hard, rigid, beaded, inelastic walls (indicate arteriosclerosis)

BOX 3-19 *Locating the Aortic, Pulmonic, Tricuspid, and Apical Areas of the Precordium*

• Locate the angle of Louis. It is felt as a prominence on the sternum.

• Move your fingertips down each side of the angle until you can feel the second intercostal spaces. The client's right second intercostal space is the *aortic area,* and the left second intercostal space is the *pulmonic area.*

• From the pulmonic area, move your fingertips down three left intercostal spaces along the side of the sternum. The left fifth intercostal space close to the sternum is the *tricuspid* or *right ventricular area.*

• From the tricuspid area, move your fingertips laterally 5 to 7 cm (2 to 3 in) to the left midclavicular line (LMCL). This is the *apical* or *mitral area, or PMI.* If you have difficulty locating the PMI, have the client roll onto the left side to move the apex closer to the chest wall.

Box 3-20 *Auscultating the Heart*

- Eliminate all sources of room noise. Heart sounds are of low intensity, and other noise hinders the nurse's ability to hear them.
- Keep the client in the supine position with head elevated 30 to 45 degrees.
- Use both the flat-disc diaphragm and the bell-shaped diaphragm to listen to all areas.
- In every area of auscultation, distinguish both S_1 and S_2 sounds.

- When auscultating, concentrate on one particular sound at a time in each area: the first heart sound, followed by systole, then the second heart sound, then diastole. Systole and diastole are normally silent intervals.
- Later, reexamine the heart while the client is in the upright sitting position. Certain sounds are more audible in certain positions.

ASSESSMENT	NORMAL FINDINGS	DEVIATIONS FROM NORMAL
Carotid Arteries *continued*		
8. Auscultate the carotid artery to determine the presence of a bruit (see Box 3-21).	No sound heard on auscultation	Presence of bruit in one or both arteries (suggests occlusive artery disease)
Jugular Veins		
9. Inspect the jugular veins for distention while the client is placed in a semi-Fowler's position (30- to 45-degree angle), with the head supported on a small pillow.	Veins not visible (indicating right side of heart is functioning normally)	Veins visibly distended (indicating advanced cardiopulmonary disease)
10. If jugular distention is present, assess the jugular venous pressure (JVP). • Locate the highest visible point of distention of the internal jugular vein. Although either the internal or the external jugular vein can be used, the internal jugular vein is more reliable. The external jugular vein is more easily affected by obstruction or kinking at the base of the neck. • Measure the vertical height of this point in centimeters from the sternal angle (the point at which the clavicles meet; Figure 3-62 ◆). • Repeat the steps above on the other side.		Bilateral measurements above 3 to 4 cm are considered elevated (may indicate right-sided heart failure) Unilateral distention (may be caused by local obstruction)

Box 3-21 *Palpating and Auscultating the Carotid Artery*

Palpation

- Palpate only one carotid artery at a time. This ensures adequate cerebral blood flow through the other and thus prevents possible ischemia. Ischemia is a deficiency of blood in a body part due to constriction or obstruction of a blood vessel.
- Avoid exerting too much pressure and massaging the area. Pressure can occlude the artery, and carotid sinus massage can precipitate bradycardia. The carotid sinus is a small dilation at the beginning of the internal carotid artery just above the bifurcation of the common carotid artery, in the upper third of the neck.
- Ask the client to turn the head slightly toward the side being examined. This makes the carotid artery more accessible.

Auscultation

- Turn the client's head slightly away from the side being examined. This facilitates the placement of the stethoscope.
- Auscultate the carotid artery on one side and then the other.
- Listen for the presence of a bruit.
- If you hear a bruit, gently palpate the artery to determine the presence of a thrill.

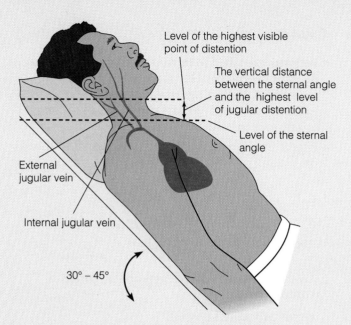

Level of the highest visible point of distention

The vertical distance between the sternal angle and the highest level of jugular distention

Level of the sternal angle

External jugular vein

Internal jugular vein

30° – 45°

FIGURE 3-62 ◆ Assessing the highest point of jugular venous distention.

11. **Document** findings in the client record using forms or checklists supplemented by narrative notes when appropriate.

Assessing the Heart and Central Vessels

Infant

- Physiological splitting of the second heart sound may be heard when the child takes a deep breath and the aortic valve closes a split second before the pulmonic valve. If splitting is heard during normal respirations, it is abnormal and may indicate an atrial-septal defect.

Child

- Heart sounds are louder because of the thinner chest wall.
- A third heart sound, best heard at the apex, is present in about one-third of all children.
- The PMI is higher and more medial in children under 8 years old.

Elders

- If no disease is present, heart size remains the same size throughout life.
- Cardiac output and strength of contraction decrease, thus lessening the older person's activity tolerance.
- The heart rate returns to its resting rate more slowly after exertion than it did when the individual was younger.
- S_4 heart sound is considered normal in older adults.
- Extrasystoles commonly occur. Ten or more extrasystoles per minute are considered abnormal.
- Sudden emotional and physical stresses may result in cardiac arrhythmias and heart failure.

EVALUATION

- Perform a detailed follow-up examination based on findings that deviated from expected or normal for the client. Relate findings to previous assessment data if available.
- Report significant deviations from normal to the physician.

Peripheral Vascular System

Assessment of the peripheral vascular system includes measurement of the blood pressure; palpation of peripheral pulses; inspection of the peripheral veins; and inspection of the skin and tissues to determine perfusion to the extremities. (Pulse sites and pulse assessments are described in Chapter 2. Figure 2-14 illustrates the sites for palpating the peripheral pulses.)

PLANNING

Delegation

Due to the substantial knowledge and skill required, assessment of the peripheral vascular system is not delegated to UAP. However, many aspects of the vascular system are observed during usual care and may be recorded by persons other than the nurse. Abnormal findings must be validated and interpreted by the nurse.

EVALUATION

- Perform a detailed follow-up examination of the heart or central vessels, integument, or other systems based on findings that deviated from expected or normal for the client. Relate findings to previous assessment data if available.

- Report significant deviations from normal to the physician.

IMPLEMENTATION:
TECHNIQUE 3-13 ASSESSING THE PERIPHERAL VASCULAR SYSTEM

Equipment

- None.

Performance

1. Explain to the client what you are going to do, why it is necessary, and how he or she can cooperate. Discuss how the results will be used in planning further care or treatments.

2. Wash hands and observe appropriate infection control procedures.

3. Provide for client privacy.

4 Inquire if the client has any history of the following: heart disorders, varicosities, arterial disease, and hypertension; lifestyle, specifically exercise patterns, activity patterns and tolerance, smoking habits, and use of alcohol.

ASSESSMENT	NORMAL FINDINGS	DEVIATIONS FROM NORMAL
Peripheral Pulses		
5. Palpate the peripheral pulses (except the carotid pulse) on both sides of the client's body individually, simultaneously, and systematically to determine the symmetry of pulse volume. If you have difficulty palpating some of the peripheral pulses, use a Doppler ultrasound probe.	Symmetric pulse volumes Full pulsations	Asymmetric volumes (indicate impaired circulation) Absence of pulsation (indicates arterial spasm or occlusion) Decreased, weak, thready pulsations (indicate impaired cardiac output) Increased pulse volume (may indicate hypertension, high cardiac output, or circulatory overload)
Peripheral Veins		
6. Inspect the peripheral veins in the arms and legs for the presence and/or appearance of superficial veins when limbs are dependent and when limbs are elevated.	In dependent position, distention and nodular bulges at calves are present When limbs are elevated, veins collapse (veins may appear tortuous or distended in older people)	Distended veins in the thigh and/or lower leg or on posterolateral part of calf from knee to ankle
7. Assess the peripheral leg veins for signs of phlebitis (see Box 3-22).	Limbs not tender Symmetric in size	Tenderness on palpation Pain in calf muscles with forceful dorsiflexion of the foot (positive Homans') Warmth and redness over vein Swelling of one calf or leg
Peripheral Perfusion		
8. Inspect the skin of the hands and feet for color, temperature, edema, and skin changes.	Skin color pink	Cyanotic (venous insufficiency) Pallor that increases with limb elevation Dusky red color when limb is lowered (arterial insufficiency) Brown pigmentation around ankles (arterial or chronic venous insufficiency)

ASSESSMENT	NORMAL FINDINGS	DEVIATIONS FROM NORMAL
Peripheral Perfusion *continued*		
8. *(continued)*	Skin temperature not excessively warm or cold No edema Skin texture resilient and moist	Skin cool (arterial insufficiency) Marked edema (venous insufficiency) Mild edema (arterial insufficiency) Skin thin and shiny or thick, waxy, shiny, and fragile, with reduced hair and ulceration (venous or arterial insufficiency)
9. Assess the adequacy of arterial flow if arterial insufficiency is suspected (see Box 3-23).	Buerger's test: Original color returns in 10 seconds; veins in feet or hands fill in about 15 seconds Capillary refill test: Immediate return of color	Delayed color return or mottled appearance; delayed venous filling; marked redness of arms or legs (indicates arterial insufficiency) Delayed return of color (arterial insufficiency)

10. **Document** findings in the client record using forms or checklists supplemented by narrative notes when appropriate.

AMBULATORY AND COMMUNITY SETTINGS

Assessing the Peripheral Vascular System

- Use the assessment as an opportunity to provide teaching regarding appropriate care of the extremities in those at high risk for or with actual vascular impairment. Educate clients and families regarding skin and nail care, exercise, and positioning to promote circulation.

AGE-RELATED CONSIDERATIONS

Assessing the Peripheral Vascular System

Infant

- Palpation of the pulses in the lower extremities (particularly the femoral pulses) is essential to screen for coarctation of the aorta.

Elders

- The overall effectiveness of blood vessels decreases as smooth muscle cells are replaced by connective tissue. The lower extremities are more likely to show signs of arterial and venous impairment because of the more distal and dependent position.
- Proximal arteries become thinner and dilate.
- Peripheral arteries become thicker and dilate less effectively because of arteriosclerotic changes in the vessel walls.

- Blood vessels lengthen and become more tortuous and prominent. Varicosities occur more frequently.
- In some instances, arteries may be palpated more easily because of the loss of supportive surrounding tissues. Often, however, the most distal pulses of the lower extremities are more difficult to palpate because of decreased arterial perfusion.
- Systolic and diastolic blood pressures increase, but the increase in the systolic pressure is greater. As a result, the pulse pressure widens. Any client with a blood pressure reading above 140/90 should be referred for follow-up assessments.
- Peripheral edema is frequently observed and is most commonly the result of chronic venous insufficiency or low protein levels in the blood (hypoproteinemia).

Breasts and Axillae

The breasts of men and women need to be inspected and palpated. Glandular tissue, a potential site for malignancy, is present throughout the breast in women and beneath the nipples in men. The largest portion of glandular breast tissue is in the upper outer quadrant of each breast, including the axillary tail of Spence (Figure 3-63 ◆). During assessment, the nurse can localize specific findings by using the division of the breast into quadrants and the axillary tail.

Clients need to be instructed to do monthly **breast self-examination (BSE)** and about breast health guidelines (see Box 3-24).

PLANNING

Delegation

Due to the substantial knowledge and skill required, assessment of the breasts and axillae is not delegated to UAP. However, persons other than the nurse may record aspects observed during usual care. Abnormal findings must be validated and interpreted by the nurse.

EVALUATION

- Perform a detailed follow-up examination based on findings that deviated from expected or normal for the client. Relate findings to previous assessment data if available.
- Report significant deviations from normal to the physician.

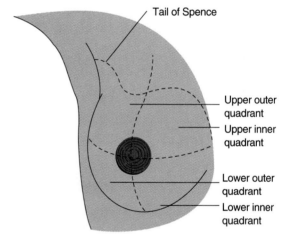

FIGURE 3-63 ◆ Four breast quadrants and tail of Spence.

Box 3-24 *Breast Health Guidelines*

Women Aged 20 to 39

- Monthly breast self-exam
- Clinical breast exam by a health professional every 3 years

Women Aged 40 and Older

- Monthly breast self-exam
- Clinical breast exam by a health professional every year
- Screening mammogram every year

Equipment

• Centimeter ruler

Performance

1. Explain to the client what you are going to do, why it is necessary, and how he or she can cooperate. Inquire whether the client has ever had a clinical breast exam. Discuss how the results will be used in planning further care or treatments.

2. Wash hands and observe appropriate infection control procedures.

3. Provide for client privacy.

4. Inquire if the client has any history of the following: breast self-examination; technique used and when performed in relation to the menstrual cycle; history of breast masses and what was done about them; any pain or tenderness in the breasts and relation to the woman's menstrual cycle; any discharge from the nipple; medication history (some medications, e.g., oral contraceptives, steroids, digitalis, and diuretics, may cause nipple discharge; estrogen replacement therapy may be associated with the development of cysts or cancer); risk factors that may be associated with development of breast cancer (e.g., mother, sister, aunt with breast cancer; alcohol consumption, high-fat diet, obesity, use of oral contraceptives, menarche before age 12, menopause after age 55, age 30 or above at first pregnancy).

ASSESSMENT	NORMAL FINDINGS	DEVIATIONS FROM NORMAL
5. Inspect the breasts for size, symmetry, and contour or shape while the client is in a sitting position.	Females: Rounded shape; slightly unequal in size; generally symmetric Males: Breasts even with the chest wall; if obese, may be similar in shape to female breasts	Recent change in breast size; swellings; marked asymmetry
6. Inspect the skin of the breast for localized discolorations or hyper-pigmentation, retraction or dimpling, localized hypervascular areas, swelling, or edema (Figure 3-64 ◆).	Skin uniform in color (same in appearance as skin of abdomen or back) Skin smooth and intact Diffuse symmetric horizontal or vertical vascular pattern in light-skinned people Striae (stretch marks); moles and nevi	Localized discolorations or hyper-pigmentation Retraction or dimpling (result of scar tissue or an invasive tumor) Unilateral, localized hypervascular areas (associated with increased blood flow) Swelling or edema appearing as pig skin or orange peel due to exaggeration of the pores
7. Emphasize any retraction by having the client: • Raise the arms above the head. • Push the hands together, with elbows flexed (Figure 3-65 ◆). • Press the hands down on the hips (Figure 3-66 ◆).		
8. Inspect the areola area for size, shape, symmetry, color, surface characteristics, and any masses or lesions.	Round or oval and bilaterally the same Color varies widely, from light pink to dark brown Irregular placement of sebaceous glands on the surface of the areola (Montgomery's tubercles)	Any asymmetry, mass, or lesion
9. Inspect the nipples for size, shape, position, color, discharge, and lesions.	Round, everted, and equal in size; similar in color; soft and smooth; both nipples point in same direction No discharge, except from pregnant or breast-feeding females Inversion of one or both nipples that is present from puberty	Asymmetrical size and color Presence of discharge, crusts, or cracks Recent inversion of one or both nipples

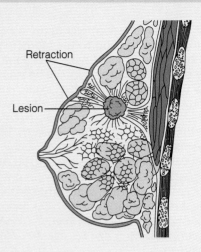

FIGURE 3-64 ◆ A lesion causing retraction of the skin.

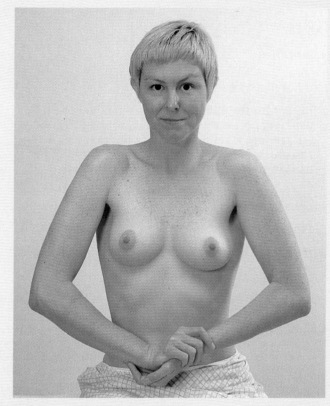

FIGURE 3-65 ◆ Pushing the hands together to accentuate retraction of breast tissues.

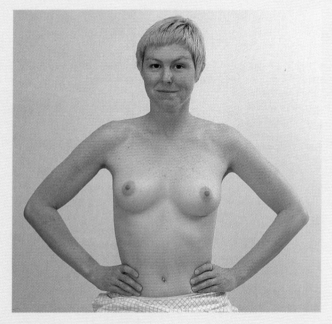

FIGURE 3-66 ◆ Pressing the hands down to accentuate retraction of breast tissues.

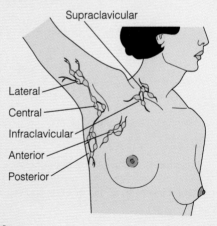

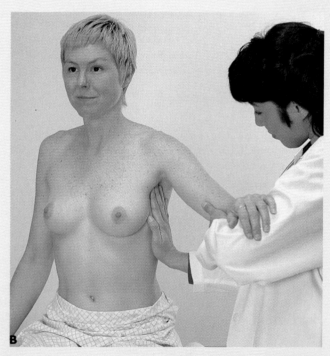

FIGURE 3-67 ◆ Location and palpation of the lymph nodes that drain the lateral breast. (A) lymph nodes; (B) palpating the axilla.

ASSESSMENT	NORMAL FINDINGS	DEVIATIONS FROM NORMAL
10. Palpate the axillary, subclavicular, and supraclavicular lymph nodes (Figure 3-67 ◆) while the client sits with the arms abducted and supported on the nurse's forearm. For palpation of clavicular lymph nodes, see page 86. Use the flat surfaces of all fingertips to palpate the four areas of the axilla: • The edge of the greater pectoral muscle (musculus pectoralis major) along the anterior axillary line • The thoracic wall in the midaxillary area • The upper part of the humerus • The anterior edge of the latissimus dorsi muscle along the posterior axillary line	No tenderness, masses, or nodules	Tenderness, masses, or nodules
11. Palpate the breast for masses, tenderness, and any discharge from the nipples. See Box 3-25 for palpation methods.	No tenderness, masses, nodules, or nipple discharge	Tenderness, masses, nodules, or nipple discharge
12. Palpate the areola and the nipples for masses. Compress each nipple to determine the presence of any discharge. If discharge is present, milk the breast along its radius to identify the discharge-producing lobe. Assess any discharge for amount, color, consistency, and odor. Note also any tenderness on palpation.	No tenderness, masses, nodules, or nipple discharge	Tenderness, masses, nodules, or nipple discharge

---

Box 3-25 *Palpating a Client's Breast*

Palpation of the breast is generally performed while the client is supine. In the supine position, the breasts flatten evenly against the chest wall, facilitating palpation. For clients who have a past history of breast masses, who are at high risk for breast cancer, or who have pendulous breasts, examination in both supine and sitting positions is recommended.

• If the client reports a breast lump, start with the "normal" breast to obtain baseline data that will serve as a comparison to the reportedly involved breast.

• To enhance flattening of the breast, instruct the client to abduct the arm and place her hand behind her head. Then place a small pillow or rolled towel under the client's shoulder.

• For palpation, use the palmar surface of the middle three fingertips (held together) and make a gentle rotary motion on the breast.

• Choose one of three patterns for palpation:
  a. Hands-of-the-clock or spokes-on-a-wheel (Figure 3-68 ◆)
  b. Concentric circles (Figure 3-69 ◆)
  c. Vertical strips pattern (Figure 3-70 ◆)

• Start at one point for palpation, and move systemati-

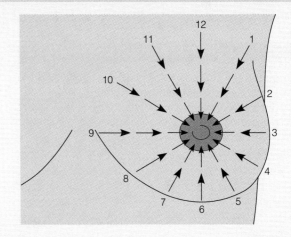

FIGURE 3-68 ◆ Hands-of-the-clock pattern of breast palpation.

cally to the end point to ensure that all breast surfaces are assessed.

• Pay particular attention to the upper outer quadrant area and the tail of Spence.

• If you detect a mass, record the following data:

Box 3-25 *Palpating a Client's Breast (continued)*

a. *Location:* The exact location relative to the quadrants and axillary tail, or the clock (as in Figure 3-68) and the distance from the nipple in centimeters.

b. *Size:* The length, width, and thickness of the mass in centimeters. If you are able to determine the discrete edges, record this fact.

c. *Shape:* Whether the mass is round, oval, lobulated, indistinct, or irregular.

d. *Consistency:* Whether the mass is hard or soft.

e. *Mobility:* Whether the mass is movable or fixed.

f. *Skin over the lump:* Whether it is reddened, dimpled, or retracted.

g. *Nipple:* Whether it is displaced or retracted.

h. *Tenderness:* Whether palpation is painful.

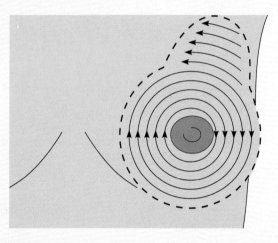

FIGURE 3-69 ◆ Concentric circles pattern of breast palpation.

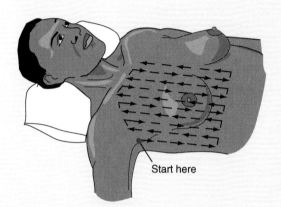

Start here

FIGURE 3-70 ◆ Vertical strips pattern of breast palpation.

Box 3-26 *Teaching Breast Self-Examination*

Inspection Before a Mirror

Look for any change in size or shape; lumps or thickenings; any rashes or other skin irritations; dimpled or puckered skin; any discharge or change in the nipples (e.g., position or asymmetry). Inspect the breasts in *all* of the following positions:

• Stand and face the mirror with your arm relaxed at your sides or hands resting on the hips; then turn to the right and the left for a side view (look for any flattening in the side view).

• Bend forward from the waist with arms raised over the head.

• Stand straight with the arms raised over the head and move the arms *slowly* up and down at the sides. (Look for free movement of the breasts over the chest wall.)

• Press your hands firmly together at chin level while the elbows are raised to shoulder level.

Palpation: Lying Position

• Place a pillow under your *right* shoulder and place the *right* hand behind your head. This position distributes breast tissue more evenly on the chest.

• Use the finger pads (tips) of the three middle fingers (held together) on your *left* hand to feel for lumps.

• Press the breast tissue against the chest wall firmly enough to know how your breast feels. A ridge of firm tissue in the lower curve of each breast is normal.

• Use small circular motions along one arrow in your chosen pattern (Figure 3-68, 3-69, or 3-70). Then move your fingers about 2 cm and feel along the next arrow. Repeat this action as many times as necessary until the entire breast is covered.

• Bring your arm down to your side and feel under your armpit, where breast tissue is also located.

• Repeat the exam on your *left* breast, using the finger pads of your *right* hand.

Palpation: Standing or Sitting

• Repeat the examination of both breasts while upright with one arm behind your head. This position makes it easier to check the area where a large percentage of breast cancers are found, the upper outer part of the breast and toward the armpit.

• *Optional:* Do the upright BSE in the shower. Soapy hands glide more easily over wet skin.

Report any changes to your health care provider promptly.

13. Teach the client the technique of breast self-examination (see Box 3-26).

 14. **Document** findings in the client record using forms or checklists supplemented by narrative notes when appropriate.

Assessing the Breasts and Axillae

Infant

- Newborns up to 2 weeks of age may have breast enlargement and white discharge from the nipples (witch's milk).

Child

- Female breast development begins between 10 and 13 years of age and occurs in five stages. One breast may develop more rapidly than the other (see Box 3-27).
- Boys may have some breast development in early adolescence.
- Gynecomastia, enlargement of breast tissue in males, can occur during puberty and may affect only one breast.

Pregnant Females

- Breast, areola, and nipple size increase.

- The areolae and nipples darken; nipples may become more erect; areolae contain small, scattered, elevated Montgomery's glands.
- Superficial veins become more prominent, and jagged, linear stretch marks may develop.
- A thick yellow fluid (colostrum) may be expressed from the nipples after the first trimester.

Elders

- In the postmenopausal female, breasts change in shape and often appear pendulous or flaccid; they lack the firmness they had in younger years.
- The presence of breast lesions may be detected more readily because of the decrease in connective tissue.
- General breast size remains the same. Although glandular tissue atrophies, the amount of fat in breasts (predominantly in the lower quadrants) increases in most women.

Box 3-27 *Five Stages of Breast Development**

- Stage 1: Elevation of the nipple
- Stage 2: Enlargement of the areola
- Stage 3: Enlargement of the breast
- Stage 4: Projection of the areola and nipple

- Stage 5: Recession of the areola by about age 14 or 15, leaving only the nipple projecting

* The 2-year transient breast growth that occurs in males reaches only the second stage.

Abdomen

The nurse locates and describes abdominal findings by using two common methods of subdividing the abdomen: quadrants and nine regions. To divide the abdomen into quadrants, the nurse imagines two lines: a vertical line from the xiphoid process to the pubic symphysis, and a horizontal line across the umbilicus (Figure 3-71 ◆). These quadrants are labeled (1) right upper quadrant, (2) left upper quadrant, (3) right lower quadrant, and (4) left lower quadrant. Using the second method, division into nine regions, the nurse imagines two vertical lines that extend superiorly from the midpoints of the inguinal ligaments, and two horizontal lines, one at the level of the edge of the lower ribs and the other at the level of the iliac crests (Figure 3-72 ◆). Specific organs or parts of

organs lie in each abdominal region. See Tables 3-9 and 3-10.

In addition, practitioners use landmarks to locate abdominal signs and symptoms. These are the xiphoid process of the sternum, the costal margins, the midline (a line drawn from the tip of the sternum through the umbilicus to the pubic symphysis), the anterosuperior iliac spine, the inguinal ligaments, and the superior margin of the pubic symphysis (Figure 3-73 ◆).

Assessment of the abdomen involves inspection, auscultation, palpation, and percussion. The nurse performs inspection first, followed by auscultation, palpation, and/or percussion. Auscultation is done before palpation and percussion because palpation and percussion cause movement or stimulation of the bowel, which can increase bowel motility and thus heighten bowel sounds, creating false results.

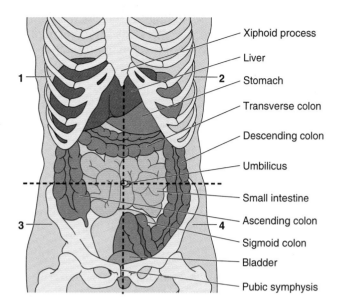

FIGURE 3-71 ◆ The four abdominal quadrants and underlying organs. (1) right upper quadrant; (2) left upper quadrant; (3) right lower quadrant; (4) left lower quadrant.

Labels for Figure 3-71:
- Xiphoid process
- Liver
- Stomach
- Transverse colon
- Descending colon
- Umbilicus
- Small intestine
- Ascending colon
- Sigmoid colon
- Bladder
- Pubic symphysis

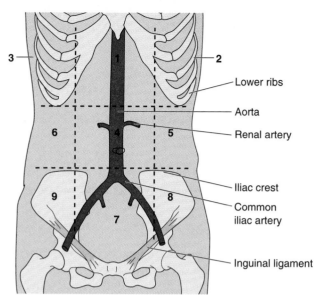

FIGURE 3-72 ◆ The nine abdominal regions. (1) epigastric; (2, 3) left and right hypochondriac; (4) umbilical; (5, 6) left and right lumbar; (7) suprapublic and hypogastric; (8, 9) left and right inguinal or iliac.

Labels for Figure 3-72:
- Lower ribs
- Aorta
- Renal artery
- Iliac crest
- Common iliac artery
- Inguinal ligament

PLANNING

Ask the client to urinate because an empty bladder makes the assessment more comfortable. Ensure that the room is warm since the client will be exposed.

TABLE 3-9	ORGANS IN THE FOUR ABDOMINAL REGIONS
Right Upper Quadrant	**Left Upper Quadrant**
Liver	Left lobe of liver
Gallbladder	Stomach
Duodenum	Spleen
Head of pancreas	Upper lobe of left kidney
Right adrenal gland	Pancreas
Upper lobe of right kidney	Left adrenal gland
Hepatic flexure of colon	Splenic flexure of colon
Section of ascending colon	Section of transverse colon
Section of transverse colon	Section of descending colon
Right Lower Quadrant	**Left Lower Quadrant**
Lower lobe of right kidney	Lower lobe of left kidney
Cecum	Sigmoid colon
Appendix	Section of descending colon
Section of ascending colon	Left ovary
Right ovary	Left fallopian tube
Right fallopian tube	Left ureter
Right ureter	Left spermatic cord
Right spermatic cord	Part of uterus
Part of uterus	

TABLE 3-10   ORGANS IN THE NINE ABDOMINAL REGIONS

Right Hypochondriac	Epigastric	Left Hypochondriac
Right lobe of liver	Aorta	Stomach
Gallbladder	Pyloric end of stomach	Spleen
Part of duodenum	Part of duodenum	Tail of pancreas
Hepatic flexure of colon	Pancreas	Splenic flexure of colon
Upper half of right kidney	Part of liver	Upper half of left kidney
Suprarenal gland		Suprarenal gland
Right Lumbar	**Umbilical**	**Left Lumbar**
Ascending colon	Omentum	Descending colon
Lower half of right kidney	Mesentery	Lower half of left kidney
Part of duodenum and jejunum	Lower part of duodenum	Part of jejunum and ileum
	Part of jejunum and ileum	
Right Inguinal	**Hypogastric (Pubic)**	**Left Inguinal**
Cecum	Ileum	Sigmoid colon
Appendix	Bladder	Left ureter
Lower end of ileum	Uterus	Left spermatic cord
Right ureter		Left ovary
Right spermatic cord		
Right ovary		

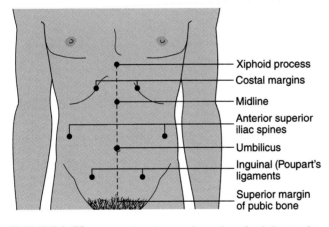

FIGURE 3-73 ◆ Landmarks used to identify abdominal areas.

Xiphoid process
Costal margins
Midline
Anterior superior iliac spines
Umbilicus
Inguinal (Poupart's ligaments
Superior margin of pubic bone

Delegation

Due to the substantial knowledge and skill required, assessment of the abdomen is not delegated to UAP. However, signs and symptoms of problems may be observed during usual care and should be recorded by those persons. Abnormal findings must be validated and interpreted by the nurse.

EVALUATION

- Perform a detailed follow-up examination of other systems based on findings that deviated from expected or normal for the client. Relate findings to previous assessment data if available.

- Report significant deviations from normal to the physician.

IMPLEMENTATION:
TECHNIQUE 3-15 ASSESSING THE ABDOMEN

Equipment

- Examining light
- Tape measure
- Water-soluble skin-marking pencil
- Stethoscope

Performance

1. Explain to the client what you are going to do, why it is necessary, and how he or she can cooperate. Discuss how the results will be used in planning further care or treatments.

2. Wash hands and observe appropriate infection control procedures.

3. Provide for client privacy.

4. Inquire if the client has any history of the following: Incidence of abdominal pain: its location, onset, sequence, and chronology; its quality (description); its frequency; associated symptoms (e.g., nausea, vomiting, diarrhea); bowel habits; incidence of constipation or diarrhea (have client describe what he or she means by these terms); change in appetite, food intolerances, and foods ingested in last 24 hours; specific signs and symptoms (e.g., heartburn, flatulence, and/or belching), difficulty swallowing, hematemesis (vomiting blood), blood or mucus in stools, and aggravating and alleviating factors; previous problems and treatment (e.g., stomach ulcer, gallbladder surgery, history of jaundice).

5. Assist the client to a supine position, with the arms placed comfortably at the sides. Place small pillows beneath the knees and the head to reduce tension in the abdominal muscles. Expose only the client's abdomen from chest line to the pubic area to avoid chilling and shivering, which can tense the abdominal muscles.

ASSESSMENT	NORMAL FINDINGS	DEVIATIONS FROM NORMAL
Inspection of the Abdomen		
6. Inspect the abdomen for skin integrity (refer to the discussion of skin assessment, earlier in this chapter).	Unblemished skin Uniform color Silver-white striae (stretch marks) or surgical scars	Presence of rash or other lesions Tense, glistening skin (may indicate ascites, edema) Purple striae (associated with Cushing's disease)
7. Inspect the abdomen for contour and symmetry		
• Observe the abdominal contour (profile line from the rib margin to the pubic bone) while standing at the client's side when the client is supine.	Flat, rounded (convex), or scaphoid (concave)	Distended
• Ask the client to take a deep breath and to hold it (*makes an enlarged liver or spleen more obvious*).	No evidence of enlargement of liver or spleen	Evidence of enlargement of liver or spleen
• Assess the symmetry of contour while standing at the foot of the bed. • If distention is present, measure the abdominal girth by placing a tape around the abdomen at the level of the umbilicus (Figure 3-74 ◆).	Symmetric contour	Asymmetric contour (e.g., localized protrusions around umbilicus, inguinal ligaments, or scars [possible hernia or tumor])
8. Observe abdominal movements associated with respiration, peristalsis, or aortic pulsations.	Symmetric movements caused by respiration Visible peristalsis in very lean people Aortic pulsations in thin persons at epigastric area	Limited movement due to pain or disease process Visible peristalsis in nonlean clients (with bowel obstruction) Marked aortic pulsations

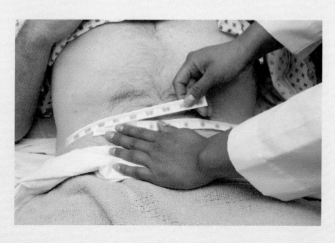

FIGURE 3-74 ◆ Measuring abdominal girth.

ASSESSMENT	NORMAL FINDINGS	DEVIATIONS FROM NORMAL

Inspection of the Abdomen *continued*

9. Observe the vascular pattern.

No visible vascular pattern

Visible venous pattern (dilated veins) is associated with liver disease, ascites, and venocaval obstruction

Auscultation of the Abdomen

10. Auscultate the abdomen for bowel sounds, vascular sounds, and peritoneal friction rubs. The auscultation procedure is shown in Box 3-28.

Audible bowel sounds
Absence of arterial bruits
Absence of friction rub

Absent, hypoactive, or hyperactive bowel sounds
Loud bruit over aortic area (possible aneurysm)
Bruit over renal or iliac arteries

Box 3-28 *Auscultating the Abdomen*

Warm the hands and the stethoscope diaphragms. Cold hands and a cold stethoscope may cause the client to contract the abdominal muscles, and these contractions may be heard during auscultation.

For Bowel Sounds

- Use the flat-disc diaphragm. Intestinal sounds are relatively high pitched and best accentuated by the flat-disc diaphragm. Light pressure with the stethoscope is adequate.

- Ask when the client last ate. Shortly after or long after eating, bowel sounds may normally increase. They are loudest when a meal is long overdue. Four to 7 hours after a meal, bowel sounds may be heard continuously over the ileocecal valve area while the digestive contents from the small intestine empty through the valve into the large intestine.

- Place the flat-disc diaphragm of the stethoscope in each of the four quadrants of the abdomen over all the auscultatory sites (Figure 3-75 ◆).

- Listen for active bowel sounds—irregular gurgling noises occurring about every 5 to 20 seconds. The duration of a single sound may range from less than a second to more than several seconds.

- Normal bowel sounds are described as audible. Alterations in sounds are described as absent, hypoactive (i.e., extremely soft and infrequent [e.g., one per minute]), or hyperactive/increased (i.e., high-pitched, loud, rushing sounds that occur frequently [e.g., every 3 seconds]) also known as borborygmi. True absence of sounds (none heard in 3 to 5 minutes) indicates a

cessation of intestinal motility. Hypoactive sounds indicate decreased motility and are usually associated with manipulation of the bowel during surgery, inflammation, paralytic ileus, or late bowel obstruction. Hyperactive sounds indicate increased intestinal motility and are usually associated with diarrhea, an early bowel obstruction, or the use of laxatives.

For Vascular Sounds

- Use the bell of the stethoscope over the aorta, renal arteries, iliac arteries, and femoral arteries (Figure 3-76 ◆).

- Listen for bruits (blowing sound due to restricted blood flow through narrowed vessels).

Peritoneal Friction Rubs

Peritoneal friction rubs are rough, grating sounds like two pieces of leather rubbing together. Friction rubs may be caused by inflammation, infection, or abnormal growths.

- To auscultate the splenic site, place the stethoscope over the left lower rib cage in the anterior axillary line, and ask the client to take a deep breath. A deep breath may accentuate the sound of a friction rub area.

- To auscultate the liver site, place the stethoscope over the lower right rib cage.

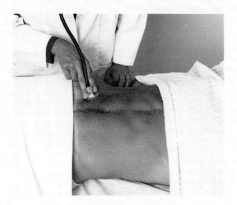

FIGURE 3-75 ◆ Auscultating the abdomen for bowel sounds.

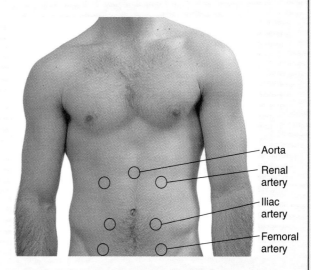

Aorta
Renal artery
Iliac artery
Femoral artery

FIGURE 3-76 ◆ Sites for auscultating the abdomen.

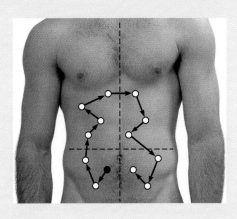

FIGURE 3-77 ◆ Systematic percussion sites for all four abdominal quadrants.

ASSESSMENT	NORMAL FINDINGS	DEVIATIONS FROM NORMAL
Percussion of the Abdomen		
11. Percuss several areas in each of the four quadrants to determine presence of tympany (gas in stomach and intestines) and dullness (decrease, absence, or flatness of resonance over solid masses or fluid). Use a systematic pattern: Begin in the lower right quadrant, proceed to the upper right quadrant, the upper left quadrant, and the lower left quadrant (Figure 3-77 ◆).	Tympany over the stomach and gas-filled bowels; dullness, especially over the liver and spleen, or a full bladder	Large dull areas (associated with presence of fluid or a tumor)
Percussion of the Liver		
12. Percuss the liver to determine its size (see Box 3-29).	6 to 12 cm (2.5 to 3.5 in) in the midclavicular line; 4 to 8 cm (1.5 to 3 in) at the midsternal line	Enlarged size (associated with liver disease)

Box 3-29 *Percussing the Liver*

Percussion to determine liver size begins in the right midclavicular line below the level of the umbilicus and proceeds as follows:

1. Percuss upward over tympanic areas until a dull percussion sound indicates the lower liver border. Mark the site with a skin-marking pencil (see Figure 3-78 ◆).

2. Then percuss downward at the right midclavicular line, beginning from an area of lung resonance and progressing downward until a dull percussion sound indicates the upper liver border (usually at the fifth to seventh interspace). Mark this site.

3. Measure the distance between the two marks (upper and lower liver borders) in centimeters to establish the liver span or size.

4. Repeat steps 1 to 3 at the midsternal line.

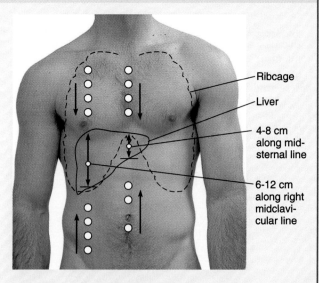

Ribcage

Liver

4-8 cm along midsternal line

6-12 cm along right midclavicular line

FIGURE 3-78 ◆ Percussion pattern to determine liver size.

Palpation of the Abdomen

13. Perform light palpation first to detect areas of tenderness and/or muscle guarding. Systematically explore all four quadrants. See Box 3-30 for palpation technique.	No tenderness; relaxed abdomen with smooth, consistent tension	Tenderness and hypersensitivity Superficial masses Localized areas of increased tension
14. Perform deep palpation over all four quadrants (see Box 3-30).	Tenderness may be present near xiphoid process, over cecum, and over sigmoid colon	Generalized or localized areas of tenderness Mobile or fixed masses

---

BOX 3-30 *Palpating the Abdomen*

Palpation is used to detect tenderness, the presence of masses or distention, and the outline and position of abdominal organs (e.g., the liver, spleen, and kidneys). Before palpation, (1) ensure that the client's position is appropriate for relaxation of the abdominal muscles, and (2) warm the hands. Cold hands can elicit muscle tension and thus impede palpatory evaluation.

Light Palpation

• Hold the palm of your hand slightly above the client's abdomen, with your fingers parallel to the abdomen.

• Depress the abdominal wall lightly, about 1 cm or to the depth of the subcutaneous tissue, with the pads of your fingers (Figure 3-79 ◆).

• Move the finger pads in a slight circular motion.

• Note areas of tenderness or superficial pain, masses, and muscle guarding. To determine areas of tenderness, ask the client to tell you about them and watch for changes in the client's facial expressions.

• If the client is excessively ticklish, begin by pressing your hand on top of the client's hand while pressing lightly. Then slide your hand off the client's and onto the abdomen to continue the examination.

Deep Palpation

• Palpate sensitive areas last.

• Press the distal half of the palmar surface of the fingers of one hand into the abdominal wall.
or
Use the bimanual method of palpation discussed earlier in this chapter on page 49.

• Depress the abdominal wall about 4 to 5 cm (1.5 to 2 in) (Figure 3-80 ◆).

• Note masses and the structure of underlying contents. If a mass is present, determine its size, location, mobility, contour, consistency, and tenderness. Normal abdominal structures that may be mistaken for masses include the lateral borders of the rectus abdominis muscles, the feces-filled colon, the aorta, and the uterus.

• Check for rebound tenderness in areas where the client complains of pain. With one hand, press slowly and deeply over the area indicated and then lift the hand quickly. If the client does not complain of pain during the deep pressure but indicates pain at the release of the pressure, rebound tenderness is present. This can indicate peritoneal inflammation and should be reported to the physician immediately.

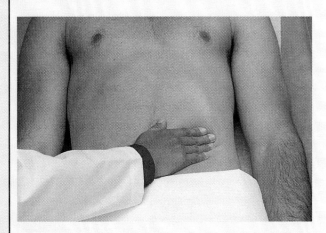

FIGURE 3-79 ◆ Light palpation of the abdomen.

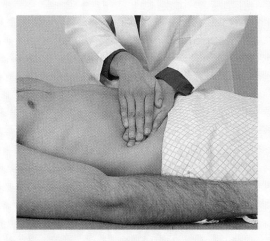

FIGURE 3-80 ◆ Deep palpation of the abdomen.

BOX 3-31 *Palpating the Liver*

Two bimanual approaches are used in palpation of the liver. In using the first method, place one hand along the anterior rib cage and the other hand on the posterior rib cage.

- Stand on the client's right side.

- Place your left hand on the posterior thorax at about the 11th or 12th rib. This hand is used to push upward and provide support of underlying structures for the subsequent anterior palpation.

- Place your right hand along the rib cage at about a 45-degree angle to the right of the rectus abdominis muscle or parallel to the rectus muscle with the fingers pointing toward the rib cage (Figure 3-81 ◆).

- While the client exhales, exert a gradual and gentle downward and forward pressure beneath the costal margin until you reach a depth of 4 to 5 cm (1.5 to 2 in). During expiration, the abdominal wall relaxes, facilitating deep palpation.

- Maintain your hand position, and ask the client to inhale deeply. This makes the liver border descend and moves the liver into a palpable position.

- While the client inhales, feel the liver border move against your hand. It should feel firm and have a regular contour. If you do not palpate the liver initially, ask the client to take two or three more deep breaths while you maintain or apply slightly more palpation

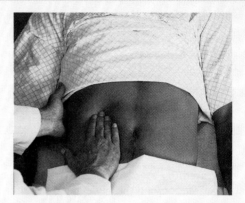

FIGURE 3-81 ◆ Palpating the liver.

pressure. Livers are harder to palpate in obese, tense, or very physically fit people.

- If the liver is enlarged (i.e., palpable below the costal margin), measure the number of centimeters it extends below the costal region.

A second method is the bimanual palpation method discussed on page 49, in which one hand is superimposed on the other (see Figure 3-2). The techniques and principles used for palpating the liver with one hand apply to the two-hand method as well.

ASSESSMENT	NORMAL FINDINGS	DEVIATIONS FROM NORMAL
Palpation of the Liver		
15. Palpate the liver to detect enlargement and tenderness. See palpation methods in Box 3-31.	May not be palpable Border feels smooth	Enlarged (abnormal finding, even if liver is smooth and not tender) Smooth but tender; nodular or hard
Palpation of the Bladder		
16. Palpate the area above the pubic symphysis if the client's history indicates possible urinary retention (Figure 3-82 ◆).	Not palpable	Distended and palpable as smooth, round, tense mass (indicates urinary retention)

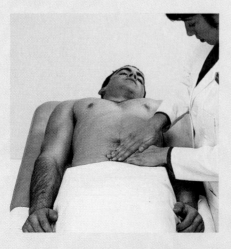

FIGURE 3-82 ◆ Palpating the bladder.

17. **Document** findings in the client record using forms or checklists supplemented by narrative notes when appropriate.

Assessing the Abdomen

- Examining the client in a clinic setting requires special attention to positioning on the examination table. Be sure safety measures are in place.
- Be sure you have the required equipment on a home visit, including a tape measure and skin-marking pen.

- Examining the client in the home may be facilitated since the setting is familiar. Use pillows to position the client.
- A complete abdominal examination may not be necessary. Focus the assessment on areas indicated by the history and present complaint.

Assessing the Abdomen

Infant

- The abdomen of the newborn and infant is round.

Child

- Toddlers have a characteristic "pot belly" appearance, which persists until about the fifth year.
- Peristaltic waves are usually more visible than in adults.
- Children may not be able to pinpoint areas of tenderness; by observing facial expressions, the examiner can determine areas of maximum tenderness.
- The liver is relatively larger than in adults. It can be palpated 1 to 2 cm below the right costal margin.
- If the child is ticklish, guarding, or fearful, use a task that requires concentration (such as squeezing the hands together) to distract the child's attention.

Elders

- The rounded abdomens of older persons are due to an increase in adipose tissue and a decrease in muscle tone.
- The abdominal wall is slacker and thinner, making palpation easier and more accurate than in younger clients. Muscle wasting and loss of fibroconnective tissue occur.
- The pain threshold in the elderly is often higher; major abdominal problems such as appendicitis or other acute emergencies may therefore go undetected.

- Gastrointestinal pain needs to be differentiated from cardiac pain. Gastrointestinal pain may be located in the chest or abdomen, whereas cardiac pain is usually located in the chest. Factors aggravating gastrointestinal pain are usually related to either ingestion or lack of food intake; gastrointestinal pain is usually relieved by antacids, food, or assuming an upright position. Common factors that can aggravate cardiac pain are activity or anxiety; rest or nitroglycerin relieves cardiac pain.
- Stool passes through the intestines at a slower rate in elderly clients, and the perception of stimuli that produce the urge to defecate often diminishes.
- Fecal incontinence may occur in confused or neurologically impaired older adults.
- Many older persons erroneously believe that the absence of a daily bowel movement signifies constipation. When assessing for constipation, the nurse must consider the client's diet, activity, medications, and characteristics and ease of passage of feces as well as the frequency of bowel movements.
- The incidence of colon cancer is higher among older adults than younger adults. Symptoms include a change in bowel function, rectal bleeding, and weight loss. Changes in bowel function, however, are associated with many factors, such as diet, exercise, and medications.
- Decreased absorption of oral medications often occurs with aging.
- In the liver, impaired metabolism of some drugs may occur with aging.

Musculoskeletal System

The musculoskeletal system encompasses the muscles, bones, and joints. The nurse assesses the musculoskeletal system for muscle strength, tone, size and symmetry of muscle development, and fasciculations and tremors. A **fasciculation** is an abnormal contraction of a bundle of muscle fibers that appears as a twitch. A **tremor** is an involuntary trembling of a limb or body part. An *intention tremor* becomes more apparent when an individual attempts a voluntary movement (e.g., holding a cup of coffee). A *resting tremor* is more apparent when the client is at rest and diminishes with activity.

Bones are assessed for normalcy of form. Joints are assessed for tenderness, swelling, thickening, crepitation (a crackling, grating sound), and range of motion. Body posture is assessed for normalcy in standing and sitting positions.

PLANNING

Delegation

Due to the substantial knowledge and skill required, assessment of the musculoskeletal system is not delegated to UAP. However, many aspects of its functioning are observed during usual care and may be recorded by persons other than the nurse. Abnormal findings must be validated and interpreted by the nurse.

EVALUATION

- Perform a detailed follow-up examination of other systems based on findings that deviated from expected or normal for the client. Relate findings to previous assessment data if available.

- Report significant deviations from normal to the physician.

IMPLEMENTATION:
TECHNIQUE 3-16 ASSESSING THE MUSCULOSKELETAL SYSTEM

Equipment

- Goniometer

Performance

1. Explain to the client what you are going to do, why it is necessary, and how he or she can cooperate. Discuss how the results will be used in planning further care or treatments.

2. Wash hands and observe appropriate infection control procedures.

3. Provide for client privacy.

4. Inquire if the client has any of the following: history or presence of muscle pain: onset, location, character, associated phenomena (e.g., redness and swelling of joints), and aggravating and alleviating factors; any limitations to movement or inability to perform activities of daily living; previous sports injuries; any loss of function without pain.

ASSESSMENT	NORMAL FINDINGS	DEVIATIONS FROM NORMAL
Muscles		
5. Inspect the muscles for size. Compare the muscles on one side of the body (e.g., of the arm, thigh, and calf) to the same muscle on the other side. For any discrepancies, measure the muscles with a tape.	Equal size on both sides of body	Atrophy (a decrease in size) or hypertrophy (an increase in size)
6. Inspect the muscles and tendons for contractures (shortening).	No contractures	Malposition of body part, for example, foot drop (foot flexed downward)
7. Inspect the muscles for fasciculations and tremors. Inspect any tremors of the hands and arms by having the client hold the arms out in front of the body.	No fasciculation or tremors	Presence of fasciculation or tremor
8. Palpate muscles at rest to determine muscle tonicity (the normal condition of tension, or tone, of a muscle at rest).	Normally firm	Atonic (lacking tone)
9. Palpate muscles while the client is active and passive for flaccidity, spasticity, and smoothness of movement.	Smooth coordinated movements	Flaccidity (weakness or laxness) or spasticity (sudden involuntary muscle contraction)
10. Test muscle strength (see tests in Box 3-32). Compare the right side with left side.	Equal strength on each body side	25 percent or less of normal strength

Box 3-32 *Testing and Grading Muscle Strength*

Muscle/Activity

Sternocleidomastoid: Client turns the head to one side against the resistance of your hand. Repeat with the other side.

Trapezius: Client shrugs the shoulders against the resistance of your hands.

Deltoid: Client holds arm up and resists while you try to push it down.

Biceps: Client fully extends each arm and tries to flex it while you attempt to hold arm in extension.

Triceps: Client flexes each arm and then tries to extend it against your attempt to keep arm in flexion.

Wrist and finger muscles: Client spreads the fingers and resists as you attempt to push the fingers together.

Grip strength: Client grasps your index and middle fingers while the you try to pull the fingers out.

Hip muscles: Client is supine, both legs extended; client raises one leg at a time while you attempt to hold it down.

Hip abduction: Client is supine, both legs extended. Place your hands on the lateral surface of each knee; client spreads the legs apart against your resistance.

Hip adduction: Client is in same position as for hip abduction. Place your hands between the knees; client brings the legs together against your resistance.

Hamstrings: Client is supine, both knees bent. Client resists while you attempt to straighten the legs.

Quadriceps: Client is supine, knee partially extended; client resists while you attempt to flex the knee.

Muscles of the ankles and feet: Client resists while you attempt to dorsiflex the foot and again resists while you attempt to flex the foot.

Grading Muscle Strength

0: 0% of normal strength; complete paralysis.

1: 10% of normal strength; no movement, contraction of muscle is palpable or visible.

2: 25% of normal strength; full muscle movement against gravity, with support.

3: 50% of normal strength; normal movement against gravity.

4: 75% of normal strength; normal full movement against gravity and against minimal resistance.

5: 100% of normal strength; normal full movement against gravity and against full resistance.

ASSESSMENT	NORMAL FINDINGS	DEVIATIONS FROM NORMAL
Bones		
11. Inspect the skeleton for normal structure and deformities.	No deformities	Bones misaligned
12. Palpate the bones to locate any areas of edema or tenderness.	No tenderness or swelling	Presence of tenderness or swelling (may indicate fracture, neoplasms, or osteoporosis)
Joints		
13. Inspect the joint for swelling Palpate each joint for tenderness, smoothness of movement, swelling, crepitation, and presence of nodules.	No swelling No tenderness, swelling, crepitation, or nodules Joints move smoothly	One or more swollen joints Presence of tenderness, swelling, crepitation, or nodules
14. Assess joint range of motion. See Chapter 8 for the types of joint movements. • Ask the client to move selected body parts. The amount of joint movement can be measured by a **goniometer,** a device that measures the angle of the joint in degrees (Figure 3-83 ◆).	Varies to some degree in accordance with person's genetic makeup and degree of physical activity	Limited range of motion in one or more joints

 15. **Document** findings in the client record using forms or checklists supplemented by narrative notes when appropriate.

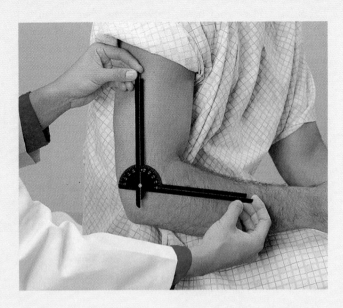

FIGURE 3-83 ◆ A goniometer used to measure joint angle.

AMBULATORY AND COMMUNITY SETTINGS

Assessing the Musculoskeletal System

- When making a home visit, observe the client in natural movement around the living area. To assess children, have them remove their clothes down to the underwear.

- A complete examination of joints, bone, and muscles may not be necessary. Focus the assessment on areas indicated by the history and present complaint.

AGE-RELATED CONSIDERATIONS

Assessing the Musculoskeletal System

Infant

- Palpate the clavicles of newborns. A mass and crepitus may indicate a fracture experienced during vaginal delivery.

- Newborns naturally return their arms and legs to the fetal position when extended and released.

- Check muscle strength by holding the infant lightly under the arms. The infant should not fall through the hands if normal muscle strength is present.

- Check infants for developmental dysplasia of the hip (congenital dislocation) by examining for asymmetric gluteal folds, asymmetric abduction of the legs, or apparent shortening of the femur.

Child

- Should be able to sit without support by 8 months of age.

- Pronation of the feet is common in children between 12 and 30 months of age.

- Genu varum (bowleg) is normal in children for 1 year after beginning to walk.

- Lordosis (swayback) is common in children before age 5.

- Observe the child in normal activities to determine motor function.

Elders

- Muscle mass decreases progressively with age, but there are wide variations among different individuals.

- The decrease in speed, strength, resistance to fatigue, reaction time, and coordination in the older person is due to a decrease in nerve conduction and muscle tone.

- The bones become more fragile and osteoporosis leads to a loss of total bone mass. As a result, elderly people are predisposed to fractures and compressed vertebrae.

- In most elderly people, osteoarthritic changes in the joints can be observed.

Neurologic System

Examination of the neurologic system includes assessment of (1) mental status, (2) level of consciousness, (3) the cranial nerves, (4) reflexes, (5) motor function, and (6) sensory function. A thorough neurologic examination may take 1 to 3 hours; however, routine screening tests are usually done first. If the results of these tests are questionable, more extensive evaluations are made. Three major considerations determine the extent of a neurologic exam: (1) the client's chief complaints; (2) the client's physical condition (i.e., level of consciousness and ability to ambulate), because many parts of the exam require movement and coordination of the extremities; and (3) the client's willingness to participate and cooperate.

PLANNING

If possible, determine whether a screening or full neurological examination is indicated. This will affect preparation of the client, equipment, and timing.

Delegation

Due to the substantial knowledge and skill required, assessment of the neurologic system is not delegated to UAP. However, many aspects of neurologic behavior are observed during usual care and may be recorded by persons other than the nurse. Abnormal findings must be validated and interpreted by the nurse.

IMPLEMENTATION:
TECHNIQUE 3-17 ASSESSING MENTAL STATUS

Equipment (depending on type of examination)

- Percussion hammer
- Tongue depressors (one broken diagonally for testing pain sensation)
- Wisps of cotton to assess light touch sensation
- Test tubes of hot and cold water for skin temperature assessment (optional)

Performance

1. Explain to the client what you are going to do, why it is necessary, and how he or she can cooperate. Discuss how the results will be used in planning further care or treatments.

2. Wash hands and observe appropriate infection control procedures.

3. Provide for client privacy.

4. Inquire if the client has any history of the following: presence of pain in the head, back, or extremities, as well as onset and aggravating and alleviating factors; disorientation to time, place, or person: speech disorder; any history of loss of consciousness, fainting, convulsions, trauma, tingling or numbness, tremors or tics, limping, paralysis, uncontrolled muscle movements, loss of memory, mood swings, or problems with smell, vision, taste, touch, or hearing.

    Assessment of mental status reveals the client's general cerebral function. These functions include intellectual (cognitive) as well as emotional (affective) functions.

    If problems with use of language, memory, concentration, thought processes, or attention span

and memory are noted during the nursing history, a more extensive examination is required during neurologic assessment. Major areas of mental status assessment include language, orientation, memory, and attention span and calculation.

Language

5. Any defects in or loss of the power to express oneself by speech, writing, or signs or to comprehend spoken or written language due to disease or injury of the cerebral cortex is called aphasia.

    If the client displays difficulty speaking,

6. Point to common objects, and ask the client to name them.

7. Ask the client to read some words and to match the printed and written words with pictures.

8. Ask the client to respond to simple verbal and written commands (e.g., "point to your toes" or "raise your left arm").

Orientation

9. Determine the client's orientation to *time, place* and *person* by tactful questioning. Ask the client the city and state or residence, time of day, date, day of the week, duration of illness, and names of family members. More direct questioning may be necessary for some people (e.g., "Where are you now?" "What day is it today?"). Most people readily accept these questions if initially the nurse asks, "Do you get confused at times?"

Memory

10. Listen for lapses in memory. Ask the client about difficulty with memory. If problems are apparent,

three categories of memory are tested: immediate recall, recent memory, and remote memory.

To assess immediate recall:

- Ask the client to repeat a series of three digits (e.g., 7-4-3), spoken slowly.

- Gradually increase the number of digits (e.g., 7-4-3-5, 7-4-3-5-6, and 7-4-3-5-6-7-2), until the client fails to repeat the series correctly.

- Start again with a series of three digits, but this time ask the client to repeat them backward. The average person can repeat a series of five to eight digits in sequence and four to six digits in reverse order.

To assess recent memory:

- Ask the client to recall the recent events of the day, such as how the client got to the clinic. This information must be validated, however.

- Ask the client to recall information given early in the interview (e.g., the name of a doctor).

- Provide the client with three facts to recall (e.g., a color, an object, an address, or a three-digit number), and ask the client to repeat all three. Later in the interview, ask the client to recall all three items.

  To assess remote memory, ask the client to describe a previous illness or surgery (e.g., 5 years ago), or a birthday or anniversary.

Attention Span and Calculation

11. Test the ability to concentrate or attention span by asking the client to recite the alphabet or to count backward from 100. Test the ability to calculate by asking the client to subtract 7 or 3 progressively from 100 (i.e., 100, 93, 86, 79, or 100, 97, 94, 91) (referred to as serial sevens or serial threes). Normally, an adult can complete serial sevens test in about 90 seconds with three or fewer errors. Educational level and language or cultural differences affect calculating ability; this test may be inappropriate for some people.

Level of consciousness (LOC) can lie anywhere along a continuum from a state of alertness to coma. A fully alert client responds to questions spontaneously; a comatose client may not respond to verbal stimuli. The Glasgow Coma Scale was originally developed to predict recovery from a head injury; however, it is used today to assess LOC.

12. Apply the Glasgow Coma Scale: eye response, motor response, and verbal response. An assessment totaling 15 points indicates the client is alert and completely oriented. A comatose client scores 7 or less (see Table 3-11).

TABLE 3-11	LEVEL OF CONSCIOUSNESS: GLASGOW COMA SCALE	
Faculty Measured	**Response**	**Score**
Eye opening	Spontaneous	4
	To verbal command	3
	To pain	2
	No response	1
Motor response	To verbal command	6
	To localized pain	5
	Flexes and withdraws	4
	Flexes abnormally	3
	Extends abnormally	2
	No response	1
Verbal response	Oriented, converses	5
	Disoriented, converses	4
	Uses inappropriate words	3
	Makes incomprehensible sounds	2
	No response	1

From *Fundamentals of nursing: Concepts, process, and practice*, 6th ed., by B. Kozier, G. Erb, A. Berman, & K. Burke, 2000, Upper Saddle River, NJ: Prentice Hall Health.

13. For the specific functions and assessment methods of each cranial nerve, see Table 3-12. The nurse needs to be aware of these functions to detect abnormalities. (The names and order of the cranial nerves can be recalled by mnemonic device: "On old Olympus's treeless top, a Finn and German viewed a hop." The first letter of each word in the sentence is the same as the first letter of the name of the cranial nerve, in order.) Test each nerve not already being evaluated in another component of the health assessment.

IMPLEMENTATION:
TECHNIQUE 3-20 ASSESSING THE REFLEXES

14. Test reflexes using a percussion hammer, comparing one side of the body with the other to evaluate the symmetry of response. The response is described on a scale of 0 to +4. See Box 3-33 for a scale describing reflex responses.

Biceps Reflex

The biceps reflex tests the spinal cord level C5, C6.

1. Partially flex the client's arm at the elbow, and rest the forearm over the thighs, placing the palm of the hand down.

2. Place the thumb of your nondominant hand horizontally over the biceps tendon.

3. Deliver a blow (slight downward thrust) with the percussion hammer to your thumb.

4. Observe the normal slight flexion of the elbow, and feel the bicep's contraction through your thumb (Figure 3-84A ◆).

Triceps Reflex

The triceps reflex tests the spinal cord level C7, C8.

1. Flex the client's arm at the elbow, and support it in the palm of your nondominant hand.

2. Palpate the triceps tendon about 2 to 5 cm (1 to 2 in) above the elbow.

3. Deliver a blow with the percussion hammer directly to the tendon (Figure 3-84B).

4. Observe the normal slight extension of the elbow.

Brachioradialis Reflex

The brachioradialis reflex tests the spinal cord level C3, C6.

1. Rest the client's arm in a relaxed position on your forearm or on the client's own leg.

2. Deliver a blow with the percussion hammer directly on the radius 2 to 5 cm (1 to 2 in) above the wrist or the styloid process, the bony prominence on the thumb side of the wrist (Figure 3-84C).

3. Observe the normal flexion and supination of the forearm. The fingers of the hand may also extend slightly.

Patellar Reflex

The patellar reflex tests the spinal cord level L2, L3, L4.

1. Ask the client to sit on the edge of the examining table so that the legs hang freely.

2. Locate the patellar tendon directly below the patella (kneecap).

3. Deliver a blow with the percussion hammer directly to the tendon (Figure 3-84D).

4. Observe the normal extension or kicking out of the leg as the quadriceps muscle contracts.

5. If no response occurs and you suspect the client is not relaxed, ask the client to interlock the fingers and pull. This action often enhances relaxation so that a more accurate response is obtained.

Achilles Reflex

The Achilles reflex tests the spinal cord level S1, S2.

1. With the client in the same position as for the patellar reflex, slightly dorsiflex the client's ankle by supporting the foot lightly in the hand.

2. Deliver a blow with the percussion hammer directly to the Achilles tendon just above the heel (Figure 3-84E).

3. Observe and feel the normal plantar flexion (downward jerk) of the foot.

Box 3-33 *Scale for Grading Reflex Responses*

- 0 No reflex response
- +1 Minimal activity (hypoactive)
- +2 Normal response
- +3 More active than normal
- +4 Maximum activity (hyperactive)

TABLE 3-12   CRANIAL NERVE FUNCTIONS AND ASSESSMENT METHODS

Cranial Nerve	Name	Type	Function	Assessment Method
I	Olfactory	Sensory	Smell	Ask client to close eyes and identify different mild aromas, such as coffee, vanilla, peanut butter, orange, lemon, lime, chocolate.
II	Optic	Sensory	Vision and visual fields	Ask client to read Snellen chart; check visual fields by confrontation; and conduct an ophthalmoscopic examination.
III	Oculomotor	Motor	Extraocular eye movement (EOM); movement of sphincter of pupil; movement of ciliary muscles of lens	Assess six ocular movements and pupil reaction
IV	Trochlear	Motor	EOM, specifically moves eyeball downward and laterally	Assess six ocular movements.
V	Trigeminal Ophthalmic branch	Sensory	Sensation of cornea, skin of face, and nasal mucosa	While client looks upward, lightly touch lateral sclera of eye to elicit blink reflex. To test light sensation, have client close eyes, wipe a wisp of cotton over client's forehead and paranasal sinuses. To test deep sensation, use alternating blunt and sharp ends of a safety pin over same areas.
	Maxillary branch	Sensory	Sensation of skin of face and anterior oral cavity (tongue and teeth)	Assess skin sensation as for ophthalmic branch above.
	Mandibular branch	Motor and sensory	Muscles of mastication; sensation of skin of face	Ask client to clench teeth.
VI	Abducens	Motor	EOM; moves eyeball laterally	Assess directions of gaze.
VII	Facial	Motor and sensory	Facial expression; taste (anterior two-thirds of tongue)	Ask client to smile, raise the eyebrows, frown, puff out cheeks, close eyes tightly. Ask client to identify various tastes placed on tip and sides of tongue: sugar (sweet), salt, lemon juice (sour), and quinine (bitter); identify areas of taste.
VIII	Auditory Vestibular branch	Sensory	Equilibrium	Assessment methods are discussed with cerebellar functions (in next section).
	Cochlear branch	Sensory	Hearing	Assess client's ability to hear spoken word and vibrations of tuning fork.
IX	Glossopharyngeal	Motor and sensory	Swallowing ability, tongue movement, taste (posterior tongue)	Apply tastes on posterior tongue for identification. Ask client to move tongue from side to side and up and down.
X	Vagus	Motor and sensory	Sensation of pharynx and larynx; swallowing; vocal cord movement	Assessed with cranial nerve IX; assess client's speech for hoarseness.
XI	Accessory	Motor	Head movement; shrugging of shoulders	Ask client to shrug shoulders against resistance from your hands and turn head to side against resistance from your hand (repeat for other side).
XII	Hypoglossal	Motor	Protrusion of tongue; moves tongue up and down and side to side	Ask client to protrude tongue at midline, then move it side to side.

From *Fundamentals of nursing: Concepts, process, and practice*, 6th ed., by B. Kozier, G. Erb, A. Berman, & K. Burke, 2000, Upper Saddle River, NJ: Prentice Hall Health.

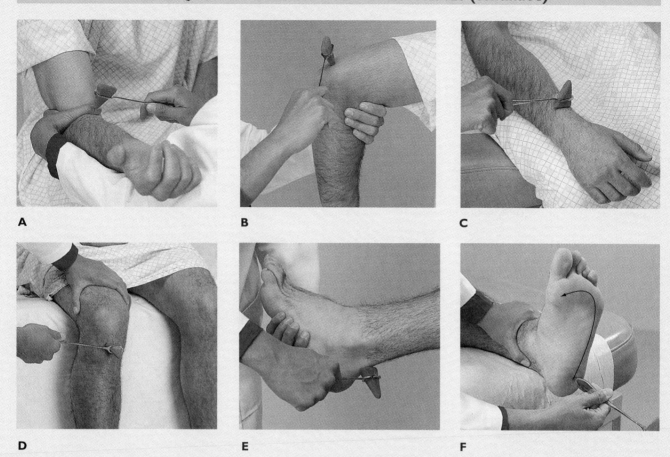

A   B   C

D   E   F

FIGURE 3-84 ◆ Testing reflexes. (A) biceps; (B) triceps; (C) brachioradialis; (D) patellar; (E) Achilles; (F) plantar (Babinski).

Plantar (Babinski) Reflex

The plantar, or Babinski, reflex is superficial. It may be absent in adults without pathology or overridden by voluntary control.

1. Use a moderately sharp object, such as the handle of the percussion hammer, a key, or the dull end of a pin or applicator stick.

2. Stroke the lateral border of the sole of the client's foot, starting at the heel, continuing to the ball of the foot, and then proceeding across the ball of the foot toward the big toe (Figure 3-84F).

3. Observe the response. Normally, all five toes bend downward; this reaction is negative Babinski. In an abnormal Babinski response, the toes spread outward and the big toe moves upward.

IMPLEMENTATION:

TECHNIQUE 3-21 ASSESSING MOTOR FUNCTION

ASSESSMENT	NORMAL FINDINGS	DEVIATIONS FROM NORMAL
15. Gross Motor and Balance Tests Generally, the Romberg test and one other gross motor function and balance test are used.		
Walking Gait		
Ask the client to walk across the room and back, and assess the client's gait.	Has upright posture and steady gait with opposing arm swing; walks unaided, maintaining balance	Has poor posture and unsteady, irregular, staggering gait with wide stance; bends legs only from hips; has rigid or no arm movements

ASSESSMENT	NORMAL FINDINGS	DEVIATIONS FROM NORMAL
Romberg Test Ask the client to stand with feet together and arms resting at the sides, first with eyes open, then closed. Stand close during this test to prevent the client from falling.	Negative Romberg: May sway slightly but is able to maintain upright posture and foot stance	Positive Romberg: cannot maintain foot stance; moves the feet apart to maintain stance If client cannot maintain balance with the eyes shut, client may have sensory ataxia If balance cannot be maintained whether the eyes are open or shut, client may have cerebellar ataxia
Standing on One Foot with Eyes Closed Ask the client to close the eyes and stand on one foot and then the other. Stand close to the client during this test.	Maintains stance for at least 5 seconds	Cannot maintain stance for 5 seconds
Heel–Toe Walking Ask the client to walk a straight line, placing the heel of one foot directly in front of the toes of the other foot.	Maintains heel–toe walking along a straight line	Assumes a wider foot gait to stay upright
Toe or Heel Walking Ask the client to walk several steps on the toes and then on the heels. 16. Fine Motor Tests for the Upper Extremities	Able to walk several steps on toes or heels	Cannot maintain balance on toes or heels
Finger-to-Nose Test Ask the client to abduct and extend the arms at shoulder height and rapidly touch the nose alternately with one index finger and then the other. The client repeats the test with the eyes closed if the test is performed easily.	Repeatedly and rhythmically touches the nose (Figure 3-85 ◆)	Misses the nose or gives lazy response
Alternating Supination and Pronation of Hands on Knees Ask the client to pat both knees with the palms of both hands and then with the backs of the hands alternately at an ever-increasing rate.	Can alternately supinate and pronate hands at rapid pace	Performs with slow, clumsy movements and irregular timing; has difficulty alternating from supination to pronation

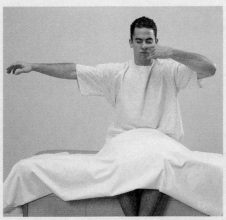

FIGURE 3-85 ◆ Finger-to-Nose Test.

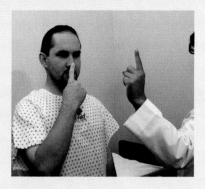 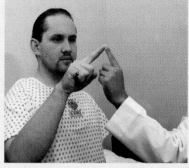

FIGURE 3-86 ◆ Finger to Nose and to the Nurse's Finger Test.

Finger to Nose and to the Nurse's Finger

Ask the client to touch the nose and then your index finger, held at a distance at about 45 cm (18 in), at a rapid and increasing rate.

Performs with coordination and rapidity (Figure 3-86 ◆)

Misses the finger and moves slowly

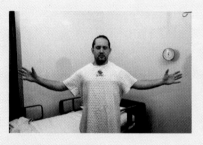 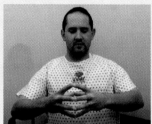

FIGURE 3-87 ◆ Fingers-to-Fingers Test.

Fingers to Fingers

Ask the client to spread the arms broadly at shoulder height and then bring the fingers together at the midline, first with the eyes open and then closed, first slowly and then rapidly.

As above (Figure 3-87 ◆)

Moves slowly and is unable to touch fingers consistently

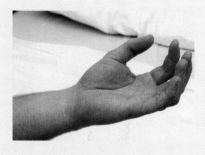 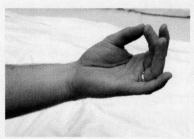

FIGURE 3-88 ◆ Fingers-to-thumb (Same Hand) Test.

Fingers to Thumb (Same Hand)

Ask the client to touch each finger of one hand to the thumb of the same hand as rapidly as possible

Rapidly touches each finger to thumb with each hand (Figure 3-88 ◆).

Cannot coordinate this fine discrete movement with either one or both hands

17. Fine Motor Tests for the Lower Extremities
Ask the client to lie supine and to perform these tests.

Heel Down Opposite Shin

Ask the client to place the heel of one foot just below the opposite knee and run the heel down the shin to the foot. Repeat with the other foot. The client may also use a sitting position for this test.

Demonstrates bilateral equal coordination (Figure 3-89 ◆).

Has tremors or is awkward; heel moves off shin

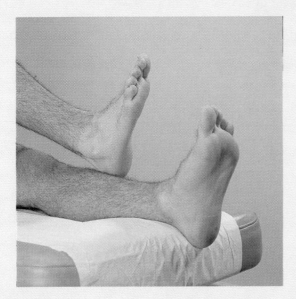

FIGURE 3-89 ◆ Heel down Opposite Shin Test.

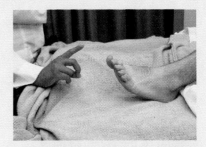

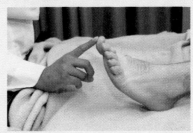

FIGURE 3-90 ◆ Toe or Ball of Foot to the Nurse's Finger Test.

Toe or Ball of Foot to the Nurse's Finger

Ask the client to touch your finger with the large toe of each foot.	Moves smoothly, with coordination (Figure 3-90 ◆).	Misses your finger; cannot coordinate movement

Sensory Function
Sensory functions include touch, pain, temperature, position, and tactile discrimination. The first three are routinely tested in a few locations. Generally, the face, arms, legs, hands, and feet are tested for touch and pain, although all parts of the body can be tested. If the client complains of numbness, peculiar sensations, or paralysis, the practitioner should check sensation more carefully over flexor and extensor surfaces of limbs, mapping out clearly any abnormality of touch or pain by examining responses in the area about every 2 cm (1 in). A more detailed neurologic examination includes position sense, temperature sense, and tactile discrimination.

ASSESSMENT	NORMAL FINDINGS	DEVIATIONS FROM NORMAL
18. Light-Touch Sensation Compare the light-touch sensation of symmetric areas of the body. *Sensitivity to touch varies among different skin areas.* • Ask the client to close the eyes and to respond by saying "yes" or "now" whenever the client feels the cotton wisp touching the skin. • With a wisp of cotton, lightly touch one specific spot and then the same spot on the other side of the body (Figure 3-91 ◆). • Test areas on the forehead, cheek, hand, lower arm, abdomen, foot, and lower leg. Check a specific area of the limb first (i.e., the hand before the arm	Light tickling or touch sensation	**Anesthesia, hyperesthesia, hypoesthesia,** and **paresthesia**

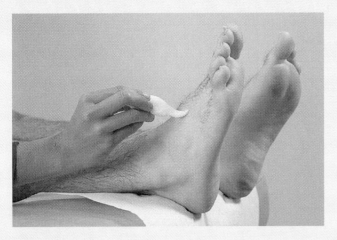

FIGURE 3-91 ◆ Assessing light-touch sensation.

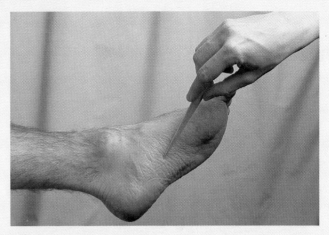

FIGURE 3-92 ◆ Assessing pain sensation using a broken tongue depressor.

ASSESSMENT	NORMAL FINDINGS	DEVIATIONS FROM NORMAL
and the foot before the leg), *because the sensory nerve may be assumed to be intact if sensation is felt at its most peripheral part.* • Ask the client to point to the spot where the touch was felt. *This demonstrates whether the client is able to determine tactile location (point localization), that is, can accurately perceive where he or she was touched.* • If areas of sensory dysfunction are found, determine the boundaries of sensation by testing responses about every 2.5 cm (1 in) in the area. Make a sketch of the sensory loss area for recording purposes.		
19. Pain Sensation Assess pain sensation as follows: • Ask the client to close the eyes and to say "sharp," "dull," or "don't know" when the sharp or dull end of the broken tongue depressor is felt. • Alternately, use the sharp and dull end of the sterile pin or needle to lightly prick designated anatomic areas at random (e.g., hand, forearm, foot, lower leg, abdomen). The face is not tested in this manner (Figure 3-92 ◆). *Alternating the sharp and dull ends of the instrument more accurately evaluates the client's response.* • Allow at least 2 seconds between each test to prevent summation effects of stimuli (i.e., several successive stimuli perceived as one stimulus)	Able to discriminate "sharp" and "dull" sensations	Areas of reduced, heightened, or absent sensation (map them out for recording purposes)
20. Temperature Sensation Temperature sensation is not routinely tested if pain sensation is found to be within normal limits. If pain sensation is not normal or is absent, testing sensitivity to temperature may prove more reliable. • Touch skin areas with test tubes filled with hot or cold water. • Have the client respond say saying "hot," "cold," or "don't know."	Able to discriminate between "hot" and "cold" sensations	Areas of dulled or lost sensation (when sensations of pain are dulled, temperature sense is usually also impaired because distribution of these nerves over the body is similar)

21. Position or Kinesthetic Sensation
Commonly, the middle fingers and the large toes are tested for the kinesthetic sensation (sense of position).
- To test the fingers, support the client's arm with one hand, and hold the client's palm in the other. To test the toes, place the client's heels on the examining table.
- Ask the client to close the eyes.
- Grasp a middle finger or a big toe firmly between your thumb and index finger, and exert the same pressure on both sides of the finger or toe while moving it.
- Move the finger or toe until it is up, down, or straight out, and ask the client to identify the position.
- Use a series of brisk up-and-down movements before bringing the finger or toe suddenly to rest in one of the three positions.

Can readily determine the position of fingers and toes

Unable to determine the position of one or more fingers or toes

22. Tactile Discrimination
For all tests, the client's eyes need to be closed.

One- and Two-Point Discrimination

Alternately stimulate the skin with two pins simultaneously and then with one pin. Ask whether the client feels one or two pinpricks.

Perception varies widely in adults over different parts of the body. Normally, a person can distinguish between a one-point and a two-point stimulus within the following minimum distances:
Fingertips, 2.8 mm
Palms of hands, 8 to 12 mm
Chest, forearm, 40 mm
Back, 50 to 70 mm
Upper arm, thigh, 75 mm
Toes, 3 to 8 mm

Unable to sense whether one or two areas of the skin are being stimulated by pressure

Stereognosis (ability to recognize objects by touching them)

Recognizes common objects

Unable to recognize common objects

Place familiar objects, such as a key, paper clip, or coin, in the client's hand, and ask the client to identify them.
If the client has a motor impairment of the hand and is unable to manipulate an object, write a number or letter on the client's palm, using a blunt instrument, and ask the client to identify it.

Able to identify numbers or letters written on palm

Unable to identify numbers or letters written on palm

Extinction Phenomenon

Simultaneously stimulate two symmetric areas of the body, such as the thighs, the cheeks, or the hands.

Both points of stimulus are felt

Failure to perceive touch on one side of the body when two symmetric areas of the body are touched simultaneously (frequently noted in clients with lesions of the sensory cortex)

23. **Document** findings in the client record using forms or checklists supplemented by narrative notes when appropriate. Describe any abnormal findings in objective terms, for example, "when asked to count backward by threes, client made seven errors and completed the task in 4 minutes."

Assessing the Neurologic System
Infant

- Reflexes commonly tested in newborns include the rooting reflex—when the baby's cheek is touched, the head turns toward that side; palmar grasp—baby's fingers curl around an object; tonic neck reflex—when the baby is supine and the head is turned to one side, the arm and leg on that side extend while those on the opposite side flex (fencing position). Most of these disappear by 6 months of age.

Child

- Present the procedures as games whenever possible.
- Positive Babinski reflex is abnormal after the child ambulates or at age 2.
- For children under age 5, the Denver Developmental Screening Test II provides a comprehensive neurologic evaluation—particularly for motor function.
- Note the child's ability to understand and follow directions.
- Assess immediate recall or recent memory by using names of cartoon characters. Normal recall in children is one less than age in years.
- Assess for signs of hyperactivity or abnormally short attention span.
- Should be able to walk backward by age 2, balance on one foot for 5 seconds by age 4, heel–toe walk by age 5, and heel–toe backward by age 6.
- Romberg test is appropriate over age 3.

Elders

- A full neurologic assessment can be lengthy. Conduct in several sessions if indicated and cease the tests if the client is noticeably fatigued.
- A decline in mental status is not a normal result of aging. Changes are more the result of physical or psychological disorders (e.g., fever, fluid and electrolyte imbalances).

- Intelligence and learning ability are unaltered with age. Many factors, however, inhibit learning (e.g., anxiety, illness, pain, cultural barrier).
- Short-term memory is often less efficient. Long-term memory is usually unaltered.
- Because old age is often associated with loss of support persons, depression is a common disorder. Mood changes, weight loss, anorexia, constipation, and early morning awakening may manifest it.
- The stress of being in unfamiliar situations can cause confusion in the elderly person.
- As a person ages reflex responses may become less intense.
- Because older clients tire more easily than younger clients, a total neurologic assessment is often done at a different time than the other parts of the physical assessment.
- Although there is a progressive decrease in the number of functioning neurons in the central nervous system and in the sense organs, the older client usually functions well because of the abundant reserves in the number of brain cells.
- Impulse transmission and reaction to stimuli are slower.
- Many elderly clients have some impairment of hearing, vision, smell, temperature and pain sensation, memory, and mental endurance.
- Coordination changes, including a reduced speed of fine finger movements. Standing balance remains intact, and Romberg's test remains negative.
- Reflex responses may slightly increase or decrease. Many show loss of Achilles reflex, and the plantar reflex may be difficult to elicit.
- When testing sensory function, the nurse needs to give the older client time to respond. Normally, older clients have unaltered perception of light touch and superficial pain, decreased perception of deep pain, and decreased perception of temperature stimuli. Many also reveal a decrease or absence of position sense in the large toes.

EVALUATION

- Perform a detailed follow-up examination of other systems based on findings that deviated from

expected or normal for the client. Relate findings to previous assessment data if available.

- Report significant deviations from normal to the physician.

Female Genitals and Inguinal Area

In adult females, the examination of the genitals and reproductive tract includes assessment of the inguinal lymph nodes and inspection and palpation of the external genitals. Extent of the assessment of the genitals and reproductive tract depends on the needs and problems of the individual client. Examination of the genitals usually creates uncertainty and apprehension and, in females, the lithotomy position required can cause embarrassment. The nurse must perform the examination in an objective and efficient manner.

PLANNING

Delegation

Due to the substantial knowledge and skill required, assessment of the female genitals and inguinal lymph nodes is not delegated to unlicensed assistive personnel. However, persons other than the nurse may record any aspect that is observed during usual care. Abnormal findings must be validated and interpreted by the nurse.

IMPLEMENTATION:
TECHNIQUE 3-23 ASSESSING THE FEMALE GENITALS AND INGUINAL LYMPH NODES

Equipment

- Examination gloves
- Drape
- Supplemental lighting, if needed

Performance

1. Explain to the client what you are going to do, why it is necessary, and how she can cooperate. Discuss how the results will be used in planning further care or treatments.

2. Wash hands, apply gloves, and observe appropriate infection control procedures.

3. Provide for client privacy.

4. Inquire if the client has any history of the following: age of onset of menstruation, last menstrual period (LMP), regularity of cycle, duration, amount of daily flow, and whether menstruation is painful; incidence of pain during intercourse; vaginal discharge; number of pregnancies, number of live births, labor or delivery complications; urgency and frequency of urination at night; blood in urine, painful urination, incontinence; history of sexually transmitted disease, past and present.

5. Position the client supine with feet elevated on the stirrups of an examination table. Alternately, assist the client into the dorsal recumbent position with knees flexed and thighs externally rotated.

ASSESSMENT	NORMAL FINDINGS	DEVIATIONS FROM NORMAL
6. Inspect the distribution, amount, and characteristics of pubic hair.	There are wide variations; generally kinky in the menstruating adult, thinner and straighter after menopause Distributed in the shape of an inverse triangle	Scant pubic hair (may indicate hormonal problem) Hair growth should not extend over the abdomen
7. Inspect the skin of the pubic area for parasites, inflammation, swelling, and lesions. To assess pubic skin adequately, separate the labia majora and labia minora.	Pubic skin intact, no lesions Skin of vulva area slightly darker than the rest of the body Labia round, full, and relatively symmetric in adult females	Lice, lesions, scars, fissures, swelling, erythema, excoriations, scars from episiotomies, varicosities, or leukoplakia
8. Inspect the clitoris, urethral orifice, and vaginal orifice when separating the labia minora.	Clitoris does not exceed 1 cm in width and 2 cm in length Urethral orifice appears as a small slit and is the same color as surrounding tissues No inflammation, swelling, or discharge	Presence of lesions Presence of inflammation, swelling, or discharge
9. Palpate the inguinal lymph nodes (Figure 3-93 ◆). Use the pads of the fingers in a rotary motion, noting any enlargement or tenderness.	No enlargement or tenderness	Enlargement and tenderness

10. **Document** findings in the client record using forms or checklists supplemented by narrative notes when appropriate.

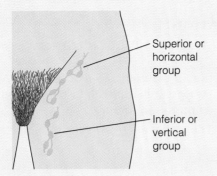

FIGURE 3-93 ◆ Lymph nodes of the groin.

Assessing the Female Genitals and Inguinal Lymph Nodes

Infant

- Infants can be held in the supine position on the mother's lap with the knees supported in a flexed position and separated.

- In newborns, in response to maternal estrogen the labia and clitoris may be edematous and enlarged, and there may be a white vaginal discharge.

Child

- Ensure that you have the parent or guardian's approval to perform the examination and then tell the child what you are going to do. Preschool children are taught to resist touching of their "private parts."

- Assessment of adolescent girls is limited to inspection of the external genitals, unless the girl is sexually active. If so, and the girl has an increased or abnormal vaginal discharge, specimens should be taken to check for sexually transmitted disease.

- Box 3-34 shows the five stages of pubic hair development during puberty.

- The clitoris is a common site for syphilitic chancres in younger females.

Box 3-34 *Five Stages of Pubic Hair Development in Females*

- Stage 1: Preadolescence. No pubic hair except for fine body hair.
- Stage 2: Usually occurs at ages 11 and 12. Sparse, long, slightly pigmented curly hair develops along the labia.
- Stage 3: Usually occurs at ages 12 and 13. Hair becomes darker in color and curlier and develops over the pubic symphysis.

- Stage 4: Usually occurs between ages 13 and 14. Hair assumes the texture and curl of the adult but is not as thick and does not appear on the thighs.
- Stage 5: Sexual maturity. Hair assumes adult appearance and appears on the inner aspect of the upper thighs (Figure 3-94 ◆)

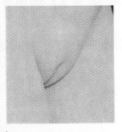
1

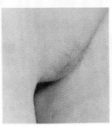
2

3

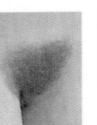
4

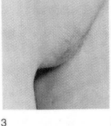
5

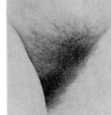
6

FIGURE 3-94 ◆ Stages of female pubic hair development.

Assessing the Female Genitals and Inguinal Lymph Nodes (continued)

Elders

- Labia atrophied and flatter in older females.

- The clitoris is a common site for cancerous lesions in older females.

- The vulva atrophies as a result of a reduction in vascularity, elasticity, adipose tissue, and estrogen levels. Because the vulva is more fragile, it is more easily irritated.

- The vaginal environment becomes drier and more alkaline, resulting in an alteration of the type of flora present and a predisposition to vaginitis. Dyspareunia (difficult or painful coitus) is also a common occurrence.

- The cervix and uterus decrease in size.

- The fallopian tubes and ovaries atrophy.

- Ovulation and estrogen production cease.

- Vaginal bleeding unrelated to estrogen therapy is abnormal in older women.

- Prolapse of the uterus occurs in older females, especially those who have had multiple pregnancies.

- Older females may be arthritic and find the examination position uncomfortable.

EVALUATION

- Perform a detailed follow-up examination based on findings that deviated from expected or normal for the client. Relate findings to previous assessment data if available.

- Report significant deviations from normal to the physician or nurse practitioner qualified to perform an internal vaginal examination.

Male Genitals and Inguinal Area

In adult males, complete examination should include assessment of the external genitals, the inguinal area, and the prostate gland. As with females, nurses in some practice settings performing routine assessment of clients may assess only the external genitals. If a female nurse does not feel comfortable about this part of the examination or if the client is reluctant to be examined by a female, the nurse should refer this part of the examination to a male practitioner.

PLANNING

Delegation

Due to the substantial knowledge and skill required, assessment of the male genitals and inguinal area is not delegated to UAP. However, persons other than the nurse may record any aspect that is observed during usual care. Abnormal findings must be validated and interpreted by the nurse.

Equipment

- Examination gloves

Performance

1. Explain to the client what you are going to do, why it is necessary, and how he can cooperate. Discuss how the results will be used in planning further care or treatments.

2. Wash hands, apply gloves, and observe appropriate infection control procedures.

3. Provide for client privacy.

4. Inquire if the client has any history of the following: usual voiding patterns and any changes, bladder control, urinary incontinence, frequency, urgency, abdominal pain; any symptoms of sexually transmitted disease; any swellings that could indicate presence of hernia; family history of nephritis, malignancy of the prostate, or malignancy of the kidney.

ASSESSMENT	NORMAL FINDINGS	DEVIATIONS FROM NORMAL
Pubic Hair		
5. Inspect the distribution, amount, and characteristics of pubic hair.	Triangular distribution, often spreading up the abdomen	Scant amount or absence of hair

ASSESSMENT	NORMAL FINDINGS	DEVIATIONS FROM NORMAL

Penis

6. Inspect the penile shaft and glans penis for lesions, nodules, swellings, and inflammation.

Penile skin intact
Appears slightly wrinkled and varies in color as widely as other body skin
Foreskin easily retractable from the glans penis
Small amount of thick white smegma between the glans and foreskin

Presence of lesions, nodules, swellings, or inflammation

7. Inspect the urethral meatus for swelling, inflammation, and discharge.
   - Compress or ask the client to compress the glans slightly to open the urethral meatus to inspect it for discharge.
   - If the client has reported a discharge, instruct the client to strip the penis from the base to the urethra (i.e., grasp the base of the penis, with the thumb at the front and fingers behind, and while applying moderate pressure, move the thumb and fingers slowly down the shaft of the penis).

Pink and slitlike appearance
Positioned at the tip of the penis

Inflammation; discharge
Variation in meatal locations (e.g., hypospadias, on the underside of the penile shaft, and epispadias, on the upper side of the penile shaft)

8. Palpate the penis for tenderness, thickening, and nodules. Use your thumb and first two fingers.

Smooth and semifirm
Is slightly movable over the underlying structures

Presence of tenderness, thickening, or nodules
Immobility

Scrotum

9. Inspect the scrotum for appearance, general size, and symmetry.
   - To facilitate inspection of the scrotum during a physical examination, ask the client to hold the penis out of the way.
   - Inspect all skin surfaces by spreading the rugated surface skin and lifting the scrotum as needed to observe posterior surfaces.

Scrotal skin is darker in color than that of the rest of the body and is loose
Size varies with temperature changes (the dartos muscles contract when the area is cold and relax when the area is warm)
Scrotum appears asymmetric (left testis is usually lower than right testis)

Discolorations; any tightening of skin (may indicate edema or mass)
Marked asymmetry in size

10. Palpate the scrotum to assess status of underlying testes, epididymis, and spermatic cord. Palpate both testes simultaneously for comparative purposes. The palpation procedure is outlined in Box 3-35.

Testicles are rubbery, smooth, and free of nodules and masses
Testis is about 2 × 4 cm (0.7 × 1.5 in)
Epididymis is resilient, normally tender, and softer than the spermatic cord
Spermatic cord is firm

Testicles are enlarged, with uneven surface (possible tumor)
Epididymis is nonresilient and painful

BOX 3-35 *Palpating the Scrotum*

- Using your first two fingers and thumb, palpate each testis for size, consistency, shape, smoothness, and presence of masses.
- Palpate the epididymis between your thumb and index finger. It is located at the top of the testis and extends behind it.
- Palpate the spermatic cord between thumb and index finger. It is usually found at the top lateral portion of the scrotum and feels firm.

- If swelling, irregularities, or nodules are detected during the scrotal examination, attempt to transilluminate the lesion. This is done by darkening the room and shining a flashlight behind the scrotum through the mass. Serous fluid causes the light to show with a red glow; tissue or blood does not transilluminate.
- Describe all scrotal masses in terms of their size, shape, placement, consistency, tenderness, and presence of transillumination.

BOX 3-36 *Palpating a Hernia*

Direct Hernia

- Using your right hand for the client's right side or left hand for the client's left side, advance your index finger into the loose scrotal skin and over the external inguinal ring.
- Instruct the client to bear down.
- If a hernia is present, a palpable bulge will appear in the area.

Indirect Hernia

- Attempt to move the index or little finger into the path of the inguinal canal while the client flexes the knee on the same side.

- When your finger has moved as far as possible, ask the client to bear down.
- If a hernia is present, it will be felt as a mass of tissue touching the finger and withdrawing from it.

Femoral Hernia

- Palpate the inguinal area directly again, first while the client is at rest and then while the client bears down.
- If a hernia is present, a bulge will be felt most prominently when the client bears down.

ASSESSMENT	NORMAL FINDINGS	DEVIATIONS FROM NORMAL
Inguinal Area		
11. Inspect both inguinal areas for bulges while the client is standing, if possible. • First, have the client remain at rest. • Next, have the client hold his breath and strain or bear down as though having a bowel movement. Bearing down may make the hernia more visible	No swelling or bulges	Swelling or bulge (possible inguinal or femoral **hernia**)
12. Palpate hernias as described in Box 3-36.	No palpable bulge	Palpable bulge in the area

  13. **Document** findings in the client record using forms or checklists supplemented by narrative notes when appropriate.

AGE-RELATED CONSIDERATIONS

Assessing the Male Genitals and Inguinal Area

Infant

- The foreskin of the uncircumcised infant is normally tight the first 2 or 3 months of life and is not readily retractable.

Child

- The scrotum is usually palpated to determine whether testes are descended.
- Ensure that you have the parent or guardian's approval to perform the examination and then tell the child what you are going to do. Preschool children are taught to resist touching of their "private parts."
- In young boys, the cremasteric reflex can cause the testes to ascend into the inguinal canal. If possible have the boy sit cross-legged, which stretches the muscle and decreases the reflex.

- Table 3-13 shows the five stages of development of pubic hair, penis, and testes/scrotum.

Elders

- The penis decreases in size with age; the size and firmness of the testes decrease.
- Testosterone is produced in smaller amounts.
- More time and direct physical stimulation are required for an older man to achieve an erection, but he can maintain the erection for a longer period before ejaculation than he could at a younger age.
- Seminal fluid is reduced in amount and viscosity.
- Urinary frequency, nocturia, dribbling, and problems with beginning and ending the stream are usually the result of prostatic enlargement.

TABLE 3-13

FIVE STAGES OF DEVELOPMENT OF PUBIC HAIR, PENIS, AND TESTES/SCROTUM

Stage	Pubic Hair	Penis	Testes/Scrotum
1 (preadolescent)	None, except for body hair like that on the abdomen	Size is relative to body size, as in childhood	Size is relative to body size, as in childhood
2	Scant, long, slightly pigmented at base of penis	Slight enlargement occurs	Becomes reddened in color and enlarged
3	Darker, begins to curl and becomes more coarse; extends over pubic symphysis	Elongation occurs	Continuing enlargement
4	Continues to darken and thicken; extends on the sides, above and below	Increase in both breadth and length; glans develops	Continuing enlargement; color darkens
5	Adult distribution that extends to inner thighs, umbilicus, and anus	Adult appearance	Adult appearance

EVALUATION

- Perform a detailed follow-up examination based on findings that deviated from expected or normal for the client. Relate findings to previous assessment data if available.
- Report significant deviations from normal to the physician.

Rectum and Anus

Rectal examination, an essential part of every comprehensive physical examination, involves inspection and palpation (digital examination). In many practice settings, the nurse performs only inspection of the anus.

A Sims' position with the upper leg acutely flexed is required for the examination. For females, a dorsal recumbent position with hips externally rotated and knees flexed or a lithotomy position may be used

(Figure 3-95 ◆). A standing position while the client bends over the examining table may also be used.

PLANNING

Delegation

Due to the substantial knowledge and skill required, assessment of the rectum and anus is not delegated to UAP. However, many aspects are observed during usual care and may be recorded by persons other than the nurse. Abnormal findings must be validated and interpreted by the nurse.

IMPLEMENTATION:
TECHNIQUE 3-25 ASSESSING THE RECTUM AND ANUS

Equipment

- Examination gloves
- Water-soluble lubricant

Performance

1. Explain to the client what you are going to do, why it is necessary, and how he or she can cooperate. Discuss how the results will be used in planning further care or treatments. Because digital examination can cause apprehension and embarrassment in the client, it is important that the nurse help the client relax by encouraging him or her to take slow, deep breaths (tension can cause spasms of the anal sphincters, making the examination uncomfortable) and informing the client about potential sensations such as feelings of defecation or passing gas.

2. Wash hands, apply gloves, and observe appropriate infection control procedures for all rectal examinations.

3. Provide for client privacy. Drape the client appropriately to prevent undue exposure of body parts.

4. Inquire if the client has any history of the following: bright blood in stools, tarry black stools, diarrhea, constipation, abdominal pain, excessive gas, hemorrhoids, or rectal pain; family history of colorectal cancer; when last stool specimen for occult blood was performed and the results; and for males, if not obtained during the genitourinary examination, any signs or symptoms of prostate enlargement (e.g., slow urinary stream, hesitance, frequency, dribbling, and nocturia).

ASSESSMENT	NORMAL FINDINGS	DEVIATIONS FROM NORMAL
5. Inspect the anus and surrounding tissue for color, integrity, and skin lesions. Then, ask the client to bear down as though defecating. Bearing down creates slight pressure on the skin that may accentuate rectal fissures, rectal prolapse, polyps, or internal hemorrhoids. Describe the location of all abnormal findings in terms of a clock, with the 12 o'clock position toward the pubic symphysis.	Intact perianal skin; usually slightly more pigmented than the skin of the buttocks Anal skin is normally more pigmented, coarser, and moister than perianal skin and is usually hairless	Presence of fissures (cracks), ulcers, excoriations, inflammations, abscesses, protruding hemorrhoids (dilated veins seen as reddened protrusions of the skin), lumps or tumors, fistula openings, or rectal prolapse (varying degrees of protrusion of the rectal mucous membrane through the anus)
6. Palpate the rectum for anal sphincter tonicity, nodules, masses, and tenderness. See Box 3-37 for palpation technique.	Anal sphincter has good tone Rectal wall is smooth and not tender	Hypertonicity of the anal sphincter (may occur in the presence of an anal fissure or other lesion that causes contraction). Hypotonicity of anal sphincter (may occur after rectal surgery or result from a neurologic deficiency) Rectal wall is tender and nodular
7. On withdrawing the finger from the rectum and anus, observe it for feces.	Brown color	Presence of mucus, blood, or black tarry stool

---

8. **Document** findings in the client record using forms or checklists supplemented by narrative notes when appropriate.

- Lubricate your gloved index finger, and instruct the client to bear downward as though having a bowel movement. This relaxes the anal sphincter.
- Slowly insert your finger into the anus and into the rectum in the direction of the umbilicus. The anal canal (distance from the anal opening to the anorectal junction) is short (less than 3 cm [about 1 in]). The posterior wall of the rectum follows the curve of the coccyx and sacrum. The nurse's finger is usually able to palpate a distance of 6 to 10 cm (2 to 4 in).

- Never force digital insertion. If lesions are painful or bleeding occurs, discontinue the examination.
- Ask the client to tighten the anal sphincter around your finger, and note the tone of the anal sphincter.
- Rotate the pad of the index finger along the anal and the rectal walls, feeling for nodules, masses, and tenderness.
- Note the location of any abnormalities of the rectum (e.g., "anterior wall, 2 cm proximal to the internal anal sphincter").

AGE-RELATED CONSIDERATIONS

Assessing the Rectum and Anus
Infant

- Lightly touching the anus should result in a brief anal contraction.
- A rectal examination is not routinely performed on children.

Child

- Erythema and scratch marks around the anus may indicate a pinworm parasite.
- A rectal examination is not routinely performed on children.

EVALUATION

- Perform a detailed follow-up examination based on findings that deviated from expected or normal for the client. Relate findings to previous assessment data if available.
- Report significant deviations from normal to the physician.

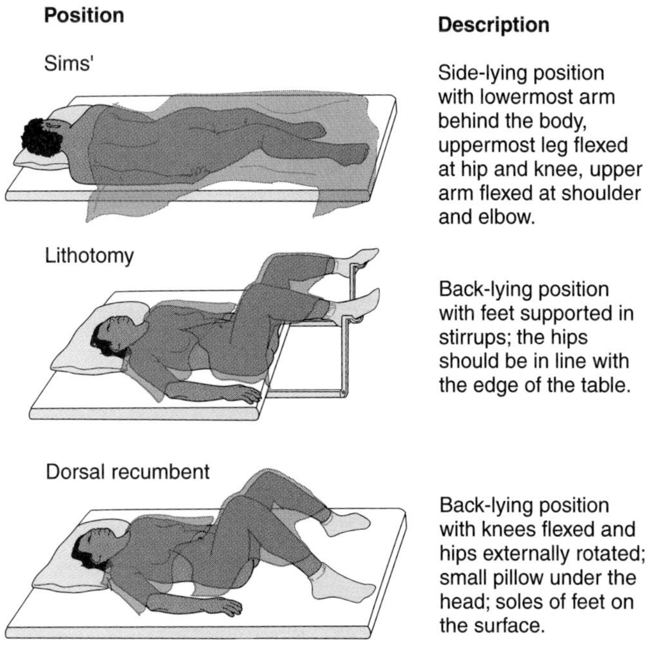

Position	Description
Sims'	Side-lying position with lowermost arm behind the body, uppermost leg flexed at hip and knee, upper arm flexed at shoulder and elbow.
Lithotomy	Back-lying position with feet supported in stirrups; the hips should be in line with the edge of the table.
Dorsal recumbent	Back-lying position with knees flexed and hips externally rotated; small pillow under the head; soles of feet on the surface.

FIGURE 3-95 ◆ Left Sims', lithotomy, and dorsal recumbent positions.

Chapter Summary

TERMINOLOGY

adventitious breath sounds
alopecia
anesthesia
anisocoria
astigmatism
auscultation
blanch test
breast self examination (BSE)
bromhidrosis
cataract
cerumen
clubbing
conjunctivitis
dacryocystitis
dullness
edema
erythema
exophthalmos
fasciculation
flatness
gingivitis
glaucoma

glossitis
goniometer
heave
hematoma
hernia
hordeolum (sty)
hyperesthesia
hyperopia
hyperpigmentation
hyperresonance
hypoesthesia
hypopigmentation
inspection
iritis
lift
miosis
mydriasis
myopia
normocephalic
otoscope
pallor
palpation

paresthesia
parotitis
percussion
pitch
plaque
pleximeter
plexor
point of maximal impulse (PMI)
presbycusis
presbyopia
resonance
sordes
stereognosis
stomatitis
tartar
tremor
tympany
visual acuity
visual fields
vitiligo

FORMING CLINICAL JUDGMENTS

Consider This:

1. What should you do if the client answers all history questions with simple one-word answers or gestures?

2. Your 78-year-old client has very thin skin with many bruises on her forearms and raised, pale, solid, soft lesions on her upper arms. What questions would you ask to help determine the cause of these lesions?

3. When speaking with the client during the nursing history, you note that one eye seems to be out of alignment with the other eye. What techniques would you use to determine that your observation is or is not valid?

4. You are performing the Rinne test on a client who has complained of difficulty hearing the television at home. The client states ability to hear the tuning fork when held next to the ear canal after ceasing to hear it while the tuning fork was

held against the mastoid process. How would you interpret this result?

5. The thyroid gland can be very difficult to feel. What aspects of the technique assist in this examination?

6. When auscultating the client's posterior chest, you hear low-pitched sighing sounds at the left base and high-pitched squeaky sounds at the right base. Are these normal or abnormal findings? If not normal, what does the sound indicate?

7. When auscultating the heart of an obese client, all sounds are extremely distant and difficult to hear. What might you do to enhance the auscultation?

8. When palpating the client's left breast, a thickened area about 1 cm wide and 2 cm long is noted in the upper outer quadrant. What actions should you take before ending this examination?

9. The client complains of constipation and vague abdominal discomfort. In listening for bowel sounds, you hear gurgling sounds about every 30 to 45 seconds. What action would you take next?

10. You are conducting a full assessment on an older client in a long-term care facility. What data would you gather from the medical record and from the usual caregivers prior to assessing the musculoskeletal system?

11. The client's spouse reports that the client has recently been irritable and forgetful. Which aspects of the neurologic examination would be most pertinent?

12. You are preparing to perform a genital and rectal examination on a client of the same gender as yourself for the first time as a nurse. What measures can you take to ensure a successful examination for both you and the client?

RELATED RESEARCH

Barton, M. B., Harris, R., & Fletcher, S. W. (1999). Does this patient have breast cancer? The screening clinical breast examination: Should it be done? How? *Journal of the American Medical Association, 282,* 1270–1280.

REFERENCES

Cox, C. L., & McGrath, A. (1999). Respiratory assessment in critical care units. *Intensive and Critical Care Nursing, 15,* 226–234.

Darovic, G. (1997). Assessing pupillary responses. *Nursing, 27*(2), 48.

Faria, S. H. (1999). Assessment of peripheral arterial pulses. *Home Care Provider, 4,* 140–141.

Fritz, D. J. (1997). Fine tune your physical assessment of the lungs and respiratory system. *Home Care Provider, 2,* 299–302.

Greenberger, N. J. (1998). Techniques for physical assessment of acute abdominal pain: Getting the most out of the history and physical exam. *Journal of Critical Illness, 13,* 735–742.

Hayko, D. M. (1998) Clinical practice: Peripheral vascular assessment of the lower extremities. *Home Health Focus, 5*(1), 1, 2, 5.

Hayko, D. M. (1999) Clinical practice: Assessing the lungs. *Home Health Focus, 5*(10), 73, 75.

Jackson, R., Alghareeb, M., Alaradi, I., & Tomi, Z. (1999). The diagnosis of skin disease. *Dermatology Nursing, 11,* 275, 278–283.

Kacker, A., Gonzales, D. A., & Selesnick, S. H. (1999). The otoscopic examination: What to look for: Where to search. *Consultant, 39,* 2397–2402, 2405–2406.

Kirton, C. A. (1997). Assessing S_3 and S_4 heart sounds. *Nursing, 27*(7), 52–53.

Klingman, L. (1999). Assessing the female reproductive system. *American Journal of Nursing, 99*(8), 37–43.

Klingman, L. (1999). Assessing the male genitalia. *American Journal of Nursing, 99*(7), 47–50.

Langan, J. C. (1998). Abdominal assessment in the home: From A to ZZZ. *Home Healthcare Nurse, 16,* 51–57.

O'Hanlon-Nichols, T. (1997). Basic assessment series: The adult cardiovascular system. *American Journal of Nursing, 97*(12), 34–40.

O'Hanlon-Nichols, T. (1998). A review of the adult musculoskeletal system. *American Journal of Nursing, 98*(6), 48–52.

O'Hanlon-Nichols, T. (1998). Basic assessment series: Gastrointestinal system. *American Journal of Nursing, 98*(4), 48–53.

O'Hanlon-Nichols, T. (1998). Basic assessment series: The adult pulmonary system. *American Journal of Nursing, 98*(2) Continuing Care Extra Ed., 39–45.

Owen, A. (1998). Respiratory assessment revisited. *Nursing, 28*(4), 48–49.

Chapter 4

Specimen Collection

Techniques

OBJECTIVES

- Discuss the nursing responsibilities for specimen collection.
- Explain the rationale for the collection of each type of specimen.
- Describe sources of fluid intake and output.
- Identify normal daily fluid intake and output.
- List factors that influence fluid balance.
- Monitor a client's fluid intake and output.
- Accurately measure blood glucose from a capillary blood specimen and using a blood glucose meter.
- State at least two reasons for testing feces.
- Effectively obtain and collect a stool specimen.
- Correctly test a stool specimen for the presence of occult blood.
- Effectively collect routine, timed, clean-catch, and sterile urine specimens.
- Correctly test urine for specific gravity, pH, glucose, ketones, and occult blood.
- Collect sputum, nose, and throat specimens.
- Identify essential steps of obtaining wound specimens.

Fluid Balance

In good health, a delicate balance of fluids, electrolytes, and acids and bases is maintained in the body. This balance, or physiologic homeostasis, depends on multiple physiologic processes that regulate fluid intake and output and the movement of water and the substances dissolved in it between the body compartments.

Almost every illness has the potential to threaten this balance. Even in normal daily living, excessive temperatures or vigorous activity can disturb the balance if adequate water and salt intake is not maintained. Therapeutic measures, such as the use of diuretics or nasogastric suction, can also disturb the body's homeostasis unless water and electrolytes are replaced.

The proportion of the human body composed of fluids is surprisingly large. About 46 to 60 percent of the average adult's weight is water, the primary body fluid. Age, gender, and body fat affect total body water. Infants have the highest proportion of water, accounting for 70 to 80 percent of their body weight. The proportion of body water decreases with aging (see Table 4-1).

Maintaining Fluid Volume

In a healthy person, the fluid volume and chemical composition of the fluid compartments stay within narrow, safe limits. Normally, fluid intake and fluid loss are balanced. Illness can upset this balance so that the body has too little or too much fluid.

Fluid Intake

During periods of moderate activity at moderate temperature, the average adult drinks about 1,500 mL per day but needs 2,500 mL per day, an additional 1,000 mL. This added volume is acquired from foods and from the oxidation of these foods during metabolic processes. Interestingly, the water content of food is relatively large, contributing about 750 mL per day. The water content of fresh vegetables is approximately 90 percent, for fresh fruits about 85 percent, and for lean meats around 60 percent. Water as a by-product of food metabolism accounts for most of the remaining fluid volume required. This quantity is approximately 200 mL per day for the average adult.

The thirst mechanism is the primary regulator of fluid intake. Thirst is normally relieved immediately after drinking a small amount of fluid, even before it is absorbed from the gastrointestinal tract. However, this relief is only temporary, and the thirst returns in about 15 minutes. The thirst is again temporarily relieved after the ingested fluid distends the upper gastrointestinal tract. These mechanisms protect the individual from drinking too much, because it takes from 30 minutes to one hour for the fluid to be absorbed and distributed throughout the body.

Fluid Output

Fluid losses from the body counterbalance the adult's 2,500-mL average daily intake of fluid. See Table 4-2 for the average daily fluid output for an adult and the four routes of fluid output. It is important to remember that daily intake equals daily output.

Urine

Urine formed by the kidneys and excreted from the urinary bladder is the major avenue of fluid output. Normal urine output for an adult is 1,400 to 1,500 mL per 24 hours, or at least 30 to 50 mL per hour. In healthy people, urine output may vary noticeably from day to day. Urine volume automatically increases as fluid intake increases. If fluid loss through perspiration is large, however, urine volume decreases to maintain fluid balance in the body.

TABLE 4-1	WATER AS PERCENTAGE OF BODY WEIGHT
Age	Percentage of Body Weight
Infant	70–80
Child	60–77
Adult female	50
Adult male	60
Elder	45–50

TABLE 4-2	AVERAGE DAILY FLUID OUTPUT FOR AN ADULT
Route	Amount (mL)
Urine	1,400 to 1,500
Insensible losses	
Lungs	350 to 400
Skin	350 to 400
Sweat	100
Feces	100 to 200
Total	2,300 to 2,600

Insensible Losses

Insensible fluid loss occurs through the skin and lungs. It is called insensible because it is usually not noticeable and cannot be measured. Insensible fluid loss through the skin occurs in two ways. Water is lost through diffusion and through perspiration (which is noticeable but not measurable). Water losses through diffusion are not noticeable but normally account for 300 to 400 mL per day. This loss can be significantly increased if the protective layer of the skin is lost as with burns or large abrasions. Perspiration varies depending on factors such as environmental temperature and metabolic activity. Fever and exercise increase metabolic activity and heat production, thereby increasing fluid losses through the skin.

Another type of insensible loss is the water in exhaled air. In an adult, this is normally 300 to 400 mL per day. When respiratory rate accelerates, for example, due to exercise or an elevated body temperature, this loss can increase.

Feces

The chyme, digested products that leave the stomach and pass from the small intestine into the large intestine, contains water and electrolytes. The volume of chyme entering the large intestine in an adult is normally about 1,500 mL per day. Of this amount, all but about 100 mL is reabsorbed in the proximal half of the large intestine.

Obligatory Fluid Losses

Certain fluid losses are required to maintain normal body function. These are known as **obligatory losses.** A minimum volume of 500 mL of fluid must be excreted through the kidneys of an adult each day to eliminate metabolic waste products from the body. Water lost through respirations, through the skin, and in **feces** also are obligatory losses, necessary for temperature regulation and elimination of waste products. The total of all these losses is approximately 1,300 mL per day.

Because the vaporized losses are not readily measured, the obligatory kidney loss becomes of prime importance in critical illness. An adult hourly urine volume of less than 30 mL or daily volume under 500 mL is serious. Clients with inadequate output require immediate attention, and such a finding by the nurse must therefore be reported promptly.

Factors Affecting Fluid Balance

Age

Infants and growing children have much greater fluid turnover than adults because their higher metabolic rate increases fluid loss. Infants lose more fluid through the kidneys because immature kidneys are less able to conserve water than adult kidneys. In addition, infants' respirations are more rapid and the body surface area is proportionately greater than adults', increasing insensible fluid losses. The more rapid turnover of fluid plus the losses produced by disease can create critical fluid imbalances in children much more rapidly than in adults.

In elderly people, the normal aging process may affect fluid balance. For example, the thirst response often is blunted and the nephrons (the functional unit of the kidney), become less able to conserve water. These normal changes of aging increase the risk of dehydration. When combined with the increased likelihood of heart diseases, impaired renal function, and multiple drug regimens, the older adult's risk for fluid and electrolyte imbalance is significant.

Gender and Body Size

Total body water also is affected by gender and body size. Because fat cells contain little or no water and lean tissue has a high water content, people with a higher percentage of body fat have less body fluid. Women have proportionately more body fat and less body water than men. Water accounts for approximately 60 percent of an adult male's weight, but only 50 percent for an adult female. In an obese individual, this may be even less, with water responsible for only 30 to 40 percent of the person's weight.

Environmental Temperature

People with an illness and those participating in strenuous activity are at risk for fluid and electrolyte imbalances when the environmental temperature is high. Fluid losses through sweating are increased in hot environments as the body attempts to dissipate heat. These losses are even greater in people who have not been acclimatized to the environment.

Lifestyle

Other factors such as diet and stress affect fluid balance. The intake of fluids and electrolytes is affected by the diet. People with anorexia nervosa or bulimia are at risk for severe fluid and electrolyte imbalances because of inadequate intake or purging regimens (e.g., induced vomiting, using diuretics and laxatives). Seriously malnourished people have decreased serum albumin levels and may develop edema because of the decreased colloid osmotic pressure (a pulling force exerted by colloids that help maintain the water content of blood).

Stress affects a person's fluid and electrolyte balance. Stress can increase cellular metabolism, blood glucose concentration, and muscle glycolysis. These mechanisms can lead to sodium and water retention. In addition, stress can increase production of the antidiuretic hormone, which in turn decreases urine production. The overall response of the body to stress is to increase the blood volume.

Monitoring Fluid Intake and Output

Intake and output monitoring is often ordered by the physician; however, it can also be an independent nursing action initiated by the nurse. The measurement and recording of all fluid intake and output (I&O) during a 24-hour period provides important data about the client's fluid and electrolyte balance. Generally, intake and output are measured for hospitalized at-risk clients (see Box 4-1).

The unit used to measure intake and output is the milliliter (mL) or cubic centimeter (cc); these are equivalent metric units of measurement. In household measures, 30 mL is roughly equivalent to one fluid ounce, 500 mL is about one pint, and 1,000 mL is about one quart. To measure fluid intake, nurses convert household measures such as a glass, cup, or soup bowl to metric units. Most agencies provide conversion tables, since the sizes of dishes vary from agency to agency. Such a table is often provided on or with the bedside I&O record. Examples of equivalents are given in Box 4-2.

Box 4-2 *Commonly Used Fluid Containers and Their Volumes*

Water glass	200 mL
Juice glass	120 mL
Cup	180 mL
Soup bowl	
Adult	180 mL
Child	100 mL
Teapot	240 mL
Creamer	
Large	90 mL
Small	30 mL
Water pitcher	1,000 mL
Jello, custard dish	100 mL
Ice cream dish	120 mL
Paper cup	
Large	200 mL
Small	120 mL

From *Fundamentals of nursing: Concepts, process, and practice,* 6th ed., by B. Kozier, G. Erb, A. Berman, & K. Burke, 2000, Upper Saddle River, NJ: Prentice Hall Health.

Box 4-1 *Common Risk Factors for Fluid, Electrolyte, and Acid–Base Imbalances*

Chronic Diseases and Conditions

- Chronic lung disease (COPD, asthma, cystic fibrosis)
- Congestive heart failure
- Kidney disease
- Diabetes mellitus
- Cushing's syndrome or Addison's disease
- Cancer
- Malnutrition, anorexia nervosa, bulimia
- Ileostomy

Acute Conditions

- Acute gastroenteritis
- Bowel obstruction
- Head injury or decreased level of consciousness
- Trauma such as burns or crushing injuries
- Surgery
- Fever, draining wounds, fistulas

Medications

- Diuretics
- Corticosteroids
- Nonsteroidal anti-inflammatory drugs (NSAIDs)

Treatments

- Chemotherapy
- IV therapy and total parenteral nutrition (TPN)
- Nasogastric suction
- Enteral feedings
- Mechanical ventilation

Other Factors

- Age: Very old or very young
- Inability to access food and fluids independently

From *Fundamentals of nursing: Concepts, process, and practice,* 6th ed., by B. Kozier, G. Erb, A. Berman, & K. Burke, 2000, Upper Saddle River, NJ: Prentice Hall Health.

BEDSIDE INTAKE-OUTPUT RECORD

Mary Brown — Name   747-2 — Room No   7/11 — Date

Time	INTAKE Liquids	Intravenous	OUTPUT Urine	Emesis	Drainage etc
8-4	0900 Juice 120		0700 - 250		
	Coffee 180		1100 - 400		
	Cream 90		1500 - 350		
	0930 Water 90				
	1200 Tea 180				
	Cream 90				
	Jello 50				
	1400 Juice 180				
Total	980		1000		
4-12					
Total					
12-8					
Total					

FIGURE 4-1 ◆ A sample bedside fluid intake and output record.

PATIENT LABEL

Intake and Output Record

INTAKE	0600-1800	1800-0600	TOTAL
Oral			
Tube feeding			
IV (primary)			
IV Meds			
TPN			
Blood			
TOTAL			24-Hour Total
OUTPUT	0600-1800	1800-0600	TOTAL
Urine			
Emesis			
G.I. Suction			
Stool			
TOTAL			24-Hour Total

FIGURE 4-2 ◆ A sample 24-hour fluid intake and output record.

Most agencies have two forms for recording I&O: (a) a bedside worksheet record on which the nurse lists all items measured and their quantities per shift (Figure 4-1 ◆) and a 24-hour permanent record on the client's chart noting the totals for each 24-hour period (see Figure 4-2 ◆). Agencies may use the same form or have another form for recording the specifics of intravenous fluids, such as the type of solution, additives, time started, amounts absorbed, and amounts remaining per shift.

Nursing Process: Monitoring Fluid Intake and Output

ASSESSMENT

- Determine if the client is receiving medications or fluids that may predispose him to fluid overload. Assess the client's risk factors for fluid loss.
- Weigh the client daily at the same time, on the same scale, and in the same clothes. Is the client maintaining his weight or is there a trend of increasing or decreasing weight? If so, assess for signs and symptoms of fluid excess or deficit.
- Determine the client and family's understanding of the purpose of I&O and willingness to cooperate and participate as both will help ensure accuracy.

PLANNING

Delegation

Measuring and recording of oral intake and urine output is often delegated to unlicensed assistive personnel (UAP). It is important for the nurse to stress the importance of accurate measuring and recording. The UAP needs to be aware of the importance of reporting any changes in a client's intake as well as changes in color, amount, and odor of output and the presence of stool and/or urine incontinence. Certain intake such as tube feedings, parenteral fluids, intravenous medications, and catheter or tube irrigants are measured and recorded by the nurse rather than the UAP because of the need to apply professional knowledge and problem solving. Likewise, the nurse measures output from tube drainage (e.g., Hemovac, Jackson–Pratt) because of the need for cleansing the drain site to minimize the introduction of microbes into the closed system.

Equipment

- I&O form at bedside
- I&O graphic record in chart
- Bedside bedpan, commode, or urinal
- A urine "hat" (a receptacle that fits inside the toilet) (Figure 4-3 ◆)
- Calibrated containers: one to measure intake and another container to measure output
- Disposable gloves
- Sign at bedside stating client is on I&O

Preparation

Check that all necessary equipment is located in the client's room.

Performance

1. Explain to the client, family members, and all caregivers that an accurate measurement of fluid intake and output is required and the reasons. Emphasize the need to use a bedpan, urinal, commode, or in-toilet collection device (unless a urinary drainage system is in place). Instruct the client not to put toilet tissue into the container with the urine. Many people wish to be involved in recording fluid intake measurements and need to be taught how to compute the values and what foods are considered fluids.

2. Wash hands and observe other appropriate infection control procedures.

3. Measure the client's fluid intake. Following meals, record on the bedside I&O form the amount of

each fluid item taken, if the client has not already done so. Specify the kind of fluid and the time. All of the following fluids need to be recorded:

- *Oral fluids.* Water, milk, juice, soft drinks, coffee, tea, cream, soup, and any other beverages. Include water taken with medications. To assess the amount of water taken from a water pitcher, measure what remains and subtract this amount from the volume of the full pitcher. Then refill the pitcher.

- *Ice chips.* Record these as fluids at approximately one-half their volume.

- *Foods that are or tend to become liquid at room temperature.* These include ice cream, sherbet, custard, and gelatin such as Jello. Do not measure foods that are pureed because purees are simply solid foods prepared in a different form.

- *Tube feedings.* Remember to include the 30- to 60-mL water rinse at the end of intermittent feedings or during continuous feedings.

- *Parenteral fluids.* The exact amount of intravenous fluid administered is to be recorded since some fluid containers may be overfilled. Blood transfusions are included.

- *Intravenous medications.* Intravenous medications that are prepared with solutions such as normal saline (NS) and are administered as an intermittent or continuous infusion must also be included (e.g., tobramycin sulfate 80 mg in 50 mL of normal saline). Most intravenous medications are mixed in 50 to 100 mL of solution.

- *Catheter or tube irrigants.* Fluid used to irrigate urinary catheters, nasogastric tubes, and intestinal tubes must be measured and recorded if not immediately withdrawn.

4. Measure the client's fluid output. Wash hands and observe other appropriate infection control procedures (e.g., gloves). Measure the following fluids:

- *Urinary output.* Following each voiding, pour the urine into a measuring container, observe the amount and record it and the time of voiding on the I&O form. For clients with retention catheters, empty the drainage bag into a measuring container at the end of the shift (or at prescribed times if output is to be measured more often). Note and record the amount of urine output. In intensive care areas, urine output often is measured hourly.

- If the client is incontinent of urine, estimate and record these outputs. For example, for an incontinent client the nurse might record "Incontinent ×3" or "Drawsheet soaked in 12-inch diameter." If urine is frequently soiled

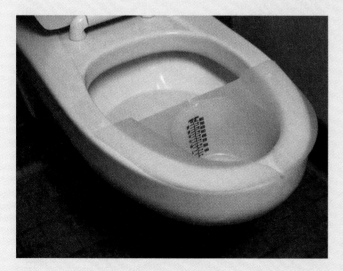

FIGURE 4-3 ◆ Urine collection device for the toilet

with feces, the number of voidings may be recorded rather than the volume of urine.

- *Vomitus and liquid feces.* The amount and type of fluid and the time need to be specified.

- *Tube drainage,* such as gastric or intestinal drainage.

- *Wound drainage* and *draining fistulas.* Wound drainage may be recorded by documenting the type and number of dressings or linen saturated with drainage or by measuring the exact amount of drainage collected in a vacuum drainage (e.g., Hemovac) or gravity drainage system.

5. Total the measurements at the end of the shift (i.e., every 8 or 12 hours).

Note: In intensive care areas, the nurse may record intake and output hourly.

 6. **Document** pertinent assessment data and the totals of the client's I&O in the client's permanent record.

AGE-RELATED CONSIDERATIONS

Intake and Output

Infant

- A more accurate estimate of the urine output of infants may be obtained by first weighing diapers that are dry, and then subtracting this weight from the weight of the soiled diaper. Each gram of weight left after subtracting is equal to 1 mL of urine.

Child

- Sudden weight gain (e.g., 0.5 kg [1 lb] in one day) in a child is due to the accumulation of fluid ver-sus normal growth. Look at the speed with which the increase develops.

Elders

- Urinary incontinence, the loss of control over voiding with continuous or intermittent leakage of urine, is a common problem among elderly clients. Age, however, is not the cause of incontinence.

EVALUATION

- Compare the total 24-hour fluid output measurement with the total fluid intake measurement and compare both to previous measurements. Urinary output is normally equivalent to the amount of fluids ingested; the usual range is 1,500 to 2,000 mL in 24 hours or 40 to 80 mL in one hour. Clients whose output substantially exceeds intake are at risk for fluid volume deficit. By contrast, clients whose intake substantially exceeds output are at risk for fluid volume excess.

- Relate 24-hour fluid I&O totals to daily weights. Is there a correlation? Remember, one liter of fluid equals 2.2 pounds or one kilogram.

- Report to the physician a significant discrepancy between intake and output or when fluid intake or output is inadequate (for example, a urine output of less than 500 mL in 24 hours or less than 30 mL per hour in an adult).

- Conduct follow-up assessments pertinent to the fluid imbalance, if appropriate. For example, if the 24-hour I&O reflects fluid overload, determine if the client also exhibits clinical signs of fluid overload. And, follow-up assessments related to fluid balance are needed after medical intervention, such as diuretics, is implemented.

Specimen Collection

The nurse contributes to the assessment of a client's health status by collecting **specimens** of body fluids. All hospitalized clients have at least one laboratory specimen collected during their stay at the health care facility. Laboratory examination of specimens such as urine, blood, stool, sputum, and wound drainage provides important adjunct information for diagnosing health care problems as well as measuring a response to therapy.

Nurses often assume the responsibility for specimen collection. Depending on the type of specimen and skill required, the nurse may be able to delegate this task to UAP under the supervision of the professional nurse.

Nursing responsibilities associated with specimen collection include the following:

- Provide client comfort, privacy, and safety. Clients may experience embarrassment or discomfort when providing a specimen. The nurse should provide the client with as much privacy as possible and handle the specimen discretely. The nurse needs to be nonjudgmental and sensitive to possible sociocultural beliefs that may affect the client's willingness to participate in the specimen collection.

- Explain the purpose of the specimen collection and the procedure for obtaining the specimen. Clients may experience anxiety about the procedure, especially if it is perceived as being intrusive or the client is afraid of an unknown test result. A clear explanation will facilitate the client's cooperation in the collection of the specimen. With proper instruction, many clients are able to collect their own specimen, which promotes independence and reduces or avoids embarrassment.

- Use the correct procedure for obtaining a specimen or ensure that the client or staff follows the correct procedure. Aseptic technique is used in specimen collection to prevent contamination, which can cause inaccurate test results. A nursing procedure or laboratory manual is often available if the nurse is unfamiliar with the procedure. If there is any question about the procedure, the nurse calls the laboratory for directions before collecting the specimen.

- Note relevant information on the laboratory requisition slip, for example, medications the client is taking that may affect the results.

- Transport the specimen to the laboratory promptly. Fresh specimens provide more accurate results.

- Report abnormal laboratory findings to the health care provider in a timely manner consistent with the severity of the abnormal results.

Capillary Blood Glucose

A capillary blood specimen is often taken to measure blood **glucose** when frequent tests are required or when a venipuncture cannot be performed. This technique is less painful than a venipuncture and easily performed. Hence, clients can perform this technique on themselves.

The development of home glucose test kits and reagent strips has simplified the testing of blood glucose and greatly facilitated the management of home

care by diabetic clients. A number of manufacturers have developed blood glucose meters (Figure 4-4 ◆). Most meters permit measurements between 20 and 600 mg per dL or 100 mL of blood. Meters differ, and with the development of new technology, it is imperative that the nurse or client review the manufacturer's operating guidelines. Being familiar with and proper use of the equipment helps ensure accurate readings.

Capillary blood specimens are commonly obtained from the lateral aspect or side of the finger in adults. This site avoids the nerve endings and calloused areas at the fingertip. The earlobe may be used if the client is in shock or the fingers are edematous.

Technique 4-2 describes how to obtain a capillary blood specimen and measure blood glucose using a portable meter.

Nursing Process: Measuring Capillary Blood Glucose

ASSESSMENT

- Before obtaining a capillary blood specimen, determine:
  - The frequency and type of testing
  - The client's understanding of the procedure
  - The client's response to previous testing
- Assess the client's skin at the puncture site to determine if it is intact and the circulation is not compromised.
- Review the client's record for medications that may prolong bleeding such as anticoagulants.
- Assess the client's self-care abilities that may affect accuracy of test results, such as visual impairment and finger dexterity.

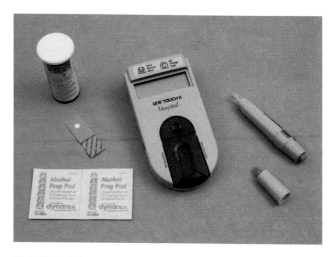

FIGURE 4-4 ◆ Blood glucose monitor, test strips, and lancet injector.

Delegation

Check the Nurse Practice Act and the facility policy and procedure manual to determine who can perform this skill. It is usually considered an invasive technique and one that requires problem solving and application of knowledge. It is the responsibility of the nurse to know the results of the test.

IMPLEMENTATION:

TECHNIQUE 4-2 OBTAINING A CAPILLARY BLOOD SPECIMEN AND MEASURING BLOOD GLUCOSE

Equipment

- **Blood glucose meter**
- Blood glucose reagent strip compatible with the meter
- Paper towel
- Warm cloth or other warming device (optional)
- Antiseptic swab
- Disposable gloves
- Sterile **lancet** or 19- or 21-gauge needle
- **Lancet injector** (optional)
- Cotton ball to wipe the glucose reagent strip (dry wipe method)

Preparation

Review type of meter and manufacturer's instructions. Assemble the equipment at the bedside.

Performance

1. Explain to the client what you are going to do, why it is necessary, and how he or she can cooperate. Discuss how the results will be used in planning further care or treatments.

2. Wash hands and observe other appropriate infection control procedures (e.g., gloves).

3. Provide for client privacy.

4. Prepare the equipment.
   - Obtain a reagent strip from the container and place it on a clean, dry paper towel. *Moisture can change the strip, thereby altering the test results.*
   - Calibrate the meter, and run a control sample according to the manufacturer's instructions.

5. Select and prepare the vascular puncture site.
   - Choose a vascular puncture site (e.g., the side of an adult's finger). Avoid sites beside bone. Wrap the finger first in a warm cloth for 30 to 60 seconds (optional), *or* hold a finger in a dependent position and massage it toward the site. If the earlobe is used, rub it gently with a small piece of gauze. *These actions increase the blood flow to the area, ensure an adequate specimen, and reduce the need for a repeat puncture.*
   - Clean the site with the antiseptic swab and allow it to dry completely as *alcohol can affect accuracy.*

6. Obtain the blood specimen.
   - Put on gloves.
   - Place the injector, if used, against the site, and release the needle, thus permitting it to pierce the skin. Make sure the lancet is perpendicular to the site. *The lancet is designed to pierce the skin at a specific depth when it is in a perpendicular position relative to the skin* (Figure 4-5 ◆).

     or

     Prick the site with a lancet or needle, using a darting motion.
   - Wipe away the first drop of blood with a cotton ball. *The first blood usually contains a greater proportion of serous fluid, which can alter test results.*
   - Gently squeeze (but do not touch) the puncture site until a large drop of blood forms.
   - Hold the reagent strip under the puncture site until enough blood covers the indicator square. The pad will absorb the blood and a chemical reaction will occur. Do not smear the blood. *This will cause an inaccurate reading* (Figure 4-6 ◆).
   - Ask the client to apply pressure to the skin puncture site with a cotton ball. *Pressure will assist hemostasis.*

7. Expose the blood to the test strip for the period and the manner specified by the manufacturer. As soon as the blood is placed on the test strip:

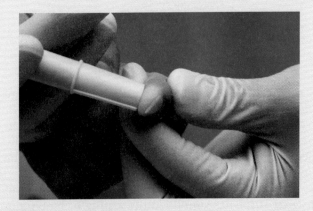

FIGURE 4-5 ◆ Place the injector against the site.

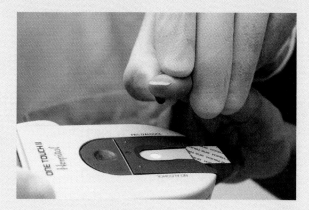

FIGURE 4-6 ◆ Gently squeeze a large drop of blood onto the reagent strip.

a. Follow the manufacturer's recommendations on the glucose meter and monitor the time as indicated by the manufacturer (e.g., 60 seconds). *The blood must remain in contact with the test pad for a prescribed time for accurate results.*

b. If indicated, lay the glucose strip on a paper towel or on the side of the timer. *The strip should be kept flat so that blood will not pool on only one part of the pad.*

8. Measure the blood glucose.

• Place the strip into the meter according to the manufacturer's instructions. Some devices require that the strip be wiped or blotted after a designated period of time before being inserted in the meter. Other strips do not require blotting or wiping. Refer to the specific manufacturer's recommendations for the specific procedure.

• After the designated time most glucose meters will display the glucose reading automatically.

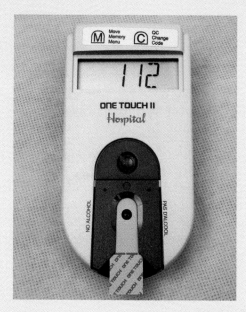

FIGURE 4-7 ◆ The glucose meter will display the glucose reading.

Correct timing ensures accurate results (Figure 4-7 ◆).

• Turn off the meter and discard the test strip and cotton balls.

9. **Document** the method of testing and results on the client's record. If appropriate, record the client's understanding and ability to demonstrate the technique. The client's record may also include a flow sheet on which **capillary blood glucose (CBG)** results and amount, type, route, and time of insulin administration is recorded.

AMBULATORY AND COMMUNITY SETTINGS

Capillary Blood Glucose

• Assess the client or caregiver's ability and willingness to perform blood glucose monitoring at home.

• Teach the proper use of the lancet and glucose monitor, and provide written guidelines. Allow time for a return demonstration. The client may need several visits to completely learn the procedure.

• Ensure the client's ability to obtain supplies and purchase reagent strips. The strips are relatively

expensive and may not be covered by the client's insurance.

• Instruct the client how to record the blood glucose levels and when to notify the health care provider.

• Diabetic children who need to perform fingersticks should be taught about safe practices for cleaning blood from surfaces (household bleach is best) and for safe storage of equipment to prevent young children from having access to it. Identify a place in the school where the child can store glucose-monitoring equipment and perform the procedure in private.

AGE-RELATED CONSIDERATIONS

Capillary Blood Glucose

Infant

• The outer aspect of the heel is the most common site for neonates and infants. Placing a warm cloth

on the infant's heel often increases the blood flow to the area.

Capillary Blood Glucose (continued)
Child

- Use a fingertip for a young client older than age 2, unless contraindicated.
- Allow the child to choose the puncture site, when possible.
- Praise the young client for cooperating and assure the child that the procedure is not a punishment.

Elders

- Older clients may have arthritic joint changes, poor vision, or hand tremors and may need assistance using the glucose meter.
- Older clients may have difficulty obtaining diabetic supplies due to financial concerns or homebound status.

EVALUATION

- Compare glucose meter reading with normal blood glucose level; status of puncture site and motivation of the client to perform the test independently.
- Relate blood glucose reading to previous readings and the client's current health status.
- Report abnormal results to the physician.
- Conduct appropriate follow-up such as asking the client to explain the meaning of the results and/or demonstrating the procedure at the next scheduled test.

Stool Specimens

Analysis of stool specimens can provide information about a client's health condition. Some of the reasons for testing feces include:

- *To determine the presence of **occult** (hidden) blood.* Bleeding can occur as a result of ulcers, inflammatory disease, or tumors. The test for occult blood, often referred to as the **guaiac** test, can be readily performed by the nurse in the clinical area or by the client at home. Guaiac paper used in the test is sensitive to fecal blood content. Certain foods, medications, and vitamin C can produce inaccurate test results. False-positive results can occur if the client has recently ingested (1) red meat; (2) raw vegetables or fruits; or (3) certain medications that irritate the gastric mucosa and cause bleeding, such as aspirin or other nonsteroidal anti-inflammatory drugs (NSAIDs), steroids, iron preparations, and anticoagulants. False-negative results can occur if the client has taken more than 250 mg per day of vitamin C from all dietary and supplemental sources up to 3 days before the test—even if bleeding is present.

- *To analyze for dietary products and digestive secretions.* For example, an excessive amount of fat in the stool **(steatorrhea)** can indicate faulty absorption of fat from the small intestine. A decreased amount of bile can indicate obstruction of bile flow from the liver and gallbladder into the intestine. For these kinds of tests, the nurse needs to collect and send the total quantity of stool expelled at one time instead of a small sample.

- *To detect the presence of **ova and parasites**.* When collecting specimens for parasites, it is important that the sample be transported immediately to the lab while it is still warm. Usually, three stool specimens are evaluated to confirm the presence of and identify the organism so that appropriate treatment can be ordered (Kee, 1999, p. 655).

- *To detect the presence of bacteria or viruses.* Only a small amount of feces is required because the specimen will be cultured. Collection containers or tubes must be sterile and aseptic technique used during collection. Stools need to be sent immediately to the laboratory. The nurse needs to note if the client is receiving any antibiotics on the lab requisition.

Nursing Process: Stool Specimens and Tests

ASSESSMENT

Assessment can include the following aspects:

- Client's need for assistance to defecate or use a bedpan
- Any abdominal discomfort before, during, or after defecation
- Status of perianal skin for any irritation, especially if the client defecates frequently and has liquid stools
- Any interventions related to the specimen collection (e.g., dietary or medication orders)

- Presence of hemorrhoids that may bleed (particularly important for clients who are constipated, because constipated stool can aggravate existing hemorrhoids and any bleeding can affect test results)
- Any interventions (e.g., medication) ordered to follow a defecation

PLANNING

Before obtaining a specimen, determine the reason for collecting the stool specimen and the correct method of obtaining and handling it (i.e., how much stool to obtain, whether a preservative needs to be added to the stool, and whether it needs to be sent immediately to the laboratory). It may be necessary to confirm this information by checking with the agency laboratory. In many situations, only a single specimen is required; in others, timed specimens are necessary, and every stool passed is collected within a designated time period. Check whether the client needs to be placed on a diet free of red meat and whether to discontinue oral iron preparations before an occult blood test.

Delegation

UAP may obtain and collect stool specimen(s). The nurse, however, needs to consider the collection process before delegating this task. For example, a random stool specimen collected in a specimen container may be delegated, but a stool culture requiring a sterile swab in a test tube should be done by the nurse. Incorrect collection technique can cause inaccurate test results.

The task of obtaining and testing a stool specimen for occult blood may be performed by UAP. It is important that the nurse instruct the UAP to tell the nurse if blood is detected and/or if the test is positive. In addition, the stool specimen should be saved to allow the nurse to repeat the test.

IMPLEMENTATION:
TECHNIQUE 4-3 OBTAINING AND TESTING A STOOL SPECIMEN

Equipment

Collecting a Stool Specimen
- Clean or sterile bedpan or bedside commode
- Disposable gloves
- Cardboard or plastic specimen container (labeled) with a lid or, for stool culture, a sterile swab in a test tube, as policy dictates
- Two tongue blades
- Paper towel
- Completed laboratory requisition
- Air freshener

Testing the Stool for Occult Blood
- Clean bedpan or bedside commode
- Disposable gloves
- Two tongue blades
- Paper towel
- Test product

Preparation

Assemble the needed equipment. Post a sign in the client's bathroom if a timed specimen is required (e.g., "Save All Stools").

Performance

1. Explain to the client what you are going to do, why it is necessary, and how he or she can cooperate. Discuss how the results will be used in planning further care or treatments.

Give ambulatory clients the following information and instructions.
- The purpose of the stool specimen and how the client can assist in collecting it.
- Defecate in a clean or sterile bedpan or bedside commode.
- Do not contaminate the specimen, if possible, with urine or menstrual discharge. Void before the specimen collection.
- Do not place toilet tissue in the bedpan after defecation, because contents of the paper can affect the laboratory analysis.
- Notify the nurse as soon as possible after defecation, particularly for specimens that need to be sent to the laboratory immediately after collection.

2. Wash hands and observe other appropriate infection control procedures.
   When obtaining stool samples, that is, when handling the client's bedpan, when transferring the stool sample to a specimen container, and when disposing of the bedpan contents, the nurse follows medical aseptic technique meticulously.

3. Provide for client privacy.

4. Assist clients who need help.
   - Assist the client to a bedside commode or a bedpan placed on a bedside chair or under the toilet seat in the bathroom.
   - After the client has defecated, cover the bedpan or commode. *Covering the bedpan reduces odor and embarrassment to the client.*

- Put on gloves to prevent hand contamination, and clean the client as required. Inspect the skin around the anus for any irritation, especially if the client defecates frequently and has liquid stools.

5. Transfer the required amount of stool to the stool specimen container.

- Use one or two tongue blades to transfer some or all of the stool to the specimen container, taking care not to contaminate the outside of the container. The amount of stool to be sent depends on the purpose for which the specimen is collected. Usually, 2.5 cm (1 in) of formed stool or 15 to 30 mL of liquid stool is adequate. For some timed specimens, however, the entire stool passed may need to be sent. Visible pus, mucus, or blood should be included in the sample.

- For a culture, dip a sterile swab into the specimen, preferably where purulent fecal matter is present in the feces. Place the swab in a sterile test tube using sterile technique.

- For an occult blood test, see step 7.

- Wrap the used tongue blades in a paper towel before disposing of them in a waste container. *These measures help prevent the spread of microorganisms by contact with other articles.*

- Place the lid on the container as soon as the specimen is in the container. *Putting the lid on immediately prevents the spread of microorganisms.*

6. Ensure client comfort.

- Empty and clean the bedpan or commode, and return it to its place.

- Remove and discard the gloves.

- Provide an air freshener for any odors unless contraindicated by the client (e.g., a spray may increase dyspnea).

7. Label and send the specimen to the laboratory.

- Ensure that the specimen label and the laboratory requisition have the correct information on them and are securely attached on the specimen container. *Inappropriate identification of the specimen can lead to errors of diagnosis or therapy for the client.*

- Arrange for the specimen to be taken to the laboratory. Specimens to be cultured or tested for parasites need to be sent immediately. If this is not possible, follow the directions on the specimen container. In some instances, refrigeration is indicated because bacteriologic changes take place in stool specimens left at room temperature. Never place a stool specimen in a refrigerator that contains food or medication *to prevent contamination.*

To test the stool for occult blood:

- Select a test product.
- Put on gloves.
- Follow the manufacturer's directions. For example:

a. For a guaiac test, smear a thin layer of feces on a paper towel or filter paper with a tongue blade, and drop reagents onto the smear as directed.

b. For a Hematest, smear a thin layer of feces on filter paper, place a tablet in the middle of the specimen, and add two drops of water as directed.

c. For a Hemoccult slide, smear a thin layer of feces over the circle inside the envelope, and drop reagent solution onto the smear (see Figure 4-8 ◆).

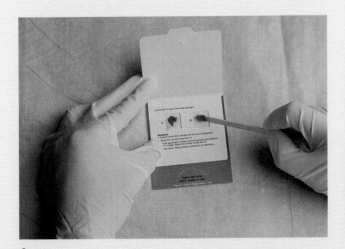

A

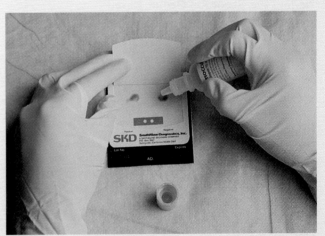

B

FIGURE 4-8 ◆ (A) Opening the front cover of a Hemoccult slide and applying a thin smear of feces on the slide. (B) Opening the flap on the back of the slide and applying two drops of developing fluid over each smear.

- Note the reaction. For all tests, a blue color indicates a positive result, that is, the presence of occult blood.

8. **Document** all relevant information.
  - Record the collection of the specimen on the client's chart and on the nursing care plan. Include in the recording the date and time of the collection and all nursing assessments (e.g., color, odor, consistency, and amount of feces); presence of abnormal constituents, such as blood or mucus; results of test for occult blood if obtained; discomfort during or after defecation; status of perianal skin; any bleeding from the anus after defecation.
  - For an occult blood test, record the type of test product used and the reaction.

AMBULATORY AND COMMUNITY SETTINGS

Stool Specimen

- Ask the client or caregiver to call when the stool specimen is obtained. If a laboratory test is needed, the nurse can pick up the specimen or a family member may take it to the laboratory.
- Place the stool specimen inside a plastic biohazard bag. Carry the bag in a sealed container marked "biohazard" and take it to the laboratory promptly. Do not expose the specimen to extreme temperatures in the car.

Specimen Collection

- If specimen collection is done on an outpatient basis or in the home, the nurse teaches the client how to obtain the specimens. Provide written instructions and specimen containers to ensure correct and safe performance of the procedure.
- Ensure that the laboratory knows where to send the test results.

AGE-RELATED CONSIDERATIONS

Stool Specimen

Infant

- To collect a stool specimen for an infant, the stool is scraped from the diaper.

Child

- A child who is toilet trained should be able to provide a fecal specimen, but may prefer being assisted by a parent.

- When explaining the procedure to the child, use words appropriate for the child's age rather than medical terms. Ask the parent what words the family normally uses to describe a bowel movement.

Elders

- Older adults may need assistance if serial stool specimens are required.

EVALUATION

- Report positive test results for occult blood to the physician.
- Conduct appropriate follow-up after stool specimen tests are completed, such as discussing with the physician any changes in the client's health care plan or need for additional testing as a result of the tests.

Urine Specimens

The nurse is responsible for collecting urine specimens for a number of tests: clean voided specimens for routine urinalysis, **clean-catch** or **midstream urine specimens** for urine culture, and timed urine specimens for a variety of tests that depend on the client's specific health problem.

Routine Urine Specimen

A clean voided specimen is usually adequate for routine examination. Many clients are able to collect a clean voided specimen and provide the specimen independently with minimal instructions. Male clients generally are able to **void** directly into the specimen container, and female clients usually sit or squat over the toilet, holding the container between their legs during voiding. Technique 4-4 describes how to collect a routine urine specimen.

Timed Urine Specimen

Some urine examinations require collection of all urine produced and voided over a specific period of time, ranging from one to two hours to 24 hours. Timed specimens generally either are refrigerated or contain a preservative to prevent bacterial growth or decomposition of urine components. Each voiding of urine is collected in a small, clean container and then emptied immediately into the large refrigerated bottle or carton. See Technique 4-5 for a detailed description. Some of the tests performed on timed urine specimens include:

- To assess the ability of the kidney to concentrate and dilute urine
- To determine disorders of glucose metabolism (e.g., diabetes mellitus)
- To determine levels of specific constituents (e.g., albumin, amylase, creatinine, urobilinogen, certain hormones such as estriol or corticosteroids) in the urine

Clean-Catch Urine Specimen

Clean-catch or midstream voided specimens are collected when a urine culture is ordered to identify microorganisms causing urinary tract infection. Care is taken to ensure that the specimen is as free as possible from contamination by microorganisms around the urinary meatus. Clean-catch specimens are collected into a sterile specimen container with a lid. Disposable clean-catch kits are available (Figure 4-9 ◆).

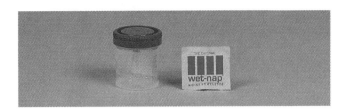

FIGURE 4-9 ◆ Disposable clean-catch specimen equipment.

Technique 4-6 explains how to collect a clean-catch urine specimen for culture.

Urine Tests

Several simple urine tests are often done by nurses on the nursing units. These include tests for specific gravity, pH, and the presence of abnormal constituents such as glucose, ketones, protein, and occult blood (see Table 4-3).

Nurses in a health care facility or clients in the home setting can use many commercially prepared kits available to test abnormal constituents in the urine. These kits contain the required equipment and an appropriate **reagent** (substance used in a chemical reaction to detect a specific substance). Reagents may be in the form of a tablet, fluid, or paper test strips or

TABLE 4-3	SIMPLE URINE TESTS DONE BY NURSES ON THE UNIT OR CLIENTS IN THE HOME			
Test	**Purpose**	**Normal**	**Equipment Used for Testing**
Specific gravity	To measure urine concentration or the amount of solutes (metabolic wastes and electrolytes) present in the urine	1.010–1.025	Urinometer or spectrometer or refractometer
Urinary pH	To measure the relative acidity or alkalinity of urine and to assess the client's acid–base status	Slightly acidic with an average pH of 6	Litmus paper
Glucose	To screen clients for diabetes mellitus and to assess clients during pregnancy for abnormal glucose tolerance	Negative	Reagent tablets or a test strip
Ketones	Type I diabetics should test urine for ketones when they are not feeling well, when blood glucose is consistently over 240 mg/dL or when they are running a fever	Negative	Reagent tablets or a test strip
Protein	Protein molecules normally are too large to escape from glomerular capillaries into the filtrate. If the glomerular membrane has been damaged, however (e.g., glomerulonephritis), it can become "leaky," allowing proteins to escape	Negative reagent strip test	Reagent test strip
Occult blood	To determine if occult (not visible) blood is present	Negative	Reagent test strip

dipsticks. When the urine contacts the reagent, a chemical reaction occurs, causing a color change that is then compared with a chart to interpret the significance of the color. Specific directions for the amount of urine needed, the time required for the chemical reaction, and the meaning of the colors produced vary among manufacturers. Thus, it is essential that nurses and clients read and follow directions supplied by each manufacturer.

Technique 4-7 describes how to test urine for specific gravity and the tests that use a reagent (e.g., pH, glucose, ketones, and occult blood).

Collecting a Routine Urine Specimen

Routine urine examination is usually done on the first voided specimen in the morning because it tends to have a higher, more uniform concentration and a more acidic pH than specimens later in the day.

Nursing Process: Urine Specimen

ASSESSMENT

- Before collecting the specimen, the nurse determines whether the client can assist with the technique or may require supervision or assistance.
- The nurse also assesses the client's medications to determine if there any medications that may discolor the urine or affect the test results.
- Often, the client is able to provide the specimen independently. About 120 mL (4 oz) of urine is generally required.

PLANNING

Delegation

UAP may be assigned to collect a routine urine specimen. Provide the UAP with clear directions on how to instruct the client to collect his or her own urine specimen or how to correctly collect the specimen for the client who may need to use a bedpan or urinal.

IMPLEMENTATION:
TECHNIQUE 4-4 COLLECTING A ROUTINE URINE SPECIMEN

Equipment

- Nonsterile gloves as needed
- Clean bedpan, urinal, or commode for clients who are unable to void directly into the specimen container
- Wide-mouthed specimen container
- Completed laboratory requisition
- Completed specimen identification label

Preparation

Obtain needed equipment. Determine if the client requires supervision or assistance in the bathroom. Clients who are seriously ill, physically incapacitated, or disoriented may need to use a bedpan or urinal in bed.

Performance

1. Explain to the client what you are going to do, why it is necessary, and how they can cooperate. Discuss how the results will be used in planning further care or treatments. Give ambulatory clients the following information and instructions:
   - Explain the purpose of the urine specimen and how the client can assist.
   - Explain that all specimens must be free of fecal contamination, so voiding needs to occur at a different time from defecation.

- Instruct female clients to discard the toilet tissue in the toilet or in a waste bag rather than in the bedpan because *tissue in the specimen makes laboratory analysis more difficult.*
   - Give the client the specimen container, and direct the client to the bathroom to void 120 mL (4 oz) into it.

2. Wash hands and observe other appropriate infection control procedures.

3. Provide for client privacy.

4. Assist clients who are seriously ill, physically incapacitated, or disoriented. Provide required assistance in the bathroom or help the client to use a bedpan or urinal in bed.

5. Ensure that the specimen is sealed and the container clean.
   - Put the lid tightly on the container. *This prevents spillage of the urine and contamination of other objects.*
   - If the outside of the container has been contaminated by urine, clean it with soap and water. *This prevents the spread of microorganisms.*

6. Label and transport the specimen to the laboratory.
   - Ensure that the specimen label and the laboratory requisition have the correct information on them. Attach them securely to the specimen con-

tainer. *Inappropriate identification of the specimen will lead to errors of diagnosis or therapy for the client.*

- Arrange for the specimen to be taken immediately to the laboratory or placed in a refrigerator. *Urine deteriorates relatively rapidly from bacterial contamination when left at room temperature; speci-*

mens should be analyzed immediately after collection.

 7. **Document** the collection of the specimen on the client's chart. Include the date and time of collection and the appearance and odor of the urine.

EVALUATION

Conduct appropriate follow-up such as checking the test results and informing the physician as needed.

Collecting a Timed Urine Specimen

For timed urine specimens, appropriate specimen containers with or without preservative in accordance with the specific test are generally obtained from the laboratory and placed in the client's bathroom or in the utility room. Signs to remind staff of the test in progress are placed in the client's room. Specimen identification labels need to indicate the date and time of each voiding in addition to the usual identification information. They may also be numbered sequentially (e.g., 1st specimen, 2nd specimen, 3rd specimen).

Nursing Process: Urine Specimen

ASSESSMENT

- Determine the client's ability to understand instructions and to provide urine samples independently. Are there any fluid or dietary requirements associated with the test?
- Are there any medication restrictions or requirements for the test?

PLANNING

Delegation

UAP may be assigned to assist in the collection of a timed urine specimen. Provide clear directions about the collection procedure, proper storage of the specimen container, and the importance of saving all of the client's urine to avoid the need to restart the collection process.

Equipment

- Appropriate specimen containers with or without preservative in accordance with the specific test
- Completed specimen identification labels
- Completed laboratory requisition
- Bedpan or urinal
- Sign on or near the bed indicating the specific times for urine collection
- Antiseptic
- Nonsterile gloves, as needed
- Ice-filled container if a refrigerator is not available

Preparation

Obtain a specimen container with preservative (if

indicated) from the laboratory. Label the container with identifying information for the client, the test to be performed, time started, and time of completion. Provide a clean receptacle to collect urine (bedpan, commode, or toilet collection device). Post signs in the client's chart, Kardex, room, and bathroom alerting personnel to save all urine during the specified time.

Performance

1. Explain to the client what you are going to do, why it is necessary, and how he or she can cooperate. Discuss how the results will be used in planning further care or treatments. Give the client the following information and instructions:
   - The purpose of the test and how the client can assist

- When the specimen collection will begin and end (for example, a 24-hour urine test commonly begins at 0700 hours and ends at the same hour the next day)
- That all urine must be saved and placed in the specimen containers once the test starts
- That the urine must be free of fecal contamination and toilet tissue
- That each specimen must be given to the nursing staff immediately so that it can be placed in the appropriate specimen bottle

2. Wash hands and observe other appropriate infection control procedures.

3. Provide for client privacy.

4. Start the collection period.
   - Ask the client to void in the toilet or bedpan or urinal. Discard this urine (check agency procedure), and document the time the test starts with this discarded specimen. Collect all subsequent urine specimens, including the one specimen collected at the end of the period.
   - Ask the client to ingest the required amount of liquid for certain tests or to restrict fluid intake. Follow the test directions.
   - Instruct the client to void all subsequent urine into the bedpan or urinal and to notify the nursing staff when each specimen is provided. Some tests require voiding at specified times.
   - Number the specimen containers sequentially (e.g., 1st specimen, 2nd specimen, 3rd specimen) if separate specimens are required.

5. Collect all of the required specimens.
   - Place each specimen into the appropriately labeled container. For some tests, each specimen is not kept separately but is poured into a large bottle.
   - If the outside of the specimen container is contaminated with urine, clean it with soap and water. *Cleaning prevents the transfer of microorganisms to others.*
   - Ensure that each specimen is refrigerated throughout the timed collection period. If not refrigerated, specimens are often kept on ice. *Refrigeration or other form of cooling prevents bacterial decomposition of the urine.*
   - Measure the amount of each urine specimen as required.
   - Ask the client to provide the last specimen 5 to 10 minutes before the end of the collection period.
   - Inform the client that the test is completed.
   - Remove the signs and the specimen equipment from the client's unit and bathroom.

6. **Document** all relevant information.
   - Record the starting time of the test and completion of the specimen collection on the client's chart. Include the date and specific time. In addition, if indicated for the specific test, note the time each urine specimen was collected, the volume of each specimen, the appearance of the urine, and other relevant data such as fluid intake or restrictions.

EVALUATION

- Conduct follow-up such as checking the test results and informing the physician as needed.
- Discuss abnormal test results with the physician to facilitate nursing interventions if appropriate.

Collecting a Urine Specimen for Culture and Sensitivity by Clean Catch

A clean-catch or midstream voided specimen is collected when a urine culture is ordered by the physician. The purpose of the specimen is to determine the presence of microorganisms, the type of organism(s), and the antibiotics to which the organisms are sensitive.

Nursing Process: Urine Specimen

ASSESSMENT

- Determine the ability of the client to provide the specimen.
- Assess the color, odor, and consistency of the urine and the presence of clinical signs of urinary tract infection (e.g., frequency, urgency, **dysuria**, **hematuria**, flank pain, cloudy urine with foul odor).

PLANNING

Delegation

UAP may perform the collection of a clean catch or midstream urine specimen. It is important, however, that the nurse inform the UAP how to instruct the client in the correct process for obtaining the specimen. Proper cleansing of the urethra should be emphasized to avoid contaminating the urine specimen.

Equipment

Equipment used varies from agency to agency. Some agencies use commercially prepared disposable clean-catch kits. Others are agency-prepared sterile trays. Both prepared trays and kits generally contain the following items:

- Disposable gloves
- Antiseptic towelette, such as povidone–iodine
- Sterile cotton balls or 2" × 2" gauze pads
- Sterile specimen container
- Specimen identification label

In addition, the nurse needs to obtain:

- Completed laboratory requisition form
- Urine receptacle, if the client is not ambulatory
- Basin of warm water, soap, washcloth, and towel for the nonambulatory client

Preparation

Collect the necessary equipment needed for the collection of the specimen. Use visual aids, if available, to assist the client to understand the midstream collection technique.

Performance

1. Explain to the client that a urine specimen is required, give the reason and explain the method to be used to collect it. Discuss how the results will be used in planning further care or treatments.

2. Wash hands and observe other appropriate infection control procedures.

3. Provide for client privacy.

4. For an ambulatory client who is able to follow directions, instruct the client how to collect the specimen.
   - Direct or assist the client to the bathroom.
   - Ask the client to wash and dry the genitals and perineal area with soap and water. *Washing the perineal area reduces the number of skin and transient bacteria, decreasing the risk of contaminating the urine specimen.*
   - Instruct the client how to clean the urinary meatus with antiseptic towelettes. *The antiseptic further reduces bacterial contamination of the urinary meatus and the risk of contaminating the specimen.*

For Female Clients

- Use each towelette only once. Clean the perineal area from front to back and discard the towelette. Use all towelettes provided (usually two or three).

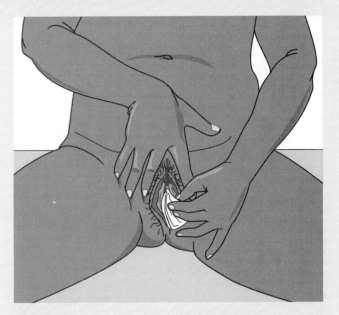

FIGURE 4-10 ◆ Cleansing the female urinary meatus. Spread the labia minora with one hand and with the other hand, cleanse perineal area from front to back.

Cleaning from front to back cleans the area of least contamination to the area of greatest contamination (see Figure 4-10 ◆).

For Male Clients

- If uncircumcised, retract the foreskin slightly to expose the urinary meatus.
- Using a circular motion, clean the urinary meatus and the distal portion of the penis. Use each towelette only once, then discard. Clean several inches down the shaft of the penis. *This cleans from the area of least contamination to the area of greatest contamination* (see Figure 4-11 ◆).

5. For a client who requires assistance, prepare the client and equipment.
   - Wash the perineal area with soap and water, rinse and dry.
   - Assist the client onto a clean commode or bedpan. If using a bedpan or urinal, position the client as upright as allowed or tolerated. *Assuming a normal anatomic position for voiding facilitates urination.*
   - Open the clean-catch kit, taking care not to contaminate the inside of the specimen container or lid. *It is important to maintain sterility of the specimen container to prevent contamination of the specimen.*
   - Put on clean gloves.
   - Clean the urinary meatus and perineal area as described in step 4.

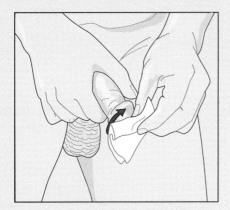

FIGURE 4-11 ◆ Cleansing the male urinary meatus. Retract the foreskin if needed. Using a towelette, cleanse the urinary meatus by moving in a circular motion from center of urethral opening around the glans and down the distal portion of the shaft of the penis.

6. Collect the specimen from a nonambulatory client or instruct an ambulatory client how to collect it.
   • Instruct the client to start voiding. *Bacteria in the distal urethra and at the urinary meatus are cleared by the first few milliliters of urine expelled.*
   • Place the specimen container into the stream of urine and collect the specimen, taking care not to touch the container to the perineum or penis. *It is important to avoid contaminating the interior of the specimen container and the specimen itself.*
   • Collect 30 to 60 mL of urine in the container.
   • Cap the container tightly, touching only the outside of the container and the cap. *This prevents contamination or spilling of the specimen.*
   • If necessary, clean the outside of the specimen container with disinfectant. *This prevents transfer of microorganisms to others.*

7. Label the specimen and transport it to the laboratory.
   • Ensure that the specimen label and the laboratory requisition carry the correct information. Attach them securely to the specimen. *Inaccurate identification or information on the specimen container can lead to errors of diagnosis or therapy.*
   • Arrange for the specimen to be sent to the laboratory immediately. *Bacterial cultures must be started immediately, before any contaminating organisms can grow, multiply, and produce false results.*

8. **Document** pertinent data.
   • Record collection of the specimen, any pertinent observations of the urine in terms of color, odor, or consistency, and any difficulty in voiding that the client experienced.
   • Indicate on the lab slip if the client is taking any current antibiotic therapy or if the client is menstruating.

Variation

Sterile urine specimens can be obtained from closed drainage systems by inserting a sterile needle attached to a syringe through a drainage port in the tubing. Aspiration of urine from catheters can be done only with self-sealing rubber catheters—not plastic, silicone, or Silastic catheters. When self-sealing rubber catheters are used, the needle is inserted just above the location where the catheter is attached to the drainage tubing. The area from which to obtain urine may be marked by a patch on the catheter (see Figure 4-12 ◆).

To collect a specimen from a Foley (retention) catheter or a drainage tube, follow these steps:

• Wash hands and observe other appropriate infection control procedures (e.g., gloves).
• If there is no urine in the catheter, clamp the drainage tubing for about 30 minutes. *This allows fresh urine to collect in the catheter.*
• Where the needle will be inserted into the catheter, wipe the area with a disinfectant swab. The site should be distal to the tube leading to the balloon to avoid puncturing this tube. *Disinfecting the needle insertion site removes any microorganisms on the surface of the catheter, thereby avoiding contamination of the needle and the entrance of microorganisms into the catheter.*
• Insert the needle at a 30- to 45-degree angle (Figure 4-12). *This angle of entrance facilitates self-sealing of the rubber.*
• Unclamp the catheter.
• Withdraw the required amount of urine, for example, 3 mL for a urine culture or 30 mL for a routine urinalysis.
• Transfer the urine to the specimen container. Make sure the needle does not touch the outside of the container if a sterile culture tube is used.
• Without recapping the needle, discard the syringe and needle into an appropriate sharps container.
• Remove gloves and discard appropriately.

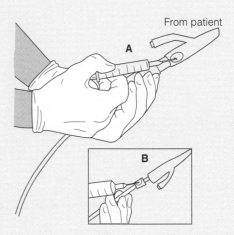

FIGURE 4-12 ◆ Obtaining a urine specimen from a retention catheter: (A) from a specific area near the end of the catheter; (B) from an access port in the tubing.

- Label the container and send the urine to the laboratory immediately for analysis or refrigeration.

- Record collection of the specimen and any pertinent observations of the urine on the appropriate records.

EVALUATION

- Report lab results to the physician.
- Discuss findings of laboratory test with physician and client.
- Conduct appropriate follow-up nursing interventions as needed, such as administering ordered medications and client teaching.

Nursing Process: Urine Testing

ASSESSMENT

- Determine the rationale for the test for each individual client, for example, to determine hydration status, acidity or alkalinity of the client's urine, the presence of glucose and ketone bodies in the urine, or the presence of occult blood in the urine.
- Testing urine for glucose is not a measure of current blood glucose level and is considered an inadequate measurement. Testing urine for glucose is *only* for people *who cannot or will not* test their blood glucose levels (American Diabetes Association, 2000, p. 66).
- Urine testing for ketone level is advised for Type I diabetics who are at home and not feeling well, running a fever, or their blood glucose is consistently over 240 mg/dL (American Diabetes Association, 2000, p. 66).

PLANNING

Delegation

Urine testing may be performed by UAP. It is important that the UAP understands the specific specimen collection procedure and reports the results of the test to the nurse. Inform the UAP to save the urine sample to allow the nurse to repeat the test if necessary.

Equipment

For All Tests
- Gloves

For Specific Gravity
- Urinometer (hydrometer) and a glass cylinder *or* spectrometer or refractometer

For Urine pH
- Litmus paper (red or blue)

For Glucose
- Reagent tablet or reagent test strip
- Appropriate color chart
- Clean test tube and a dropper, if a tablet is used

For Ketone Bodies
- Reagent tablet or test strip

For Occult Blood
- Reagent strip

Preparation

- Use a fresh urine sample.
- Determine the appropriate equipment and testing product for the client.
- Follow the manufacturer's instructions.

Performance

1. Explain to the client what you are going to do, why it is necessary, and how they can cooperate. Discuss how the results will be used in planning further care or treatments.

2. Wash hands and observe other appropriate infection control procedures.

3. Provide for client privacy.

4. Measuring specific gravity:
- To measure with a **urinometer:**
  a. Put on gloves and pour at least 20 mL of a fresh urine sample into the glass cylinder, or fill the cylinder three-quarters full.
  b. Place the urinometer into the cylinder, and give it a gentle spin to prevent it from adhering to the sides of the cylinder.
  c. Hold the urinometer at eye level, and read the measurement at the base of the meniscus at the surface of the urine (Figure 4-13 ◆). The concentration of the urine affects the degree to which the urinometer will float. The depth to which it sinks indicates the specific gravity.
- To measure with a **spectrometer** or **refractometer:**
  a. Be sure to follow the manufacturer's directions.
  b. Put on gloves, and place one or two drops of urine on the slide.
  c. Turn on the instrument light and look into the instrument. The specific gravity will appear on a scope.
  d. Write down the number, then turn off the instrument.
  e. Remove the urine with a damp towel or gauze.

5. To measure pH:
- Put on a glove and dip a strip of either red or blue litmus paper into the urine specimen.
- Observe the color of the litmus paper and compare it to a standardized color chart on the bottle. The blue litmus paper, more commonly used, remains blue if the urine is alkaline and turns red if it is acidic. The red litmus paper remains red in the presence of acidic urine and turns blue if the urine is alkaline. Whichever litmus strip is used, red always indicates acidic urine and blue always indicates alkaline urine.

6. To test for glucose:
- Obtain a freshly voided specimen. Most agencies require a **second-voided specimen:** Ask the client to void, and in 30 minutes to void again, providing a specimen for the test this time. *A second-voided specimen more accurately reflects the present condition of the body.* Urine that has accumulated in the bladder (e.g., overnight) reflects the condition of the body at the time the urine was produced (e.g., 0300 hours).
- To carry out the test, put on gloves and follow the directions specified by the manufacturer. If Clinitest tablets are used, be careful not to touch the bottom of the test tube because it becomes extremely hot when the tablet boils in the presence of urine and water.

7. To test for ketone bodies:
- Put on a glove and place one or two drops of urine on a reagent tablet (e.g., an Acetest tablet) or dip a reagent test strip (e.g., Ketostix) into the urine.
- Observe and compare the results with the appropriate color chart to determine the quantity of ketones present (see Figure 4-14 ◆).

8. To test for occult blood:
- Put on a glove, and dip the reagent strip (e.g., Hemastix) into a sample of urine.
- Compare the color change with a color chart in the same manner as with other reagent strips.

9. For all tests:
- Discard the urine following the tests. Clean the equipment with soap and water. Remove gloves.

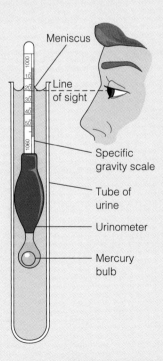

FIGURE 4-13 ◆ A urinometer measurement of the specific gravity of the urine is taken at the base of the meniscus.

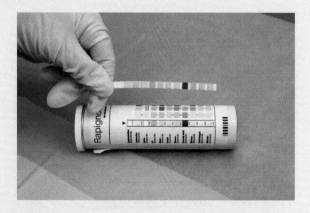

FIGURE 4-14 ◆ After dipping the reagent strip into fresh urine, wait the stated time period and compare the results to the color chart.

10. **Document** the results in accordance with the product used and agency practice.

AMBULATORY AND COMMUNITY SETTINGS

Urine Specimen

- Assess the client's ability and willingness to collect a timed urine specimen. If poor eyesight or hand tremors are a problem, suggest using a clean funnel to pour the urine into the container.
- Always wash hands well with warm, soapy water before and after collecting urine samples.

- Always wear gloves if handling another person's urine.

The home should have a refrigerator or other method for cooling the urine samples. Tell the client to keep the specimen container in a plastic or paper bag in the refrigerator, separate from other refrigerator contents. The client may also use a cooler with ice.

AGE-RELATED CONSIDERATIONS

Urine Specimen

Infant

- The process for cleaning the perineal area and the urethral opening is similar to the process for an adult. A specimen bag, however, is used to collect the urine specimen. The specimen bag has an adhesive backing that attaches to the skin. After the infant has voided a desired amount, gently remove the bag from the skin.
- If you are having trouble obtaining a bagged urine specimen from an infant, try cutting a hole in the diaper (front for a boy and middle for a girl) and pulling part of the bag through. You can see when urine is collected without having to untape the diaper (Lindemann, 2000).

Child

- When collecting a routine urine specimen, explain the procedure in simple, nonmedical terms to the child and ask the child to void using a potty chair or a bedpan placed inside the toilet.
- Give the child a clean specimen container to play with.
- Allow a parent to assist the child, if possible. The child may feel more comfortable with a parent.

Elders

- For a clean-catch urine specimen, an older adult may have difficulty controlling the stream of urine.
- An older adult with arthritis may have difficulty holding the labia apart during the collection of a clean-catch urine specimen.

EVALUATION

- Relate test results to client's health status and nursing assessments.
- Compare test results to prior results. Is there a pattern developing? Is the pattern reflective of a positive or negative outcome for the client?
- Report abnormal results to the physician.

Sputum, Nose, and Throat Specimens

Sputum is the mucous secretion from the lungs, bronchi, and trachea. It is important to differentiate it from **saliva**, the clear liquid secreted by the salivary glands in the mouth, sometimes referred to as "spit." Healthy individuals do not produce sputum.

Sputum specimens are ordered for culture and sensitivity to identify a specific microorganism and its drug sensitivities. Cytology studies of the respiratory system often require serial collection of three early morning specimens, which are tested to identify cancer in the lung and its specific cell type. Tests to determine the presence of **acid-fast bacillus (AFB)** also require serial collection of sputum specimens, often for 3 consecutive days, to identify the presence of **tuberculosis (TB)**. Some agencies use a special glass container when the presence of AFB is suspected.

Clients need to cough to bring sputum up from the lungs, bronchi, and trachea into the mouth and expectorate it into a collecting container. Sputum specimens are often collected in the morning. On awakening, the client can cough up the secretions that have accumulated during the night. Technique 4-8 describes how to collect a sputum specimen. Sometimes, specimens are collected during **postural drainage**, when the client can usually produce sputum. When a client cannot cough, the nurse must sometimes use pharyngeal suctioning (see Chapter 21) to obtain a specimen.

Nursing Process: Sputum Specimens

ASSESSMENT

- Determine the client's ability to cough and expectorate secretions. What type of assistance is required to produce the specimen, for example, the need to splint an abdominal incision, the need to be placed in postural drainage position beforehand, or the need to perform deep-breathing exercises beforehand?

- Assess baseline data such as skin color and rate, depth, and pattern of respiration.

PLANNING

Before collecting a sputum specimen, identify the purpose for which it is to be obtained. This often determines the number of specimens to obtain and the time of day to obtain them.

Delegation

UAP can obtain a sputum specimen that is expectorated by a client. It is important to instruct the UAP as to when to collect the specimen, how to position the client, and how to correctly collect the specimen. Obtaining a sputum specimen by use of pharyngeal suctioning, however, should be performed by the nurse because it is an invasive, sterile process and requires knowledge application and problem solving.

IMPLEMENTATION:
TECHNIQUE 4-8 COLLECTING A SPUTUM SPECIMEN

Equipment

- Sterile specimen container with a cover
- Disposable gloves (if assisting the client)
- Disinfectant and swabs, or liquid soap and water
- Paper towels
- Completed label
- Completed laboratory requisition
- Mouthwash

Preparation

Determine the method of collection and gather the appropriate equipment.

Performance

1. Explain to the client what you are going to do, why it is necessary, and how he or she can cooperate. Discuss how the results will be used in planning further care or treatments. Give the client the following information and instructions:
   - The purpose of the test, the difference between sputum and saliva, and how to provide the sputum specimen
   - Not to touch the inside of the sputum container
   - To expectorate the sputum directly into the sputum container
   - To keep the outside of the container free of sputum, if possible

   - How to hold a pillow firmly against an abdominal incision if the client finds it painful to cough
   - The amount of sputum required (usually, 1 to 2 tsp [5 to 10 mL] of sputum is sufficient for analysis)

2. Wash hands and observe other appropriate infection control procedures.

3. Provide for client privacy.

4. Provide necessary assistance to collect the specimen.
   - Assist the client to a standing or a sitting position (e.g., high- or semi-Fowler's position or on the edge of a bed or in a chair). *These positions allow maximum lung ventilation and expansion.*
   - Ask the client to hold the sputum cup on the outside, or, for a client who is not able to do so, put on gloves and hold the cup for the client (Figure 4-15 ◆).
   - Ask the client to breathe deeply and then cough up secretions. *A deep inhalation provides sufficient air to force secretions out of the airways and into the pharynx.*
   - Hold the sputum cup so that the client can expectorate into it, making sure that the sputum does not come in contact with the outside of the container. *Containing the sputum within the cup restricts the spread of microorganisms to others.*
   - Assist the client to repeat coughing until a sufficient amount of sputum has been collected.
   - Cover the container with the lid immediately after the sputum is in the container. *Covering the*

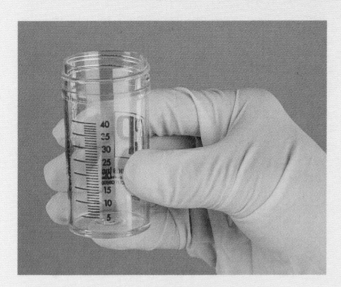

FIGURE 4-15 ◆ Sputum specimen container.

container prevents the inadvertent spread of microorganisms to others.

- If spillage occurs on the outside of the container, clean the outer surface with a disinfectant. Some agencies recommend washing the outside of all containers with liquid soap and water and then drying with a paper towel.
- Remove and discard the gloves.

5. Ensure client comfort.
   - Assist the client to rinse his or her mouth with a mouthwash as needed.
   - Assist the client to a position of comfort that allows maximum lung expansion as required.

6. Label and transport the specimen to the laboratory.
   - Ensure that the specimen label and the laboratory requisition contain the correct information. Attach the label and requisition securely to the specimen. *Inaccurate identification and/or information on the specimen container can lead to errors of diagnosis or therapy.*
   - Arrange for the specimen to be sent to the laboratory immediately or refrigerated. *Bacterial cultures must be started immediately before any contaminating organisms can grow, multiply, and produce false results.*

7. **Document** all relevant information.
   - Document the collection of the sputum specimen on the client's chart. Include the amount, color, consistency (thick, tenacious, watery), presence of hemoptysis (blood in the sputum), odor of the sputum, any measures needed to obtain the specimen (e.g., postural drainage), the general amount of sputum produced, and any discomfort experienced by the client.

EVALUATION

- In addition to assessing the client's sputum, relate respiration rate and any abnormalities or difficulty breathing after the specimen collection to your baseline data. For example, assess the color of the client's skin and mucous membranes, especially any cyanosis, which can indicate impaired blood oxygenation. Monitor vital signs and pulse oximetry if appropriate.
- Report the lab results of the sputum specimen(s) to the physician.

Nose and Throat Specimens

A **throat culture** sample is collected from the mucosa of the oropharynx and tonsillar regions using a culture swab. The sample is then cultured and examined for the presence of disease-producing microorganisms. A **nose culture** sample is collected from the mucosa of the nasal passages using a culture swab.

Technique 4-9 describes how to obtain nose and throat specimens.

Nursing Process: Nose and Throat Specimens

ASSESSMENT

- Before collecting a nose or throat specimen, determine (1) whether the client is suspected of having a contagious disease (e.g., diptheria), which requires special precautions; and (2) whether a specimen is required from the nasal cavity as well as from the pharynx and/or the tonsils.
- Assess the nasal mucosa and throat noting in particular areas of inflammation and purulent drainage.
- Ask if the client has any complaints of soreness or tenderness.
- Determine the presence of clinical signs of infection (e.g., fever, chills, fatigue).

Delegation

Obtaining nose and throat cultures is an invasive technique that requires the application of scientific knowledge and potential problem solving to ensure client safety. Thus, it is best for the nurse to perform this skill.

IMPLEMENTATION:
TECHNIQUE 4-9 OBTAINING NOSE AND THROAT SPECIMENS

Equipment

- Gloves
- Two sterile cotton-tipped swabs in sterile culture tubes with transport medium
- Penlight
- Tongue blade (optional)
- Otoscope with a nasal speculum (optional)
- Container for the used nasal speculum
- Completed labels for each specimen container
- Completed laboratory requisition

Preparation

Prepare the client and the equipment.

- Assist the client to a sitting position. *This is the most comfortable position for many people and the one in which the pharynx is most readily visible.*
- Put on gloves if the client's mucosa will be touched.
- Open the culture tube and place it on the sterile wrapper. *This prevents microorganisms from entering the tube.*
- Remove one sterile applicator and hold it carefully by the stick end keeping the remainder sterile. The swab end is kept from touching any objects that could contaminate it.

Performance

1. Explain to the client what you are going to do, why it is necessary, and how he or she can cooperate. Discuss how the results will be used in planning further care or treatments. Inform the client that he may gag while swabbing the throat or feel like sneezing during the swabbing of the nose; however, the procedure will take less than one minute.

2. Wash hands and observe other appropriate infection control procedures.

3. Provide for client privacy.

4. Collect the specimen.

For a Throat Specimen

- Ask the client to tilt the head back, open the mouth, extend the tongue, and say "ah." *When the tongue is extended, the pharynx is exposed. Saying "ah" relaxes the throat muscles and helps minimize contraction of the constriction muscle of the pharynx (the gag reflex).*
- Use the penlight to illuminate the posterior pharynx while depressing the tongue with a tongue blade. Depress the anterior third of tongue firmly without touching the throat (Figure 4-16 ◆). *Touching the throat stimulates the gag reflex.* Check for inflamed areas.
- Insert a swab into the mouth without touching any part of the mouth or tongue. *The swab should not pick up microorganisms in the mouth.*
- Gently and quickly, swab along the tonsils making sure to contact any areas on the pharynx that are particularly **erythematous** (reddened) or that contain exudate. *By moving the swab quickly, you can avoid initiating the gag reflex or causing discomfort. Erythematous areas and areas with exudate will likely have the most microorganisms.*
- Remove the swab without touching the mouth or lips. *This prevents the swab from transmitting microorganisms to the mouth.*
- Crush the ampule of culture medium at the bottom of the tube.

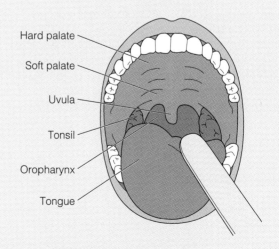

Hard palate

Soft palate

Uvula

Tonsil

Oropharynx

Tongue

FIGURE 4-16 ◆ Diagram of the mouth.

For a Throat Specimen continued

- Insert the swab into the sterile tube without allowing it to touch the outside of the container. Push the tip of the swab into the liquid medium. Make sure the swab is placed in the correctly labeled tube. *Touching the outside of the tube could transmit microorganisms to it and then to others.*

- Place the top securely on the tube, taking care not to touch the inside of the cap. *Touching the inside of the cap could transmit additional microorganisms into the tube.*

- Repeat the above steps with the second swab.

- Discard the tongue blade in the waste container.

- Discard gloves.

For a Nasal Specimen

- Ask the client to blow his nose to clear his nasal passages. Check nostrils with penlight to check for patency.

- If using a nasal speculum, gently insert the lighted nasal speculum up one nostril.

- Insert the sterile swab carefully through the speculum, without touching the edges. *This prevents the swab from picking up microorganisms from the speculum.* When working without a speculum, pass the swab along the septum and the floor of the nose.

- When reaching the area of mucosa that is reddened or contains exudate, rotate the swab quickly.

- Remove the swab without touching the speculum.

- Remove the nasal speculum if used.

- Insert the swab into the culture tube. Crush the ampule at the bottom of the tube and push the tip of the swab into the liquid medium.

- Repeat the above steps for the other nostril.

5. Label and transport the specimens to the laboratory.
   - See Technique 4-6, step 6.

6. **Document** all relevant information.
   - Record the collection of the nose and/or throat specimens on the client's chart. Include the assessments of the nasal mucosa and pharynx, and any discomfort the client experienced.

Variation

A **nasopharyngeal** culture uses the same steps as a nasal culture with the following exceptions: A special cotton-tipped swab on a flexible wire is used. While this swab is still in the package, bend the sterile swab in a curve and then open the package without contaminating the swab. Gently pass the swab through the more patent nostril about three to four inches into the nasopharynx.

AGE-RELATED CONSIDERATIONS

Sputum, Nose, and Throat Specimens

Infant

- Avoid occluding an infant's nose because infants normally breathe only through the nose.

Child

- The young child will need to be restrained gently while the throat or nasal specimen is collected. Allow the parents to assist, and explain that the procedure will be over quickly.

- Cooperative children can be asked to put their hands under their buttocks, open their mouth, and laugh or pant like a dog (Ball & Bindler, 1999).

- Observe for signs of an ear infection (e.g., rubbing the ears). A child's short respiratory tract allows bacteria to migrate easily to the ears.

Elders

- The older client may need encouragement to cough as a decreased cough reflex occurs with aging.

- Allow time for the older client to rest and recover between coughs when obtaining a sputum specimen.

EVALUATION

- While taking the specimen, assess the pharynx, tonsils, and nares for appearance, color, and

amount and consistency of any exudate. Compare this information to future assessment data.

- Report lab results to the physician

TABLE 4-4 KINDS OF WOUND DRAINAGE

Type of Exudate	Description	Constituents
Serous	Watery, clear	Serum, few cells
Purulent	Thicker because of the presence of pus; varies in color (e.g., tinges of blue, green, or yellow). The color may depend on the causative organism.	Leukocytes, liquefied dead tissue debris, and dead and living bacteria
Sanguineous (hemorrhagic)	Dark or bright red. A bright sanguineous exudate indicates fresh bleeding, whereas dark sanguineous exudate denotes older bleeding.	Red blood cells
Serosanguineous	Clear and blood-tinged drainage. Commonly seen in surgical incisions.	Serum and red blood cells
Purosanguineous	Pus and blood. Often seen in a new wound that is infected.	Leukocytes, liquefied dead tissue debris, bacteria, and red blood cells

Wound Drainage Specimen

Kinds of Wound Drainage

Fluid containing cells that has escaped from blood vessels during the inflammatory phase of wound healing and is deposited in tissue or on tissue surfaces is called **exudate**. The nature and amount of exudates vary according to the tissue involved, the intensity and duration of the inflammation, and the presence of microorganisms. There are three major types of exudates: serous, purulent, and sanguineous (hemorrhagic). Descriptions of these exudates are provided in Table 4-4.

One complication of wound healing is infection. A wound can be infected with microorganisms at the time of injury, during surgery, or postoperatively. Wounds that occur as a result of injury (e.g., bullet and knife wounds) are most likely to be contaminated at the time of injury. Surgery involving the intestines can also result in infection from the microorganisms inside the intestine. Surgical infection is most likely to become apparent 2 to 11 days postoperatively.

Wound cultures can either confirm or rule out the presence of infection. Sensitivity studies are helpful in the selection of appropriate antibiotic therapy. The nurse obtains a wound culture whenever an infection is suspected. Technique 4-10 describes how to obtain a specimen of wound drainage.

Nursing Process: Wound Drainage Specimen

ASSESSMENT

- Assess the appearance of the wound and surrounding tissue. Check the character and amount of wound drainage. Is the client complaining of pain at the wound site?
- Assess for signs of infection such as fever, chills, or elevated white blood cell count (WBC).

PLANNING

Before obtaining a specimen of wound drainage determine (1) whether the wound should be cleaned before taking the specimen, and (2) whether the site from which to take the specimen has been specified.

Delegation

Obtaining a wound culture is an invasive procedure that requires the application of sterile technique, knowledge of wound healing, and potential problem solving to ensure client safety, and therefore the nurse needs to perform this skill.

IMPLEMENTATION:
TECHNIQUE 4-10 OBTAINING A WOUND DRAINAGE SPECIMEN

Equipment

- Disposable gloves
- Sterile gloves
- Moisture-resistant bag

- Sterile dressing set
- Normal saline and irrigating syringe
- Culture tube with swab and culture medium (aerobic and anaerobic tubes are available) and/or sterile syringe with needle for anaerobic culture

- Completed labels for each container
- Completed requisition to accompany the specimens to the laboratory

Preparation

Check the medical orders to determine if the specimen is to be collected for an **aerobic** or **anaerobic** culture. Administer an analgesic 30 minutes before the procedure if the client is complaining of pain at the wound site.

Performance

1. Explain to the client what you are going to do, why it is necessary, and how he or she can cooperate. Discuss how the results will be used in planning further care or treatments.

2. Wash hands and observe other appropriate infection control procedures (e.g., gloves).

3. Provide for client privacy.

4. Remove any moist outer dressings that cover the wound.
   - Put on disposable gloves.
   - Remove the outer dressing, and observe any drainage on the dressing. Hold the dressing so that the client does not see the drainage as *the appearance of the drainage could upset the client.*
   - Determine the amount of the drainage, for example, one 2″ × 2″ gauze saturated with pale yellow drainage.
   - Discard the dressing in the moisture-resistant bag. Handle it carefully so that the dressing does not touch the outside of the bag. *Touching the outside of the bag will contaminate it.*
   - Remove your gloves and dispose of them properly.

5. Open the sterile dressing set using sterile technique.
   - See Technique 12-1.

6. Assess the wound.
   - Put on sterile gloves.
   - Assess the appearance of the tissues in and around the wound and the drainage. Infection can cause reddened tissues with a thick discharge, which may be foul-smelling, whitish, or colored.

7. Clean the wound.
   - Irrigate the wound with normal saline until all visible exudates have been washed away. See Technique 30-4.
   - After irrigating, apply a sterile gauze pad to the wound. *This absorbs excess saline.*

- If a topical antimicrobial ointment or cream is being used to treat the wound, use a swab to remove it. *Residual antiseptic must be removed prior to culture.*
- Remove and discard sterile gloves.

8. Obtain the aerobic culture.
   - Open a specimen tube and place the cap upside down on a firm, dry surface so that the inside will not become contaminated, or if the swab is attached to the lid, twist the cap to loosen the swab. Hold the tube in one hand and take out the swab in the other (Figure 4-17 ◆).
   - Rotate the swab back and forth over clean areas of granulation tissue from the sides or base of the wound. *Microorganisms most likely to be responsible for a wound infection reside in viable tissue.*
   - Do not use **pus** or pooled exudates to culture. *These secretions contain a mixture of contaminants that are not the same as those causing the infection.*
   - Avoid touching the swab to intact skin at the wound edges. *This prevents the introduction of superficial skin organisms into the culture.*
   - Return the swab to the culture tube, taking care not to touch the top or the outside of the tube. *The outside of the container must remain free of pathogenic microorganisms to prevent their spread to others.*
   - Crush the inner ampule containing the medium for organism growth at the bottom of the tube. *This ensures that the swab with the specimen is surrounded by culture medium.*
   - Twist the cap to secure.
   - If a specimen is required from another site, repeat the steps. Specify the exact site (e.g., inferior drain site or lower aspect of incision) on the label of each container. Be sure to put each swab in the appropriately labeled tube.

9. Dress the wound.
   - Apply any ordered medication to the wound.

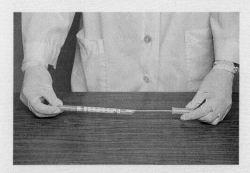

FIGURE 4-17 ◆ A culturette tube for a wound specimen.

- Cover the wound with a sterile moist transparent wound dressing. See Technique 30-7.

10. Arrange for the specimen to be transported to the laboratory immediately. Be sure to include the completed requisition.

11. **Document** all relevant information.
- Record on the client's chart the taking of the specimen and source.
- Include the date and time; the appearance of the wound; the color, consistency, amount, and odor of any drainage; the type of culture collected; and any discomfort experienced by the client.

Variation: Obtaining a Specimen for Anaerobic Culture Using a Sterile Syringe and Needle

- Insert a sterile 10-mL syringe (without needle) into the wound, and aspirate 1 to 5 mL of drainage into the syringe.
- Attach the 21-gauge needle to the syringe, and expel all air from the syringe and needle.
- Immediately inject the drainage into the anaerobic culture tube.
  or
  If a rubber stopper or cork is available, insert the needle into the rubber stopper or cork to prevent the entry of air.
- Label the tube or syringe appropriately.
- Send the tube or syringe of drainage to the laboratory immediately. Do not refrigerate the specimen.

EVALUATION

- Compare findings of wound assessment and drainage to previous assessments to determine any changes.
- Report the culture results to the physician.
- Conduct appropriate follow-up such as administering medications as ordered.

Chapter Summary

TERMINOLOGY

acid-fast bacillus (AFB)	lancet	saliva
aerobic	lancet injector	sanguineous
anaerobic	midstream urine specimen	second-voided specimen
blood glucose meter	nasopharyngeal	serosanguineous
capillary blood glucose (CBG)	nose culture	serous
clean catch	obligatory losses	specimen
dysuria	occult	spectrometer
erythematous	ova and parasites	sputum
exudate	postural drainage	steatorrhea
feces	purosanguineous	throat culture
glucose	purulent	tuberculosis (TB)
guaiac	pus	urinometer
hematuria	reagent	void
insensible fluid loss	refractometer	

Forming Clinical Judgments

Consider This:

1. What should you do if I&O has been ordered for a client and the client informs you that he voided but forgot to use the urinal?

2. What if, when measuring CBG, you do not obtain enough blood to cover the indicator square on the reagent strip?

3. What should you do if the stool becomes contaminated with urine or toilet paper when collecting a stool specimen?

4. What should you do if the client or staff forgot and discarded the client's urine during the collection of a timed 24-hour urine specimen?

5. What if your assessments clearly indicate a wound infection but the culture results return indicating no growth?

Related Research

Barton, S. J., & Holmes, S. S. (1998). Practice applications of research. A comparison of reagent strips and the refractometer for measurement of urine specific gravity in hospitalized children. *Pediatric Nursing, 24*(5), 480–482.

Brenton, S. (1997). RSV specimen collection methods: Nasal vs nasopharyngeal. *Pediatric Nursing, 11*(21), 621–623.

References

____(2000). Shopping around for the perfect blood glucose meter. *Nursing, 30*(8), 60–61.

Altman, G. B., Buschsel, P., & Coxon, V. (2000). *Fundamental and Advanced Nursing Skills*. Albany, NY: Delmar.

American Diabetes Association. (2000, January). Resource Guide 2000: Urine testing. *Diabetes Forecast Supplement,* 66–67.

American Diabetes Association. (2000, January). Resource Guide 2000: Blood glucose monitors and data management. *Diabetes Forecast Supplement,* 42–56.

Ball, J., & Bindler, R. (1999). *Pediatric Nursing, Caring for Children*, 2nd ed. Stamford, CT: Appleton & Lange.

Ball, J., & Bindler, R. (1999). *Pediatric Clinical Skills*. Stamford, CT: Appleton & Lange.

Brazier, A. M., & Palmer, M. H. (1995). Collecting clean-catch urine in the nursing home: Obtaining the uncontaminated specimen. *Geriatric Nursing: American Journal of Care for the Aging, 16*(5), 217–224.

Cook, R. (1996). Urinalysis: Ensuring accurate urine testing. *Nursing Standard, 10*, 45, 49–52.

Dammel, T. (1997). Fecal occult blood testing: Looking for hidden danger. *Nursing, 27*(7), 44–45.

Elkin, M. K., Perry, A. G., & Potter, P. A. (2000). *Nursing Interventions & Clinical Skills*, 2nd ed. St. Louis: Mosby.

Fann, B. D. (1998). Fluid and electrolyte balance in the pediatric patient. *Journal of Intravenous Nursing, 21*(3), 153–159.

Frizzell, J. (1998). Avoiding lab test pitfalls. *American Journal of Nursing, 98*(2), 34–37.

Halloran, S., & Bennitt, W. (1999). Urine reagent strips: An MDA evaluation. *Professional Nurse, 14*(11), 791–792, 794–796.

Kee, J. L., (1999). *Laboratory & Diagnostic Tests with Nursing Implications*, 5th ed. Stamford, CT: Appleton & Lange.

Lindemann, M. (2000). Tips & Timesavers. *Nursing, 30*(3), 70.

Metheny, N. M. (1996). *Fluid and Electrolyte Balance: Nursing Considerations* (3rd ed.). Philadelphia: Lippincott.

Papasian, C. J., & Kragel, P. J. (1997). The microbiology laboratory's role in life-threatening infections. *Critical Care Nursing Quarterly, 20*, 44–60.

Parini, S. (2000). How to collect specimens. *Nursing, 30*(5), 66–67.

Semple, M., & Elley, K. (1998). Practical procedures for nurses. Collecting a sputum specimen. *Nursing Times, 94*(48), 2–8.

Smith, S. F., Duell, D. J., & Martin, B. C. (2000). *Clinical Nursing Skills Basic to Advanced Skills*. Upper Saddle River, NJ: Prentice Hall Health.

Wells, M. (1997). Urinalysis. *Professional Nurse, 13*(2), S11–13, S15.

Chapter 5

Positioning the Client

Techniques

OBJECTIVES

- Identify essential guidelines for safe and efficient body movements.
- Use correct body mechanics when assisting clients to move.
- Describe essential steps and rationale of techniques to position, move, and turn clients in bed and to transfer clients from bed to chair or stretcher.
- Effectively support and maintain proper alignment of clients for the described bed positions included in this chapter.
- Position, move, turn, and transfer clients safely.

Body Mechanics

Body mechanics is the term used to describe the efficient, coordinated, and safe use of the body to move objects and carry out the activities of daily living. The major purpose of body mechanics is to facilitate the safe and efficient use of appropriate muscle groups to maintain balance, reduce the energy required, reduce fatigue, and decrease the risk of injury. Good body mechanics is essential to both clients and nurses. Back injuries affect up to 38 percent of all nurses (American Nurses Association, 2000). Therefore, it is imperative that nurses know and use proper technique when moving and turning clients in bed and transferring clients between beds, wheelchairs, and stretchers. One way to help prevent back injury is to use correct body mechanics.

Elements of Body Mechanics

Body Alignment (Posture)

Body **alignment** is the geometric arrangement of body parts in relation to each other. Good alignment promotes optimal balance and maximal body function in whatever position the client assumes: standing, sitting, or lying down. Good body alignment and good **posture** are synonymous terms. When the body is well aligned, it achieves balance without undue strain on the joints, muscles, tendons, or ligaments.

Balance

Balance is a state of equilibrium in which opposing forces counteract each other. Good body alignment is essential to body balance. It is difficult to differentiate balance from body alignment, although balance is the result of proper alignment. A person maintains balance as long as the **line of gravity** (an imaginary vertical line drawn through an object's center of gravity) passes through the **center of gravity** (the point at which all of the mass of an object is centered) and the **base of support** (the foundation on which an object rests).

The center of gravity of a well-aligned standing adult is located slightly anterior to the upper part of the sacrum (see Figure 5-1 ◆). For greatest balance and stability, a standing adult must center body weight symmetrically along the line of gravity.

In a well-aligned standing person, the center of gravity remains fairly stable. When a person moves, however, the center of gravity shifts continuously in the direction of the moving body parts. Balance depends on the interrelationship of the center of gravity, the line of gravity, and the base of support. When a person moves, the closer the line of gravity is to the center of the base of support, the greater the person's stability (Figure 5-2A ◆). Conversely, the closer the line of gravity is to the edge of the base of support, the

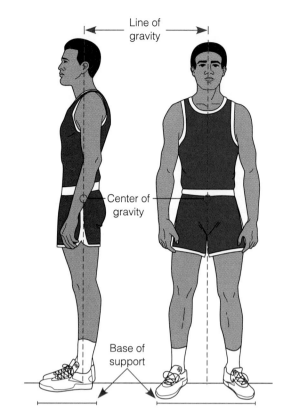

FIGURE 5-1 ◆ The center of gravity and the line of gravity influence standing alignment.

more precarious the balance (Figure 5-2B). If the line of gravity falls outside the base of support, the person falls (Figure 5-2C).

The broader the base of support and the lower the center of gravity, the greater the stability and balance. Body balance, therefore, can be greatly enhanced by (1) widening the base of support and (2) lowering the center of gravity, bringing it closer to the base of support. The base of support is easily widened by spreading the feet farther apart. The center of gravity is readily lowered by flexing the hips and knees until a squatting position is achieved. The importance of a balanced center of gravity promoting effective body mechanics cannot be overemphasized for nurses.

Coordinated Body Movement

Body mechanics involves the integrated functioning of the musculoskeletal and nervous systems. Muscle tone, the neuromuscular reflexes, and the coordinated movements of opposing voluntary muscle groups play important roles in producing balanced, smooth, purposeful movement.

Principles of Body Mechanics

Lifting

Nursing personnel often lift objects from the floor and assume a bending position, for example, when help-

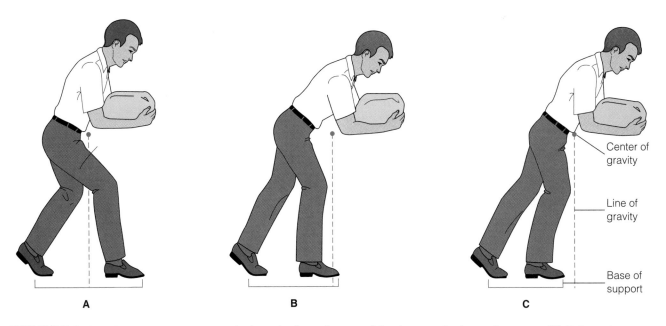

FIGURE 5-2 ◆ (A) Balance is maintained when the line of gravity falls close to the base of support. (B) Balance is precarious when the line of gravity falls at the edge of the base of support. (C) Balance cannot be maintained when the line of gravity falls outside the base of support.

ing clients to put on slippers, placing foot pedals down on wheelchairs, picking up laundry, and lifting supplies from the bottom shelves of carts. When a person lifts or carries an object, the weight of the object becomes part of the person's body weight and affects the location of the person's center of gravity. By holding the lifted object as close as possible to the body's center of gravity, the lifter avoids undue displacement of the center of gravity and achieves greater stability.

People can lift more weight when they use a lever than when they do not. In the body, the bones of the skeleton act as levers, a joint is a fulcrum (fixed point about which a lever moves), and the muscles exert the force. When the nurse lifts objects, the resisting force or weight is held in the hands or on the forearms, the fulcrum is the elbow, and the force is applied by contraction of the flexor muscles of the forearm (Figure 5-3 ◆). The lifting power is increased when the elbow (fulcrum) is supported on a bed surface or a countertop. Use of the arms as levers is often applied in clinical practice when the nurse needs to raise a client's head off the bed, for example, or give back care to a client in traction.

Because lifting involves movement against gravity, the nurse must use major muscle groups of the thighs, knees, upper and lower arms, abdomen, and pelvis to prevent back strain. The nurse can increase overall muscle strength by the synchronized use of as many muscle groups as possible during an activity. For instance, when the arms are used in an activity, dividing the work between the arms and legs helps to prevent back strain. Lifting power is further enhanced by using the nurse's body weight to counteract the client's

weight. The nurse increases hip and knee flexion to lower the center of gravity. As the nurse does so, the forearms and hands supporting the client automatically rise.

Another technique based on the principle of leverage can be used when lifting objects from the floor to waist level. In this technique, the back and knees are flexed until the load is at thigh level, at which point the person flexes the knees more to provide thrust as the back begins to straighten. This technique provides for balance, leverage, and synchronized use of muscles, which help to avoid back pain and injury. When one lifts an object to knee level, the shoulder and arm muscles pull, the abdominal and lumbar muscles contract for leverage and pull, and the thigh and leg mus-

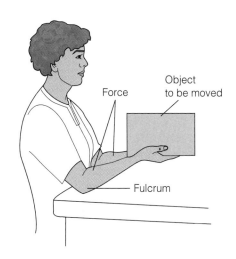

FIGURE 5-3 ◆ Using the arm as a lever.

cles exert the upward thrust to bring the object off the floor. When one lifts an object from midthigh to waist level, force is provided essentially by the leg and thigh muscle groups, but the back and lumbar muscles remain contracted.

In all positions, it is important to maintain a distance of at least 30 cm (12 in) between the feet and to keep the load close to the body, especially when it is at knee level. Before attempting the lift, the nurse must ensure that there are no hazards on the floor, that there is a clear path for moving the object, and that the nurse's base of support is secure.

Pulling and Pushing

When pulling or pushing an object, a person maintains balance with least effort when the base of support is enlarged in the direction in which the movement is to be produced or opposed. When pushing an object, for example, a person can enlarge the base of support by moving the front foot forward. When pulling an object, a person can enlarge the base of support by (1) moving the rear leg back if the person is facing the object; or (2) moving the front foot forward if the person is facing away from the object. It is easier and safer to pull an object toward one's own center of gravity than to push it away, as the person can exert more control of the object's movement when pulling it.

Pivoting

Pivoting is a technique in which the body is turned in a way that avoids twisting of the spine. To **pivot**, place one foot ahead of the other, raise the heels very slightly, and put the body weight on the balls of the feet. When the weight is off the heels, the frictional surface is decreased and the knees are not twisted when the body turns. Keeping the body aligned, turn (pivot) about 90 degrees in the desired direction. The foot that was forward will now be behind.

A summary of principles and guidelines related to body mechanics is shown in Table 5-1.

Preventing Back Injury

Nurses provide clients the opportunity for position change, lung expansion, and a change in environment as appropriate. It is important, however, that nurses not jeopardize their own health while caring for clients. Client positioning, lifting, and transferring are significant risk factors for back injuries. The National Institute of Occupational Safety and Health (NIOSH) says that a 51-pound stable object with handles is the maximum amount anyone should lift (American Nurses Association, 2000).

Two movements to avoid because of their potential for causing back injury are twisting (rotation) of the thoracolumbar spine and acute flexion of the back with hips and knees straight (stooping). Undesirable

twisting of the back can be prevented by squarely facing the direction of movement, whether pushing, pulling, or sliding and moving the object directly toward or away from one's center of gravity.

Lower back injuries are preventable. Some guidelines for preventing back injuries are presented in Box 5-1.

Positioning Clients in Bed

Positioning a client in good body alignment and changing the position regularly and systematically are essential aspects of nursing practice. Clients who can move easily automatically reposition themselves for comfort. Such people generally require minimal positioning assistance from nurses, other than guidance about ways to maintain body alignment and to exercise their joints. People who are weak, frail, in pain, paralyzed, or unconscious, however, rely on nurses to provide or assist with position changes. For all clients, it is important to assess the skin and provide skin care before and after a position change.

Any position, correct or incorrect, can be detrimental if maintained for a prolonged period. Frequent change of position helps to prevent muscle discomfort, undue pressure resulting in pressure ulcers, damage to superficial nerves and blood vessels, and **contractures.** Position changes also maintain muscle tone and stimulate postural reflexes.

When the client is not able to move independently or assist with moving, the *preferred method is to use two or more nurses to move or turn the client.* Appropriate assistance reduces the risk of muscle strain and body injury to both the client and nurse.

When positioning clients in bed, the nurse can do a number of things to ensure proper alignment and promote client comfort and safety:

- Make sure the mattress is firm and level, yet has enough give to fill in and support natural body curvatures.

- Ensure that the bed is kept clean and dry. Less friction between the object moved and the surface on which it is moved requires less energy for the nurse. Make sure the client's extremities can move freely whenever possible.

- Place support devices in specified areas according to the client's position. (See Box 5-2 for commonly used support devices.) Use only those support devices needed to maintain alignment and to prevent stress on the client's muscles and joints. If the person is capable of movement, too many devices limit mobility and increase the potential for muscle weakness and atrophy. Common alignment prob-

TABLE 5-1	SUMMARY OF GUIDELINES AND PRINCIPLES RELATED TO BODY MECHANICS	

Guidelines	Principles
Plan the move or transfer carefully. Free the surrounding area of obstacles.	Appropriate preparation prevents potential falls and injury.
Obtain the assistance of other people or use mechanical devices to move objects that are too heavy. Encourage clients to assist as much as possible. Use arms as levers whenever possible to increase lifting power.	The heavier an object, the greater the force needed to move the object.
Adjust the working area to waist level and keep the body close to the area. Elevate adjustable beds and overbed tables or lower the bedside rails to prevent stretching and reaching.	Objects that are close to the center of gravity are moved with the least effort.
Use proper alignment. Stand as close as possible to the object to be moved. Avoid stretching, reaching, and twisting, which may place the line of gravity outside the base of support.	Balance is maintained and muscle strain is avoided as long as the line of gravity passes through the base of support.
Before moving an object, widen your stance and flex your knees, hips, and ankles.	The wider the base of support and the lower the center of gravity, the greater the stability.
Before moving an object, contract your gluteal, abdominal, leg, and arm muscles to prepare them for action.	The greater the preparatory contraction of muscles before moving an object, the less the energy required to move it, and the less likelihood of musculoskeletal strain and injury.
Always face the direction of the movement.	Ineffective use of major muscle groups occurs when the spine is rotated or twisted.
Avoid working against gravity. Pull, push, roll, or turn objects instead of lifting them. Lower the head of the client's bed before moving the client up in bed.	Moving an object along a level surface requires less energy than moving an object up an inclined surface or lifting it against the force of gravity. Pulling creates less friction than pushing.
Use your gluteal and leg muscles rather than the sacrospinal muscles of your back to exert an upward thrust when lifting. Distribute the workload between both arms and legs to prevent back strain.	The synchronized use of as many large muscle groups as possible during an activity increases overall strength and prevents muscle fatigue and injury.
When *pushing* an object, enlarge the base of support by moving the front foot forward. When *pulling* an object, enlarge the base of support by either moving the rear leg back if facing the object or moving the front foot forward if facing away from the object.	Balance is maintained with minimal effort when the base of support is enlarged in the direction in which the movement will occur.
When moving or carrying objects, hold them as close as possible to your center of gravity.	The closer the line of gravity to the center of the base of support, the greater the stability.
Use the weight of the body as a force for pulling or pushing, by rocking on the feet or leaning forward or backward.	Body weight adds force to counteract the weight of the object and reduces the amount of strain on the arms and back.

lems that can be corrected with support devices include:

Flexion of the neck

Internal rotation of the shoulder

Adduction of the shoulder

Flexion of the wrist

Anterior convexity of the lumbar spine

External rotation of the hips

Hyperextension of the knees

Plantar flexion of the ankle

• Avoid placing one body part, particularly one with bony prominences, directly on top of another body part. Excessive pressure can damage veins and pre-dispose the client to thrombus formation. Pressure against the popliteal space may damage nerves and blood vessels in this area.

• Plan a *systematic 24-hour schedule* for position changes. Frequent position changes are essential to prevent pressure ulcers in immobilized clients. Such clients should be repositioned every 2 hours throughout the day and night and more frequently when there is a risk for skin breakdown. This schedule is usually outlined on the client's nursing care plan.

• Always obtain information from the client to determine which position is most comfortable and appropriate. Seeking information from the client about what feels best is a useful guide when align-

Box 5-1 *Preventing Back Injuries*

- Become consciously aware of your posture and body mechanics.
- Make it a habit to review the principles of good body mechanics. Ask the physical therapy department to provide in-service education on transfer techniques.
- Exercise regularly to maintain overall physical condition. Include exercises that strengthen the pelvic, abdominal, and lumbar muscles.
- Ask others to assist you when moving a client who cannot move independently and has limited mobility.

- When moving an object, spread your feet apart to provide a wide base of support.
- When lifting an object, distribute the weight between large muscles of the legs and arms.
- Use mechanical lifting devices, transfer boards, and other tools to promote client safety and healthy backs.
- Inform those you supervise that using mechanical transfer devices consistently is the expected practice.

ing persons and is an essential aspect of evaluating the effectiveness of an alignment intervention. Sometimes, a person who appears well aligned may be experiencing real discomfort. Both appearance, in relation to alignment criteria, and comfort are important in achieving effective alignment.

Fowler's Position

Fowler's position, or a semisitting position, is a bed position in which the head and trunk are raised and the knees may or may not be flexed. Nurses, therefore, need to clarify the meaning of the term *Fowler's position* in a particular agency. For example, Fowler's position may refer to elevation of the upper part of the body without knee flexion and the term *semi-Fowler's* may refer to the sitting position with knee flexion.

The most common Fowler's position is **semi-Fowler's position** in which the head and trunk are raised 45 to 60 degrees. Clients are in **low-Fowler's position** when their head and trunk are raised 15 to 45 degrees. In **high-Fowler's position**, the client's head and torso are raised 60 to 90 degrees. See Box 5-3 and Technique 5-1 for information about positioning a client in semi-Fowler's position. Fowler's position is the position of choice for people who have difficulty breathing and for some people with heart problems. Gravity pulls the diaphragm downward allowing greater lung expansion when the client is in semi- or high-Fowler's position. Clients who are confined to bed but are capable of eating, reading, watching television, or visiting find this position comfortable.

Box 5-2 *Support Devices*

- *Pillows.* Different sizes are available. Used for support or elevation of an arm or leg. Specially designed dense pillows can be used to elevate the upper body.
- *Mattresses.* There are two types of mattresses: ones that fit on the bed frame (e.g., standard bed mattress) and mattresses that fit on the standard bed mattress (e.g., egg crate mattress). Mattresses should be evenly supportive.
- *Foot boot.* These are made of a variety of substances. They usually have a firm exterior and padding of foam to protect the skin. They provide support to the feet in a natural position and keep the weight of covers off the toes.
- *Footboard.* A flat panel often made of plastic or wood. It keeps the feet in dorsiflexion to prevent plantar flexion.
- *Trochanter roll.* Usually made by rolling a towel or bath blanket. Placed from the client's iliac crest to midthigh. Prevents external rotation of leg when client is in a supine position.
- *Hand roll.* Can be made by rolling a washcloth. Purpose is to keep hand in a functional position and prevent finger contractures.

- *Abduction pillow.* A triangular shaped foam pillow that maintains hip abduction to prevent hip dislocation following total hip replacement (see figure).

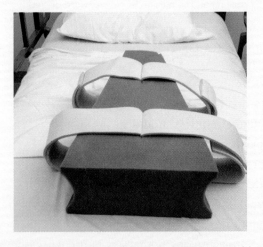

Maintaining postoperative abduction following total hip replacement.

Box 5-3 *Semi-Fowler's Position (Supported)*

Bed-sitting position with upper part of body elevated 45 to 60 degrees commencing at hips.

Measures to Promote Alignment and Comfort*

- Pillow at lower back to support lumbar region and prevent posterior flexion of lumbar curvature.

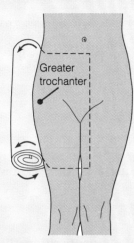

Making a trochanter roll: (1) Fold the towel in half lengthwise. (2) Roll the towel tightly, starting at one narrow edge and rolling within approximately 30 cm (1 ft) of the other edge. (3) Invert the roll. Then palpate the greater trochanter of the femur and place the roll with the center at the level of the greater trochanter; place the flat part of towel under the client; then roll the towel snugly against the hip.

* The amount of support depends on the needs of the individual client.

- Pillow to support head, neck, and upper back to prevent hyperextension of neck. Avoid too large a pillow or too many pillows as they may cause neck flexion contractures.
- Pillow under forearms to eliminate pull on shoulder and assist venous blood flow from hands and lower arms.
- Small pillow under thighs to flex knees to prevent hyperextension of knees.
- Trochanter roll lateral to femur to prevent external rotation of hips (see figure at left).
- Footboard to provide support for dorsiflexion and prevent plantar flexion of feet (footdrop).

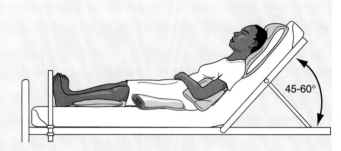

Semi-Fowler's position (supported).

Orthopneic Position

An adaptation of high-Fowler's position is the **orthopneic position**. The client sits either in bed or on the side of the bed with an overbed table across the lap (Figure 5-4 ◆). This position facilitates respiration by allowing maximum chest expansion. It is particularly helpful to clients who have problems exhaling because they can press the lower part of the chest against the edge of the overbed table.

Dorsal Recumbent Position

In the **dorsal recumbent (back-lying) position**, the client's head and shoulders are slightly elevated on a small pillow. In some agencies, the terms *dorsal recumbent* and *supine* are used interchangeably. Strictly speaking, however, in the supine or dorsal position, the head and shoulders are not elevated. The dorsal recumbent position is used to provide comfort and to facilitate healing following certain surgeries or anesthetics (e.g., spinal). See Box 5-4 and Technique 5-1 for

information about positioning a client in dorsal recumbent position.

Prone Position

In the **prone position**, the client lies on his or her abdomen with the head turned to one side. The hips are not flexed. Both children and adults sleep in this

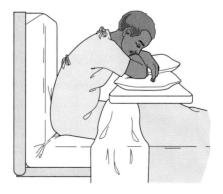

FIGURE 5-4 ◆ Orthopneic position.

Box 5-4 *Dorsal Recumbent Position (Supported)*

Measures to Promote Alignment and Support*

- Pillow of suitable thickness under head and shoulders if necessary for alignment and to prevent hyperextension of neck in thick-chested person.
- Roll or small pillow under lumbar curvature to prevent posterior flexion of lumbar curvature.
- Roll or sandbag placed laterally to trochanter of femur to prevent external rotation of legs.
- Small pillow under thigh to flex knee slightly and prevent hyperextension of knees.

* Amount of support depends on the needs of the individual client.

- Footboard or rolled pillow to support feet in dorsiflexion and to prevent plantar flexion (footdrop).
- Pillow under lower legs to prevent pressure on heels.

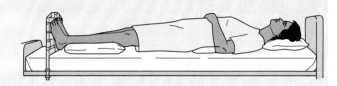

Dorsal recumbent position (supported).

position, sometimes with one or both arms flexed over their heads (see figure in Box 5-5). This position has several advantages. It is the only bed position that allows full extension of the hip and knee joints. When used periodically, the prone position helps to prevent flexion contractures of the hips and knees, thereby counteracting a problem caused by all other bed positions. The prone position also promotes drainage from the mouth and is especially useful for clients recovering from surgery of the mouth or throat.

The prone position also poses some distinct disadvantages. The pull of gravity on the trunk produces a marked lordosis (forward curvature of the lumbar spine) in most persons, and the neck is rotated laterally to a significant degree. For this reason, physicians may not recommend this position, especially for persons with problems of the cervical or lumbar spine. This position also causes plantar flexion. Some clients with cardiac or respiratory problems find the prone position confining and suffocating, because chest expansion is inhibited during respirations. The prone position should be used only when the client's back is properly aligned, only for short periods, and only for persons with no evidence of spinal abnormalities. Box 5-5 and Technique 5-1 describe how to support a client in the prone position.

Lateral Position

In the **lateral (side-lying) position**, the person lies on one side of the body (see figure in Box 5-6). Flexing the top hip and knee and placing this leg in front of the body creates a wider, triangular base of support and achieves greater stability. The greater the flexion of the top hip and knee, the greater the stability and balance in this position. This flexion reduces lordosis and promotes good back alignment. For this reason, the lateral position is good for resting and sleeping clients. The lateral position helps to relieve pressure on the sacrum and heels in persons who sit for much of the day or who are confined to bed and rest in the Fowler's or dorsal recumbent position much of the time. In the lateral position, most of the body's weight is borne by the lateral aspect of the lower scapula, the lateral aspect of the ilium, and the greater trochanter of

Box 5-5 *Prone Position (Supported)*

Measures to Promote Alignment and Support*

- Small pillow under head unless contraindicated because of promotion of mucous drainage from mouth—prevents flexion or hyperextension of neck.
- Small pillow or roll under abdomen just below diaphragm to prevent hyperextension of lumbar curvature; difficulty breathing; pressure on breasts (women); pressure on genitals (men).
- Allow feet to fall naturally over end of mattress or

support lower legs on a pillow so that toes do not touch the bed to prevent plantar flexion (footdrop).

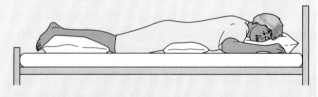

Prone position (supported).

* Amount of support depends on the needs of the individual client.

Box 5-6 *Lateral Position (Supported)*

Measures to Promote Alignment and Support*

- Pillow under head and neck to provide good alignment and prevent lateral flexion and fatigue of sternocleidomastoid muscles.
- Pillow under upper arm to place it in good alignment; lower arm should be flexed comfortably. Avoids internal rotation and adduction of shoulder that could cause subsequent limited function, and prevents impaired chest expansion.
- Pillow under leg and thigh to place them in good alignment. Check that shoulders and hips are in straight

* Amount of support depends on the needs of the individual client.

alignment. These measures prevent internal rotation and adduction of femur and twisting of the spine.

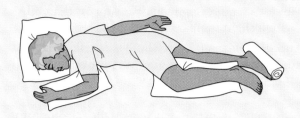

Lateral position (supported).

the femur. Persons who have sensory or motor deficits on one side of the body usually find that lying on the uninvolved side is more comfortable. Box 5-6 and Technique 5-1 describe how to support a client in the lateral position.

Sims' Position

In **Sims' (semiprone) position,** the client assumes a posture halfway between the lateral and the prone positions. The lower arm is positioned behind the client and the upper arm is flexed at the shoulder and the elbow. Both legs are flexed in front of the client. The upper leg is more acutely flexed at both the hip and the knee than the lower leg.

Sims' position is occasionally used for unconscious clients because it facilitates drainage from the mouth and prevents aspiration of fluids. It is also used for paralyzed (paraplegic or hemiplegic) clients because it

reduces pressure over the sacrum and greater trochanter of the hip. It is often used for clients receiving enemas and occasionally for clients undergoing examinations or treatments of the perineal area. Many people, especially pregnant women, find the Sims' position comfortable for sleeping. Persons with sensory or motor deficits on one side of the body usually find that lying on the uninvolved side is more comfortable. Box 5-7 and Technique 5-1 describe how to support a client in the Sims' position.

Nursing Process: Positioning Clients in Bed

ASSESSMENT

Assess the client's strength and ability to move before the change of position. Factors to assess include:

- *Adipose tissue.* A client who has ample adipose (fatty) tissue generally requires less support and

Box 5-7 *Sims' (Semiprone) Position (Supported)*

Measures to Promote Alignment and Support*

- Pillow to support head, maintaining it in good alignment unless drainage from the mouth is required.
- Pillow under upper arm to prevent internal rotation of shoulder and arm.
- Pillow under upper leg to support it in alignment and to prevent internal rotation and adduction of hip and leg.
- Sandbags (or rolled towels) to support feet in dorsiflexion to prevent footdrop.

* Amount of support depends on the needs of the individual client.

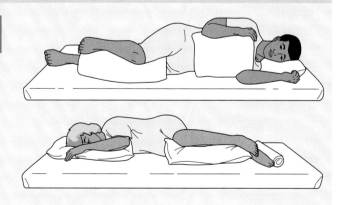

Sims' position (supported).

cushioning than the emaciated person while in a back-lying position, but greater support to maintain a lateral position.

- *Skeletal structure.* Both the amount and the type of support needed vary according to the individual's skeletal structure. A person with a marked lumbar lordosis requires more lumbar support than one with a slight lumbar curvature.
- *Health status.* A person who has flaccid (weak, soft) or spastic paralysis requires supportive devices. The support differs with the client's specific health status.
- *Discomfort.* A person who experiences pain during movement requires more support to prevent movement than one who can move without pain. A person who is unconscious is unable to indicate discomfort and will need appropriate support and change of position.
- *Skin condition.* People who have nutrition problems and/or impaired circulation require more cushioning of the pressure points to prevent skin breakdown than do healthy people.
- *Ability to move.* People who can move in bed can change position frequently. The client who is unable to move (e.g., the unconscious client) requires support so that muscles do not become strained.

- *Hydration.* Dehydrated clients are at greater risk of pressure ulcer formation than well-hydrated clients and therefore need more support under pressure areas.

PLANNING

- Determine the client's need for supportive devices, such as pillows, rolled or folded towels, foam rubber supports, footboard, hand rolls, wrist splints, or sandbags.
- Determine the amount of assistance required to position the client. The risk of muscle strain and body injury, to both the client and nurse, is lowered when appropriate assistance is provided.

Delegation

Positioning clients in bed can be delegated to unlicensed assistive personnel (UAP). The nurse must give specific directions to the UAP about the appropriate positions for the client and the reporting of any changes in skin integrity. The UAP should be encouraged to have the client participate as much as possible in the position change. The nurse is responsible for evaluating the client's comfort and alignment after the repositioning and for assessing skin integrity, particularly at pressure points.

IMPLEMENTATION:
TECHNIQUE 5-1 SUPPORTING THE CLIENT'S POSITION IN BED

Equipment

The following equipment can be used when positioning clients:

- Pillows—one to six depending on client need
- Trochanter rolls
- Footboard
- Hand rolls or wrist splints, if needed
- Folded towel
- Sandbag or rolled towel

Preparation

- Check the position-change schedule for the next time and type of position change.
- Administer an analgesic, if appropriate, before changing the client's position.
- Obtain required assistance, as needed.

Performance

1. Explain to the client what you are going to do, why it is necessary, and how he or she can cooper-

ate. Discuss how the results will be used in planning further care or treatments.

2. Wash hands and observe other appropriate infection control procedures.

3. Provide for client privacy.

Supporting a Client in Fowler's Position

1. Position the client.
   - Have the client flex the knees slightly before raising the head of the bed. *Slight knee flexion prevents the person from sliding toward the foot of the bed as the bed is raised.* Be certain the client's hips are positioned directly over the point where the bed will bend when the head is raised. *An appropriate hip position ensures that the client will be sitting upright when the head of the bed is raised.*
   - Raise the head of the bed to 45° or the angle required by or ordered for the client.

2. Provide supportive devices to align the client appropriately (see Box 5-3).
   - Place a small pillow or roll under the lumbar region of the back if you feel a space in the lumbar curvature. *The pillow supports the natural lum-*

bar curvature and prevents flexion of the lumbar spine.

- Place a small pillow under the client's head. *The pillow supports the cervical curvature of the vertebral column.* Alternatively, have the client rest the head against the mattress. *Too many pillows beneath the head can cause neck flexion contracture.*

- Place one or two pillows under the lower legs from below the knees to the ankles. *The pillows provide a broad base of support that is soft and flexible, prevent uncomfortable hyperextension of the knees, and reduce pressure on the heels.* Make sure that no pressure is exerted on the popliteal space and that the knees are flexed. *Pressure against the popliteal space can damage nerves and vein walls, predisposing the client to thrombus formation. Keeping the knees slightly flexed also prevents the person from sliding down in the bed.*

- Avoid using the knee gatch of a hospital bed to flex the client's knees. *The position of the knee gatch rarely coincides with the position of the client's knees. Even when the knee gatch does bend at the client's knees, considerable pressure (due to the narrow base of support beneath the knees and the firm, unyielding mattress) can be exerted against the popliteal space and beneath the client's calves.*

- Put a trochanter roll lateral to each femur (optional). *This prevents external rotation of the hips.*

- Support the client's feet with a footboard. *This prevents plantar flexion.* The footboard should protrude several inches above the toes. *This protects the toes from pressure exerted by the top bedding.* The footboard should be placed 1 inch away from the heels. *This prevents undue pull on the Achilles tendon and discomfort.*

- Place pillows to support both arms and hands if the client does not have normal use of them. *These pillows prevent shoulder and muscle strain from the effects of downward gravitational pull, dislocation of the shoulder in paralyzed persons, edema of the hands and arms, and flexion contracture of the wrist.* Arrange the pillows to support only the forearms and hands, up to the elbow. In this way, the pillows support the shoulder girdle.

Supporting a Client in the Dorsal Recumbent Position

1. Assist the client to the supine position.

2. Provide supportive devices to align the client appropriately (see Box 5-4).

- Place a pillow of suitable thickness under the client's head and shoulders as needed. *This prevents hyperextension of the neck. Too many pillows beneath the head may cause or worsen neck flexion contracture.*

- Place a pillow under the lower legs from below the knees to the ankles. *This prevents hyperextension of the knees, keeps the heels off the bed, and reduces lumbar lordosis.*

- Place trochanter rolls laterally against the femurs (optional). *These prevent external rotation of the hips.*

- Place a rolled towel or small pillow under the lumbar curvature if you feel a space between the lumbar area and the bed. *This pillow supports the lumbar curvature and prevents flexion of the lumbar spine.*

- Put a footboard or rolled pillow on the bed to support the feet. *This prevents plantar flexion (footdrop).*

- If the client is unconscious or has paralysis of the upper extremities, elevate the forearms and hands (*not* the upper arm) on pillows. *This position promotes comfort and prevents edema. Pillows are not placed under the upper arms because they can cause shoulder flexion.*

- If the client has actual or potential finger and wrist flexion deformities, use handrolls or wrist/hand splints. *This prevents flexion contractures of the fingers.* Handrolls, having a circumference of 13 to 15 cm (5 to 6 in) exert even pressure over the entire flexor surface of the palm and fingers (Figure 5-5 ◆).

Supporting a Client in the Prone Position

1. Assist the client to a prone position.
- See Technique 5-3.

2. Provide supportive devices to position the client appropriately (see Box 5-5).

- Turn the client's head to one side, and either omit the pillow entirely if drainage from the mouth is being encouraged, or place a small pillow under the head to align the head with the trunk. *This prevents flexion of the neck laterally.* Avoid placing the pillow under the shoulders. *A pillow placed under the shoulders increases lumbar lordosis.*

- Place a small pillow or roll under the abdomen in the space between the diaphragm (or the breasts

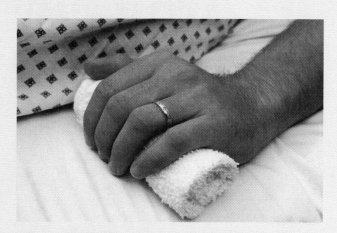

FIGURE 5-5 ◆ A hand roll may be made from a folded and rolled washcloth. It is used to maintain functional position of the wrist and fingers and to prevent contractures.

Supporting a Client in the Prone Position continued

of a woman) and the iliac crests. *The pillow prevents hyperextension of the lumbar curvature, difficulty breathing, and, for some women, pressure on the breasts. Supports placed too low can increase lumbar lordosis and pressure on bony prominences.*

- Place a pillow under the lower legs from below the knees to just above the ankles. *This raises the toes off the bed surface and reduces plantar flexion. This pillow also flexes the knees slightly for comfort and prevents excessive pressure on the patellae.* Or, position the client on the bed so that the feet are extended in a normal anatomic position over the lower edge of the mattress. *There should be no pressure on the toes.*

Supporting a Client in the Lateral Position

1. Assist the client to a lateral position.
   - See Technique 5-3.

2. Provide supportive devices to align the client appropriately (see Box 5-6).
   - Place a pillow under the client's head so that the head and neck are aligned with the trunk. *The pillow prevents lateral flexion and discomfort of the major neck muscles (e.g., the sternocleidomastoid muscles).*
   - Have the client flex the lower shoulder and position it forward so that the body does not rest on it. Rotate it into any position of comfort. *In this way, circulation is not disrupted.*
   - Place a pillow under the upper arm. *This prevents internal rotation and adduction of the shoulder and downward pressure on the chest that could interfere with chest expansion during respiration.* If the client has respiratory difficulty, increase the shoulder flexion and position the upper arm in front of the body off the chest.
   - Place two or more pillows under the upper leg and thigh so that the extremity lies in a plane parallel to the surface of the bed. *A position parallel to the bed most closely approximates correct standing alignment and prevents internal rotation of the thigh and adduction of the leg. The pillow also prevents pressure caused by the weight of the top leg resting on the lower leg. Such pressure can damage the vein walls in the lower leg and predispose the client to thrombus formation.*
   - Ensure that the two shoulders are aligned in the same plane as the two hips. If they are not, pull one shoulder or hip forward or backward until all four joints are aligned in the same plane. *Proper alignment prevents twisting of the spine.*
   - Place a folded towel under the natural hollow at the waistline (optional). *This prevents postural sco-

liosis of the lumbar spine. Take care to fill in only the space at the waistline. A towel support that extends too high or too low creates undue pressure against the rib cage or iliac crests.

- Place a rolled pillow alongside the client's back to stabilize the position (optional). This pillow is not usually needed when the client's upper hip and knee are appropriately flexed.

Supporting a Client in Sims' Position

1. Turn the client as for the prone position.

2. Provide supportive devices to align the client appropriately (see Box 5-7).
   - Place a small pillow under the client's head, unless drainage from the mouth is being encouraged. *The pillow prevents lateral flexion of the neck and cushions the cranial and facial bones and the ear.* It is contraindicated if drainage of mucus is required. *Too large a pillow produces an uncomfortable lateral flexion of the neck.*
   - Place the lower arm behind and away from the client's body in a position that is comfortable and does not disrupt circulation. *This position prevents damage to the nerves and blood vessels in the axillae.*
   - Position the upper shoulder so that it is abducted slightly from the body and the shoulder and elbow are flexed. Place a pillow in the space between the chest and abdomen and the upper arm and bed. *This position and support prevent internal shoulder rotation and adduction and maintain alignment of the upper trunk.*
   - Place a pillow in the space between the abdomen and pelvis and the upper thigh and bed. *This position prevents internal rotation and adduction of the hip and also reduces lumbar lordosis.*
   - Ensure that the two shoulders are aligned in the same plane as the two hips. If they are not, pull one shoulder or hip forward or backward until all four joints are aligned in the same plane. *This prevents twisting of the spine.*
   - Place a support device (e.g., a sandbag or rolled towel) against the lower foot. *This device may prevent footdrop.* Efforts to correct plantar flexion in this position, however, are usually unsuccessful.

Document:
- Time and change of position moved from and to, according to agency protocol
- Any signs of pressure areas or contractures
- Any difficulty client has with breathing (Fowler's, prone, and Sims' positions)
- Use of support devices

- Check the skin integrity of the pressure areas from the previous position. Relate findings to previous assessment data if available. Conduct follow-up assessment for previous and/or new skin breakdown areas.
- Check for proper alignment after the position change. Do a visual check and ask the client for a comfort assessment.
- Determine that all required safety precautions (e.g., side rails) are in place.
- Report significant changes to the physician.

Moving and Turning Clients in Bed

Although healthy people usually take for granted that they can change body position and go from one place to another with little effort, ill people may have difficulty moving even in bed. How much assistance clients require depends on their own ability to move and their health status. In general, nurses should be sensitive to both the need of people to function independently and their need for assistance to move.

When assisting a person to move, the nurse needs to employ correct body mechanics to avoid injury. Actions and rationales common to the lifting and moving procedures that follow are outlined in Box 5-8. Correct body alignment for the client must also be

maintained so that undue stress is not placed on the musculoskeletal system.

See Techniques 5-2 through 5-5 on moving and turning clients in bed and helping them sit up on the edge of the bed.

Nursing Process: Moving and Turning Clients in Bed

ASSESSMENT

Before moving a client, assess the following:

- The client's physical abilities (e.g., muscle strength, presence of paralysis)
- Ability to understand instructions
- Degree of comfort or discomfort when moving
- Client's weight
- Presence of orthostatic hypotension (particularly important when client will be standing)
- Your own strength and ability to move the client

PLANNING

Delegation

The skills of moving and turning clients in bed can be delegated to UAP. The nurse may wish to review proper body mechanics with the UAP to protect the UAP from injury. Emphasize the need for the UAP to report changes in the client's condition that require assessment and intervention by the nurse.

BOX 5-8 *Actions and Rationales Applicable to Moving and Lifting Clients*

- Raise the height of the bed to bring the client close to your center of gravity.
- Lock the wheels on the bed and raise the rail on the side of the bed opposite you to ensure client safety.
- Face in the direction of the movement to prevent spinal twisting.
- Assume a broad stance to increase stability and provide balance.
- Incline your trunk forward and flex your hips, knees, and ankles to lower your center of gravity, increase

stability, and ensure use of large muscle groups during movements.
- Tighten your gluteal, abdominal, leg, and arm muscles to prepare them for action and prevent injury.
- Rock from the front leg to the back leg when pulling or from the back leg to the front leg when pushing to overcome inertia, counteract the client's weight, and help attain a balanced, smooth motion.

IMPLEMENTATION:
TECHNIQUE 5-2 MOVING A CLIENT UP IN BED

Clients who have slid down in bed from Fowler's position or been pulled down by traction often need assistance to move up in bed.

Equipment

- Assistive devices such as overhead trapeze, pull and/or turn sheet, and transfer or sliding bar.

Preparation

Determine:

- Assistive devices that will be required
- Encumbrances to movement such as an IV or a heavy cast on one leg

- Medications the client is receiving, as certain medications may hamper movement or alertness of the client
- Assistance required from other health care personnel

Performance

1. Explain to the client what you are going to do, why it is necessary, and how he or she can cooperate. Listen to any suggestions made by the client or support people. Discuss how the results will be used in planning further care or treatments.

2. Wash hands and observe other appropriate infection control procedures.

3. Provide for client privacy.

4. Adjust the bed and the client's position.
   - Adjust the head of the bed to a flat position or as low as the client can tolerate. *Moving the client upward against gravity requires more force and can cause back strain.*
   - Raise the bed to the height of your center of gravity.
   - Lock the wheels on the bed and raise the rail on the side of the bed opposite you.
   - Remove all pillows, then place one against the head of the bed. *This pillow protects the client's head from inadvertent injury against the top of the bed during the upward move.*

5. Elicit the client's help in lessening your workload.
   - Ask the client to flex the hips and knees and position the feet so that they can be used effectively for pushing. *Flexing the hips and knees keeps the entire lower leg off the bed surface preventing friction during movement, and ensures use of the large muscle groups in the client's legs when pushing, thus increasing the force of movement.*
   - Ask the client to
     a. Grasp the head of the bed with both hands and pull during the move.
       or
     b. Raise the upper part of the body on the elbows and push with the hands and forearms during the move.
       or
     c. Grasp the overhead trapeze with both hands and lift and pull during the move. *Client assistance provides additional power to overcome inertia and friction during the move. These actions also keep the client's arms partially off the bed surface, reducing friction during movement, and make use of the large muscle groups of the client's arms to increase the force during movement.*

6. Position yourself appropriately, and move the client.

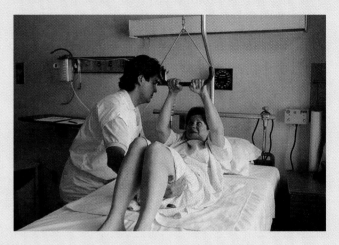

FIGURE 5-6 ◆ Moving a client up in bed.

- Face the direction of the movement, and then assume a broad stance with the foot nearest the bed behind the forward foot and weight on the forward foot. Incline your trunk forward from the hips. Flex hips, knees, and ankles.
- Place your near arm under the client's thighs (Figure 5-6 ◆). *This supports the heaviest part of the body (the buttocks). Push down on the mattress with the far arm. The far arm acts as a lever during the move.*
- Tighten your gluteal, abdominal, leg, and arm muscles and rock from the back leg to the front leg and back again. Then, shift your weight to the front leg as the client pushes with the heels and pulls with the arms so that the client moves toward the head of the bed.

7. Ensure client comfort.
   - Elevate the head of the bed and provide appropriate support devices for the client's new position.
   - See the sections on positioning clients earlier in this chapter.

Variation: A Client Who Has Limited Strength of the Upper Extremities

- Assist the client to flex the hips and knees as in step 5 previously. Place the client's arms across the chest. *This keeps them off the bed surface and minimizes friction during movement.* Ask the client to flex the neck during the move and keep the head off the bed surface.
- Position yourself as in step 6 and place one arm under the client's back and shoulders and the other arm under the client's thighs. *This placement of the arms distributes the client's weight and supports the heaviest part of the body (the buttocks).* Shift your weight as in step 6.

Variation: Two Nurses Using a Hand–Forearm Interlock

Two people are required to move clients who are unable to assist because of their condition or weight. Using the technique described in step 6, with the second staff member on the opposite side of the bed, both of you interlock your forearms under the client's thighs and shoulders and lift the client up in bed (Figure 5-7 ◆).

Variation: Two Nurses Using a Turn Sheet

Two nurses can use a turn sheet to move a client up in bed. *A turn sheet distributes the client's weight more evenly, decreases friction, and exerts a more even force on the client during the move. In addition, it prevents injury of the client's skin, because the friction created between two sheets when one is moved is less than that created by the client's body moving over the sheet.*

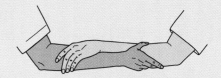

FIGURE 5-7 ◆ Two nurses using a hand–forearm interlock.

- Place a drawsheet or a full sheet folded in half under the client, extending from the shoulders to the thighs. Each person rolls up or fanfolds the turn sheet close to the client's body on either side.
- Both individuals grasp the sheet close to the shoulders and buttocks of the client. *This draws the weight closer to the nurses' center of gravity and increases the nurses' balance and stability, permitting a smoother movement.* Follow the method of moving clients with limited upper extremity strength as described earlier.

IMPLEMENTATION:
TECHNIQUE 5-3 TURNING A CLIENT TO THE LATERAL OR PRONE POSITION IN BED

Movement to the lateral (side-lying) position may be necessary when placing a bedpan beneath the client, when changing the client's bed linen, or when repositioning the client.

Performance

1. Explain to the client what you are going to do, why it is necessary, and how he or she can cooperate. Discuss how the results will be used in planning further care or treatments.

2. Wash hands and observe other appropriate infection control procedures.

3. Provide for client privacy.

4. Position yourself and the client appropriately before performing the move.

   - Move the client closer to the side of the bed opposite the side the client will face when turned. *This ensures that the client will be positioned safely in the center of the bed after turning.* Use a pull sheet beneath the client's trunk and thighs to pull the client to the side of the bed. Roll up the sheet as close as possible to the client's body and pull the client to the side of the bed. Adjust the client's head and reposition the legs appropriately.

   - While standing on the side of the bed nearest the client, place the client's near arm across the chest. Abduct the client's far shoulder slightly from the side of the body and externally rotate the shoulder (Figure 5-8 ◆). *Pulling the one arm forward facilitates the turning motion. Pulling the other arm away from the body and externally rotating the shoulder prevents that arm from being caught beneath the client's body during the roll.*

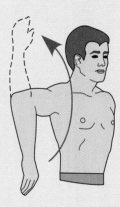

FIGURE 5-8 ◆ External rotation of the shoulder prevents the arm from being caught beneath the client's body when the client is turned.

   - Place the client's near ankle and foot across the far ankle and foot. *This facilitates the turning motion. Making these preparations on the side of the bed closest to the client helps prevent unnecessary reaching.*

   - Raise the side rail next to the client before going to the other side of the bed. *This ensures that the client, who is close to the edge of the mattress, will not fall.*

   - Position yourself on the side of the bed toward which the client will turn, directly in line with the client's waistline and as close to the bed as possible.

   - Incline your trunk forward from the hips. Flex your hips, knees, and ankles. Assume a broad stance with one foot forward and the weight placed on this forward foot.

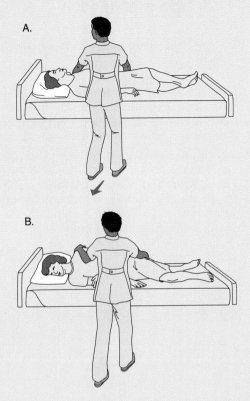

FIGURE 5-9 ◆ Moving a client to a lateral position.

5. Pull or roll the client toward you to the lateral position.

- Place one hand on the client's far hip and the other hand on the client's far shoulder (Figure 5-9A ◆). *This position of the hands supports the client at the two heaviest parts of the body, providing greater control in movement during the roll.*
- Tighten your gluteal, abdominal, leg, and arm muscles; rock backward, shifting your weight from the forward to the backward foot, and roll the client onto the side of the body to face you (Figure 5-9B). *Turning the client toward you promotes the client's sense of security.*
- Position the client on his or her side with the top hip and knee flexed. Move the top leg forward. Place one or two pillows under top leg. The top leg should be parallel to the mattress (Figure 5-10 ◆).
- Place a flat, firm pillow under the client's head and neck so they are aligned with the trunk.

Align shoulders with the hips *to avoid twisting of the spine.*

- Bring the bottom shoulder blade forward *to prevent the client's weight from resting directly on the shoulder joint.* Position both arms in flexed position. Support the upper arm with a pillow *to prevent wristdrop and pull on the shoulder.*
- Place a pillow that has been folded lengthwise with the smooth side tucked behind the client's back *to stabilize and support the client's lateral position.*
- Support the client's feet with sandbags, a firm pillow, or a footboard if necessary. *Maintaining dorsiflexion prevents footdrop.*

Variation: Turning the Client to a Prone Position

To turn a client to the prone position, follow the preceding steps, with two exceptions:

- Instead of abducting the far arm, keep the client's arm alongside the body for the client to roll over. *Keeping the arm alongside the body prevents it from being pinned under the client when the client is rolled.*
- Roll the client completely onto the abdomen. *It is essential to move the client as close as possible to the edge of the bed before the turn so that the client will be lying on the center of the bed after rolling.* Never pull a client across the bed while the client is in the prone position. *Doing so can injure a woman's breasts or a man's genitals.*

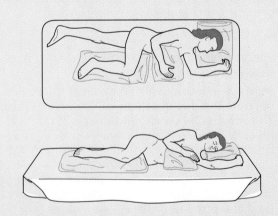

FIGURE 5-10 ◆ Lateral position with pillows in place.

Logrolling is a technique used to turn a client whose body must at all times be kept in straight alignment (like a log). An example is the client with a spinal injury. Considerable care must be taken to prevent additional injury. This technique requires two nurses or, if the client is large, three nurses. For the client who has a cervical injury, one nurse must maintain the client's head and neck alignment.

Performance

1. Explain to the client what you are going to do, why it is necessary, and how they can cooperate. Discuss how the results will be used in planning further care or treatments.

2. Wash hands and observe other appropriate infection control procedures.

3. Provide for client privacy.

4. Position yourselves and the client appropriately before the move.
   - Stand on the same side of the bed, and assume a broad stance with one foot ahead of the other.
   - Place the client's arms across the chest. *Doing so ensures that they will not be injured or become trapped under the body when the body is turned.*
   - Incline your trunk, and flex your hips, knees, and ankles.
   - Place your arms under the client as shown in Figure 5-11 ◆ or Figure 5-12 ◆, depending on the client's size. *Each staff member then has a major weight area of the client centered between the arms.*
   - Tighten your gluteal, abdominal, leg, and arm muscles.

5. Pull the client to the side of the bed.
   - One nurse counts, "One, two, three, go." Then, at the same time, all staff members pull the client to the side of the bed by shifting their weight to the back foot. *Moving the client in unison maintains the client's body alignment.*
   - Elevate the side rail on this side of the bed. *This prevents the client from falling while lying so close to the edge of the bed.*

6. Move to the other side of the bed, and place supportive devices for the client when turned.
   - Place a pillow where it will support the client's head after the turn. *The pillow prevents lateral flexion of the neck and ensures alignment of the cervical spine.*
   - Place one or two pillows between the client's legs to support the upper leg when the client is

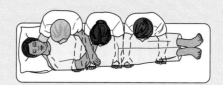

FIGURE 5-12 ◆ Correct arm placement for moving a client to the side of the bed: three nurses.

turned. *This pillow prevents adduction of the upper leg and keeps the legs parallel and aligned.*

7. Roll and position the client in proper alignment.
   - All nurses flex their hips, knees, and ankles and assume a broad stance with one foot forward.
   - All nurses reach over the client and place hands as shown in Figure 5-13 ◆. *Doing so centers a major weight area of the client between each nurse's arms.*
   - One nurse counts, "One, two, three, go." Then, at the same time, all nurses roll the client to a lateral position.
   - Support the client's head, back, and upper and lower extremities with pillows.
   - Raise the side rails and place the call bell within the client's reach.

Variation: Using a Turn or Lift Sheet

- Use a turn sheet to facilitate logrolling. First, stand with another nurse on the same side of the bed. Assume a broad stance with one foot forward, and grasp half of the fanfolded or rolled edge of the turn sheet. On a signal, pull the client toward both of you (Figure 5-14 ◆).

- Before turning the client, place pillow supports for the head and legs, as described in step 6. This helps maintain the client's alignment when turning. Then, go to the other side of the bed (farthest from the client), and assume a stable stance. Reaching over the client, grasp the far edges of the turn sheet, and roll the client toward you (Figure 5-15 ◆). The second nurse (behind the client) helps turn the client and provides pillow supports to ensure good alignment in the lateral position.

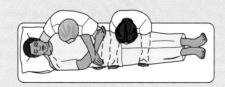

FIGURE 5-11 ◆ Correct arm placement for moving a client to the side of the bed: two nurses.

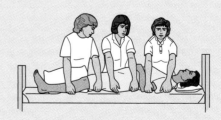

FIGURE 5-13 ◆ Correct hand placement for logrolling a client.

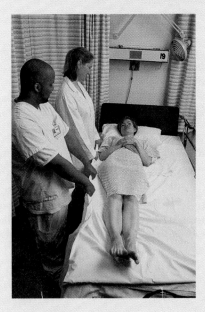

FIGURE 5-14 ◆ Using a turn sheet, the nurses pull the sheet with the client on it to the edge of the bed.

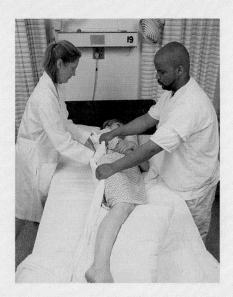

FIGURE 5-15 ◆ The nurse on the right uses the far edge of the sheet to roll the client toward him; the nurse on the left remains behind the client and assists with turning.

IMPLEMENTATION:
TECHNIQUE 5-5 ASSISTING THE CLIENT TO SIT ON THE SIDE OF THE BED (DANGLING)

The client assumes a sitting position on the edge of the bed before walking, moving to a chair or wheelchair, eating, or performing other activities.

Performance

1. Explain to the client what you are going to do, why it is necessary, and how he or she can cooperate. Discuss how the results will be used in planning further care or treatments.

2. Wash hands and observe appropriate other infection control procedures.

3. Provide for client privacy.

4. Position yourself and the client appropriately before performing the move.
   - Assist the client to a lateral position facing you.
   - Raise the head of the bed slowly to its highest position. *This decreases the distance that the client needs to move to sit up on the side of the bed.*
   - Position the client's feet and lower legs at the edge of the bed. *This enables the client's feet to move easily off the bed during the movement, and the client is aided by gravity into a sitting position.*
   - Stand beside the client's hips and face the far corner of the bottom of the bed (the angle in which movement will occur). Assume a broad stance, placing the foot nearest the client forward.

Incline your trunk forward from the hips. Flex your hips, knees, and ankles (Figure 5-16A ◆).

5. Move the client to a sitting position.
   - Place one arm around the client's shoulders and the other arm beneath both of the client's thighs near the knees (Figure 5-16A). *Supporting the client's shoulders prevents the client from falling backward during the movement. Supporting the client's thighs reduces friction of the thighs against the bed surface during the move and increases the force of the movement.*
   - Tighten your gluteal, abdominal, leg, and arm muscles.
   - Lift the client's thighs slightly. *This reduces the friction of the client's thighs and the nurse's arm against the bed surface.*
   - Pivot on the balls of your feet in the desired direction facing the foot of the bed while pulling the client's feet and legs off the bed (Figure 5-16B). *Pivoting prevents twisting of the nurse's spine. The weight of the client's legs swinging downward increases downward movement of the lower body and helps make the client's upper body vertical.*
   - Keep supporting the client until the client is well balanced and comfortable. *This movement may cause some clients to faint.*
   - Assess vital signs (e.g., pulse, respirations, and blood pressure) as indicated by the client's health status.

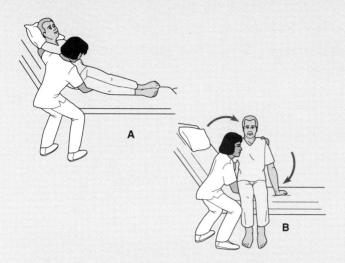

FIGURE 5-16 ◆ Assisting a client to a sitting position on the edge of the bed.

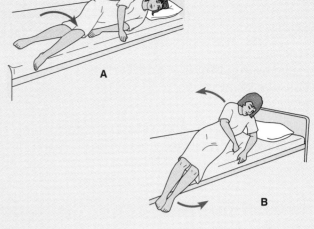

FIGURE 5-17 ◆ Moving to a sitting position independently.

Variation: Teaching a Client How to Sit on the Side of the Bed Independently

A client who has had recent abdominal surgery or who is weak may have too much abdominal pain or too little strength to sit straight up in bed. This person can be taught to assume a "dangle" position without assistance. Instruct the client to:

- Roll to the side and lift the far leg over the near leg (Figure 5-17A ◆).
- Grasp the mattress edge with the lower arm and push the fist of the upper arm into the mattress (Figure 5-17B).

- Push up with the arms as the heels and legs slide over the mattress edge (Figure 5-17B).
- Maintain the sitting position by pushing both fists into the mattress behind and to the sides of the buttocks.

 Document all relevant information. Record:
- Time and change of position moved from and position moved to
- Any signs of pressure areas
- Use of support devices
- Ability of client to assist in moving and turning
- Response of client to moving and turning (e.g., anxiety, discomfort, dizziness)

AMBULATORY AND COMMUNITY SETTINGS

Positioning, Moving, and Turning Clients

- When making a home visit, it is particularly important to inspect the mattress for support. A sagging mattress, a mattress that is too soft, or an underfilled waterbed used over a prolonged period can contribute to the development of hip flexion contractures and low back strain and pain. Bed boards made of plywood and placed beneath a sagging mattress are increasingly recommended for clients who have back problems or are prone to them.
- Assess the caregiver's knowledge and application of body mechanics to prevent injury.

- Demonstrate how to turn and position the client in bed. Observe the caregiver performing a return demonstration.
- Teach caregivers the basic principles of body alignment and how to check for proper alignment after the client has been changed to a new position.
- Teach the caregiver to check the client's skin for redness and integrity after repositioning the client. Stress the importance of informing the nurse about the length of time skin redness remains over pressure areas after the person has been repositioned. Emphasize that reddened areas should not be massaged as it may lead to tissue trauma.

AGE-RELATED CONSIDERATIONS

Positioning, Moving, and Turning Clients

Infant

- Position infants on their side for sleep, particularly after feeding.

Child

- Carefully inspect the dependent skin surfaces of all infants and children confined to bed at least three times in each 24-hour period (Ball & Bindler, p. 929).

Positioning, Moving, and Turning Clients (continued)

Elders

- Decreased subcutaneous fat and thinning of the skin place older clients at risk for skin breakdown.

Repositioning at least every 2 hours helps reduce pressure on bony prominences and avoid skin trauma.

EVALUATION

- Check the skin integrity of the pressure areas from the previous position. Relate findings to previous assessment data if available. Conduct follow-up assessment for previous and/or new skin breakdown areas.
- Check for proper alignment after the position change. Do a visual check and ask the client for a comfort assessment.
- Determine that all required safety precautions (e.g., side rails) are in place.
- Determine client's tolerance of the activity (e.g., vital signs before and after dangling) particularly the first time client dangles
- Report significant changes to the physician.

Transferring Clients

Many clients require some assistance in transferring between bed and chair or wheelchair, between wheelchair and toilet, and between bed and stretcher. Because wheelchairs and stretchers are unstable, they can predispose the client to falls and injury. Guidelines for the safe use of wheelchairs and stretchers are shown in Boxes 5-9 and 5-10.

Transfer (walking) belts provide the greatest safety. This belt has a handle that allows the nurse to control movement of the client during the transfer. An increasing number of hospitals and nursing homes are requiring that personnel use the transfer belt to ambulate or move clients. See Technique 5-6 for transferring a client between a bed and a chair and Technique 5-7 for transferring a client between a bed and a stretcher.

Nursing Process: Transferring Clients

ASSESSMENT

Assess:

- The client's body size
- Ability to follow instructions

BOX 5-9 *Wheelchair Safety*

- Always lock the brakes on both wheels of the wheelchair when the client transfers in or out of it.
- Raise the footplates before transferring the client into the wheelchair.
- Lower the footplates after the transfer, and place the client's feet on them.
- Ensure the client is positioned well back in the seat of the wheelchair.
- Use seat belts that fasten behind the wheelchair to protect confused clients from falls.
- Back the wheelchair into or out of an elevator, rear large wheels first.
- Place your body between the wheelchair and the bottom of an incline.

BOX 5-10 *Safe Use of Stretchers*

- Lock the wheels of the bed and stretcher before the client transfers in or out of them.
- Fasten safety straps across the client on a stretcher, and raise the side rails.
- Never leave a client unattended on a stretcher unless the wheels are locked and the side rails are raised on both sides and/or the safety straps are securely fastened across the client.
- Always push a stretcher from the end where the client's head is positioned. This position protects the client's head in the event of a collision.
- If the stretcher has two swivel wheels and two stationary wheels:
  a. Always position the client's head at the end with the stationary wheels *and*
  b. Push the stretcher from the end with the stationary wheels. The stretcher is maneuvered more easily when pushed from this end.
- Maneuver the stretcher when entering the elevator so that the client's head goes in first.

- Activity tolerance
- Muscle strength
- Joint mobility
- Presence of paralysis
- Level of comfort
- Presence of orthostatic hypotension
- The technique with which the client is familiar
- The space in which the transfer is maneuvered (bathrooms, for example, are usually cramped)
- The number of assistants (one or two) needed to accomplish the transfer safely
- The skill and strength of the nurse(s)

Delegation

The skill of transferring a client can be delegated to UAP who have demonstrated good body mechanics and safe transfer technique for the involved client. It is important that the nurse assesses the client's capabilities and communicates specific information about what the UAP should report back to the nurse.

IMPLEMENTATION:
TECHNIQUE 5-6 TRANSFERRING BETWEEN BED AND CHAIR

Equipment

- Robe or appropriate clothing
- Slippers or shoes with nonskid soles
- Transfer (walking) belt
- Chair, commode, wheelchair, or stretcher as appropriate to client need
- Sliding board

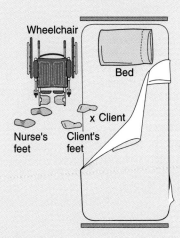

FIGURE 5-18 ◆ The wheelchair is placed parallel to the bed as close to the bed as possible. Note that placement of the nurse's feet mirrors that of the client's feet.

Preparation

- Plan what to do and how to do it.
- Obtain essential equipment before starting (e.g., transfer belt, wheelchair), and check that it is functioning correctly.
- Remove obstacles from the area used for the transfer.

Performance

1. Explain the transfer process to the client, including what the client should do. During the transfer, explain step-by-step what the client should do, for example, "Move your right foot forward."

2. Wash hands and observe other appropriate infection control procedures.

3. Provide for client privacy.

4. Position the equipment appropriately.
   - Lower the bed to its lowest position so that the client's feet will rest flat on the floor. Lock the wheels of the bed.
   - Place the wheelchair parallel to the bed as close to the bed as possible (Figure 5-18 ◆). Put the wheelchair on the side of the bed that allows the client to move toward his or her stronger

side. Lock the wheels of the wheelchair and raise the footplate.

5. Prepare and assess the client.
   - Assist the client to a sitting position on the side of the bed (see Technique 5-5).
   - Assess the client for orthostatic hypotension before moving the client from the bed.
   - Assist the client in putting on a bathrobe and nonskid slippers or shoes.
   - Place a transfer belt snugly around the client's waist. Check to be certain that the belt is securely fastened.

6. Give explicit instructions to the client. Ask the client to:
   - Move forward and sit on the edge of the bed. *This brings the client's center of gravity closer to the nurse's.*

- Lean forward slightly from the hips. *This brings the client's center of gravity more directly over the base of support and positions the head and trunk in the direction of the movement.*
- Place the foot of the stronger leg beneath the edge of the bed and put the other foot forward. *In this way, the client can use the stronger leg muscles to stand and power the movement. A broader base of support makes the client more stable during the transfer.*
- Place the client's hands on the bed surface or on your shoulders so that the client can push while standing. *This provides additional force for the movement and reduces the potential for strain on the nurse's back.* The client should not grasp your neck for support. *Doing so can injure the nurse.*

7. Position yourself correctly.
- Stand directly in front of the client. Incline the trunk forward from the hips. Flex the hips, knees, and ankles. Assume a broad stance, placing one foot forward and one back. Mirror the placement of the client's feet, if possible. *This helps prevent loss of balance during the transfer.*
- Encircle the client's waist with your arms, and grasp the transfer belt at the client's back (Figure 5-19 ◆) with thumbs pointing downward. *The belt provides a secure handle for holding on to the client and controlling the movement. Downward placement of the thumbs prevents potential wrist*

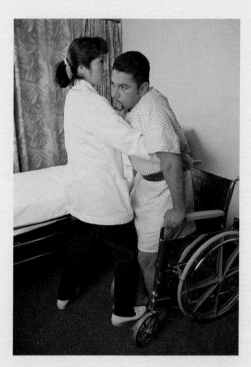

FIGURE 5-19 ◆ Using a transfer (walking) belt.

injury as the nurse lifts. By supporting the client in this manner, you keep the client from tilting backward during the transfer.
- Tighten your gluteal, abdominal, leg, and arm muscles.

8. Assist the client to stand, and then move together toward the wheelchair.
- On the count of three, ask the client to push with the back foot, rock to the forward foot, and extend (straighten) the joints of the lower extremities. Push or pull up with the hands, while pushing with the forward foot, rock to the back foot, extend the joints of the lower extremities, and pull the client (directly toward your center of gravity) into a standing position.
- Support the client in an upright standing position for a few moments. *This allows the nurse and the client to extend the joints and provides the nurse with an opportunity to ensure that the client is stable before moving away from the bed.*
- Together, pivot or take a few steps toward the wheelchair.

9. Assist the client to sit.
- Ask the client to:
  a. Back up to the wheelchair and place the legs against the seat. *Having the client place the legs against the wheelchair seat minimizes the risk of the client's falling when sitting down.*
  b. Place the foot of the stronger leg slightly behind the other. *This supports body weight during the movement.*
  c. Keep the other foot forward. *This provides a broad base of support.*
  d. Place both hands on the wheelchair arms or on your shoulders. *This increases stability and lessens the strain on the nurse.*
- Stand directly in front of the client. Place one foot forward and one back.
- Tighten your grasp on the transfer belt, and tighten your gluteal, abdominal, leg, and arm muscles.
- On the count of three, have the client shift the body weight by rocking to the back foot, lower the body onto the edge of the wheelchair seat by flexing the joints of the legs and arms. Place some body weight on the arms, while shifting your body weight by stepping back with the forward foot and pivoting toward the chair while lowering the client onto the wheelchair seat.

10. Ensure client safety.
- Ask the client to push back into the wheelchair seat. *Sitting well back on the seat provides a broader base of support and greater stability and minimizes*

the risk of falling from the wheelchair. A wheelchair can topple forward when the client sits on the edge of the seat and leans far forward.

- Lower the footplates, and place the client's feet on them.
- Apply a seat belt as required.

11. **Document** relevant information:
- Client's ability to bear weight and pivot
- Number of staff needed for transfer
- Length of time up in chair
- Client response to transfer and being up in chair or wheelchair

Variation: Angling the Wheelchair

For clients who have difficulty walking, place the wheelchair at a 45-degree angle to the bed. *This enables the client to pivot into the chair and lessens the amount of body rotation required.*

Variation: Transferring Without a Belt

- For clients who need minimal assistance, place the hands against the sides of the client's chest (not at the axillae) during the transfer (Figure 5-20 ◆). For clients who require more assistance, reach through the client's axillae and place the hands on the client's scapulae during the transfer. Avoid placing hands or pressure on the axillae, especially for clients who have upper extremity paralysis or paresis.
- Follow the steps described previously.

Variation: Transferring with a Belt and Two Nurses

- When the client is able to stand, position yourselves on both sides of the client, facing the same direction as the client. Flex your hips, knees, and ankle. Grasp the client's transfer belt with the hand closest to the client, and with the other hand support the client's elbows.
- Coordinating your efforts, all three of you stand simultaneously, pivot, and move to the wheelchair. Reverse the process to lower the client onto the wheelchair seat.

Variation: Transferring a Client with an Injured Lower Extremity

When the client has an injured lower extremity, movement should always occur toward the client's unaffected (strong) side. For example, if the client's right leg is injured and the client is sitting on the edge of the bed preparing to transfer to a wheelchair, position the wheelchair on the client's left side. In this way, the client can use the unaffected leg most effectively and safely.

Variation: Using a Sliding Board

For a client who cannot stand, use a sliding board to move without nursing assistance. This method not only promotes the client's sense of independence but preserves your energy (Figure 5-21 ◆).

FIGURE 5-20 ◆ Transferring without a belt.

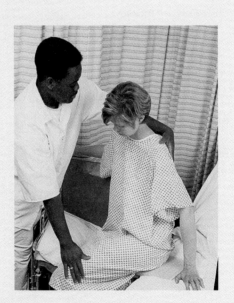

FIGURE 5-21 ◆ Using a sliding board.

- Compare client capabilities such as weight bearing, pivoting ability and strength and control to previous transfers.

- Report any significant deviations from normal to the physician.

- Note use of appropriate safety measures (e.g., transfer belt, locking wheels of bed and wheelchair) by UAP during transfer process.

IMPLEMENTATION:
TECHNIQUE 5-7 TRANSFERRING BETWEEN BED AND STRETCHER

The stretcher, or gurney, is used to transfer supine clients from one location to another. Whenever the client is capable of accomplishing the transfer from bed to stretcher independently, either by lifting onto it or by rolling onto it, the client should be encouraged to do so. If the client cannot move onto the stretcher independently, at least two nurses are needed to assist with the transfer; more are needed if the client is totally helpless or is heavy.

Preparation

Obtain the necessary equipment and nursing personnel to assist in the transfer.

Performance

1. Explain to the client what you are going to do, why it is necessary, and how he or she can cooperate. Explain the transfer to the nursing personnel who are helping and specify who will give directions (one person needs to be in charge).

2. Wash hands and observe other appropriate infection control procedures.

3. Provide for client privacy.

4. Adjust the client's bed in preparation for the transfer.
   - Lower the head of the bed until it is flat or as low as the client can tolerate.
   - Raise the bed so that it is slightly higher than the surface of the stretcher. *It is easier for the client to move down an incline.*
   - Ensure that the wheels on the bed are locked.
   - Pull the drawsheet out from both sides of the bed.

5. Move the client to the edge of the bed and position the stretcher.
   - Roll the drawsheet as close to the client's side as possible.
   - Pull the client to the edge of the bed and cover the client with a sheet or bath blanket to maintain comfort.
   - Place the stretcher parallel to the bed next to the client and lock the stretcher's wheels.
   - Fill the gap that exists between the bed and the

stretcher loosely with the bath blankets (optional).

6. Transfer the client securely to the stretcher.
   - In unison with the other staff members press your body tightly against the stretcher. *This prevents the stretcher from moving.*
   - Roll the pull sheet tightly against the client. *This achieves better control over client movement.*
   - Flex your hips and pull the client on the pull sheet in unison directly toward you and onto the stretcher. *Pulling downward requires less force than pulling along a flat surface.*
   - Ask the client to flex the neck during the move, if possible, and place the arms across the chest. *This prevents injury to these body parts.*

7. Ensure client comfort and safety.
   - Make the client comfortable, unlock the stretcher wheels, and move the stretcher away from the bed.
   - Immediately raise the stretcher side rails and/or fasten the safety straps across the client. *Because the stretcher is high and narrow, the client is in danger of falling unless these safety precautions are taken.*

8. **Document** relevant information:
   - Equipment used
   - Number of people needed for transfer
- Destination if reason for transfer is transport from one location to another

---

Variation: Using a Roller Bar
During the Transfer

A roller bar is a metal frame covered with longitudinal rollers. Place the bar over the gap between the bed and the stretcher. Using a pull sheet, pull the client onto the roller bar, and roll the client easily onto the stretcher.

Variation: Using a Long or Sliding Board

The long board, which may be referred to as the Smooth Mover or Easyglide, is a lacquered or smooth polyethylene board measuring 45 to 55 cm (18 to 22 in) by 182 cm (72 in) with handholds along its edges. This device may be used by one nurse alone or up to four nurses together. Turn the client to a lateral position away from you, position the board close to the client's back, and roll the client onto the board. Pull the client and board across the bed to the stretcher. Safety belts may be placed over the chest, abdomen, and legs.

Variation: Using a Three-Person Carry
(Use Caution)

Three people of about equal height stand side-by-side facing the client. Recommendations vary as to which staff member lifts a specific area of the client. Often, the strongest person supports the heaviest part of the client or the tallest person with the longest reach supports the head and shoulders. The stretcher or bed to which the client will be moved is placed at a right angle at the foot of the bed. The wheels of the bed and stretcher are locked. Each person flexes the knees and places the foot nearest to the stretcher slightly forward.

The arms of the lifters are put under the client at the head and shoulders, hips and thighs, and upper and lower legs. On the count of 3, the lifters roll the

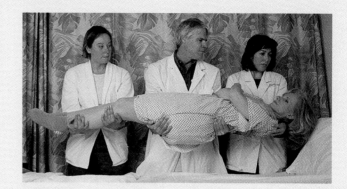

FIGURE 5-22 ◆ The three carrier lift.

client onto their chests and step back in unison (see Figure 5-22 ◆). They then pivot around to the stretcher and lower the client by flexing their knees and hips until their elbows are on the surface of the stretcher. The client is then released on the stretcher surface and is aligned and covered and the stretcher side rails are raised.

AMBULATORY AND COMMUNITY SETTINGS

Transferring from Bed to a Chair

- The caretaker and client should practice transfer technique(s) in the hospital or long-term care setting before being discharged.
- Assess furniture in the home. Does the client's

favorite chair have arms for ease of using and sitting? Examine the fabric—is it rough? Will it cause skin abrasions? If the client will be using a wheelchair, is there enough space in the bedroom and bathroom for a safe transfer?

AGE-RELATED CONSIDERATIONS

Transferring Clients
Infant

- The infant who is lying down, either on the side or supine, can be placed in a bassinet or crib for transport. If the bassinet has a bottom shelf, it can be used for carrying the IV pump or monitor.

Child

- The toddler should be transported in a high-top crib with the side rails up and the protective top in

place. Stretchers should not be used because the mobile toddler may roll or fall off.

Elders

- Use special caution with older clients to prevent skin tears or bruising during a transfer or using a hydraulic lift.

EVALUATION

Focus on client safety and comfort. Report any significant deviations from normal to the physician.

Hydraulic Lifts

Hydraulic lifts, such as the Hoyer lift, are used primarily for clients who cannot help themselves or who are

too heavy for others to lift safely. The lift can be used in transferring the client between the bed and a wheelchair, the bed and the bathtub, and the bed and a stretcher. The Hoyer lift consists of a base on casters, a hydraulic mechanical pump, a mast boom, and a sling (Figure 5-23 ◆). The sling may consist of a one- or two-piece canvas seat. The one-piece seat stretches from the client's head to the knees. The two-piece seat has one canvas strap to support the client's buttocks and

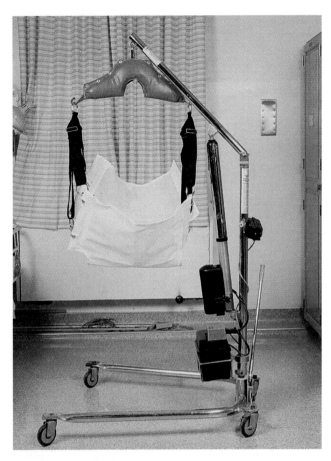

FIGURE 5-23 ◆ A one-piece seat hydraulic lift.

thighs and a second strap extending up to the axillae to support the back. It is important to be familiar with the model used and the practices that accompany use of that model. Before using the lift, ensure that it is in working order and that the hooks, chains, straps, and canvas seat are in good repair. *Most agencies recommend that two nurses operate a lift.* Check agency policy.

Nursing Process: Hydraulic Lifts

ASSESSMENT

Determine the following before the transfer:

- Client's ability to comprehend instructions
- Degree of physical disability
- Weight of the client (to ensure that the lift can safely move the client)
- Presence of orthostatic hypotension
- Pulse rate

PLANNING

Delegation

The skill of using a hydraulic lift can be delegated to UAP who have demonstrated competent use of the equipment for the involved client.

IMPLEMENTATION:
TECHNIQUE 5-8 USING A HYDRAULIC LIFT

Equipment

- Hoyer lift with slings and canvas straps

Preparation

Obtain the lift and put in the client's room. Arrange for assistance from others at a designated time.

Performance

1. Explain the procedure and demonstrate the lift. *Some clients are afraid of being lifted and will be reassured by a demonstration.* Discuss how the lift will be used in planning further care or treatments.

2. Wash hands and observe other appropriate infection control procedures.

3. Provide for client privacy.

4. Prepare the equipment.
   - Lock the wheels of the client's bed and raise the bed to the high position.
   - Put up the side rail on the opposite side of the bed and lower the side rail near you.
   - Position the lift so that it is close to the client.
   - Place the chair that is to receive the client beside the bed. Allow adequate space to maneuver the lift.
   - Lock the wheels, if a chair with wheels is used.

5. Position the client on the sling.
   - Roll the client away from you.
   - Place the canvas seat or sling under the client with the wide lower edge under the client's thighs to the knees and the more narrow upper edge up under the client's shoulders. *This places the sling under the client's center of gravity and greatest part of body weight. Correct placement permits the client to be lifted evenly, with minimal shifting.*
   - Raise the bed rail on your side of the bed, and go to the opposite side of the bed. Lower this side rail.
   - Roll the client to the opposite side, and pull the canvas sling through.

- Roll the client to the supine position and center the client on top of the canvas sling.

6. Attach the sling to the swivel bar.
   - Wheel the lift into position, with the footbars under the bed on the side where the chair is positioned. Set the adjustable base at the widest position to ensure stability. Lock the wheels of the lifter.
   - Lower the side rail.
   - Move the lift arms directly over the client and lower the horizontal bar by releasing the hydraulic valve. Lock the valve.
   - Attach the lifter straps or hooks to the corresponding openings in the canvas seat. Check that the hooks are correctly placed and that matching straps or chains are of equal length. Face the hooks away from the client. *This prevents the hooks from injuring the client.*

7. Lift the client gradually.
   - Elevate the head of the bed to place the client in a sitting position.
   - Ask the client to remove eyeglasses and put them in a safe place. *The swivel bar may come close to the face and cause breakage of eyeglasses.*
   - *Nurse 1:* Close the pressure valve, and gradually pump the jack handle until the client is above the bed surface. *Gradual elevation of the lift is less frightening to the client than a rapid rise.*
   - *Nurse 2:* Assume a broad stance, and guide the client with your hands as the client is lifted. *This prepares to hold the client and provide control during the movement.*

- Check the placement of the sling before moving the client away from the bed.

8. Move the client over the chair.
   - *Nurse 1:* With the pressure valve securely closed, slowly roll the lift until the client is over the chair. Use the steering handle to maneuver the lift.
   - *Nurse 2:* Guide movement by hand until the client is directly over the chair. *Slow movement decreases swaying and is less frightening. Guidance also decreases swaying and gives a sense of security.*

9. Lower the client into the chair.
   - *Nurse 1:* Release the pressure valve very gradually. *Gradual release is less frightening than a quick descent.*
   - *Nurse 2:* Guide the client into the chair.

10. Ensure client comfort and safety.
    - Remove the hooks from the canvas seat. Leave the seat in place. *The seat is left in place in preparation for the lift back to bed.*
    - Align the client appropriately in a sitting position and return the client's eyeglasses, if appropriate.
    - Apply a seat belt or other restraint as needed.
    - Place the call bell within reach.

 11. **Document** the type of equipment, number of assistants needed, and the client's physiological and psychological response.

EVALUATION

- Note safety precautions required for clients during and after the transfer.
- Check body alignment of client in the sitting position.

- Relate vital signs, especially pulse rate and blood pressure to determine response to the transfer.
- Compare client's current response to previous responses to use of hydraulic lift.
- Report any significant deviations from normal to physician.

Chapter Summary

TERMINOLOGY

alignment	hand roll	posture
balance	high-Fowler's position	prone position
base of support	hydraulic lift	semi-Fowler's position
body mechanics	lateral (side-lying) position	Sims' (semiprone) position
center of gravity	line of gravity	sliding board
contractures	logrolling	transfer (walking) belt
dorsal recumbent (back-lying) position	low-Fowler's position	trochanter roll
Fowler's position	orthopneic position	
	pivot	

FORMING CLINICAL JUDGMENTS

Consider This:

1. As a nurse, what assessments and interventions can you do to promote good body mechanics and prevent back injury for yourself and others?

2. You are providing nursing care for a client who has the following equipment: two IVs (one inserted into a central line and the other in a peripheral line), a Foley catheter, a nasogastric tube connected to suction, and a hemovac. The client is scheduled to go to the radiology department via gurney. How will you facilitate the client being moved to the gurney without injury to the client or yourself?

3. You and another nursing student have turned a client with right-sided paralysis to a left semi-prone position. The client can understand what you say to him but he cannot express himself verbally. He can appropriately move his head for "yes" and "no." How will you determine that the client is comfortable and in correct alignment after positioning him?

4. What would you do if a client who needs to be transferred from the bed to a chair exhibits the following: expresses fear of falling, does not want to move because "it will hurt," and states "you are new and don't know what to do"?

RELATED RESEARCH

Colin, D., Abraham, P., Preault, L., Bregeon, C., & Saumet, J. L. (1996). Comparison of 90° and 30° laterally inclined positions in the prevention of pressure ulcers using transcutaneous oxygen and carbon dioxide pressures. *Advances in Wound Care, 9*(3), 35–38.

Smedley, J., & Egger, P. (1997). Prospective cohort study of predictors of incident low back pain in nurses. *British Medical Journal, 314*(7089), 1225–1229.

Goodridge, D., & Laurila, B. (1997). Minimizing transfer injuries. *Canadian Nurse, 93*(7), 38–40.

REFERENCES

Altman, G. B., Buschsel, P., & Coxon, V. (2000). *Fundamental & Advanced Nursing Skills*. Albany, NY: Delmar.

American Nurses Association. (2000, May/June). ANA calls for publication of ergonomics standard. *The American Nurse, 29.*

Bindler, R., & Ball, J. (1999). *Pediatric Clinical Skills*. Stamford, CT: Appleton & Lange.

Elkin, M. K., Perry, A. G., & Potter, P. A. (2000). *Nursing Interventions and Clinical Skills,* 2nd ed. St. Louis: Mosby.

Lannon, B. P., & Reichelt, P. A. (1998). Nurse managers' role in injury preventions. *Nursing Management, 29*(8), 70–75.

McConnell, E. A. (1990). Clinical do's & don'ts: Placing your patient in the lateral position. *Nursing, 20*(7), 65

McConnell, E. A. (1994). Clinical do's & don'ts: Logrolling a patient safely. *Nursing, 24*(9), 16.

McConnell, E. A. (1995). Clinical do's & don'ts: Transferring a patient from bed to chair. *Nursing, 25*(11), 30.

Metzler, D. J., & Harr, J. (1996). Positioning your patient properly. *American Journal of Nursing, 96*(3), 33–37.

Minter, S. G. (1999). Is healthcare safety being neglected? *Occupational Hazards, 61*(4), 37–41.

Peck, R. L. (1996). Patient-handling equipment: How to get value. *Nursing Homes Long Term Care Management, 45*(1), 34–36.

Schuldenfrei, P. (1998). No heavy lifting: Making safety work. *American Journal of Nursing, 98*(9), 46–48.

Smith, S. F., Duell, D. J., & Martin, B. C. (2000). *Clinical Nursing Skills Basic to Advanced Skills.* Upper Saddle River, NJ: Prentice Hall Health.

Chapter 6

Mobilizing the Client

Techniques

OBJECTIVES

- Discuss differentiated care of clients using various specialized beds.
- Describe the technique of turning a client in a Stryker wedge frame.
- List clinical guidelines for wheelchair safety.
- Describe safety measures appropriate when assisting clients to ambulate.
- Identify the steps in proper use of crutches, canes, and walkers.

TABLE 6-1

COMMONLY USED THERAPEUTIC BEDS

Type	Description	Brand Name	Indicated Use
Air-fluidized (AF) beds	Forced temperature-controlled air is circulated around millions of tiny silicone-coated beads.	Clinitron	Pressure relief (Figure 6-1 ◆) Treatment of pressure sores, burns
Spinal stabilization	Permits frequent turning while maintaining spinal alignment.	Stryker-Wedge Frame CircOlectric Bed	Spinal injury Immobilized clients
Static **low-air-loss (LAL)**	Consists of many air-filled cushions divided into 4 or 5 sections. Separate controls permit each section to be inflated to a different level of firmness.	Mediscus KinAir IV	Pressure relief on bony prominences and/or compromised areas (Figure 6-2 ◆)
Active or second-generation low-air-loss	Like the static LAL but in addition gently pulsates or rotates from side to side, thus stimulating capillary blood flow and facilitating movement of pulmonary secretions.	Therapulse Rescue BioDyne	Immobilized clients who have pulmonary problems and compromised skin integrity
Special feature beds	*Obesity beds* permit care of obese clients. Some can assume sitting and Trendelenburg positions.	Magnum	For clients over 300 lbs (some beds accommodate up to 800 lbs) (Figure 6-3 ◆)
	Orthopedic beds can be used as a tilt table, recliner, or chair.	Nelson Bed	Immobilized clients

Adapted from "Understanding Therapeutic Beds," by C. M. Ceccio, 1990, *Orthopaedic Nursing, 9*, pp. 57–70; and "Put Your Patient on the Right Bed," by M. Martes, 1984, *Orthopaedic Nursing, 3*, pp. 51–54.

Mobility

The importance of movement to a person's health cannot be overemphasized. The overall benefits of exercise and the ability to carry out the activities of daily living (ADL) by walking and moving are often taken for granted by a healthy person. Being ill and confined to bed weakens the body and can result in serious impairments not only to movement but also to the functioning of other body systems. Persons not required to be confined to bed may require assistance with mobility though the use of wheelchairs or other assistive devices.

Specialized Beds

Therapeutic beds, also referred to as specialized or specialty beds, are bed units that provide a healing environment. They are used primarily to stabilize the spine, treat the complications of immobility (e.g., pulmonary congestion), and to relieve pressure and/or subsequent skin breakdown. Five major types of therapeutic beds are commonly used today (see Table 6-1).

Nurses should understand how to operate therapeutic beds before providing care. Operating instructions should be attached to the bed in a prominent place. Controls should be conveniently located for both the client and the nurse and have a lockout mechanism to prevent accidental activation. Mattress sections of therapeutic beds often require special sheets.

Spinal immobilization beds such as the Stryker frame consist of two removable metal frames (anterior and posterior) with canvas stretched across them. The current adaptation of the Stryker frame is the **Stryker wedge frame** that requires only one nurse to turn the client (Figure 6-4 ◆). Thin, sponge-rubber mattresses, covered with special sheets with ties, are placed over the canvas.

Nursing Process: Specialized Beds

ASSESSMENT

Inquire if the client has any recent complaints of the following: skin irritation or pressure areas; discomfort; numbness or tingling in the extremities; change in ability to move or motor strength of extremities.

PLANNING

Review the features and use of the frame prior to approaching the client. Review the client's needs to ensure that all care that should be provided while the client is in the current position has been accomplished. Determine whether restraining straps are applied continuously or only at night; the client's previous tolerance for specific positions; and which positioning supports are required. Ascertain the availability of other assistants, if required.

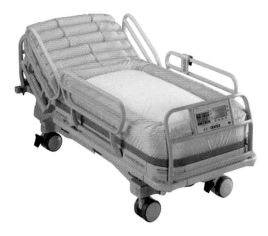

FIGURE 6-1 ◆ Air-fluidized bed (Clinitron).

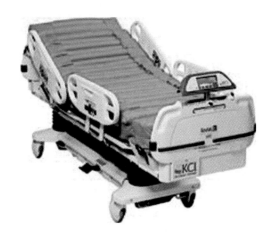

FIGURE 6-2 ◆ Low-air-loss bed (Therapulse II).

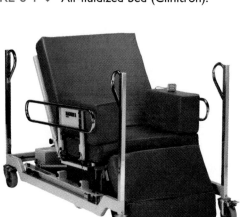

FIGURE 6-3 ◆ Magnum bed.

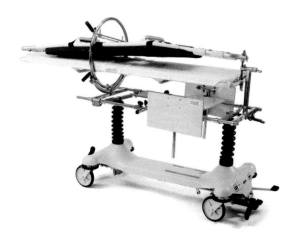

FIGURE 6-4 ◆ A Stryker wedge frame.

Delegation

Turning and positioning of clients in special beds requires training. Unlicensed assistive personnel (UAP) and other care providers who have been trained may perform these procedures for stable clients. The nurse should perform the first few turns when a client is newly placed on a special bed. The nurse also ensures that the UAP knows how to handle catheters and other tubing or equipment involved. In some particularly unstable situations, two persons should perform the turn. If the UAP turns the client without a nurse, any abnormal findings must be reported immediately to the nurse.

IMPLEMENTATION:
TECHNIQUE 6-1 TURNING THE CLIENT ON A STRYKER WEDGE FRAME

Equipment

- Anterior or posterior frame, depending on the turn (these are usually kept at the bedside)
- Clean linen for the frame, as required
- Positioning devices (e.g., pillow supports, footboards)
- Restraining straps
- Protective devices for the skin (e.g., sheepskin)
- Incontinence pads, if required

Performance

1. Explain to the client what you are going to do, why it is necessary, and how he or she can cooperate. Discuss how the results will be used in planning further care or treatments.

2. Wash hands and observe appropriate infection control procedures.

3. Provide for client privacy.

4. Prepare the client.

- Before turning, ensure that all nursing care is completed. For example, if the client is on the posterior frame, bathe all but the back, and place a clean gown on the person.
- Explain the direction in which the turn will take place (e.g., to the client's right or left).
- Place any suction or drainage tubes at the head of the bed. Be sure that the tubing is long enough to accommodate the turn. *This will avoid pulling or tangling the tubing.* Place urinary drainage bags on the side of the mattress the client will turn toward; they must not pass above the client during the turn.

5. Prepare the equipment.
   - Ensure that the wheels of the frame are locked.
   - Remove the armboards and bed linen or bath blanket. If the client is unconscious, do not remove the armboards until the arms are secured with straps.
   - Ensure that the frame to be applied has clean linen on it.

6. Position the client.
   - Make sure the client's arms are not extended beyond the turning radius.
   - Place a pillow lengthwise over the lower legs *to provide security during the turn and maintain alignment of the feet and legs.*

Turning from Supine to Prone Position

- Place the anterior frame over the client, and tighten the knurled nut at the head of the frame (Figure 6-5 ◆). The anterior frame will be angled with the posterior frame to form a wedge.
- Ensure that the forehead and chin bands are placed appropriately, that is, that they do not obstruct the nose, mouth, and eyes. A pillow may be placed beside the head to prevent lateral movement during the turn.

Turning from Prone to Supine Position

- Place incontinence pads or sheepskins over the client's sacrum, if necessary, and put a small pillow under the lumbar curvature, if required.
- Place the posterior frame over the client, and tighten the knurled nut at the head of the frame (Figure 6-5). The posterior frame will be angled with the anterior frame to form a wedge.

7. Close the turning ring over the frame, making sure that it is locked securely and that the frame fits snugly over the client. The nuts on the turning ring can be adjusted to tighten the frame against the client. Directions for doing this are written on the frame.
   - Place the two restraining straps around both the frame and the client's legs and chest. Buckle the straps at the side of the client *to make them easier to open after the turn.*

8. Turn the client.

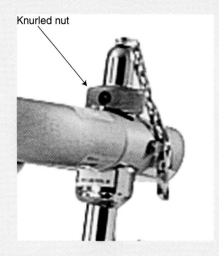

Knurled nut

FIGURE 6-5 ◆ Knurled nut at the head of the frame.

- Ask the client to wrap both arms around the anterior frame, if able. Otherwise, make sure that the arms are restrained.
- Pull out the positive lock pin at the head of the frame (Figure 6-6 ◆). *The frame can pivot when this pin is out.*
- Pull out the red turning lock knob on the turning ring (Figure 6-7 ◆). *This allows the frame to turn.*
- Grasp the handle on the turning ring, and inform the client that you will turn on the count of three. When two nurses are present, the nurse at the head of the bed usually gives the directions for turning.
- Count to three, and turn the frame toward you, using a smooth, gradual motion. *People feel more secure when turned toward the nurse.*

9. Secure the frame.
   - Replace the positive lock pin. The pin stabilizes the frame and prevents it from pivoting.

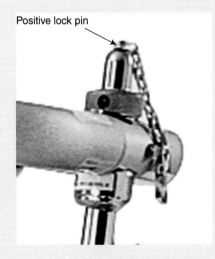

Positive lock pin

FIGURE 6-6 ◆ Lock pin at the head of the frame.

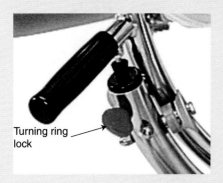

FIGURE 6-7 ◆ Lock knob on the turning ring.

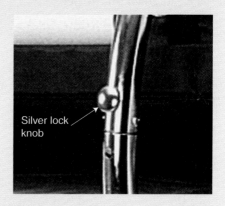

Silver lock knob

FIGURE 6-8 ◆ Silver lock knob.

- Push in the circular silver lock knob (Figure 6-8 ◆). *This opens the turning ring.*
- Release the knurled nut, and remove the uppermost frame.

10. Provide necessary care, and position the client.
   - Provide skin care to pressure areas as required.
   - Position the client in correct body alignment.
   - Attach the armboards, and position the client's arms appropriately *to prevent adduction contractures of the shoulders and flexion contractures of the elbows.* The armboards should be slightly below the level of the frame when the client is in the prone position and level with the frame when the client is in the supine position.

- Cover the client appropriately for warmth.
- Place restraining straps around the client as a protective measure if required. Generally, one restraining strap is placed around the hips for clients receiving narcotics or sedatives and for all people at bedtime.
- Instruct the client about foot or leg exercises, for example, dorsiflexion and plantar flexion, inversion and eversion of the foot, if health indicates.

 11. **Document** the turn in the client record using forms or checklists supplemented by narrative notes when appropriate.

AMBULATORY AND COMMUNITY SETTINGS

Specialized Beds

- Some clients with long-term disabilities may have specialized beds in the home. Ensure that all family and caregivers have been instructed in proper use of the bed and can demonstrate appropriate level of care.

- If the bed is electric, assess adequacy and safety of the wiring in the home.
- Confirm that the caregivers are aware of emergency measures should the client arrest, there be a fire in the home, or the electricity fail.

AGE-RELATED CONSIDERATIONS

Specialized Beds

Child

- Spinal cord and other injuries requiring therapeutic beds are rare in children. Most orthopedic conditions can be treated with body casts and external braces.

Elders

- Elders are at increased risk for skin and neurological impairments. They may be less aware of or less able to report complications related to pressure areas.

- Perform a detailed follow-up based on findings that deviated from expected or normal for the client. Relate findings to previous assessment data if available.

- Report significant deviations from normal to the physician.

Using a Wheelchair

Some clients may require the use of a wheelchair for a short or an extended period of time. Depending on the purpose of the wheelchair, the client and family may also need to learn how to use the equipment.

Types of Wheelchairs and Wheelchair Components

There are two general types of wheelchairs: manual and electric/power. This chapter focuses on manual wheelchairs since there is significant variation in the design and operation of power wheelchairs. Manual wheelchairs may be either folding or rigid framed. Folding wheelchairs have an "X"-shaped brace under the seat that allows the seat to fold arm to arm. Although the ability to fold the wheelchair for placement in a car or for compact storage may be desirable, there are also drawbacks to the folding wheelchair. The brace makes the wheelchair heavy and possibly too heavy for one person to lift. In addition, the frame is not as strong as the rigid frame and the moving joints are subject to wear. The rigid frame usually has a seatback that folds down and easily removable wheels. Since it weights about 10 to 20 pounds, it can be easily lifted without the wheels. Armrests can be removed from most wheelchairs.

Footrests and legrests may be rigid or adjustable. Adjustable legrests are more common in wheelchairs found in hospitals since they are used when the feet need to be raised to aid in circulation or for persons who cannot bend their knees.

Wheel locks are generally side mounted with short or long lever arms used to manually move the brake arm against the wheel. The size and type of the wheelchair's smaller front caster wheels are selected according to the expected use. Larger caster wheels roll over bumps more easily but are heavier, are harder to turn, and take more room to turn. Tires may be air filled (pneumatic), which are light, smooth, and durable or solid (airless), which, since they do not go flat, are more reliable for power wheelchairs when the extra weight is less of a concern.

For persons who spend a great deal of time in a wheelchair, proper seating is of utmost importance. If the seat does not adequately support the client, skin breakdown and adverse effects of poor posture can result. For temporary use, the sling seat that comes with most wheelchairs is acceptable. However, it can cause internal rotation of the hips, flexion of the pelvis, and inadequate neck support. In long-term use, a rigid back plus a solid seat platform with foam, air, gel, or honeycomb cushion is required.

Nursing Process: Wheelchairs

ASSESSMENT

Determine the client's body size, ability to follow instructions, activity tolerance, muscle strength, joint mobility, presence of paralysis, level of comfort, and experience with the use of a wheelchair.

PLANNING

Review the client's needs and the types of wheelchairs available. Wheelchairs vary in the ability to adjust the chair back, arms, legs, and foot supports, and to carry an IV pole, oxygen tank, or other supplies. Wheelchairs also come in a variety of sizes (see Figure 6-9 ◆).

Delegation

UAP are qualified to transfer clients into and out of wheelchairs and to transport clients in wheelchairs if the client is in stable condition. If it is the first time the client has transferred into or out of the wheelchair, the nurse should observe, provide assistance as needed, and reinforce proper technique with both the client and the UAP.

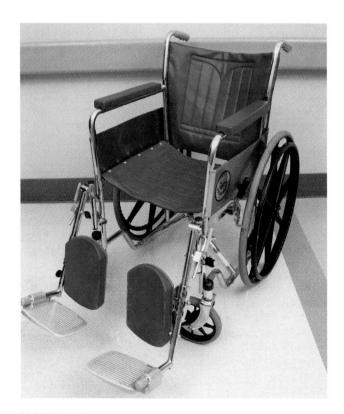

FIGURE 6-9 ◆ Standard wheelchair.

Equipment

- Wheelchair
- Pillows and soft restraints (as needed)

Performance

1. Explain to the client what you are going to do, why it is necessary, and how he or she can cooperate. Discuss how the results will be used in planning further care or treatments.

2. Wash hands and observe appropriate infection control procedures.

3. Provide for client privacy.

4. Lock the wheels of the wheelchair, raise the footplate, and transfer the client into the wheelchair (Technique 5-6).

5. Examine the client's body alignment and provide support if the client cannot maintain proper alignment independently.

6. Place equipment (e.g., urinary catheter bags and oxygen tubing) safely on the wheelchair where they cannot get caught in the wheels.

7. Instruct the client in the importance of periodic shifting of body weight *to reduce pressure on bony prominences.* If the client cannot perform these movements independently, establish a routine for assisting the client at least every hour.

8. Ensure client safety.

- Ask the client to sit far back into the wheelchair seat. *A wheelchair can topple forward when the client sits on the edge of the seat and leans far forward.*

- Do not put overly heavy items on the back of the wheelchair.

- Position the calf supports. Lower the footplates, and place the client's feet on them. Adjust the leg height if needed.

- Apply a seat belt as required.

- Release the brakes and transport the client (see Box 6-1).

- Do not leave the client unattended if the client cannot mobilize the wheelchair independently.

9. **Document** the transfer and client teaching in the client record using forms or checklists supplemented by narrative notes when appropriate. If necessary, include a description of the positioning aids used.

Box 6-1 *Transporting a Client in a Wheelchair*

- Lock the wheels whenever the client is not moving.

- Recognize that the wheel locks are not brakes. They will not stop a rolling wheelchair and may not prevent sliding.

- Wheel the client backwards into an elevator. This allows the client to see the door and makes exiting the elevator easier.

- When wheeling the client down a steep ramp or curb, proceed backwards, using your body weight as a brake if needed.

- If it is appropriate to take a rest while going up or down a long slope, turn the wheelchair sideways, perpendicular to the slope.

- When wheeling the client up or down steps both the helper and the client should be facing up the steps. *Note:* Clients should be wheeled up or down only long-tread, low-rise steps. Since adequate control cannot be ensured on steps where the entire back wheel cannot rest, the client must be carried up or down regular-sized steps.

AMBULATORY AND COMMUNITY SETTINGS

Using a Wheelchair

- Many homes are not constructed to permit wheelchair access. Arrange for a home assessment prior to discharging a client who will need to use a wheelchair inside the home. Modifications may be necessary especially for use of bathrooms.

- Teach the client and family how to use the wheelchair appropriately. This includes collapsing the wheelchair for transport in a car, proper wheeling down sidewalks and ramps, and public transportation services (e.g., buses that accept wheelchairs, elevator access to transit loading areas).

Using a Wheelchair

Child

- Children learn quickly how to maneuver themselves in an appropriate-sized wheelchair. Ensure that all safety procedures are in place.

Elders

- Some elders may have incomplete sensation or control in their extremities. Ensure that arms and legs are appropriately supported and protected from injury.

EVALUATION

- Perform a detailed follow-up based on findings that deviated from expected or normal for the client. Relate findings to previous assessment data if available.

- Report significant deviations from normal to the physician.

Ambulation

Ambulation (the act of walking) is a function that most people take for granted. However, when people are ill, they are often confined to bed and are nonambulatory. The longer clients are in bed, the more difficulty they have walking. Even 1 or 2 days of bed rest can make a person feel weak, unsteady, and shaky when first getting out of bed. A client who has had surgery, is elderly, or has been immobilized for a longer time will feel more pronounced weakness. The potential problems of immobility are far less likely to occur when clients become ambulatory as soon as possible. The nurse can assist clients to prepare for ambulation by helping them become as independent as possible while in bed. Nurses should encourage clients to perform ADL, maintain good body alignment, and carry out active range-of-motion exercises to the maximum degree possible yet within the limitations imposed by their illness and recovery program (see Chapter 8).

Common problems that affect walking include pathology of the muscles, disease or injury of the bones of the lower extremities, and impaired balance—such as from an inner ear infection or due to a cerebrovascular accident (CVA) that produces **hemiplegia** (loss of movement on one side of the body). Nurses frequently need to assist clients in walking, and with a variety of such devices as **canes**, **walkers**, and **crutches**.

Nursing Process: Ambulation

ASSESSMENT

Inquire about the client history of the following: length of time in bed and time up previously; baseline pulse rate, respiratory rate, and blood pressure; range-of-motion of joints needed for ambulating (e.g., hips, knees, ankles); muscle strength of lower extremities; need for ambulation aids (e.g., cane, walker, crutches); client's intake of medications (e.g., narcotics, sedatives, tranquilizers, and antihistamines) that may cause drowsiness, dizziness, weakness, and orthostatic hypotension and seriously hinder the client's ability to walk safely; presence of joint inflammation, fractures, muscle weakness, or other conditions that impair physical mobility; ability to understand directions; need for the assistance of another nurse.

PLANNING

The amount of assistance ambulating will depend on the client's condition, for example, age, health status, length of inactivity, and emotional readiness. Review any previous experiences with ambulation and the success of such efforts. Plan the length of the walk with the client, in light of the nursing or physician's orders. Be prepared to shorten the walk according to the person's activity tolerance.

Delegation

Ambulation of clients is frequently delegated to UAP. However, the nurse should conduct an initial assessment of the client's abilities in order to direct other personnel in providing appropriate assistance. Any unusual events that arise from assisting the client in ambulation must be validated and interpreted by the nurse.

IMPLEMENTATION:
TECHNIQUE 6-3 ASSISTING THE CLIENT TO AMBULATE

Equipment

- Transfer belt if the client is known to be unsteady

Performance

1. Explain to the client how you are going to assist, why ambulation is necessary, and how he or she

can cooperate. Discuss how this activity relates to the overall plan of care.

2. Wash hands and observe appropriate infection control procedures.

3. Ensure that the client is appropriately dressed to walk and has shoes or slippers with nonskid soles.

4. Prepare the client for ambulation.
   - Apply elastic (antiemboli) stockings as required (see Technique 19-1).
   - Assist the client to sit on the edge of the bed.
   - Assess the client carefully for signs and symptoms of orthostatic hypotension (dizziness, light-headedness, or a sudden increase in heart rate) prior to leaving the bedside.
   - Assist the client to stand by the side of the bed until he or she feels secure.

5. Ensure client safety while assisting the client to ambulate.
   - Encourage the client to ambulate independently if he or she is able, but walk beside the client.
   - Remain physically close to the client in case assistance is needed at any point.
   - Use a transfer or walking belt if the client is slightly weak and unstable. Make sure the belt is pulled snugly around the client's waist and fastened securely. Grasp the belt at the client's back, and walk behind and slightly to one side of the client (Figure 6-10 ◆).
   - If it is the client's first time out of bed following surgery, injury, or an extended period of immobility, or if the client is quite weak or unstable, have an assistant follow you and the client with a wheelchair in the event that it is needed quickly.
   - If the client is moderately weak and unstable, walk on the client's weaker side and interlock your forearm with the client's closest forearm. Encourage the client to press the forearm against your hip or waist for stability if desired. In addition, have the client wear a transfer or walking belt *so that you can quickly grab the belt and prevent a fall if the client feels faint.*
   - If the client is very weak and unstable, place your near arm around the client's waist, and with your other arm support the client's near arm at the elbow. Walk on the client's stronger side. Again, have the client wear a transfer or walking belt in case of an emergency.
   - Encourage the client to assume a normal walking stance and gait as much as possible.

6. Protect the client who begins to fall while ambulating.

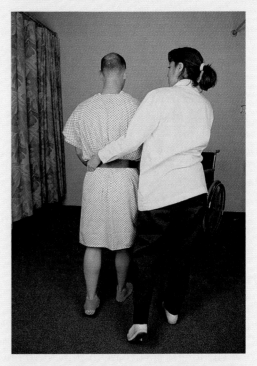

FIGURE 6-10 ◆ Using a transfer (walking) belt to support the client.

- If a client begins to experience the signs and symptoms of orthostatic hypotension or extreme weakness, quickly assist the client into a nearby wheelchair or other chair, and help the client to lower the head between the knees.
- Stay with the client. *A client who faints while in this position could fall head first out of the chair.*
- When the weakness subsides, assist the client back to bed.
- If a chair is not close by, assist the client to a horizontal position on the floor before fainting occurs (Figure 6-11 ◆).
   a. Assume a broad stance with one foot in front of the other. *A broad stance widens your base of support. Placing one foot behind the other allows you to rock backward and use the femoral muscles when supporting the client's weight and lowering the center of gravity (see the next step), thus preventing back strain.*
   b. Bring the client backward so that your body supports the person. *Clients who faint or start to fall usually pitch slightly forward because of the momentum of ambulating. Bringing the client's weight backward against your body allows gradual movement to the floor without injury to the client.*
   c. Allow the client to slide down your leg, and lower the person gently to the floor, making sure the client's head does not hit any objects.

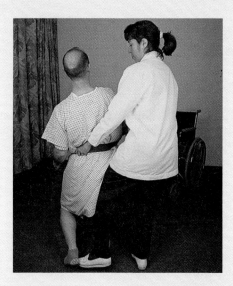

FIGURE 6-11 ◆ Lowering a fainting client to the floor.

Variation: Two Nurses

- After the client stands, assume a position with one nurse at either side. Grasp the inferior aspect of the client's upper arm with your nearest hand and the client's lower arm or hand with your other hand (Figure 6-12 ◆). *This provides a secure grip for each nurse.*

- *Optional:* Place a walking belt around the client's waist. Each nurse grasps the side handle with the near hand and the lower aspect of the client's upper arm with the other hand.

- Walk in unison with the client, using a smooth, even gait, at the same speed and with steps the same size as the client's. *This gives the client a greater feeling of security.*

- If the client starts to fall and cannot regain strength or balance, slip your arms under the client's axillae, grasp the client's hands, and lower the person gently to the floor or to a nearby chair (Figure 6-13 ◆). *Placing the nurse's arms under the client's axillae evenly balances the client's weight between the two nurses, preventing injury to both the nurses and the client.*

7. **Document** distance and duration of ambulation in the client record using forms or checklists supplemented by narrative notes when appropriate. Include description of the client's gait (including body alignment) when walking; pace; activity tolerance when walking (e.g., pulse rate, facial color, any shortness of breath, feelings of dizziness, or weakness); degree of support required; and respiratory rate and blood pressure after initial ambulation to compare with baseline data.

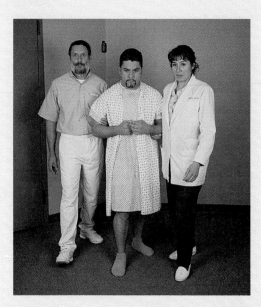

FIGURE 6-12 ◆ Two nurses supporting an ambulatory client.

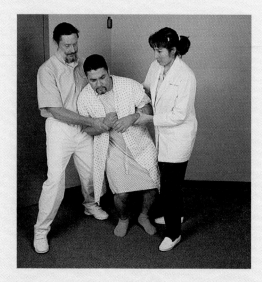

FIGURE 6-13 ◆ Two nurses lowering a fainting client to the floor.

AMBULATORY AND COMMUNITY SETTINGS

Assisting the Client to Ambulate

- When making a home visit, assess carefully for safety issues for ambulation. Counsel the client and family about unfastened rugs, slippery floors, and loose objects on the floors.

- Check the surroundings for adequate supports such as railings and grab bars.

- Recommend that nonskid strips be placed on outside steps and inside stairs that are not carpeted.

AGE-RELATED CONSIDERATIONS

Assisting the Client to Ambulate

Elders

- Inquire how the client has ambulated previously and modify assistance accordingly.

- Take into account a decrease in speed, strength, resistance to fatigue, reaction time, and coordination due to a decrease in nerve conduction.

EVALUATION

- Establish a plan for continued ambulation based on expected or normal ability for the client.

- Report significant deviations from normal to the physician.

Assisting Clients to Use Mechanical Aids for Walking

Mechanical aids for walking include canes, crutches, and walkers. Three types of canes are commonly used: the standard straight-legged cane; the tripod or crab cane, which has three feet; and the **quad cane**, which has four feet (Figure 6-14 ◆). Cane tips should have rubber caps to improve traction and prevent slipping. The standard cane is 91 cm (36 in) long; some alu-minum canes can be adjusted from 56 to 97 cm (22 to 38 inches). The length should permit the elbow to be slightly flexed. Clients may use either one or two canes, depending on how much support they require.

Walkers are for clients who need more support than a cane provides. The standard type is made of polished aluminum. It has four legs with rubber tips and plastic hand grips (Figure 6-15A ◆). The standard walker requires partial strength in both hands and wrists; strong elbow extensors, and strong shoulder depressors. The client also needs the ability to bear at least partial weight on both legs. Four-wheeled or roller walkers do not need to be picked up to be moved, but they are less stable than the standard walker. Some roller walkers have a seat at the back so the client can sit down to rest when desired. Another walker has two tips and two wheels (Figure 6-15B). The client tilts the walker, lifting the tips while the wheels remain on the ground, then pushes the walker forward. The nurse may need to adjust the height of a client's walker so that the hand bar is below the client's waist and the client's elbows are slightly flexed. A walker that is too low causes the client to stoop; one that is too high makes the client stretch and reach. Instructions for using walkers are provided in Box 6-2.

Crutches may be a temporary need for some people and a permanent one for others. Crutches should enable a person to ambulate independently; therefore, it is important to learn to use them properly. The most frequently used kinds of crutches are the underarm crutch, or **axillary crutch** with hand bars, and the **Lofstrand crutch**, which extends only to the forearm (Figure 6-16 ◆). The metal cuff around the forearm and the metal bar stabilize the wrists and thus make walking safer and easier. The platform, or elbow extensor crutch also has a cuff for the upper arm (Figure 6-16). All crutches require suction tips, usually made of rubber, which help to prevent slipping on a floor surface.

Nursing Process: Assisting Clients to Use Mechanical Aids for Walking

ASSESSMENT

Inquire about the following: client's physical strength of the lower extremities, arms, and hands; ability to

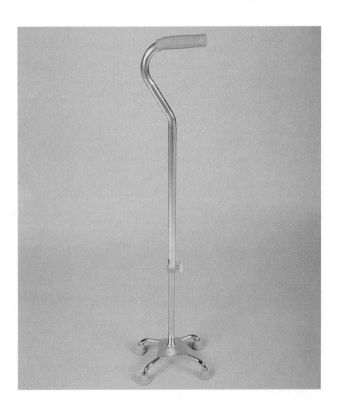

FIGURE 6-14 ◆ Quad cane

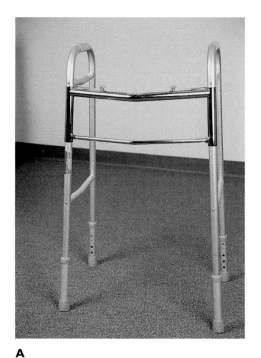

A

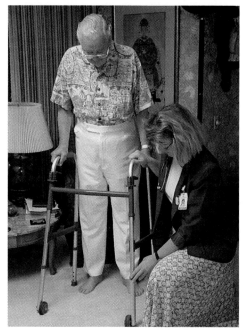

B

FIGURE 6-15 ◆ (A) Standard walker. (B) Two-wheeled walker.

bear body weight; ability to keep balance in a standing position on one or both legs; ability to hold the body erect.

PLANNING

Determine what type of ambulatory assistive device is most appropriate for the client. The physician or physical therapist may specify this information.

Box 6-2 *Using Walkers*

When Maximum Support Is Required

- Move the walker ahead about 15 cm (6 in) while body weight is borne by both legs.
- Then, move the right foot up to the walker while body weight is borne by the left leg and both arms.
- Next, move the left foot up to the right foot while body weight is borne by the right leg and both arms.

If One Leg Is Weaker Than the Other

- Move the walker and the weak leg ahead together about 15 cm (6 in) while weight is borne by the stronger leg.
- Then, move the stronger leg ahead while weight is borne by the affected leg and both arms.

Delegation

Due to the extent of knowledge required, teaching the client to use assistive devices is not delegated to UAP. The nurse or the physical therapist does the teaching. However, once the client has demonstrated adequate skill, UAP may assist the client in ambulating with this equipment.

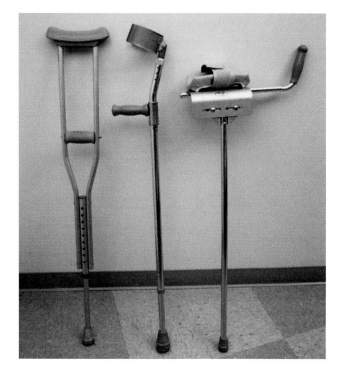

FIGURE 6-16 ◆ Types of crutches: axillary, Lofstrand, platform.

Equipment

• Cane with rubber tips.

Performance

1. Explain to the client what you are going to do, why it is necessary, and how he or she can cooperate. Discuss how the results will be used in planning further care or treatments.

2. Wash hands and observe appropriate infection control procedures.

3. Provide for client privacy.

4. Prepare the client for walking.

   • Ask the client to hold the cane on the stronger side of the body. *This provides support and body alignment when walking. The arm opposite the advancing foot normally swings forward when walking, so the hand holding the cane will come forward and the cane will support the weaker leg.*

   • Position the tip of a standard cane (and the nearest tip of other canes) about 15 cm (6 in) to the side and 15 cm (6 in) in front of the near foot, so that the elbow is slightly flexed. *This provides the best balance and prevents the person from leaning on the cane. In this position, the client stands erect, with the center of gravity within the base of support.*

5. When maximum support is required, instruct the client to move as follows:

   • Move the cane forward about 30 cm (1 ft), or a distance that is comfortable while the body weight is borne by both legs (Figure 6-17A ◆).

   • Then, move the affected (weak) leg forward to the cane while the weight is borne by the cane and stronger leg (Figure 6-17B).

   • Next, move the unaffected (stronger) leg forward ahead of the cane and weak leg while the weight is borne by the cane and weak leg (Figure 6-17C).

   • Repeat the above three steps. *This pattern of moving provides at least two points of support on the floor at all times.*

6. When the client becomes stronger and requires less support, instruct the client to follow these steps:

   • Move the cane and weak leg forward at the same time, while the weight is borne by the stronger leg (Figure 6-18A ◆).

   • Move the stronger leg forward while the weight is borne by the cane and the weak leg (Figure 6-18B).

7. Ensure client safety.

   • Walk beside the client on the affected side. *The client is most likely to fall toward the affected side.*

   • Walk the client for the time or distance indicated in the plan of care.

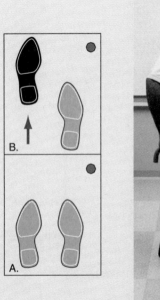
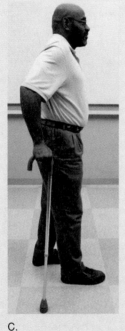

C.

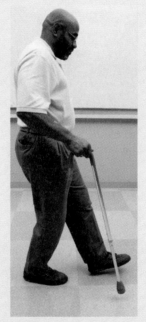
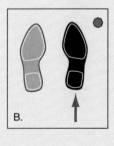

A.

FIGURE 6-17 ◆ Steps involved in using a cane to provide maximum support.

FIGURE 6-18 ◆ Steps involved in using a cane when less than maximum support is required.

- If the client loses balance or strength and is unable to regain it, slide your hand up to the client's axilla, and take a broad stance to provide a base of support. Have the client rest against your hip until assistance arrives, or gently lower yourself and the client to the floor.

8. **Document** the client's progress in the client record using forms or checklists supplemented by narrative notes when appropriate. Describe the distance ambulated and any difficulties the client experienced.

1. Ensure that the crutches are the proper length (see Box 6-3).

2. Assist the client to assume the tripod (triangle) position, the basic crutch stance used before crutch walking.

   - Ask the client to stand and place the tips of the crutches 15 cm (6 in) in front of the feet and out laterally about 15 cm (6 in). See Figure 6-20 ◆. *The tripod position provides a wide base of support and enhances both stability and balance.*

   - Make sure the feet are slightly apart. A tall person requires a wider base than a short person.

   - Ensure that posture is erect, that is, the hips and knees are extended, the back is straight, and the head is held straight and high. There should be no hunch to the shoulders and thus no weight borne by the axillae. The elbows should be extended sufficiently to allow weight bearing on the hands.

- Stand slightly behind and on the client's affected side. *By standing behind the client and toward the affected side, the nurse can provide support if the client loses balance.*

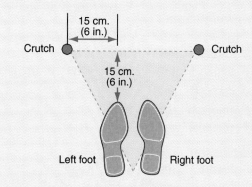

FIGURE 6-20 ◆ The tripod position.

Box 6-3 *Measuring Clients for Crutches*

When nurses measure clients for axillary crutches, it is most important to obtain the correct length for the crutches and the correct placement of the hand piece. There are two methods of measuring crutch length:

1. The client lies in the supine position, and the nurse measures from the anterior fold of the axilla to a point 10 cm (4 in) lateral from the heel of the foot.

2. The client stands erect and positions the crutch tips 5 cm (2 in) in front of and 15 cm (6 in) to the side of the feet (Figure 6-19 ◆). The nurse makes sure the shoulder rest of the crutch is at least three finger widths, that is, 2.5 to 5 cm (1 to 2 in), below the axilla.

To determine the correct placement of the hand bar:

1. The client stands upright and supports the body weight by the hand grips of the crutches.

2. The nurse measures the angle of elbow flexion. It should be about 30 degrees. A goniometer (see Figure 3-83) may be used to verify the correct angle.

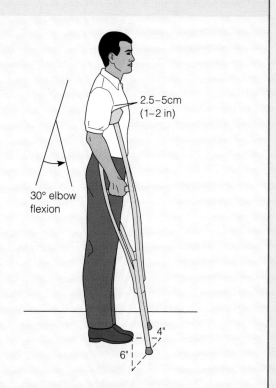

FIGURE 6-19 ◆ Standing position for measuring crutches.

- If the client is unsteady, place a walking belt around the client's waist, and grasp the belt from above, not from below. *A fall can be prevented more effectively if the belt is held from above.*

3. Teach the client the appropriate crutch gait.

Four-Point Alternate Gait

This is the most elementary and safest gait, providing at least three points of support at all times, but it requires coordination. It can be used when walking in crowds because it does not require much space. To use this gait, the client has to be able to bear some weight on both legs (Figure 6-21 ◆, reading from bottom to top). Ask the client to:

- Move the right crutch ahead a suitable distance (e.g., 10 to 15 cm [4 to 6 in]).
- Move the left foot forward, preferably to the level of the crutch.
- Move the left crutch forward.
- Move the right foot forward.

Three-Point Gait

To use this gait, the person must be able to bear entire body weight on the unaffected leg. The two crutches and the unaffected leg bear weight alternately (Figure 6-22 ◆, reading from bottom to top). Ask the client to:

- Move both crutches and the weaker leg forward.
- Move the stronger leg forward.

Two-Point Alternate Gait

This gait is faster than the four-point gait. It requires more balance, because only two points support the body at one time; it also requires at least partial weight bearing on each foot. In this gait, arm movements with the crutches are similar to the arm movements during normal walking (Figure 6-23 ◆, reading from bottom to top). Ask the client to:

- Move the left crutch and the right foot forward together.
- Move the right crutch and the left foot ahead together.

Swing-To Gait

People with paralysis of the legs and hips use the swing gaits. Prolonged use of these gaits results in atrophy of the unused muscles. The swing-to gait is the easier of these two gaits (Figure 6-24 ◆). Ask the client to:

- Move both crutches ahead together.
- Lift body weight by the arms and swing *to* the crutches.

Swing-Through Gait

This gait requires considerable client skill, strength, and coordination (Figure 6-25 ◆). Ask the client to:

- Move both crutches forward together.

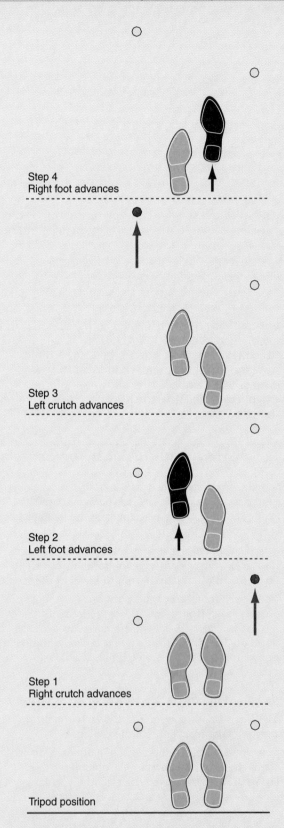

Step 4
Right foot advances

Step 3
Left crutch advances

Step 2
Left foot advances

Step 1
Right crutch advances

Tripod position

FIGURE 6-21 ◆ The four-point alternate crutch gait.

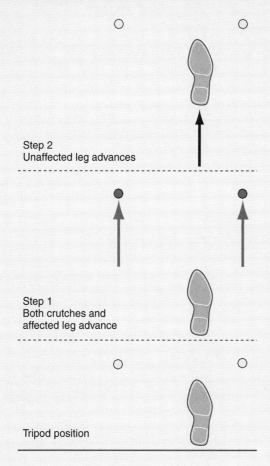

Step 2
Unaffected leg advances

Step 1
Both crutches and
affected leg advance

Tripod position

FIGURE 6-22 ◆ The three-point crutch gait.

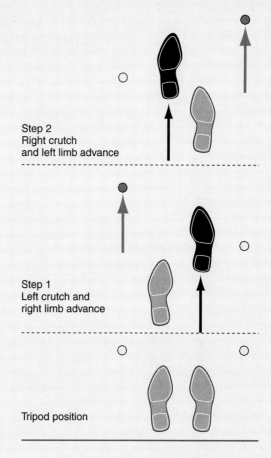

Step 2
Right crutch
and left limb advance

Step 1
Left crutch and
right limb advance

Tripod position

FIGURE 6-23 ◆ The two-point alternate crutch gait.

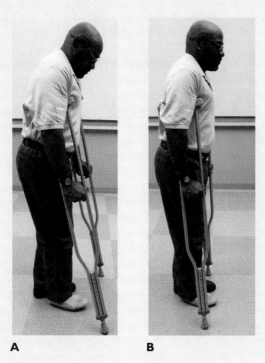

A   B

FIGURE 6-24 ◆ The swing-to crutch gait.

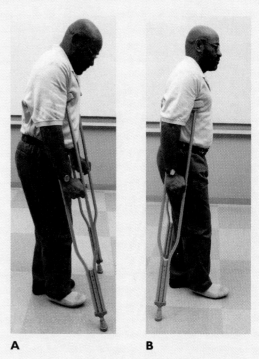

A   B

FIGURE 6-25 ◆ The swing-through crutch gait.

• Lift body weight by the arms and swing through and beyond the crutches.

4. Teach the client to get into and out of a chair.

Getting Into a Chair

• Ensure that the chair has armrests and is secure or braced against a wall.

• Instruct the client to:

a. Stand with the back of the unaffected leg centered against the chair.

b. Transfer the crutches to the hand on the affected side, hold the crutches by the hand bars, and then grasp the arm of the chair with the hand on the unaffected side (Figure 6-26 ◆). *This allows the client to support the body weight on the arms and the unaffected leg.*

c. Lean forward, flex the knees and hips, and lower into the chair.

Getting Out of a Chair

• Instruct the client to:

a. Move forward to the edge of the chair and place the unaffected leg slightly under or at the edge of the chair. *This position helps the client stand up from the chair and achieve balance, because the unaffected leg is supported against the edge of the chair.*

b. Grasp the crutches by the hand bars in the hand on the affected side, and grasp the arm of the chair by the hand on the unaffected side. *The body weight is placed on the crutches and the hand on the armrest to support the unaffected leg when the client rises to stand.*

c. Push down on the crutches and the chair armrest while elevating the body out of the chair.

d. Assume the tripod position before moving.

5. Teach the client to go up and down stairs.

Going Up Stairs

• Stand behind the client and slightly to the affected side.

• Ask the client to:

a. Assume the tripod position at the bottom of the stairs.

b. Transfer the body weight to the crutches and move the unaffected leg onto the step (Figure 6-27 ◆).

c. Transfer the body weight to the unaffected leg on the step and move the crutches and affected leg up to the step. The crutches always support the affected leg.

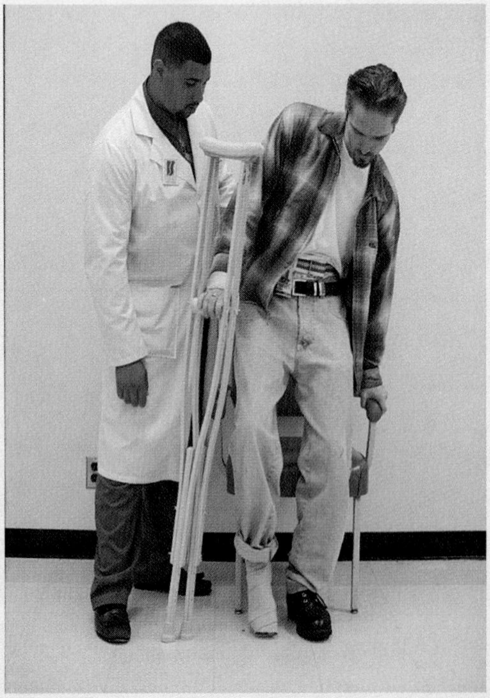

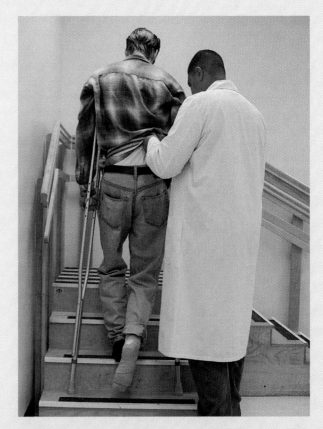

FIGURE 6-26 ◆ A client using crutches getting into a chair.

FIGURE 6-27 ◆ Climbing stairs; placing weight on the crutches while first moving the unaffected leg onto a step.

- Repeat steps b and c until the top of the stairs is reached.

Going Down Stairs

- Stand one step below the person on the affected side.
- Ask the client to:
  a. Assume the tripod position at the top of the stairs.
  b. Shift the body weight to the unaffected leg, and move the crutches and affected leg down onto the next step (Figure 6-28 ◆).
  c. Transfer the body weight to the crutches, and move the unaffected leg to that step. The crutches always support the affected leg.

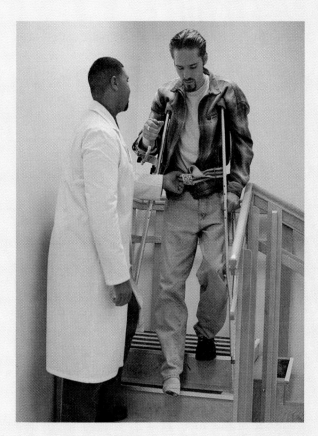

FIGURE 6-28 ◆ Descending stairs; moving the crutches and affected leg to the next step.

  d. Repeat steps b and c until the bottom of the stairs is reached.

or

- Ask the client to:
  a. Hold both crutches in the outside hand and grasp the hand rail with the other hand for support.
  b. Move as in steps b and c, above.

6. Reinforce client teaching. See Box 6-4.

 7. **Document** the client's progress in the client record using forms or checklists supplemented by narrative notes when appropriate.

Box 6-4 *Teaching the Client to Use Crutches*

- Follow the plan of exercises developed for you to strengthen your arm muscles before beginning crutch walking.
- Have a health care professional establish the correct length for your crutches and the correct placement of the handpieces. Crutches that are too long force your shoulders upward and make it difficult for you to push your body off the ground. Crutches that are too short will make you hunch over and develop an improper body stance.
- The weight of your body should be borne by the arms rather than the axillae (armpits). Continual pressure on the axillae can injure the radial nerve and eventually cause crutch palsy, a weakness of the muscles of the forearm, wrist, and hand.
- Maintain an erect posture as much as possible to prevent strain on muscles and joints and to maintain balance.
- Each step taken with crutches should be a comfortable distance for you. It is wise to start with a small rather than a large step.
- Inspect the crutch tips regularly, and replace them if worn.
- Keep the crutch tips dry to maintain their surface friction. If the tips become wet, dry them well before use.

AMBULATORY AND COMMUNITY SETTINGS

Assisting Clients to Use Mechanical Aids for Walking

- When making a home visit, assess carefully for safety issues for ambulation with mechanical devices. Counsel the client and family about unfastened rugs, slippery floors, and loose objects on the floors.
- Recommend nonskid strips be placed on outside steps and inside stairs that are not carpeted.

- Check that appropriate chairs are available.
- Reinforce client teaching about proper gaits with canes, crutches, and walkers.
- Ensure that the equipment is properly maintained and stored out of the way when not in use.
- Tennis balls with a cross cut in them may be applied over walker tips to make sliding easier.

AGE-RELATED CONSIDERATIONS

Assisting Clients to Use Mechanical Aids for Walking

Child

- Children learn and adapt quickly to the use of assistive devices. Care should be taken to check regularly that they are using proper technique.

Elders

- Elders' condition can change rapidly. Check regularly to see that the current assistive device is the most appropriate one and that it fits the client properly.
- Reinforce teaching regarding proper use of mechanical aids. Clients can easily fall into bad habits such as leaning the axillae on the crutches.

EVALUATION

- Perform a detailed follow-up based on findings that deviated from expected or normal for the client.
- Relate findings to previous assessment data if available.
- Report significant deviations from normal to the physician.

Chapter Summary

TERMINOLOGY

air-fluidized (AF) bed
ambulation
axillary crutch
cane

hemiplegia
Lofstrand crutch
low-air-loss (LAL) bed
quad cane

Stryker wedge frame
walker

FORMING CLINICAL JUDGMENTS

Consider This:

1. A client with a spinal cord injury has been placed on a spinal stabilization bed to facilitate care. When you prepare to turn him from the supine to the prone position, what signs would indicate that he is anxious? If he is anxious, how will you respond?

2. Your client has a weak right leg and arm secondary to a stroke. What modifications in usual techniques would be appropriate in assisting this client in using a wheelchair?

3. An 84-year-old client is recovering from a severe episode of the flu and is very weak. The physician has ordered that the client be ambulated in the hall three times a day. The client complains of dizziness when standing and is fearful of falling. What may be causing the dizziness? What precautions should you take?

4. A client who uses a walker lives in a two-story house. What advice would you provide regarding how to use the walker at home?

Related Research

Ferrell, B. A., Osterweil, D., & Christenson, P. (1993). A randomized trial of low-air-loss beds for treatment of pressure ulcers. *Journal of the American Medical Association, 269*, 494–497.

Foley, M. P., Prax, B., Crowell, R., & Boone, T. (1996). Effects of assistive devices on cardiorespiratory demands in older adults. *Physical Therapy, 76*, 1313–1319.

References

____(1999). Canes, walkers and crutches: Don't let choosing one throw you off balance. *Mayo Clinic Health Letter, 17*(1), 4–5.

Carroll, P. (1995). Bed selection: Help patients rest easy. *RN, 58*(5), 44–50.

Jay, R. (1997). Other considerations in selecting a support surface. *Advances in Wound Care: The Journal for Prevention and Healing, 10*(7), 37–42.

Rush, K. L., & Ouellet, L. L. (1997). Mobility aids and the elderly client. *Journal of Gerontological Nursing, 23*(1), 7–15.

Smith, R. (1999). Increasing independence . . . rolling walkers. *Rehab Management: The Interdisciplinary Journal of Rehabilitation, 12*(5), 62.

Wells, J. A., & Karr, D. (1998). Interface pressure, wound healing, and satisfaction in the evaluation of a non-powered fluid mattress. *Ostomy Wound Management, 44*(2), 38–40, 42, 44–46.

Wolfe, S. (2000). Support surfaces and specialty beds: Part 2—aggressive pressure relief. *RN, 63*(4), 65–67.

Chapter 7

Fall Prevention and Restraints

Techniques

OBJECTIVES

- Describe the characteristics of a safe physical environment.
- Explain measures to prevent falls in hospitals and ambulatory settings.
- Describe various kinds of restraints and how each may be used.
- Discuss implementation of seizure precautions.

A safe physical environment is one in which people can function without injury and feel a sense of security. Box 7-1 delineates areas of particular importance for the nurse to assess in order to assure a safe environment. The techniques in this chapter focus on those measures the nurse can take to reduce the risk of client injury as a result of unsafe movement within and out of a bed or chair. These include measures that are taken in anticipation of and in the event of a seizure during which the client cannot control physical movement and is at risk of sustaining an injury.

Preventing Falls

Falls are common among the elderly, ill, or injured who are weak. To prevent falls and subsequent injury of clients, the nurse should consider the guidelines in Box 7-2. Some agencies have a protocol to help prevent client falls. Although it may seem that raising the

Box 7-1 *Safety Assessment*

Assess the client by determining the following:

- Level of awareness or consciousness, specifically, orientation to time, place, and person; ability to concentrate and make judgments; ability to assimilate many kinds of information at one time; ability to perceive reality accurately and act on those perceptions. Consider clients whose judgment is altered by medications, such as narcotics, tranquilizers, hypnotics, and sedatives.
- Lifestyle factors, such as risk-taking behavior and use of safety equipment.
- Sensory alterations, such as impaired vision, hearing, smell, tactile perception, and taste.
- Mobility status. Note in particular individuals who have muscle weakness, poor balance or coordination, or paralysis; those weakened by illness or surgery; and those who use ambulatory aids.
- Emotional state, which can alter the ability to perceive environmental hazards. Persons who are acutely anxious, angry, or depressed may have reduced perceptual awareness or may think and react to environmental stimuli more slowly.
- Ability to communicate. Individuals with diminished ability to receive and convey information (e.g., aphasic clients) and those with language barriers may not be able to read such safety signs as "Wet Floor" or "Out of Order."
- Previous accidents and frequency or predisposition to accidents.
- Safety knowledge about use of potentially dangerous equipment and precautions to take to prevent injury (e.g., fire safety, water safety, oxygen precautions, radiation protection, accident prevention).

Box 7-2 *Preventing Falls in Health Care Settings*

- On admission, orient clients to their surroundings and explain the call system.
- Carefully assess the client's ability to ambulate and transfer. Provide walking aids and assistance as required.
- Closely supervise the clients at risk for falls, especially at night.
- Encourage the client to use call bell to request assistance. Ensure that the bell is within easy reach.
- Place beside tables and overbed tables near the bed or chair so that clients do not overreach and consequently lose their balance.
- Always keep hospital beds in the low position and wheels locked when not providing care so that clients can move in or out of bed easily.
- Encourage clients to use grab bars mounted in toilet and bathing areas and railings along corridors.
- Make sure nonskid bath mats are available in tubs and showers.
- Encourage the client to wear nonskid footwear.
- Keep the environment tidy; especially keep light cords from underfoot and furniture out of the way.
- Attach side rails to the beds of confused, sedated, restless, and unconscious clients, and keep the rails in place when the client is unattended. Consider use of half-rails if a full rail seems to make the client more agitated.

side rails on a bed is an effective method of preventing falls, rails should not be raised routinely for this purpose. Research has shown that persons with memory impairment, altered mobility, nocturia, and other sleep disorders are prone to becoming entrapped in siderails and may, in fact, be more likely to fall trying to get out around raised rails (Capezuti et al., 1999).

Electronic devices are available to detect that clients are attempting to move or get out of bed. A bed or chair safety monitor has a position-sensitive switch that triggers an audio alarm when the client attempts to get out of the bed or chair.

Nursing Process: Preventing Falls

ASSESSMENT

Determine the client's mobility status; judgment about ability to get out of bed safely; proximity of client's room to nurses' station; position of side rails; and functioning status of call light.

PLANNING

Determine the appropriate location for the device. If the device will be applied to a thigh, ensure that the location has intact skin.

Delegation

Risk factors for falls may be observed and recorded by persons other than the nurse. The nurse is responsible for assessing the client and confirming that there is a risk of the client falling when getting out of a chair or bed unassisted. The nurse develops a plan of care that includes a variety of interventions that will protect the client. If indicated, use of a **safety monitoring device** may be delegated to unlicensed assistive personnel (UAP) who have been trained in their application and monitoring.

Equipment

- Alarm and control device
- Sensor
- Connection to nurse call system (optional)

Performance

1. Explain to the client what you are going to do, why it is necessary, and how he or she can cooperate. Discuss how the results will be used in planning further care or treatments.

2. Wash hands and observe appropriate infection control procedures.

3. Provide for client privacy.

4. Explain to client and support persons the purpose and procedure of using safety monitoring device.
   - Explain that the device does not limit mobility in any manner; rather, it alerts the staff when the client is about to get out of bed.
   - Explain that the nurse must be called when the client needs to get out of bed.

5. Test the battery device and alarm sound. *This ensures that the device is functioning properly prior to use.*

6. Apply the sensor pad or leg band.
   - Place the leg band according to the manufacturer's recommendation. (Figure 7-1 ◆). Place the client's leg in a straight horizontal position. *The alarm device is position sensitive; that is, when it approaches a near-vertical position (such as in walking, crawling, or kneeling as the client attempts to get out of bed), the audio alarm will be triggered.*
   - For the bed or chair device, the sensor is usually placed under the buttocks area (Figure 7-2 ◆).
   - For a bed or chair device, set the time delay for determining the client's movement patterns from 1 to 12 seconds.
   - Connect the sensor pad to the control unit and the nurse call system.

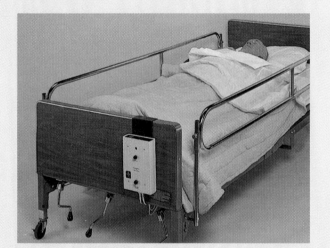

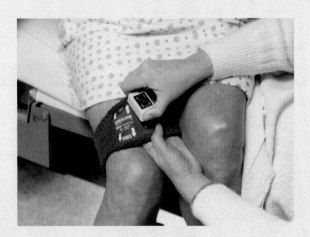

FIGURE 7-1 ◆ Placing the leg band alarm.

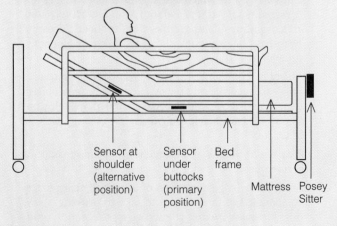

FIGURE 7-2 ◆ Placement of a bed exit monitoring device.

7. Instruct the client to call the nurse when the client wants or needs to get up, and assist as required.
   - When assisting the client up, deactivate the alarm.
   - Assist the client back to bed, and reattach the alarm device.
8. Ensure client safety with additional safety precautions.
   - Place call light within client reach, lift all side rails, and lower the bed to its lowest position.

The alarm device is not a substitute for other precautionary measures.
   - Place ambulation monitoring stickers on the client's door, chart, and Kardex.

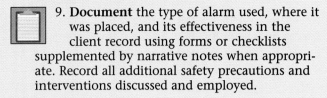 9. **Document** the type of alarm used, where it was placed, and its effectiveness in the client record using forms or checklists supplemented by narrative notes when appropriate. Record all additional safety precautions and interventions discussed and employed.

AMBULATORY AND COMMUNITY SETTINGS

Using a Bed or Chair Exit Safety Monitoring Device

- If the device is used in the home, instruct caregivers to:
  - Test the monitoring device every 12 to 24 hours to ensure that it is working.

- Check the volume of the alarm to ascertain they can hear it.
- Use of the device does not take the place of proper supervision of clients at risk for falling. Assessment of the reasons for falling, especially among elders, can lead to effective prevention.

AGE-RELATED CONSIDERATIONS

Preventing Falls

Elders

- Assess for potential personal causes of falls: hypotension, unsteady gait, altered mental responsiveness (such as from medications), poor vision, foot pathology, cognitive changes, and fear.
- In the home or community setting, assess for potential environmental causes of falls:
  - *Lighting:* inadequate amount, inaccessible or inconvenient switches
  - *Floors:* presence of electrical cords, loose rugs, clutter, slippery surfaces

- *Stairs:* absent or unsteady railings, uneven step height or surfaces
- *Furniture:* unsteady base, lack of armrests, cabinets too high or too low
- *Bathroom:* inappropriate toilet height, slippery floors or tub, absence of grab bars
- In the home, consider alternatives to hospital or regular bed if client is extremely prone to fall out of bed:
  - Place the mattress directly onto the floor
  - Use a water mattress
  - Place padding on floor next to bed or between client and side rails

EVALUATION

If the alarm is too sensitive to client movement that is not an attempt to move from bed or chair, reassess and modify accordingly. Report any difficulties using the device or any falls to the physician.

Restraining Clients

Restraints are protective devices used to limit the physical activity of the client or a part of the body. Restraints can be classified as physical or chemical. **Physical restraints** are any manual method or physical or mechanical device, material, or equipment attached to the client's body. They cannot be removed easily and they restrict the client's movement. **Chemical restraints** are medications such as neuroleptics, anxiolytics, sedatives, and psychotropic agents used to control socially disruptive behavior. The purpose of restraints is to prevent the client from injuring self or others.

Increasingly, determining the need for safety measures is viewed as an independent nursing function. However, because restraints restrict the individual's freedom, their use has legal implications. Nurses need to know their agency's policies and the state or provincial laws about restraining clients. The United States Health Care Financing Agency (HCFA) published revised standards for use of restraints in the United States in 1999. These standards apply to all health care organizations and specify two standards for applying restraints: the behavior management standard (client is a danger to self or others) and the acute medical and surgical care standard (temporary immobilization of a client related to a procedure). In the case of the behavior management standard, the nurse may apply restraints but the physician or other licensed independent practitioner must see the client within 1 hour for evaluation. A restraint order for an adult written following evaluation is valid for only 4 hours. If the client must be restrained and secluded, there must be continual visual and audio monitoring of the client's status. The medical–surgical care standard permits up to 12 hours for obtaining the physician's written order for the restraints. All orders must be renewed daily.

Standards require that a physician's order for restraints delineate the reason and time period and prohibit the use of a PRN order for restraints. In all cases, restraints should be used only after every other possible means of insuring safety have been tried (and this is documented). See alternatives to the use of restraints in Box 7-3. Restrained clients often become (more) restless and anxious as a result of the loss of self-control. Nurses must document that the need for the restraint was made clear both to the client and to support persons.

Selecting a Restraint

There are several kinds of restraints. Among the most common are **jacket restraints**, belt restraints, **mitt or hand restraints**, limb restraints, and elbow restraints. Chairs, wheelchairs, and bedsheets used to confine client activity can also be considered restraints. When using restraints, the nurse may find the guidelines in Box 7-4 helpful. Before selecting a restraint, nurses need to understand its purpose clearly and measure it against the following five criteria:

1. It restricts the client's movement as little as possible. If a client needs to have one arm restrained, do not restrain the entire body.

2. It is the least obvious to others. Both clients and visitors are often embarrassed by a restraint, even though they understand why it is being used. The less obvious the restraint, the more comfortable people feel.

3. It does not interfere with the client's treatment or health problem. If a client has poor blood circulation to the hands, apply a restraint that will not aggravate that circulatory problem.

4. It is readily changeable. Restraints need to be changed frequently, especially if they become soiled. Keeping other guidelines in mind, choose a restraint that can be changed with minimal disturbance to the client.

5. It is safe for the particular client. Choose a restraint with which the client cannot self-inflict injury. For example, a physically restrained person could incur injury trying to climb out of bed if one wrist is tied to the bed frame. A jacket restraint would restrain the person more safely.

Nursing Process: Restraining Clients

ASSESSMENT

Examine the behavior indicating the possible need for a restraint; underlying cause for assessed behavior (to ascertain what other protective measures may be

---

Box 7-3 *Alternatives to Restraints*

- Assign nurses in pairs to act as "buddies" so that one nurse can observe the client when the other leaves the unit.
- Place unstable clients in an area that is constantly or closely supervised.
- Prepare clients before a move to limit relocation shock and resultant confusion.
- Stay with a client using a bedside commode or bathroom if the client is confused or sedated or has a gait disturbance or a high risk score for falling.
- Monitor all the client's medications and if possible, attempt to lower or eliminate dosages of sedatives or psychotropics.
- Position beds at their lowest level from the floor to facilitate getting in and out of bed.
- Replace full-length side rails with half- or three-quarter-length rails to prevent confused clients from climbing over rails or falling from the end of the bed.
- Use rocking chairs to help confused clients expend some of their energy so that they will be less inclined to wander.

- Wedge pillows or pads against the sides of wheelchairs to keep clients well positioned.
- Place a removable lap tray on a wheelchair to provide support and help keep the client in place.
- To quiet agitated clients, try a warm beverage, soft lights, a back rub, or a walk.
- Use "environmental restraints," such as pieces of furniture or large plants as barriers, to keep clients from wandering beyond appropriate areas.
- Place a picture or other personal item on the door to clients' rooms to help them identify their room.
- Try to determine the causes of the client's *sundowner's syndrome* (nocturnal wandering and disorientation as darkness falls, associated with dementia). Possible causes include poor hearing, poor eyesight, or pain.
- Establish ongoing assessment to monitor changes in physical and cognitive functional abilities and risk factors.

Box 7-4 *Guidelines to Applying Restraints*

- Assure the client and the client's support persons that the restraint is temporary and protective. A restraint must never be applied as punishment for any behavior or merely for the nurse's convenience.

- Apply the restraint in such a way that the client can move as freely as possible without defeating the purpose of the restraint.

- Ensure that limb restraints are applied securely but not so tightly that they impede blood circulation to any body area or extremity.

- Pad bony prominences (e.g., wrists and ankles) before applying a restraint over them. The movement of a restraint without padding over such prominences can quickly abrade the skin.

- Always tie a limb restraint with a knot that will not tighten when pulled (e.g., a clove hitch).

- Tie the ends of a body restraint to the part of the bed that moves when the head is elevated. Never tie the ends to a side rail or to the fixed frame of the bed if the bed position is to be changed.

- Assess the restraint every 30 minutes. Some facilities have specific forms to be used to record ongoing assessment.

- Release all restraints at least every 2 to 4 hours, and provide range-of-motion (ROM) exercises (see Chapter 8) and skin care (see Chapter 10).

- Reassess the continued need for the restraint every 8 hours. Include an assessment of the underlying cause of the behavior necessitating use of the restraints.

- When a restraint is temporarily removed, do not leave the client unattended.

- Immediately report and record on the client's chart any persistent reddened or broken skin areas under the restraint.

- At the first indication of cyanosis or pallor, coldness of a skin area, or a client's complaint of a tingling sensation, pain, or numbness, loosen the restraint and exercise the limb.

- Apply a restraint with the body part in a normal anatomic position so that it can be released quickly in case of an emergency.

- Provide emotional support verbally and through touch.

---

implemented before applying a restraint); status of skin to which restraint is to be applied; circulatory status distal to restraints and of extremities; and effectiveness of other available safety precautions.

PLANNING

Review institutional policy for restraints and seek consultation as appropriate before independently deciding to apply a restraint. All other possible interventions that are less restrictive must have been tried. The physician must be notified prior to using a restraint, unless there is an emergency.

Delegation

The nurse must make the determination that restraints are appropriate in the specific situation, select the proper type of restraints, evaluate the effectiveness of the restraints, and assess for potential complications from their use. Application of ordered restraints and their temporary removal for skin assessment and care may be delegated to UAP who have been trained in their use.

IMPLEMENTATION:
TECHNIQUE 7-2 APPLYING RESTRAINTS

Equipment

- Appropriate type and size of restraint

Performance

1. Explain to the client and family what you are going to do, why it is necessary, and how they can cooperate. Discuss how the results will be used in planning further care or treatments. Allow time for the client to express feelings about being restrained. Provide needed emotional reassurance that the restraints will be used only when absolutely necessary and that there will be close contact with the client in case assistance is required.

2. Wash hands and observe appropriate infection control procedures.

3. Provide for client privacy if indicated.

4. Apply the selected restraint.

Belt Restraint (Safety Belt)

- Determine that the **safety belt** is in good order. If a Velcro safety belt is to be used, make sure that both pieces of Velcro are intact.

- If the belt has a long portion and a shorter portion, place the long portion of the belt behind (under) the bedridden client and secure it to the movable part of the bed frame. *The long attached portion will then move up when the head of the bed is elevated and will not tighten around the client.* Place the shorter portion of the belt around the client's waist, over the gown. There should be a finger's width between the belt and the client.

    or

- Attach the belt around the client's waist, and fasten it at the back of the chair.

    or

- If the belt is attached to a stretcher, secure the belt firmly over the client's hips or abdomen. *Belt restraints need to be applied to all clients on stretchers even when the side rails are up.*

Jacket Restraint

- Place vest on client, with opening at the front or the back, depending on the type.
- Pull the tie on the end of the vest flap across the chest, and place it through the slit in the opposite side of the chest.
- Repeat for the other tie.
- Use a half-bow knot to secure each tie around the movable bed frame or behind the chair to a chair leg (Figure 7-3 ◆). *A half-bow knot does not tighten or slip when the attached end is pulled but unties easily when the loose end is pulled.*

    or

- Fasten the ties together behind the chair using a square (reef) knot (Figure 7-4 ◆). *This knot does not tighten with pulling and does not slip when pressure is released.*
- Ensure that the client is positioned appropriately to enable maximum chest expansion for breathing.

Mitt Restraint

- Apply the commercial thumbless mitt (Figure 7-5 ◆)

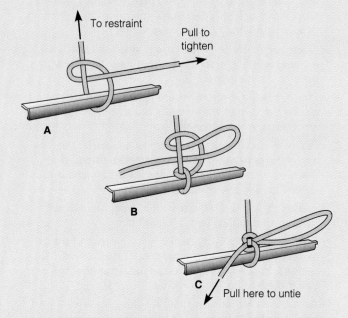

FIGURE 7-3 ◆ To make a half-bow knot (quick-release knot), first place the restraint tie under the side frame of the bed (or around a chair leg). (A) Bring the free end up, around, under, and over the attached end of the tie and pull it tight. (B) Again take the free end over and under the attached end of the tie, but this time make a half-bow loop. (C) Tighten the free end of the tie and the bow until the knot is secure. To untie the knot, pull the end of the tie and then loosen the first cross over the tie.

to the hand to be restrained. Make sure the fingers can be slightly flexed and are not caught under the hand.

- Follow the manufacturer's directions for securing the mitt.
- If a mitt is to be worn for several days, remove it at least every 2 to 4 hours. Wash and exercise the client's hand, then reapply the mitt. Check agency practices about recommended intervals for removal.

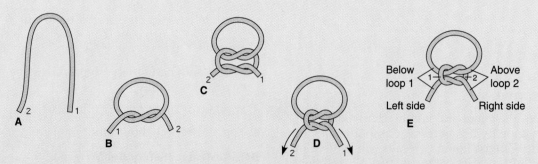

FIGURE 7-4 ◆ To make a square (reef) knot: (A) Form a "U" loop. (B) Pass one end (1) over and under the other. (C) Take the same end (1), and pass it over, under, and over the other. (D) Pull knot tight. (E) When the knot is tied correctly, the ties on each side are both either above or below the loop.

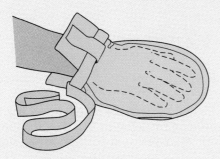

FIGURE 7-5 ◆ A mitt restraint.

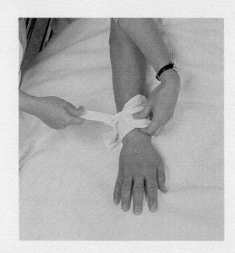

FIGURE 7-6 ◆ Make sure that two fingers can be inserted between the restraint and the wrist or ankle.

- Assess the client's circulation to the hands shortly after the mitt is applied and at regular intervals. *Feelings of numbness or discomfort or inability to move the fingers could indicate impaired circulation to the hand.*

Wrist or Ankle Restraint

- Pad bony prominences on the wrist or ankle if needed to prevent skin breakdown.
- Apply the padded portion of the restraint around the ankle or wrist.
- Pull the tie of the restraint through the slit in the wrist portion or through the buckle (see Figure 7-6 ◆).
- Using a half-bow knot (quick release knot) or a square knot as appropriate, attach the other end of the restraint to the movable portion of the bed frame. *If the ties are attached to the movable portion, the wrist or ankle will not be pulled when the bed position is changed.*

5. Record on the client's chart behavior indicating the need for the restraint, all other interventions implemented in attempt to avoid the use of restraints and their outcomes, and the time the

physician was notified of the need for restraint. Also record:

- The type of restraint applied, the time it was applied, the goal for its application
- The client's response to the restraint
- The times that the restraints were removed and skin care given
- Any other assessments and interventions
- Explanations given to the client and significant others

Adjust the plan of care as required, for example, to include releasing the restraint every 2 hours, providing skin care, and providing range-of-motion exercises.

AMBULATORY AND COMMUNITY SETTINGS

Applying Restraints

Restraints may be necessary for clients in wheelchairs or in the home. Safety guidelines apply in all cases. Assess the knowledge and skill of all caregivers in the use of restraints and educate as indicated.

- Use means other than restraints as much as possible, and stay with the client.
- Pad bony prominences, such as wrists and ankles, if needed before applying a restraint over them.

- Tie restraints with knots that will not tighten when pulled and to parts of the wheelchair that do not move.
- Assess restrained limbs for signs of impaired blood circulation.
- Always stay with a client whose restraint is temporarily removed.

AGE-RELATED CONSIDERATIONS

Applying Restraints

Infant

Elbow restraints (Figure 7-7 ◆) are used to prevent infants or small children from flexing their elbows to

touch or scratch a skin lesion or to reach the head when a scalp vein infusion is in place. This restraint consists of a piece of material with pockets into which plastic or wooden tongue depressors are inserted to provide rigidity.

- Examine the restraint to make sure that the tongue depressors are intact (i.e., all in place and not broken).
- Place the infant's elbow in the center of the restraint. Make sure that the padded material covers the ends of the tongue depressors. This prevents them from irritating the skin.
- Wrap the restraint smoothly around the arm.
- Secure the restraint, using safety pins, ties, or tape. Ensure that it is not so tight that it obstructs blood circulation.
- *Optional:* After the restraint is applied, pin it to the child's shirt. This prevents is from sliding down the arm.

A mummy restraint (Figure 7-8 ◆) is a special folding of a blanket or sheet around the infant to prevent movement during a procedure such as gastric washing, eye irrigation, or collection of a blood specimen.

- Obtain a blanket or sheet large enough so that the distance between opposite corners is about twice the length of the infant's body. Lay the blanket or sheet on a flat, dry surface.

- Fold down one corner, and place the baby on it in the supine position.
- Fold the right side of the blanket over the infant's body, leaving the left arm free (Figure 7-8A). The right arm is in a natural position at the side.
- Fold the excess blanket at the bottom up under the infant (Figure 7-8B2).
- With the left arm in a natural position at the baby's side, fold the left side of the blanket over the infant, including the arm, and tuck the blanket under the body (Figure 7-8B3).
- Remain with the infant who is in a mummy restraint until the specific procedure is completed.

Child

A crib net is simply a device placed over the top of a crib to prevent active young children from climbing out of the crib. At the same time, it allows them freedom to move about in the crib. The crib net or dome is not attached to the movable parts of the crib so that the caregiver can have access to the child without removing the dome or net.

- Place the net over the sides and ends of the crib.
- Secure the ties to the springs or frame of the crib. The crib sides can then be freely lowered without removing the net.
- Test with your hand that the net will stretch if the child stands in the crib against it.

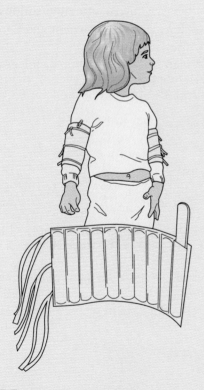

FIGURE 7-7 ◆ An elbow restraint.

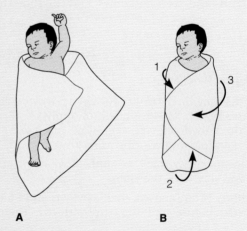

A   B

FIGURE 7-8 ◆ Making a mummy restraint.

EVALUATION

- Perform a detailed follow-up of the need for the restraints and the client's response. Relate these findings to previous data if available.

- Remove the restraints as soon as they are no longer needed and document this.
- Report significant deviations from normal to the physician.

Seizure Precautions

Clients may be prone to **seizures** due to permanent or temporary medical conditions such as drug reactions, epilepsy, or extreme fever. They are at risk for injury if they experience seizures that involve the entire body such as grand mal (tonic–clonic) seizures or any seizure that includes loss of consciousness.

Nursing Process: Seizure Precautions

ASSESSMENT

Include questions about a history of seizures during the admission assessment. If the client has experienced a seizure previously, ask for detailed information, including characteristics of an aura or premonitory symptoms that indicate the seizure is beginning, duration and frequency of the seizures, consequences of the seizures (e.g., incontinence or difficulty breathing), and actions that should be taken to prevent or reduce seizure activity.

PLANNING

Review emergency procedures since the client could have a respiratory arrest or other injury as a result of a seizure.

Delegation

UAP should be familiar with establishing and implementing **seizure precautions** and methods of obtaining assistance during a client's seizure. Care of the client during a seizure is the responsibility of the nurse due to the importance of careful assessment of respiratory status and potential need for intervention.

IMPLEMENTATION:
TECHNIQUE 7-3 IMPLEMENTING SEIZURE PRECAUTIONS

Equipment

- Blankets or other linens to pad side rails
- Oral suction equipment
- Oral airway or padded tongue depressor (according to agency policy)
- Oxygen equipment

Performance

1. Explain to the client what you are going to do, why it is necessary, and how he or she can cooperate.

2. Wash hands and observe appropriate infection control procedures. If the client is actively seizing, apply clean gloves in preparation for performing respiratory care measures.

3. Provide for client privacy.

4. Pad the bed. Secure blankets or other linens around the head, foot, and side rails of the bed (Figure 7-9 ◆).

5. Place oral suction equipment in place and test to ensure that it is functional.

6. If agency policy prescribes, tape the tongue depressor that has been wrapped with gauze padding or an oral airway within reach of the head of the bed (Figure 7-10 ◆).

7. If a seizure occurs:
   - Remain with the client and call for assistance if needed.
   - If the client is not in bed, assist client to the floor and protect the head in your lap or on a pillow.

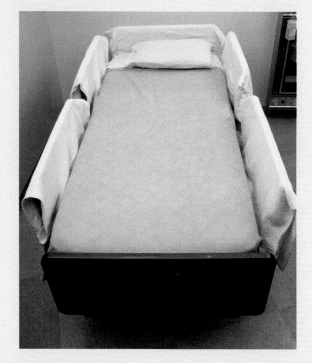

FIGURE 7-9 ◆ Padding a bed for seizure precautions.

- According to policy, insert the airway or tongue depressor between the client's upper and lower teeth. *Never force the insertion as this can cause damage.* In many agencies, an oral airway is used only for situations in which the client is having continuous seizures **(status epilepticus)**. Never place your fingers inside the client's mouth. Loosen any clothing around the neck and chest.
- Apply oxygen by mask.
- Turn the client to a lateral position if possible.

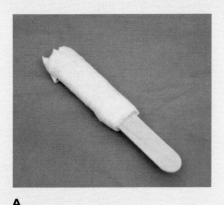

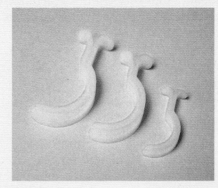

A   **B**

FIGURE 7-10 ◆ (A) Padded tongue blade and (B) oral airway.

- Time the seizure duration.
- Move items in the environment to ensure the client does not experience an injury.
- Observe the progression of the seizure, noting the sequence and type of limb involvement. Observe skin color. When the seizure allows, check pulse and respirations.
- Administer ordered anticonvulsant medications.
- Use equipment to suction the oral airway if the client vomits or has excessive oral secretions.

- When the seizure has finished, assist client to a comfortable position. Provide hygiene as necessary. Allow the client to verbalize feelings about the seizure.

 8. When the seizure has subsided, document it in the client record using forms or checklists supplemented by narrative notes when appropriate.

AMBULATORY AND COMMUNITY SETTINGS

Implementing Seizure Precautions

- If clients have frequent or recurrent seizures or take anticonvulsant medications, they should wear a medical identification tag (bracelet or necklace) and carry a card delineating any medications they take.
- When making home visits, inspect anticonvulsant medications and confirm that clients are taking them correctly. Blood level measurements may be required periodically.
- Assist the client in determining which persons in the community should/must be informed of their

seizure disorder (e.g., employers, health care providers such as dentists, motor vehicle department if driving, companions).
- Discuss safety precautions for inside and out of the home. If seizures are not well controlled, activities that may require restriction or direct supervision by others include tub bathing, swimming, cooking, using electric equipment or machinery, and driving.
- Discuss with the client and family factors that may precipitate a seizure.

AGE-RELATED CONSIDERATIONS

Implementing Seizure Precautions
Infant

- About 5 percent of children experience seizures, most while infants (Ball & Bindler, 1999).

Child

- Febrile seizures occur more commonly than in adults and are usually preventable through antipyretics and tepid baths.

- Determine oxygenation. Apply oxygen if pulse oximetry reading is less than 95 percent (see Chapter 2).
- Children who have frequent seizures may need to wear helmets for protection.
- Children on anticonvulsant medications should wear a medical identification tag (bracelet or necklace).

- Perform a detailed follow-up examination of the client. Administer medications if indicated.

- Report significant deviations from normal to the physician.

Chapter Summary

TERMINOLOGY

chemical restraints
jacket restraints
mitt (hand) restraints
physical restraints

restraints
safety belt
safety monitoring device
seizures

seizure precautions
status epilepticus
wrist (ankle) restraint

FORMING CLINICAL JUDGMENTS

Consider This:

1. In spite of repeated reminders to ask a family member for assistance before trying to go to the bathroom at night at home, your unsteady client insists on attempting the trip alone. The physician suggests trying an activity monitoring device. How would you explain this device to the client and family?

2. Your elderly client picks at her IV line and dressings. When you remind her not to touch them, she sweetly replies: "I just forgot." You are consid-

ering applying a mitt restraint to the one hand she uses for these activities. What safety measures would be needed in using such as restraint?

3. When you walk into the client's room, you find the client alternately flexing and extending the arms but the rest of the body is not moving. The head is arched back and the client does not appear to be conscious. There is an oral airway, a suction machine, and oxygen equipment in the room. What are the most important things you should do at this time?

RELATED RESEARCH

Arbesman, M. C., & Wright, C. (1999). Mechanical restraints, rehabilitation therapies, and staffing adequacy as risk factors for falls in an elderly hospitalized population. *Rehabilitation Nursing, 24*(3), 122–128, 135.

Cruz, V., Abdul-Hamid, M., & Heater, B. (1997). Research-based practice: Reducing restraints in an acute care setting—phase I. *Journal of Gerontological Nursing, 23*, 31–40, 54–55.

Mayhew, P. A., Christy, K., Berkebile, J., Miller, C., & Farrish, A. (1999). Restraint reduction: Research utilization and case study with cognitive impairment. *Geriatric Nursing: American Journal of Care for the Aging, 20*, 305–308.

REFERENCES

Ball, J., & Bindler, R. (1999). *Pediatric nursing: Caring for children.* Stamford, CT: Appleton & Lange.

Bezon, J., Echevarria, K. H., & Smith, G. B. (1999). Nursing outcome indicator: Preventing falls for elderly people.

Outcomes Management for Nursing Practice, 3, 112–117.

Brenner, Z. R. (1998). Toward restraint-free care. *American Journal of Nursing, 98*(12), 16F–16I.

Capezuti, E., Talerico, K. A., Cochran, I., Becker, H., Strumpf, N., & Evans, L. (1999). Individualized interventions to prevent bed-related falls and reduce siderail use. *Journal of Gerontological Nursing, 25*(11), 26–34, 52–53.

REFERENCES (continued)

Gardner, M. M., Robertson, M. C., & Campbell, A. J. (2000). Exercise in preventing falls and fall related injuries in older people: A review of randomised controlled trials. *British Journal of Sports Medicine, 34*(1), 7–17, 76.

Godkin, M. D., & Onyskiw, J. E. (1999). A systematic overview of interventions to reduce physical restraint use in long-term care settings. *Online Journal of Knowledge Synthesis for Nursing 6*(Document 6).

Hammond, M., & Levine, J. M. (1999). Bedrails: Choosing the best alternative. *Geriatric Nursing: American Journal of Care for the Aging, 20*, 297–301.

Health Care Financing Agency. (1999). Hospital interpretive guidelines: Patients rights. In *Comprehensive accreditation manual for hospitals.* Oakbrook Terrace, IL: Author [available: http://www.hcfa.gov/quality/4b2.htm].

Kobs, A. (1998). Questions and answers from JCAHO. Restraints revisited. *Nursing Management, 29*(1), 17–18.

Mosley, A., Galindo-Ciocon, D., Peak, N., & West, M. J. (1998). Initiation and evaluation of a research-based fall prevention program. *Journal of Nursing Care Quality, 13*(2), 38–44.

Rawsky, E. (1998). Review of literature on falls among the elderly. *Image: Journal of Nursing Scholarship, 30*, 47–52.

Resnick, B. (1999). Falls in a community of older adults: Putting research into practice. *Clinical Nursing Research, 8*, 251–266.

Rigler, S. K. (1999). Clinical experience: Preventing falls in older adults. *Hospital Practice, 34*, 117–120.

Rogers, P. D., & Bocchino, N. L. (1999). Restraint-free care: Is it possible? *American Journal of Nursing, 99*(10), 26–34.

Rutledge, D. N., Donaldson, N. E., & Pravikoff, D. S. (1998). Fall risk assessment and prevention in healthcare facilities. *Online Journal of Clinical Innovations, 1*(9), 1–33.

Walker, A. (1999). Preventing falls at home. *Nursing, 29*(4), 64hh1–2, 64hh4.

Winston, P. A., Morelli, P., Bramble, J., Friday, A., & Sanders, J. B. (1999). Improving patient care through implementation of nurse-driven restraint protocols. *Journal of Nursing Care Quality, 13*(6), 32–46.

Chapter 8

Maintaining Joint Mobility
Techniques

OBJECTIVES

- Compare and contrast the three variations of range-of-motion (ROM) exercises.
- Perform passive ROM exercises correctly and safely.
- Describe the purpose of a continuous passive motion (CPM) mechanical device.
- Use the nursing process when applying a CPM device.

8-1 Performing Passive Range-of-Motion Exercises

8-2 Using a Continuous Passive Motion Device

Joint Mobility

Promoting exercise to maintain a client's muscle tone and joint mobility is an essential function of nursing personnel. Joints are the functional units of the musculoskeletal system. The bones of the skeleton articulate at the joints and most of the skeletal muscles attach to the two bones at the joint. These muscles are categorized according to the type of joint movement they produce on contraction (e.g., flexors and extensors). The flexor muscles are stronger than the extensor muscles. Thus, when a person is inactive, the joints are pulled into a flexed (bent) position. If this tendency is not counteracted with exercise and position changes, the muscles permanently shorten and the joint becomes fixed in a flexed position. The types of joint movement are shown in Table 8-1.

The **range of motion (ROM)** of a joint is the maximum movement that is possible for that joint. Joint ROM varies from individual to individual and is determined by genetic makeup, developmental patterns, the presence or absence of disease, and the amount of physical activity in which the person normally engages.

Range-of-Motion Exercises

When people are ill, they often need to perform ROM exercises until they regain their normal activity levels. Range-of-motion exercises may be active, passive, or active–assistive.

Active Range of Motion

Active range-of-motion exercises are isotonic exercises in which the client independently moves each

joint in the body through its complete range of movement, maximally stretching all muscle groups within each plane over the joint. These exercises maintain or increase muscle strength and endurance and help to maintain cardiorespiratory function in an immobilized client. They also prevent deterioration of joint capsules, ankylosis, and **contractures**. Instructions for the client performing active ROM exercises are shown in Box 8-1.

Full ROM does not occur spontaneously in the immobilized individual who independently achieves activities of daily living (ADL), independently moves about in bed, independently transfers between bed and wheelchair or chair, or independently ambulates a short distance because only a few muscle groups are

TABLE 8-1	TYPES OF JOINT MOVEMENTS
Movement	**Action**
Flexion	Decreasing the angle of the joint (e.g., bending the elbow)
Extension	Increasing the angle of the joint (e.g., straightening the arm at the elbow)
Hyperextension	Further extension or straightening of a joint (e.g., bending the head backward)
Abduction	Movement of the bone *away from* the midline of the body
Adduction	Movement of the bone *toward* the midline of the body
Rotation	Movement of the bone around its central axis
Circumduction	Movement of the distal part of the bone in a circle while the proximal end remains fixed
Eversion	Turning the sole of the foot outward by moving the ankle joint
Inversion	Turning the sole of the foot inward by moving the ankle joint
Pronation	Moving the bones of the forearm so that the palm of the hand faces downward when held in front of the body
Supination	Moving the bones of the forearm so that the palm of the hand faces upward when held in front of the body

maximally stretched during these activities. Although clients may successfully achieve some active ROM movements of the upper extremities while combing their hair, bathing, and dressing, the immobilized client is very unlikely to achieve any active ROM movements of the lower extremities because he or she is not doing the normal functions of standing and walking. For this reason, most wheelchair and many ambulatory clients need active ROM exercises until they regain their normal activity levels. At first, the nurse may need to teach the client to perform the needed ROM exercises. Eventually, the client may be able to accomplish these exercises independently.

Passive Range of Motion

During **passive range-of-motion exercises,** *another* person moves each of the client's joints through their complete range of movement and maximally stretches all muscle groups within each plane over each joint. Because the client does not contract the muscles, passive ROM exercises are of no value in maintaining muscle strength but are useful in maintaining joint flexibility. For this reason, passive ROM exercises should be performed only when the client is unable to accomplish the movements actively.

Passive ROM exercises should be accomplished for each movement of the arms, legs, and neck *that the client is unable to achieve actively.* As with active ROM exercises, passive ROM exercises should be accomplished to the point of slight resistance, but not beyond, and never to the point of discomfort. The movements should be systematic and the same sequence should be followed during each exercise session. Each exercise should be repeated, at the client's tolerance, to a maximum of five times. Each exercise should be done twice daily. Performing one series of exercises along with the bath is helpful. Passive ROM exercises are accomplished most effectively when the client lies supine in bed.

General guidelines for providing passive exercises are shown in Box 8-2. Technique 8-1 explains how to perform these exercises.

Box 8-2 *Guidelines for Providing Passive Exercises*

- Ensure that the client understands the reason for doing ROM exercises.
- If there is a possibility of hand swelling, make sure rings are removed.
- Clothe the client in a loose gown, and cover the body with a bath blanket.
- Use correct body mechanics when providing ROM exercises to avoid muscle strain or injury to both yourself and the client.
- Position the bed at an appropriate height.
- Expose only the limb being exercised to avoid embarrassing the client.
- Support the client's limbs above and below the joint as needed to prevent muscle strain or injury (see figure). This may also be done by cupping joints in the palm of the hand or cradling limbs along the nurse's forearm as shown in the figures. If a joint is painful (e.g., arthritic), support the limb in the muscular areas above and below the joint).

- Use a firm, comfortable grip when handling the limb.
- Move the body parts smoothly, slowly, and rhythmically. Jerky movements cause discomfort and possible injury. Fast movements can cause **spasticity** (sudden, prolonged involuntary muscle contraction) or **rigidity** (stiffness or inflexibility).
- Avoid moving or forcing a body part beyond the existing range of motion. Muscle strain, pain, and injury can result. This is particularly important for people with flaccid (limp) paralysis, whose muscles can be stretched and joints dislocated without their awareness.
- If muscle spasticity occurs during movement, stop the movement temporarily, but continue to apply slow, gentle pressure on the part until the muscle relaxes; then proceed with the motion.

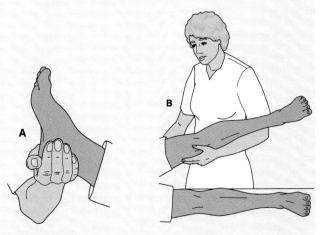

Supporting the client's arm.

Holding limbs for support during passive exercise: (A) cupping; (B) cradling.

Active–Assistive Range of Motion

During **active–assistive range-of-motion exercises**, the client uses a stronger, opposite arm or leg to move each of the joints of a limb incapable of active motion. The client learns to support and move the weak arm or leg with the strong arm or leg as far as possible. Then the nurse continues the movement passively to its maximal degree. This activity increases active movement on the strong side of the client's body and maintains joint flexibility on the weak side. Such exercise is especially useful for stroke victims who are hemiplegic (paralyzed on one half of the body). Some clients who begin with passive ROM exercises after a disability progress to active–assistive ROM exercises and, finally, to active ROM exercises.

Nursing Process: Range-of-Motion Exercises

ASSESSMENT

- Review the client's chart for nursing assessment on admission, physician's orders, medical diagnosis, physical examination, and physician progress notes to determine limitations to joint mobility.

- Determine the client's ability to perform active, passive, or active–assistive ROM exercises (e.g., level of consciousness, cognitive function, and ability to move independently).

- Assess current ROM as baseline data.

- Note the presence of any joint contractures, swelling, redness, or pain that may limit the client's range of motion.

PLANNING

Delegation

Performing passive ROM exercises can be delegated to unlicensed assistive personnel (UAP). Some agencies may have specially trained nursing assistants who perform restorative activities, such as range of motion, for clients. For UAPs who do not have this special training, however, it is important that the nurse review the general guidelines for performing passive ROM exercises (see Box 8-2) to avoid injury to the UAP or client. Encourage the UAP to perform ROM during the bath. Emphasize the importance of the UAP's reporting anything unusual to the nurse. If a client has a recent spinal cord injury or some form of orthopedic trauma, the nurse or a physical therapist should do the ROM.

IMPLEMENTATION:
TECHNIQUE 8-1 PERFORMING PASSIVE RANGE-OF-MOTION EXERCISES

Equipment

- No special equipment is needed other than a bed.

Preparation

Prior to initiating the exercises, review any possible restrictions with the physician or physical therapist. Also refer to the agency's protocol.

Performance

1. Explain to the client what you are going to do, why it is necessary, and how he or she can cooperate. Discuss the importance of ROM exercises in their plan of care.

2. Wash hands and observe other appropriate infection control procedures.

3. Provide for client privacy.

4. Assist the client to a supine position near you and expose the body parts requiring exercise.
   - Place the client's feet together, place the arms at the sides, and leave space around the head and the feet. *Positioning the client close to you prevents excessive reaching.*

5. Perform exercises in a head-to-toe format. Follow

a repetitive pattern and return to the starting position after each motion. Repeat each motion three to five times on the affected limb. To reduce discomfort, support the joint being exercised. Observe the client for nonverbal cues of discomfort or pain.

6. Neck (pivot joint)
   - Remove the client's pillow
   - Flex and extend the neck (ROM: 45 degrees from midline).
     - Place the palm of one hand under the client's head and the palm of the other hand on the client's chin.
     - Move the head from the upright midline position forward until the chin rests on the chest (Figure 8-1 ◆)
     - Move the head from the flexed position back to the resting supine position without the head pillow (Figure 8-1).
   - Lateral flexion of the neck (ROM: 40 degrees from midline)
     - Place the heels of the hands on each side of the client's cheeks
     - Move the head laterally toward the right and left shoulders (Figure 8-2 ◆).

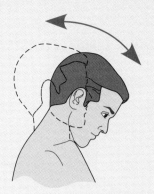

FIGURE 8-1 ◆ Flexion/extension of neck.

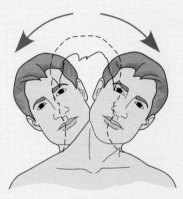

FIGURE 8-2 ◆ Lateral flexion of neck.

- Rotation (ROM: 70 degrees from midline)
  - Place the heels of the hands on each side of the client's cheeks
  - Turn the face as far as possible to the right and left (Figure 8-3 ◆).
7. Shoulder (ball-and-socket joint)
  - Flexion (ROM: 180 degrees from the side)
  - Begin with the client's arm at the side. Grasp the arm beneath the elbow with one hand and beneath the wrist with the other hand unless otherwise indicated.

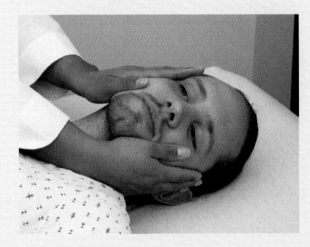

FIGURE 8-3 ◆ Rotation of the neck.

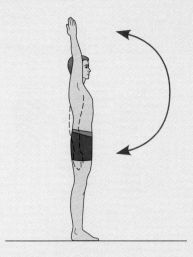

FIGURE 8-4 ◆ Flexion/extension of shoulder.

- Raise the arm from a position by the side forward and upward to a position beside the head (Figure 8-4 ◆). The elbow may need to be flexed if the headboard is in the way.
- Extension (ROM: 180 degrees from vertical position beside the head)
  - Move the arm from a vertical position beside the head forward and down to a resting position at the side of the body (Figure 8-4).
- Abduction (ROM: 180 degrees)
  - Move the arm laterally from the resting position at the side to a side position above the head, palm of the hand away from the head (Figure 8-5 ◆).
- Adduction (ROM: 230 degrees)
  - Move the arm laterally from the position beside the head downward laterally and across the front of the body as far as possible (Figure 8-6 ◆).
- External rotation (ROM: 90 degrees)
  - With arm held out to the side at shoulder level and the elbow bent to a right angle, fingers pointing down, move the arm upward so that

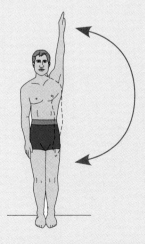

FIGURE 8-5 ◆ Abducting the shoulder.

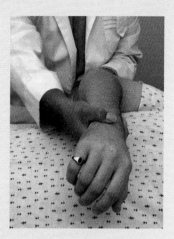

FIGURE 8-6 ◆ Adducting the shoulder.

the fingers point up and the back of the hand touches the mattress (Figure 8-7 ◆).

• Internal rotation (ROM: 90 degrees)
   • With the arm held out to the side at shoulder level and the elbow bent to a right angle, fingers pointing up, bring the arm forward and down so that the palm touches the mattress (Figure 8-7).
• Circumduction (ROM: 360 degrees)
   • Move the arm forward, up, back and down in a full circle (Figure 8-8 ◆).

8. Elbow (hinge joint)
   • Flexion (ROM: 150 degrees)
      • Bring the lower arm forward and upward so that the hand is level with the shoulder (Figure 8-9 ◆).
   • Extension (ROM: 150 degrees)
      • Bring the lower arm forward and downward, straightening the arm (Figure 8-9).
   • Rotation for supination (ROM: 70 to 90 degrees)

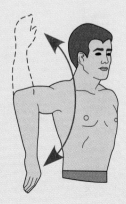

FIGURE 8-7 ◆ External/internal rotation of shoulder.

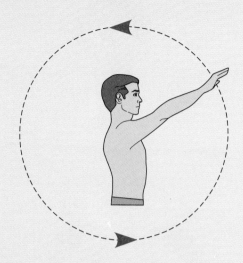

FIGURE 8-8 ◆ Circumduction of shoulder.

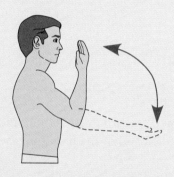

FIGURE 8-9 ◆ Flexion/extension of elbow.

• Grasp the client's hand as for a handshake and turn the palm upward (Figure 8-10 ◆). Make sure that only the forearm (not the shoulder) moves.
• Rotation for pronation (ROM: 70 to 90 degrees)
• Grasp the client's hand as for a handshake and turn the palm downward (Figure 8-11 ◆). Make sure that only the forearm (not the shoulder) moves.

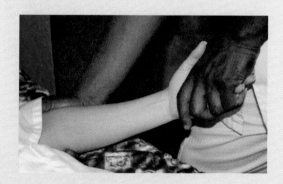

FIGURE 8-10 ◆ Supinating the forearm.

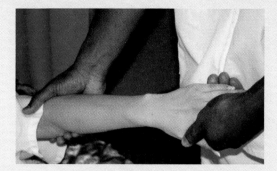

FIGURE 8-11 ◆ Pronating the forearm.

9. Wrist (condyloid joint)
   • Flexion (ROM: 80 to 90 degrees)
   • Flex the client's arm at the elbow until the forearm is at a right angle to the mattress. Support the wrist joint with one hand while your other hand manipulates the joint.
   • Bring the fingers of the hand toward the inner aspect of the forearm (Figure 8-12 ◆).

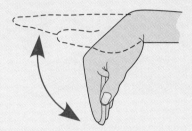

FIGURE 8-12 ◆ Flexion/extension of wrist.

   • Extension (ROM: 80 to 90 degrees)
   • Straighten the hand to the same plane as the arm (Figure 8-12).

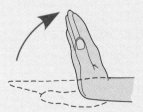

FIGURE 8-13 ◆ Hyperextension of wrist.

   • Hyperextension (ROM 70 to 90 degrees)
   • Bend the fingers of the hand back as far as possible (Figure 8-13 ◆).
   • Radial flexion (abduction) (ROM: 0 to 20 degrees)
   • Bend the wrist laterally toward the thumb side (Figure 8-14 ◆).
   • Ulnar flexion (adduction) (ROM: 30 to 50 degrees)

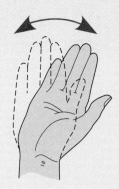

FIGURE 8-14 ◆ Radial and ulnar flexion.

   • Bend the wrist laterally toward the fifth finger (Figure 8-14).

10. Hand and fingers (metacarpophalangeal joints—condyloid; interphalangeal joints—hinge)
   • Flexion (ROM: 90 degrees)
   • Make a fist (Figure 8-15 ◆).
   • Extension (ROM: 90 degrees)
   • Straighten the fingers (Figure 8-15).

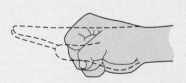

FIGURE 8-15 ◆ Flexion/extension of fingers.

   • Hyperextension (ROM: 30 degrees)
   • Gently bend fingers back.
   • Abduction (ROM: 20 degrees)
   • Spread the fingers of the hand apart (Figure 8-16 ◆).
   • Adduction (ROM: 20 degrees)
   • Bring fingers together (Figure 8-16).

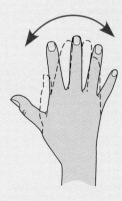

FIGURE 8-16 ◆ Abduction/adduction of fingers.

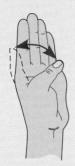

FIGURE 8-17 ◆ Flexion/extension of thumb.

11. Thumb (saddle joint)
- Flexion (ROM: 90 degrees)
  - Move the thumb across the palmar surface of the hand toward the fifth finger (Figure 8-17 ◆).
- Extension (ROM: 90 degrees)
  - Move the thumb away from the hand (Figure 8-17).
- Abduction (ROM: 30 degrees)
  - Extend the thumb laterally (can be done when placing fingers in abduction and adduction) (Figure 8-18 ◆).
- Adduction (ROM: 30 degrees)
  - Move the thumb back to the hand (Figure 8-18).

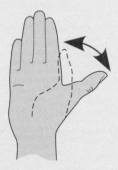

FIGURE 8-18 ◆ Abduction/adduction of thumb.

- Opposition
  - Touch thumb to the top of each finger of the same hand. The thumb joint movements involved are abduction, rotation, and flexion (Figure 8-19 ◆).

12. Hip (ball-and-socket joint)
- To carry out hip and leg exercises, place one hand under the client's knee and the other under the ankle (Figure 8-20 ◆).
- Flexion (ROM: knee extended, 90 degrees; knee flexed, 120 degrees)

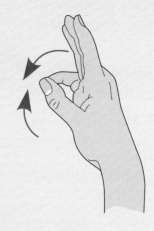

FIGURE 8-19 ◆ Opposition.

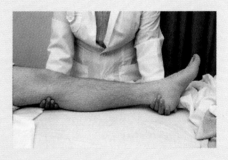

FIGURE 8-20 ◆ Position for knee and hip movements.

- Lift the leg and bend the knee moving the knee up toward the chest as far as possible (Figure 8-21 ◆).
- Extension (ROM: 90 to 120 degrees)
  - Bring the leg down, straighten the knee, and lower the leg to the bed.
- Abduction (ROM: 45 to 50 degrees)
  - Move the leg to the side away from the client (Figure 8-22 ◆).
- Adduction (ROM: 20 to 30 degrees beyond other leg)

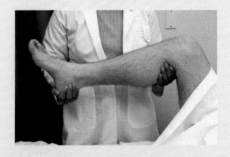

FIGURE 8-21 ◆ Flexing the knee and the hip.

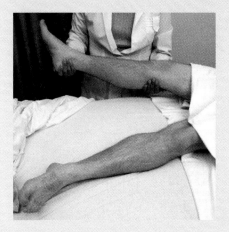

FIGURE 8-22 ◆ Abducting the leg.

• Move the leg back across and in front of the other leg (Figure 8-23 ◆).

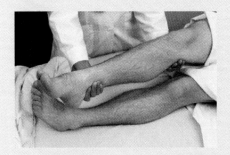

FIGURE 8-23 ◆ Adducting the leg.

• Circumduction (ROM: 360 degrees)
    • Move the leg in a circle (Figure 8-24 ◆)

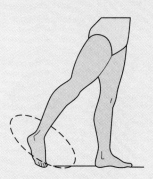

FIGURE 8-24 ◆ Circumduction of hip.

• Internal rotation (ROM: 90 degrees)
    • Roll the foot and leg inward (Figure 8-25 ◆).
• External rotation (ROM: 90 degrees)
    • Roll the foot and leg outward (Figure 8-26 ◆).

13. Knee (hinge joint)
    • Flexion (ROM: 120 to 130 degrees)
        • Bend the leg, bringing the heel toward the back of the thigh (done with hip flexion) (Figure 8-27 ◆).

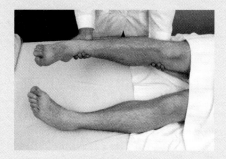

FIGURE 8-25 ◆ Internal rotation of hip.

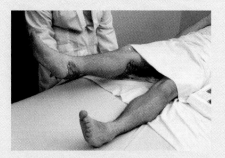

FIGURE 8-26 ◆ External rotation of hip.

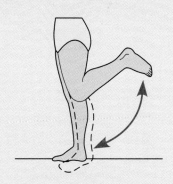

FIGURE 8-27 ◆ Flexion/extension of knee.

• Extension (ROM: 120 to 130 degrees)
    • Straighten the leg, returning the foot to the bed

14. Ankle (hinge joint)
    • Extension (plantar flexion) (ROM: 45 to 50 degrees)
        • Move the foot so the toes are pointed downward (Figure 8-28 ◆).

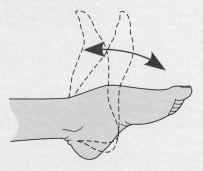

FIGURE 8-28 ◆ Extension/flexion of ankle.

• Flexion (dorsiflexion) (ROM: 20 degrees)
  • Move foot so toes are pointed upward (Figure 8-28).

15. Foot (gliding)
  • Eversion (ROM: 5 degrees)
    • Place one hand under the client's ankle and the other over the arch of the foot.
    • Turn the whole foot outward (Figure 8-29 ◆).

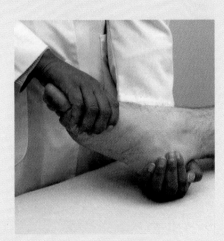

FIGURE 8-29 ◆ Everting the foot.

• Inversion (ROM: 5 degrees)
  • Using the same hand placement as above, turn the whole foot inward (Figure 8-30 ◆).

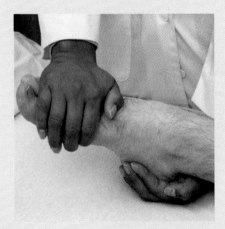

FIGURE 8-30 ◆ Inverting the foot.

16. Toes (interphalangeal joints—hinge; metatarsophalangeal joints—hinge; intertarsal joints—gliding)
  • Flexion (ROM: 35 to 60 degrees)
    • Place one hand over the arch of the foot

• Place the fingers of the other hand over the toes to curl the toes downward (Figure 8-31 ◆)

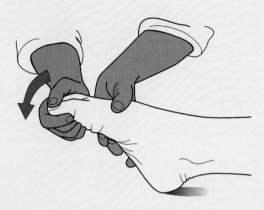

FIGURE 8-31 ◆ Flexing the toes.

• Extension (ROM: 35 to 60 degrees)
  • Place one hand over the arch of the foot
  • Place the fingers of the other hand under the toes to bend the toes upward (Figure 8-32 ◆).

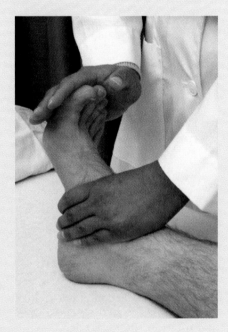

FIGURE 8-32 ◆ Extending the toes.

• Abduction (ROM: 0 to 15 degrees)
  • Spread the toes apart.
• Adduction (ROM: 0 to 15 degrees)
  • Bring the toes together.

17. Move to the other side of the bed and repeat exercises for other arm and leg.

Variation: Hyperextension Movements

- Assist the client to a prone or lateral position on the side of the bed nearest you but facing away from you.
- Hyperextend the shoulder.
  - Place one hand on the shoulder to keep it from lifting off the bed and the other under the client's elbow.
  - Pull the upper arm up and backward (Figure 8-33 ◆).

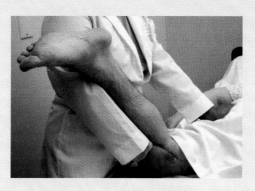

FIGURE 8-34 ◆ Hyperextending the hip.

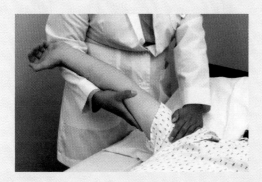

FIGURE 8-33 ◆ Hyperextending the shoulder.

- Hyperextend the hip.
  - Place one hand on the hip to stabilize it and keep it from lifting off the bed. With the other arm and hand, cradle the lower leg in the forearm, and cup the knee joint with the hand.
  - Move the leg backward from the hip joint (Figure 8-34 ◆).
- Hyperextend the neck.
  - Remove the pillow. With the client's face down, place one hand on the forehead and the other on the back of the skull.
  - Move the head backward (Figure 8-35 ◆).
  - Avoid hyperextending the neck of the immobilized elderly client, because such movements can cause painful nerve damage.

18. **Document**
  - Type of ROM exercise (e.g., active, passive, active–assistive)
- Joints exercised and their degree of joint motion
- Length of exercise
- Client's tolerance level to the activity
- Any abnormalities

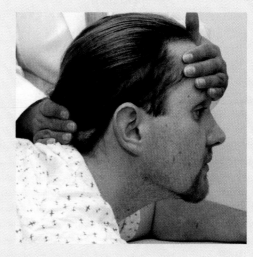

FIGURE 8-35 ◆ Hyperextending the neck.

AMBULATORY AND COMMUNITY SETTINGS

Range of Motion

Teach the client's caregiver:

- The purpose and importance of performing ROM exercises at home
- To perform the exercises at least twice daily
- How to use correct body mechanics to prevent muscle strain while performing the exercises

---

AGE-RELATED CONSIDERATIONS

Range of Motion

Elders

- Avoid hyperextending the joints of older clients. *Such movements can cause pain or nerve damage because joints become less flexible with age.*
- Work slowly and assess for pain when working

with older clients, especially those who have arthritis. *Arthritis changes can cause contractures and enlarged, painful joints.*

- Assess for skin breakdown or reddened areas during the range-of-motion procedure. *Older clients are at risk for skin breakdown due to decreased subcutaneous fat and increased thinning of the skin.*

- Relate current ROM of joints to baseline ROM: Is there a pattern of improvement? Determine the client's pulse and endurance for the exercise. Is the client progressing from passive ROM to active ROM? If so, ask the client to demonstrate active ROM exercises.

- Observe UAP performing passive ROM exercises. Provide appropriate feedback.

- Report unexpected or notable changes (e.g., resistance to ROM, pain, redness, swelling of joint, rigidity, contractures) to the physician.

Continuous Passive Motion (CPM) Devices

Continuous passive motion (CPM) is a postoperative treatment method that is used to promote recovery after joint surgery. CPM devices are available for the shoulder, elbow, wrist, hand, knee, ankle, and toe. The CPM machine is most frequently used on clients undergoing total knee replacement.

After extensive joint surgery, joint motion usually causes pain in most clients and, as a result, they fail to move the joint. With CPM, however, a machine is providing the joint motion passively and the client's muscle is not actively contracting. As a result, the client can experience decreased edema and pain, maintenance of ROM, and hopefully an accelerated recovery period.

Because the motion is provided mechanically and passively, there is no fatigue factor. The machine flexes and extends the limb continuously—usually 12 to 14 hours a day. In addition to being used postoperatively in hospitals, CPM machines are also used in outpatient and home settings.

CPM machines consist of a motorized base with a nonslip surface and a movable cradle that guides the extremity through the prescribed range of motion. A control device (Figure 8-36 ◆) gives the operator or client access to an on/off switch. Three adjustable controls set the degree of joint flexion, the degree of joint extension, and the speed of movement as ordered by the physician.

Technique 8-2 explains the steps involved in applying a continuous passive motion device for the knee.

Nursing Process: Continuous Passive Motion (CPM) Devices

ASSESSMENT

- Assess client's complaints of discomfort.
- Assess the appearance of the client's joint (e.g., size and color, character, and amount of drainage.

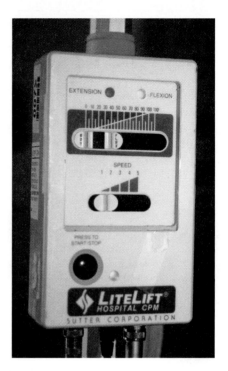

FIGURE 8-36 ◆ CPM control device.

- Determine client's baseline range of motion.
- Assess client's ability and willingness to learn about and use the CPM device.
- Check the safety test date. Note the date the machine was tested for electrical safety and ensure that it is within the guidelines established at the agency.

PLANNING

Delegation

The initial application and setting up of the CPM device should not be delegated to unlicensed assistive personnel (UAP) as application of scientific and nursing knowledge and potential problem solving is needed. The UAP, however, can assist the client with ADL (e.g., bathing) while the CPM device is being used. The nurse needs to discuss with the UAP what observations to report to the nurse (e.g., client complaint of increased pain, swelling, and/or skin breakdown).

Equipment

- CPM device
- Padding for the cradle
- Restraining straps
- Goniometer

Preparation

Verify the physician's orders and agency protocol. Determine the degrees of flexion, extension, and speed initially prescribed. Check agency protocol and physician's orders about increases in degrees and speed for subsequent treatments.

Performance

1. Explain to the client what you are going to do, why it is necessary, and how he or she can cooperate. Discuss how this treatment will be used in planning further care.

2. Wash hands and observe other appropriate infection control procedures.

3. Provide for client privacy.

4. Set up the machine.
   - Place the machine on the bed. Remove an egg crate mattress, if indicated. *This provides a stable surface.*
   - Connect the control box to the CPM machine.

5. Set the prescribed levels of flexion, extension, and speed.
   - Most postoperative clients are started on 10 to 45 degrees of flexion and 0 to 10 degrees of extension.
   - Adjust the speed control to the slow to moderate range for the first postoperative day, and then increase the speed as ordered and tolerated.
   - Place padding on the CPM cradle.
   - Run machine through a complete cycle *to check that the machine is functioning properly.*
   - Stop the machine in full extension.

6. Position the client and place the leg in the machine.
   - Place the client in a supine position with the head of the bed slightly elevated.
   - Support the leg and, with the client's help, lift the leg and place it in the padded cradle.
   - Adjust the device to the client's extremity. Lengthen or shorten appropriate sections of the frame to fit the machine to the client.

- Center client's leg on the frame *to avoid the development of pressure areas.*
- Align the client's knee joint with the hinged joint of the machine.
- Adjust the foot support so that the foot is supported in either a neutral position or slight dorsiflexion (e.g., 20 degrees) *to prevent footdrop.* Check agency protocol.
- Ensure that the leg is neither internally nor externally rotated.
- Secure straps around the thigh and top of the foot and cradle to allow enough space to fit several fingers under the strap (Figure 8-37 ◆).

7. Start the machine.
   - When the machine reaches the fully flexed position, stop the machine, and verify the degree of flexion with a goniometer. *This is a double check of the setting and helps prevent possible complications.*
   - Restart the machine, and observe a few cycles of flexion and extension to ensure proper functioning.

8. Ensure continued client safety and comfort.
   - Make sure that the client is comfortable. Observe for nonverbal signs of discomfort.
   - Place within the client's reach: the call light, bedside table, and any items frequently used by the client.
   - Turn off electric bed controls *to prevent client from inadvertently changing alignment of extremity.*
   - Instruct a mentally alert client how to operate the on/off switch.
   - Loosen the straps and check the client's skin at least twice per shift.

9. **Document** the degree of flexion, the degree of extension, the speed, the duration of the therapy, and the client's activity tolerance.

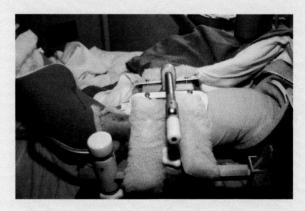

FIGURE 8-37 ◆ Extremity secured with straps.

AMBULATORY AND COMMUNITY SETTINGS

CPM Device

- The CPM machine can be used at home if the client or caregiver demonstrates competence.
- Teach the client or caregiver:
  - How to set the controls and progressively increase the adjustment as the client's tolerance builds.
  - To report excessive pain, swelling, or redness of the affected joints.
  - To provide skin care and check for skin breakdown every 4 hours.
  - How to clean and care for the equipment.

AGE-RELATED CONSIDERATIONS

CPM Device

Child

- Explain the use of the CPM device in terms that the child will understand and will not increase his or her anxiety. Use of dolls or stuffed animals may help.
- Arrange for social or creative activities that are developmentally appropriate for the child during the CPM treatment.

Elders

- Older clients may have limited joint flexibility.
- Older clients may need to balance periods of activity with periods of rest.
- If the older client is apprehensive, teach techniques for muscle relaxation and pain control such as guided imagery and progressive relaxation.

EVALUATION

- Conduct appropriate follow-up: increase in tolerance and current range of motion, degree of discomfort, and skin integrity of feet, elbow, sacrum, and groin.
- Relate baseline ROM data to the client's response to therapy.
- Report any resistance to joint motion, increased pain with CPM, or joint abnormality to the physician.

Chapter Summary

TERMINOLOGY

active range-of-motion exercises
active–assistive range-of-motion
  exercises
continuous passive motion (CPM)

contractures
goniometer
passive range-of-motion exercises
range of motion (ROM)

rigidity
spasticity

FORMING CLINICAL JUDGMENTS

Consider This:

1. The nursing assistant reports to you that an elder client is complaining of pain during the passive ROM exercises. What will you do?

2. After the nursing report, the UAP tells you that she has never taken care of a client who is on a CPM device. She is clearly nervous about the machine and says she is "afraid she will hurt the client." What actions will you take?

RELATED RESEARCH

Pope, R. O., Corcoran, S., McCaul, K., & Howie, D. W. (1997). Continuous passive motion after primary total knee arthroplasty. Does it offer any benefits? *Journal of Bone and Joint Surgery (British), 79*(6), 914–917.

Remsburg, R. E., Armacost, K. A., Radu, C., & Bennett, R. G. (1999). Two models of restorative nursing care in the nursing home: Designated versus integrated restorative nursing assistants. *Geriatric Nursing, 20*(6), 321–326.

Worland, R. L., Arredondo, J., Angles, F., Lopez-Jimenez, F., & Jessup, D. E. (1998). Home continuous passive motion machine versus professional physical therapy following total knee replacement. *Journal of Arthroplasty, 13*(7), 784–787.

Yashar, A. A., Venn-Watson, E., Welsh, T., Colwell, C. W., & Lotke, P. (1997). Continuous passive motion with accelerated flexion after total knee arthroplasty. *Clinical Orthopedics, 345*(12), 38–43.

REFERENCES

Altman, G. B., Buschsel, P., & Coxon, V. (2000). *Fundamental and Advanced Nursing Skills.* Albany, New York: Delmar.

Bonn, K. L. (1999). Restorative: The basis of nursing care. *Nursing Homes Long Term Care Management, 48*(9), 72.

Elkin, M. K., Perry, A. G., & Potter, P. A. (2000). *Nursing Interventions and Clinical Skills,* 2nd ed. St. Louis: Mosby.

Smith, S. F., Duell, D. J., & Martin, B. C. (2000). *Clinical Nursing Skills Basic to Advanced Skills.* Upper Saddle River, NJ: Prentice Hall Health.

Spencer, G. (1999). The role of exercise in successful ageing. *Professional Nurse, 15*(2), 105–108.

Chapter 9

Care of the Client in Traction

Techniques

OBJECTIVES

- Identify types of skin and skeletal traction
- List nursing measures to care for and prevent problems for clients with selected tractions

Traction is a means of immobilization using a pulling force applied to a part of the body while a second force, called **countertraction**, pulls in the opposite direction. The pulling force is provided through a system of pulleys, ropes, and weights attached to the client. The countertraction is often achieved by elevating the foot or head of the bed and therefore is supplied by the client's body. People who are in traction are often confined to bed for weeks or even months. Nursing implementation therefore involves activities of daily living (ADL), maintenance of the traction, and the prevention of problems related to immobility such as pressure sores.

Purposes of Traction

Traction is applied for several purposes:

- To reduce and/or immobilize a bone fracture for healing
- To maintain proper bone alignment
- To prevent soft tissue injury
- To correct, reduce, or prevent deformities
- To decrease muscle spasm and pain
- To treat inflammatory conditions by immobilizing a joint (e.g., for arthritis or tuberculosis of a joint)

Types of Traction

There are two major types of traction: skin and skeletal.

1. Skin traction is a pulling force applied to the skin and soft tissues through the use of tape or traction straps and a system of ropes, pulleys, and weights. The traction tape or strap is often made of vented foam rubber or cloth, and it may have either an adhesive or nonadhesive backing. Adhesive skin traction is used for continuous traction. Nonadhesive skin traction is used intermittently; it can easily be removed and reapplied.

2. Skeletal traction is applied by inserting metal pins, wires, or tongs directly into or through a bone. The metal device is then attached to a system of ropes, pulleys, and weights by means of a metal frame attached to the bed.

Traction can be either continuous or intermittent. Continuous traction (skeletal or skin) is applied and released by a specially trained practitioner who is responsible for handling the affected part when it is not in traction. Intermittent traction (nonadhesive skin traction) can be applied and released by nursing personnel with the appropriate order. However, the physician prescribes the amount of weight to be applied.

Traction setups are often named after their inventors. Figure 9-1 ◆ shows the most common varieties.

Traction Equipment

The following equipment is used for most skin and skeletal tractions:

- *Overhead frame:* This frame is attached to the hospital bed and provides a means for attachment of the traction apparatus. Each frame has at least two upright bars (one at each end of the bed) and one overhead bar.
- *Trapeze:* Attached to the overhead frame, the trapeze can be used by the client for moving in bed, unless contraindicated by the client's health.
- *Firm mattress:* To maintain body alignment and the efficiency of the traction, a firm mattress is essential. Some beds are manufactured with a solid bottom instead of springs, to provide firm support. If a firm bed is not available, a bedboard can be used to provide the needed support.
- *Ropes, pulleys, weight hangers, and weights.*

Nursing Process: Care of the Patient in Traction

ASSESSMENT

Assess:

- The neurovascular status of the affected extremity, that is, the status of peripheral pulses, color, amount of movement, temperature, capillary filling, edema, numbness, sensation.
- The presence of pain in the area: exact location, degree, duration, and description of the pain (e.g., sharp, needlelike) and identification of any movement or activity that would initiate the pain.
- Clinical signs of thrombi and emboli: Regularly assess the client's pulse, blood pressure, respirations, mental status, and breath sounds for evidence of emboli. Inspect the client's involved extremity for redness, swelling, and pain.
- Pressure areas for signs of skin irritation or breakdown. Note in particular (1) bony prominences (e.g., the heels, ankles, sacrum, elbows, chin, and shoulders) and (2) areas susceptible to pressure from the traction (e.g., the tibia for **Buck's extension**).
- Inflammation and drainage at the pin sites for skeletal traction.
- Presence of skin allergies.
- Skin for signs of infection or injury.

PLANNING

A physical therapist or orthopedic technician generally performs initial setup of traction. The nurse is responsible for caring for the client in traction and ensuring that the traction is functioning properly. If necessary, review the principles that apply to the specific type of traction. In particular, determine if the

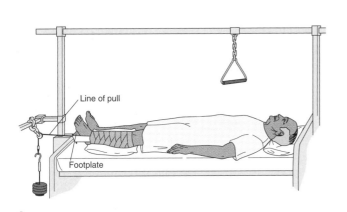

A

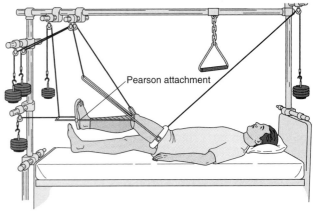

Pearson attachment

B

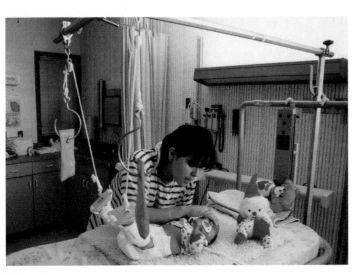

C

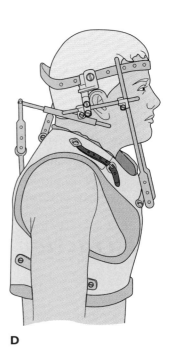

D

E

FIGURE 9-1 ◆ (A) Buck's extension. Skin traction. Immobilizes hip fractures. The knee of the bed is flexed 20 to 30 degrees. The standard foam boot cannot be used with a calf compression device for prevention of vascular problems. If the device must be used with Buck's traction, adhesive traction straps must be used instead. (B) Thomas splint with Pearson attachment for fracture of the femur. Balanced suspension skeletal traction. (C) Gardner–Wells skull tongs. Skeletal traction. Immobilizes fractures of cervical and upper thoracic vertebrae. (D) Halo-thoracic vest (external fixation) traction. Circular metal band secured by pins that penetrate the skull a fraction of an inch. Halo is attached to vest by metal rods. The vest supports and suspends the weight of the entire apparatus around the chest. Advantage over other types of head and neck traction is that client can sit, stand, and walk, thus decreasing problems associated with prolonged immobility. Keep a wrench of the appropriate type/size near the client at all times in case of emergency. (E) Bryant's traction. Ensure that the sacrum is elevated sufficiently to allow the nurse to slip a hand between the child's buttocks and the bed.

traction is continuous or intermittent and what client positions are permitted.

Delegation

Care of the client in traction may be delegated to unlicensed assistive personnel (UAP). However, the nurse or physical therapist should be the person who sets up and applies the traction initially, assesses proper functioning of the traction, and makes required modifications.

Equipment

- Trapeze
- Protective skin devices (e.g., heel protectors)

Performance

1. Explain to the client what you are going to do, why it is necessary, and how he or she can cooperate. Discuss how the results will be used in planning further care or treatments.

2. Wash hands and observe appropriate infection control procedures.

3. Provide for client privacy.

4. Determine the following: Bruises and abrasions in the area where the traction is to be applied; any history of circulatory problems and skin allergies; mental and emotional status and ability to understand activity restrictions.

5. Note the type of traction, and inspect the traction apparatus regularly, that is, whenever you are at the bedside or at prescribed intervals, such as every 2 hours.

   - Is the appropriate countertraction provided? For example, elevating the foot of the bed 1 inch for every pound of traction (Mellett, 1998) or flexing the knee of the bed 20 to 30 degrees.
   - Are the correct weights applied? For example, Buck's traction should have no more than 5 pounds (Byrne, 1999).
   - Is there free play of the ropes on the pulleys; that is, does the groove of the pulley support the rope? Are the knots positioned no closer than 12 inches to the nearest pulley?
   - Do all weights hang freely and not rest against or on the bed or floor when the bed is in the lowest position?
   - Are the ropes intact, that is, not frayed, knotted, or kinked between their points of attachment?
   - Are the ropes securely attached with slipknots and the short ends of ropes attached with tape?
   - Is the line of the traction straight and in the same plane as the long axis of the bone?
   - Do bedclothes and other objects not impinge on the traction?
   - Is the spreader bar wide enough to prevent the traction tape from rubbing on bony prominences?

6. Maintain the client in the appropriate traction position.

   - Maintain the client in the supine position unless there are other orders. *Changing position can change the body alignment and the amount of force supplied by the traction.*
   - Maintain body alignment when turning the client. In some cases, the person can turn to a lateral position if a pillow placed between the legs maintains body alignment. Refer to the client's record for information about permitted movement.
   - Provide a trapeze to assist the client to move and lift the body for back care if he or she is unable to turn.
   - Provide a fracture or slipper bedpan as required to minimize the client's movement.

7. Assess the neurovascular status of the affected extremity.

   - Conduct a neurovascular assessment 30 minutes following reapplication of the bandage, then every 2 hours for the first 24 hours. If the client's status is "normal," then assess every 4 hours during the traction. If the client's status is not normal, continue hourly assessments.

8. Provide protective devices and measures to safeguard the skin.

   - Place heel protectors or sheepskins under the heels, sacrum, shoulders, and other pressure areas. See Table 9-1.
   - Change or clean the sheepskin lining at least weekly.
   - Massage the skin with rubbing alcohol or lotion every 4 hours, or if redness and signs of pressure appear, every 2 hours. *Alcohol tends to toughen the skin and leave it less vulnerable to breakdown. Because alcohol is drying to the skin, however, lotion may be preferred for those who have dry skin (e.g., elderly people).*
   - Make sure the spreader bar is wide enough to prevent the traction tape from rubbing on the client's bony prominences.

9. Remove only intermittent nonadhesive skin traction in accordance with agency protocol or orders.

  • To remove a nonadhesive skin traction:

   a. Remove the weights first.

   b. Unwrap the bandage and provide skin care.

   c. Rewrap the limb and slowly reattach the weights.

10. Teach the client ways to prevent problems associated with immobility.

  • Teach the client deep-breathing and coughing exercises to prevent hypostatic pneumonia (see Chapter 20, pages 427–428).

  • Teach the client appropriate exercises to maintain and develop muscle tone, prevent muscle contracture and atrophy, and promote blood circulation:

   a. Range-of-motion exercises (discussed in Chapter 8).

   b. Isometric exercises to strengthen the quadricep muscles include tightening the knees. By pushing the knees down without moving them, the hamstring muscles are also strengthened. Tensing the buttocks and the inner thighs promotes stabilization of the hips. Tensing the inner thighs also helps stabilize the knees.

   c. Circulation to the extremities can be promoted by encouraging the client to flex and extend the feet as well as to perform the isometric exercises.

   d. Specific exercises to strengthen the bicep and tricep muscles in preparation for using crutches can be taught as indicated. For example, raising the buttocks off the bed by pushing down with the arms develops the triceps, and pulling the body up with a trapeze develops the biceps.

 11. **Document** findings in the client record using forms or checklists supplemented by narrative notes when appropriate.

EVALUATION

• Perform a detailed follow-up examination based on findings that deviated from expected or normal for the client. The client should be able to demonstrate usual range of motion in all unaffected body joints; move all fingers or toes of the affected extremity; feel normal sensation and have normal skin color and temperature in all fingers or toes of the affected extremity; and be free of pressure signs (pallor, redness, increased warmth or tenderness) over pressure areas.

• Relate findings to previous assessment data if available.

• Report significant deviations from normal to the physician.

Skeletal Traction

Assessment and delegation related to the client in skeletal traction are the same as those for a client in skin traction.

PLANNING

Verify the physician's orders. Determine the degree of movement permitted and any special precautions (e.g., bed positions permitted).

TABLE 9-1	TRACTION PRESSURE AREAS
Traction	**Pressure Areas**
Buck's extension	Skin over the tibia, if bandage slips; malleoli, hamstring tendon; heels; back
Russell traction	As above for Buck's extension; popliteal space due to sling; sole of foot due to footplate
Cervical head halter	Chin; occiput; ears; mandible
Thomas leg splint and Pearson attachment	Groin, popliteal space; Achilles tendon; heel; perineal nerve if splint misplaced
Halo-thoracic vest	Areas where jacket edges touch the skin; skin under vest

Equipment

- Supplies for providing pin site care according to agency policy (e.g., normal saline, cotton-tipped swabs, gauze dressings)

Performance

1. Explain to the client what you are going to do, why it is necessary, and how he or she can cooperate. Discuss how the results will be used in planning further care or treatments.

2. Wash hands and observe appropriate infection control procedures.

3. Provide for client privacy.

4. Inspect the traction apparatus. See Technique 9-1, step 5. Skeletal traction can be applied to the skull, the proximal end of the ulna, the distal end of the femur, the proximal and distal ends of the tibia, and the calcaneus (heel bone). *Because bone withstands greater stress than skin, heavier weights can be used (e.g., up to 35 pounds).* Metal pins, wires, or tongs are inserted into the bone to which the traction is applied. Common examples are the Steinmann pin and the Kirschner wire.

   - The distal end of a **Thomas leg splint** and **Pearson attachment** is attached to a weighted rope for suspension. The Pearson attachment supports the lower leg off the bed and permits the knee to be flexed (Figure 9-1B). The pin or wire drilled through the bone is attached to a spreader, which in turn is attached to ropes, pulleys, and weights. Countertraction is supplied mostly by the body's weight. A weighted rope attached to the proximal end of the Thomas splint, however, counterbalances the suspension weight. To prevent footdrop, a footplate is attached to the Pearson apparatus. To prevent skin breakdown, the ischial ring of the Thomas splint is padded. Sheepskin slings are positioned along the Pearson attachment.
   - **Skull tongs** (e.g., **Crutchfield**, Burton, Gardner-Wells, or Vinke) are secured to each side of the skull. The center metal bar is attached to ropes, pulleys, and weights and creates a traction pull along the long axis of the spine (Figure 9-1C).

5. Maintain the client in the appropriate traction position. Check that the head, knee, and foot of the bed are properly elevated.

   - For clients with skull tongs or a halo ring, turn the client as a unit. Do not allow the neck to twist. A special bed may be required (see Chapter 6).

- If skull tongs or pins become dislodged, support the head, remove the weights, place sandbags or liter fluid bags on either side of the head to maintain alignment, and notify the physician immediately.

6. Assess the neurovascular status of the affected extremity.

   - Conduct a neurovascular assessment every hour for the first 24 hours. If the client's status is "normal," then assess every 4 hours during the traction. If the client's status is not normal, continue hourly assessments.

7. Provide pin site care daily if indicated by the physician's orders and agency protocol.

   - Carefully inspect the site. Regular inspection of the pin site ensures early detection of minor infections, as manifested by signs of serosanguineous drainage, crusting, swelling, and erythema.
   - Use clean or sterile technique as agency protocol dictates. *Sterile technique is most often used in the hospital setting, clean technique in the ambulatory setting.*
   - According to agency policy, remove crusts using normal saline or other agent recommended by the agency on cotton-tipped swabs. Use a gentle, rolling technique to reduce irritation to the tissue. *Removing crusted secretions permits the pin site to drain freely. Initial crusts around pins do not create a problem and can serve as a barrier to infection, but accumulated crusts around external fixator pins may cause secondary infection.*
   - Apply sterile ointment if ordered. Determine agency practices regarding pin site care. Ointment could interfere with proper drainage (McKenzie, 1999).
   - Loosely apply gauze dressing around pin site.
   - Adjust frequency of care according to the amount of drainage. If no drainage is present, daily site care is adequate. If drainage is present, perform site care every 8 hours.
   - If purulent (containing pus) drainage is present, notify the physician and obtain specimens for culture and sensitivity.

8. Teach the client ways to prevent problems associated with immobility. (See Technique 9-1, step 10.)

9. **Document** findings in the client record using forms or checklists supplemented by narrative notes when appropriate.

AMBULATORY AND COMMUNITY SETTINGS

Traction

- Cervical traction may be done in the home setting using electrical systems or over-the-door mechanical systems. Clients may be instructed to use the system several times a day for up to 30 minutes at a time. A physical therapist should establish the system and conduct initial client and family teaching.

The nurse should reinforce proper technique and assess effectiveness during home or clinic visits.

- Clients in **halo-thoracic vest** traction are ambulatory and need not be hospitalized. Client and family teaching regarding hygiene, care of the device, and when to contact health care providers must be reinforced.

AGE-RELATED CONSIDERATIONS

Traction

Infant/Child

- **Bryant's traction** (Figure 9-1E) is an adaptation of a bilateral Buck's extension. It is used to stabilize fractured femurs or correct congenital hip dislocations in young children under 17.5 kg (35 lbs). The skin traction is applied to both the affected and the unaffected leg to maintain the position of the affected leg. A spreader bar attached to the strips or positioning of the pulleys maintains leg alignment. Unless otherwise ordered, the hips are flexed at

right angles (90 degrees) to the body with the knees extended, and the buttocks raised about 2.5 cm (1 in). Pressure areas include skin over the tibia; malleoli; hamstring tendon; soles of feet; upper back.

Elders

- Adhesive skin traction should not be used due to the fragility of elders' skin.
- Skin breakdown can occur more easily with any form of traction in the elderly than with younger clients.

EVALUATION

- Perform follow-up based on findings that deviated from expected or normal for the client.

- Relate findings to previous assessment data if available.
- Report significant deviations from normal to the physician.

Chapter Summary

TERMINOLOGY

Bryant's traction

Buck's extension

countertraction

Crutchfield tongs

halo-thoracic vest

Pearson attachment

skull tongs

Thomas leg splint

traction

FORMING CLINICAL JUDGMENTS

Consider This:

1. Your young client has been placed in Buck's traction. While assessing her response to treatment, she tells you she is "bored lying flat on her back all day" and wants you to remove the apparatus. What will you say? What will you do?

2. The hospitalized client in skeletal traction for a fractured femur has slid down to the end of the bed. Describe how you would reposition the client.

RELATED RESEARCH

Draper, P., & Scott, F. (1998). Using traction: Hamilton–Russell traction. *Nursing Times, 94*(12), 31–32.

Parker, M. J., & Handoll, H. H. G. (2000). Pre-operative traction for fractures of the proximal femur. *The Cochrane Library, 1* [CD-ROM Abstract].

REFERENCES

Ball, J., & Bindler, R. (1999). *Pediatric nursing: Caring for children.* Stamford, CT: Appleton & Lange.

Byrne, T. (1999). Orthopaedic essentials: The setup and care of a patient in Buck's traction. *Orthopaedic Nursing, 18*(2), 79–83.

McCarthy, L. (1998). Safe handling of patients on cervical traction. *Nursing Times, 94*(14), 57–59.

McKenzie, L. L. (1999). In search of a standard for pin site care. *Orthopaedic Nursing, 18*(2), 73–78.

Mellett, S. (1998). Care of the orthopaedic patient with traction. *Nursing Times, 94*(22), 52–54.

Chapter 10

Client Hygiene

Techniques

OBJECTIVES

- Describe kinds of hygienic care nurses provide to clients.
- Describe various types of baths.
- Describe steps in perineal–genital care.
- Explain specific ways in which nurses help hospitalized clients with oral hygiene.
- Perform techniques for bathing, back massage, hair care, and foot care safely and effectively.
- Describe steps for removing, cleaning, and inserting hearing aids.

10-1 Bathing the Adult Client

10-2 Providing Perineal–Genital Care

10-3 Performing a Back Massage

10-4 Brushing and Flossing the Teeth

10-5 Providing Special Oral Care

10-6 Providing Hair Care

10-7 Providing Foot Care

10-8 Removing, Cleaning, and Inserting a Hearing Aid

Hygienic Care

Hygiene is the science of health and its mainte-nance. Personal hygiene is the self-care by which people attend to such functions as bathing, toileting, general body hygiene, and grooming. Hygiene is a highly personal matter determined by various factors, including individual values and practices (see Table 10-1). It involves care of the skin, hair, nails, teeth, oral and nasal cavities, eyes, ears, and perineal–genital areas.

It is important for nurses to know exactly how much assistance a client needs for hygienic care. Clients may require help after urinating or defecating, after vomiting, and whenever they become soiled, for example, from wound drainage or from profuse per-spiration.

Nurses commonly use the following terms to describe the kinds of hygienic care:

- **Early morning care** is provided to clients as they awaken in the morning. This care consists of pro-viding a urinal or bedpan to the client confined to bed, washing the face and hands, and giving oral care.

- **Morning care** is often provided after clients have breakfast, although it may be provided before breakfast. It usually includes the provision of a uri-nal or bedpan (to clients who are not ambulatory), a bath or shower, perineal care, back massages, and oral, nail, and hair care. Making the client's bed is part of morning care.

- **Afternoon care** often includes providing a bedpan or urinal, washing the hands and face, and assist-ing with oral care to refresh clients.

- **Hour of sleep (HS) care** is provided to clients before they retire for the night. It usually involves providing for elimination needs, washing face and hands, giving oral care, and giving a back massage.

- **As-needed (prn) care** is provided as required by the client. For example, a client who is diaphoretic (sweating profusely) may need bathing and a change of clothes and linen frequently.

Bathing and Skin Care

Bathing removes accumulated oil, perspiration, dead skin cells, and some bacteria. The nurse can appreciate the quantity of oil and dead skin cells produced when observing the skin of a person after the removal of a cast that has been on for 6 weeks. The skin is crusty, flaky, and dry underneath the cast. Applications of oil over several days are usually necessary to remove the debris. Excessive bathing, however, can interfere with the intended lubricating effect of the sebum, causing dryness of the skin. This is an important consideration of the elderly, who produce limited sebum (fatty secre-tions of the sebaceous glands).

In addition to cleaning the skin, bathing also stim-ulates circulation. A warm or hot bath dilates superfi-cial arterioles, bringing more blood and nourishment to the skin. Vigorous rubbing has the same effect. Rubbing with long smooth strokes from the distal to proximal parts of extremities (from the point farthest from the body to the point closest) is particularly effective in facilitating venous blood flow.

Bathing also produces a sense of well-being. It is refreshing and relaxing and frequently improves morale, appearance, and self-respect. Some people take a morning shower for its refreshing, stimulating

TABLE 10-1	FACTORS INFLUENCING INDIVIDUAL HYGIENIC PRACTICES
Factor	**Variables**
Culture	North American culture places a high value on cleanliness. Many North Americans bathe or shower once or twice a day, whereas people from some other cultures bathe once a week. Some cultures consider privacy essential for bathing, whereas others practice communal bathing. Body odor is offensive in some cultures and accepted as normal in others.
Religion	Ceremonial washings are practiced by some religions.
Environment	Finances may affect the availability of facilities for bathing. For example, homeless people may not have warm water available; soap, shampoo, shaving lotion, and deodorants may be too expensive for people who have limited resources.
Developmental level	Children learn hygiene in the home. Practices vary according to the individual's age; for example, preschoolers can carry out most tasks independently with encouragement.
Health and energy	Ill people may not have the motivation or energy to attend to hygiene. Some clients who have neuromuscular impairments may be unable to perform hygienic care.
Personal preferences	Some people prefer a shower to a tub bath.

effect. Others prefer an evening bath because it is relaxing. These effects are more evident when a person is ill. For example, it is not uncommon for clients who have had a restless or sleepless night to feel relaxed, comfortable, and sleepy after a morning bath.

Bathing offers an excellent opportunity for the nurse to assess ill clients. The nurse can observe the condition of the client's skin and physical conditions such as reddened pressure areas over bony prominences. While assisting a client with a bath, the nurse can also assess the client's psychosocial needs (e.g., orientation to time and ability to cope with the illness). Learning needs, such as a diabetic client's need to learn foot care, can also be assessed.

It is important for the nurse to apply knowledge of the client's cultural preferences for bathing. For example, North Americans place a high value on cleanliness, with many bathing daily and using products such as deodorant, perfume, and lotions. Other cultures, however, may bathe weekly and see no need for deodorant or perfumed products (Skewes, 1997).

Categories of Baths

Two categories of baths are given to clients: cleaning and therapeutic. **Cleaning baths** are given chiefly for hygienic purposes and include these types:

- **Complete bed bath.** The nurse washes the entire body of a dependent client in bed.

- **Self-help bed bath.** Clients confined to bed are able to bathe themselves with help from the nurse for washing the back and perhaps the feet.

- **Partial (abbreviated) bath.** Only parts of the client's body that might cause discomfort or odor, if neglected, are washed: the face, hands, axillae, perineal area, and back. Omitted are the arms, chest, abdomen, legs, and feet. The nurse provides this care for dependent clients and assists self-sufficient clients confined to bed by washing their backs. Some ambulatory clients prefer to take a partial bath at the sink. The nurse can assist them by washing their backs.

- **Towel bath.** The towel bath is an in-bed bath that uses a quick-drying solution containing a disinfectant, a cleaning agent, and a softening agent mixed with water. This commercially prepared solution is used at a temperature of 43.3 to 48.0°C (110 to 120°F). The solution dries in a few seconds, avoiding the need to dry the client and thereby speeding the bathing process.

- **Bag bath.** The bag bath is an adaptation of the towel bath. The equipment needed is a plastic bag, 10 to 12 washcloths, and a nonrinsable cleaner and water mixture. The solution and washcloths are warmed in a microwave. The warming time is about 1 minute, but the nurse needs to determine how long it takes to attain a desirable temperature. Each area of the body is cleaned with a different cloth and then air dried. Because the body is not rubbed dry, the emollient in the solution remains on the skin.

- **Tub bath.** Tub baths are preferred to bed baths because it is easier to wash and rinse in a tub. Tubs are also used for therapeutic baths. The amount of assistance the nurse offers depends on the abilities of the client. There are specially designed tubs for dependent clients. These tubs greatly reduce the work of the nurse in lifting clients in and out of the tub and offer greater benefits than a sponge bath in bed.

- **Shower.** Many ambulatory clients are able to use shower facilities and require only minimal assistance from the nurse. Clients in long-term care settings are often given showers. The wheels on the shower chair allow clients to be transported from their room to the shower. The shower chair also has a commode seat to facilitate cleansing of the client's perineal area during the shower process (see Figure 10-1 ◆).

Therapeutic baths are given for physical effects, such as to soothe irritated skin or to treat an area (e.g.,

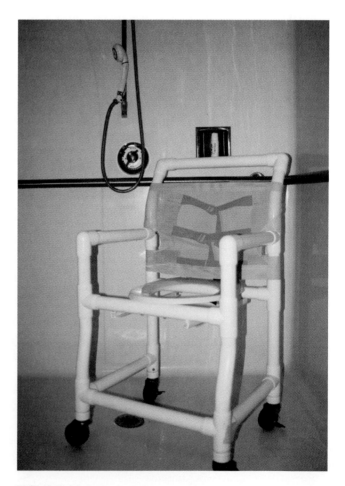

FIGURE 10-1 ◆ A shower chair.

the perineum). Medications may be placed in the water. A therapeutic bath is generally taken in a tub one-third or one-half full, about 114 L (30 gal). The client remains in the bath for a designated time, often 20 to 30 minutes. If the client's back, chest, and arms are to be treated, these areas need to be immersed in the solution. The bath temperature is generally included in the order; 37.7 to 46°C (100 to 115°F) may be ordered for adults and 40.5°C (105°F) is usually ordered for infants.

Technique 10-1 provides guidelines for bathing the adult client in bed.

Long-Term Care Setting

From a historical perspective, the bath has always been a part of nursing care and considered a component of the "art" of nursing. In today's nursing world, however, the bath is seen as "basic" and often delegated to nonprofessionals (Hektor & Touhy, 1997).

In spite of the previously listed therapeutic values associated with bathing, the choice of bathing procedure often depends on the amount of time available to the nurse or unlicensed assistive personnel (UAP) and the client's self-care ability. Nursing authors (Rader, Lavelle, Hoeffer, & McKenzie, 1996; Skewes, 1997; Hektor & Touhy, 1997) challenge nurses to switch from a task-centered approach to an individualized and aesthetic approach to bathing, especially for the older person in a long-term care setting.

The bath routine (e.g., day, time, and number/week) for clients in health care settings is often determined by agency policy, making the bath routine and depersonalized versus a therapeutic, satisfying, and person-focused approach. An individualized approach focusing on therapeutic and comforting outcomes of bathing is especially important for clients with dementia. Miller (1997) found that hygienic care (in the form of showering) of persons with cognitive impairment could cause client distress and precipitate physically aggressive behavior toward staff.

Rader and colleagues (1996) encourage nurses in the long-term care setting to view the bath from the individual's perspective. For example, what is their usual method of maintaining cleanliness? Are there any past negative experiences related to bathing? Are factors such as pain or fatigue increasing the client's difficulty with the demands and stimuli associated with bathing or showering? A client's resistance to the bathing experience can be a cue to the nurse to consider other methods of maintaining cleanliness. For example, if the shower causes distress, is there another form of bathing (such as the towel bath) that may be more therapeutic and comforting?

Collaboration between the nurse and UAP is a critical element to implementing the individualized person-focused approach for cognitively impaired clients who exhibit aggressive behavior during bathing. The nurse should observe the difficult bathing situation followed by the nurse and UAP discussing possible alternative strategies or methods during the bathing process for the client. Hoeffer and colleagues (1997) point out that nursing assistants are concerned that they may be perceived as not doing their job if they vary from the standard routine of the agency. Validation and support by the nurse is critical to the willingness of the UAP to try new approaches.

Nursing Process: Bathing and Skin Care

ASSESSMENT

Assess:

- Condition of the skin (color, texture and turgor, presence of pigmented spots, temperature, lesions, excoriations, and abrasions)
- Fatigue
- Presence of pain and need for adjunctive measures (e.g., an analgesic) before the bath
- Range of motion of the joints and any other aspect of health that may affect the client's bathing process
- Need for use of disposable gloves during the bath

PLANNING

Delegation

The nurse often delegates the skill of bathing to certified nursing assistant or UAP. However, the nurse remains responsible for assessment and client care. The nurse needs to:

- Inform the UAP of the type of bath appropriate for the client and precautions, if any, specific to the needs of the client.
- Remind the UAP to notify the nurse of any concerns or changes (e.g., redness, skin breakdown, rash) so the nurse can assess, intervene if needed, and document.
- Instruct the UAP to encourage the client to perform as much self-care as appropriate in order to promote independence and self-esteem.
- Obtain a complete report from the staff person assigned to the client.

Equipment

- Basin or sink with warm water (between 43 and 46°C or 110 and 115°F)
- Soap and soap dish
- Linens: bath blanket, two bath towels, washcloth, clean gown or pajamas or clothes as needed, additional bed linen and towels, if required
- Gloves, if appropriate (e.g., giving perineal care)
- Personal hygiene articles (e.g., deodorant, powder, lotions)
- Shaving equipment for male clients
- Table for bathing equipment
- Laundry hamper

Preparation

Before bathing a client, determine: (1) the purpose and type of bath the client needs; (2) self-care ability of the client; (3) any movement or positioning precautions specific to the client; (4) other care the client may be receiving, such as physical therapy or x-rays, in order to coordinate all aspects of health care and prevent unnecessary fatigue; (5) client's comfort level with being bathed by someone else; and (6) necessary bath equipment and linens.

Caution is needed when bathing clients who are receiving intravenous therapy. Easy-to-remove gowns that have Velcro or snap fasteners along the sleeves may be used. If a special gown is not available, the nurse needs to pay special attention when changing the client's gown after the bath (or whenever the gown becomes soiled). General guidelines are provided in Box 10-1. These guidelines do not apply if the client has an IV pump or controller. In this situation, either use a special gown or do not put the sleeve of a gown over the client's involved arm.

Performance

1. Explain to the client what you are going to do, why it is necessary, and how he or she can coop-erate. Discuss with the client the plan for bathing and explain any unfamiliar procedures to the client.

2. Wash hands and observe other appropriate infection control procedures.

3. Provide for client privacy by drawing the curtains around the bed or closing the door to the room. Some agencies provide signs indicating the need for privacy. *Hygiene is a personal matter.*

4. Prepare the client and the environment.

- Invite a family member or significant other to participate if desired.
- Close windows and doors to ensure the room is a comfortable temperature. *Air currents increase loss of heat from the body by convection.*
- Offer the client a bedpan or urinal or ask whether the client wishes to use the toilet or commode. *Warm water and activity can stimulate the need to void. The client will be more comfortable after voiding, and voiding before cleaning the perineum is advisable.*
- Encourage the client to perform as much personal self-care as possible. *This promotes independence, exercise, and self-esteem.*
- During the bath, assess each area of the skin carefully.

For a Bed Bath

5. Prepare the bed and position the client appropriately.

- Position the bed at a comfortable working height. Lower side rail on the side close to you. Keep the other side rail UP. Assist the client to move near you. *This avoids undue reaching and straining and promotes good body mechanics.*
- Place bath blanket over top sheet. Remove the top sheet from under the bath blanket by starting at client's shoulders and moving linen down towards client's feet. Ask the client to grasp and hold the top of the bath blanket while pulling

---

BOX 10-1 *Changing a Hospital Gown for a Client with an Intravenous Infusion*

- Slip the gown completely off the arm without the infusion and onto the tubing connected to the arm with the infusion.
- Holding the container above the client's arm, slide the sleeve up over the container to remove the used gown.
- Place the clean gown sleeve for the arm with the infusion over the container as if it were an extension of the client's arm, from the inside of the gown to the sleeve cuff.

- Rehang the container. Slide the gown carefully over the tubing toward the client's hand.
- Guide the client's arm and tubing into the sleeve, taking care not to pull on the tubing.
- Assist the client to put the other arm into the second sleeve of the gown, and fasten as usual.
- Count the rate of flow of the infusion to make sure it is correct before leaving the bedside.

linen to the foot of the bed. *The bath blanket provides comfort, warmth, and privacy. Note: If the bed linen is to be reused place it over the bedside chair. If it is to be changed, place it in the linen hamper.*

- Remove client's gown while keeping the client covered with the bath blanket. Place gown in linen hamper.

6. Make a bath mitt with the washcloth (Figure 10-2 ◆). *A bath mitt retains water and heat better than a cloth loosely held and prevents ends of washcloth from dragging across the skin.*

- Triangular method: (1) Lay your hand on the washcloth; (2) fold the top corner over your hand; (3, 4) fold the side corners over your hand; (5) tuck the second corner under the cloth on the palm side to secure the mitt.

- Rectangular method: (1) Lay your hand on the washcloth and fold one side over your hand; (2) fold the second side over your hand; (3) fold the top of the cloth down; and (4) tuck it under the folded side against your palm to secure the mitt.

7. Wash the face. *Begin the bath at the cleanest area and work downward toward the feet.*

- Place towel under client's head.
- Wash the client's eyes with water only and dry

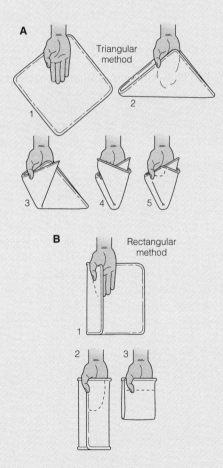

FIGURE 10-2 ◆ Making a bath mitt: (A) triangular method; (B) rectangular method.

them well. Use a separate corner of the washcloth for each eye. *Using separate corners prevents transmitting microorganisms from one eye to the other.* Wipe from the inner to the outer canthus. *This prevents secretions from entering the naso-lacrimal ducts.*

- Ask whether the client wants soap used on the face. *Soap has a drying effect, and the face, which is exposed to the air more than other body parts, tends to be drier.*

- Wash, rinse, and dry the client's face, ears, and neck.

- Remove the towel from under the client's head.

8. Wash the arms and hands. (Omit the arms for a partial bath.)

- Place a towel lengthwise under the arm away from you. *It protects the bed from becoming wet.*

- Wash, rinse, and dry the arm by elevating the client's arm and supporting the client's wrist and elbow. Use long, firm strokes from wrist to shoulder, including the axillary area. *Firm strokes from distal to proximal areas promote circulation by increasing venous blood return.*

- Apply deodorant or powder if desired.

- *Optional:* Place a towel on the bed and put a washbasin on it. Place the client's hands in the basin. *Many clients enjoy immersing their hands in the basin and washing themselves. Soaking loosens dirt under the nails.* Assist the client as needed to wash, rinse, and dry their hands, paying particular attention to the spaces between their fingers.

- Repeat for hand and arm nearest you. Exercise caution if an intravenous infusion is present, and check its flow after moving the arm.

9. Wash the chest and abdomen. (Omit the chest and abdomen for a partial bath. However, the areas under a woman's breasts may require bathing if this area is irritated.)

- Place bath towel lengthwise over chest. Fold bath blanket down to the client's pubic area. *Keeps the client warm while preventing unnecessary exposure of the chest.*

- Lift the bath towel off the chest, and bathe the chest and abdomen with your mitted hand using long, firm strokes. Give special attention to the skin under the breasts and any other skin folds, particularly if the client is overweight. Rinse and dry well.

- Replace the bath blanket when the areas have been dried.

10. Wash the legs and feet. (Omit legs and feet for a partial bath.)

- Expose the leg farthest from you by folding the bath blanket toward the other leg, being careful to keep the perineum covered. *Covering the perineum promotes privacy and maintains the client's dignity.*

- Lift leg and place the bath towel lengthwise under the leg. Wash, rinse, and dry the leg using long, smooth, firm strokes from the ankle to the knee to the thigh. *Washing from the distal to proximal areas promotes circulation by stimulating venous blood flow.*

- Reverse the coverings and repeat for the other leg.

- Wash the feet by placing them in the basin of water (Figure 10-3 ◆).

- Dry each foot. Pay particular attention to the spaces between the toes. If you prefer, wash one foot after that leg before washing the other leg.

- Obtain fresh, warm bathwater now or when necessary. *Water may become dirty or cold.* Because surface skin cells are removed with washing, the bathwater from dark-skinned clients may be dark, however, this does not mean the client is dirty. Raise side rails when refilling basin. *This ensures the safety of the client.*

11. Wash the back and then the perineum.

- Assist the client into a prone or side-lying position facing away from you. Place the bath towel lengthwise alongside the back and buttocks while keeping the client covered with the bath blanket as much as possible. *This provides warmth and undue exposure.*

- Wash and dry the client's back, moving from the shoulders to the buttocks, and upper thighs, paying attention to the gluteal folds.

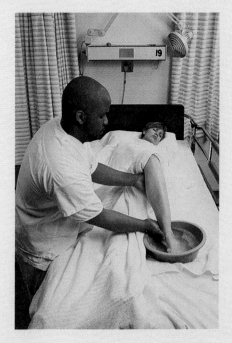

FIGURE 10-3 ◆ Soaking a foot in a basin.

- Perform a back massage now or after completion of bath. (See Technique 10-3 Performing a Back Massage).

- Assist the client to the supine position and determine whether the client can wash the perineal area independently. If the client cannot do so, drape the client as shown in Technique 10-2 and wash the area.

12. Assist the client with grooming aids such as powder, lotion, or deodorant.

- Use powder sparingly. Release as little as possible into the atmosphere. *This will avoid irritation of the respiratory tract by powder inhalation. Excessive powder can cause caking, which leads to skin irritation.*

- Help the client put on a clean gown or pajamas.

- Assist the client to care for hair, mouth, and nails. Some people prefer or need mouth care prior to their bath.

For a Tub Bath or Shower

13. Prepare the client and the tub.

- Fill the tub about one-third to one-half full of water at 43 to 46°C (110 to 115°F). *Sufficient water is needed to cover the perineal area.*

- Cover all intravenous catheters or wound dressings with plastic coverings, and instruct the client to prevent wetting these areas if possible.

- Put a rubber bath mat or towel on the floor of the tub if safety strips are not on the tub floor. *These prevent slippage of the client during the bath or shower.*

14. Assist the client into the shower or tub.

- Assist the client taking a standing shower with the initial adjustment of the water temperature and water flow pressure, as needed. Some clients need a chair to sit in the shower because of weakness. Hot water can cause elderly people to feel faint.

- If the client requires considerable assistance with a tub bath, a hydraulic bathtub chair may be required (see variations).

- Explain how the client can signal for help, leave the client for two to five minutes, and place an "occupied" sign on the door.

15. Assist the client with washing and getting out of the tub.

- Wash the client's back, lower legs, and feet, if necessary.

- Assist the client out of the tub. If the client is unsteady, place a bath towel over the client's shoulders and drain the tub of water before the client attempts to get out of it. *Draining the water first lessens the likelihood of a fall. The towel prevents chilling.*

16. Dry the client, and assist with follow-up care.
    - Follow step 12.
    - Assist the client back to his or her room.
    - Clean the tub or shower in accordance with agency practice, discard the used linen in the laundry hamper, and place the "unoccupied" sign on the door.

17. **Document**
    - Type of bath given (i.e., complete, partial, or self-help). This is usually recorded on a flow sheet.
    - Skin assessment, such as excoriation, erythema, exudates, rashes, drainage, or skin breakdown.
    - Nursing interventions related to skin integrity.
    - Ability of the client to assist or cooperate with bathing.
    - Client response to bathing.
    - Educational needs regarding hygiene.
    - Information or teaching shared with the client or their family.

Variation: Towel Bath

- Fold a large terry cloth towel in a plastic bag and saturate it with the solution provided.
- Wring out the towel, and then unroll it over the client, while at the same time moving the top bed linen off the client.
- Fold excess towel under the client's chin for subsequent use.
- Use a gentle massaging motion to clean the body, starting at the feet and working toward the head.
- Fold the towel upward after the massage and replace it with a clean sheet.

- Use the part of the towel folded under the chin to clean the client's face, neck, and ears.
- Remove the towel. Roll the client to one side and apply the clean side of the towel to the back of the neck, back, and buttocks.
- Remove the towel.
- Place clean linen on the bed, dress the client, and position the client appropriately.

Variation: Bathing Using a Hydraulic Bathtub Chair

A hydraulic lift, often used in a long-term care or rehabilitation setting, can facilitate the transfer of a client who is unable to ambulate to a tub. The lift also helps eliminate strain on the nurse's back.

- Bring the client to the tub room in a wheelchair or shower chair.
- Fill the tub and check the water temperature with a bath thermometer *to avoid thermal injury to the client.*
- Lower the hydraulic chair lift to its lowest point, outside the tub.
- Transfer the client to the chair lift and secure the seat belt.
- Raise the chair lift above the tub.
- Support the client's legs as the chair is moved over the tub *to avoid injury to the legs.*
- Position the client's legs down into the water and slowly lower the chair lift into the tub.
- Assist bathing the client, if appropriate.
- Reverse the procedure when taking the client out of the tub.
- Dry the client and transport him or her to his or her room.

AMBULATORY AND COMMUNITY SETTINGS

Bathing

- Focus on promoting function, independence, and autonomy during the bathing process. This will help clients avoid dependence on caretakers in the long-term care setting.
- The type of bath chosen depends on assessment of the home, caregiver, availability of running water, and condition of bathing facilities.
- Suggestions for bathing in the home setting:
    - Purchase a bath seat that fits in the tub or shower.
    - Install a hand shower for use with a bath seat and shampooing.
    - Use a nonskid surface on the tub or shower.

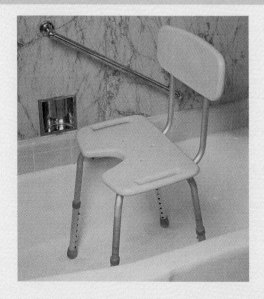

Bathing (*continued*)

- Install hand bars on both sides of the tub or shower to facilitate transfers in and out of the tub or shower.
- Monitor the temperature of the water.
- Apply lotion and oil *after* a bath because these solutions can make a tub surface slippery.

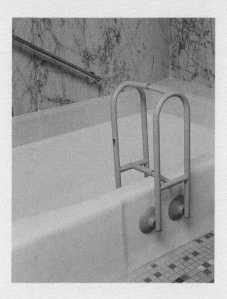

Bathing

Infant

- Sponge baths are suggested for the newborn because daily tub baths are not considered necessary. After the bath, the infant should be immediately dried and wrapped. Parents need to be advised that the infant's ability to regulate body temperature has not yet fully developed and their body loses heat readily.

Child

- Encourage a child's participation appropriate for developmental level.
- Closely supervise children in the bathtub. Do not leave them unattended.

- Assist adolescents as needed to choose deodorants and antiperspirants. Secretions from newly active sweat glands react with bacteria on the skin, causing a pungent odor.

Elders

- To minimize skin dryness in older adults, avoid excessive use of soap. The ideal time to moisturize the skin is immediately after bathing.
- Avoid powder as it causes moisture loss and is a hazardous inhalant. Cornstarch should also be avoided because in the presence of moisture it breaks down into glucose supporting the growth of organisms (Skewes, 1997).
- Protect older adults and children from injury related to hot water burns.

EVALUATION

- Note the client's tolerance of the procedure (e.g., respiratory rate and effort, pulse rate, signs of resistance)
- Conduct appropriate follow up, such as:
  - Condition and integrity of skin (dryness, turgor, redness, lesions, etc.)
  - Client strength
  - Percentage of bath done without assistance
- Relate to prior assessment data, if available.

Perineal–Genital Care

Perineal–genital care is also referred to as **perineal care** or **peri-care**. Perineal care as part of the bed bath is embarrassing for many clients. Nurses also may find it embarrassing initially, particularly with clients of the opposite sex. Most clients who require a bed bath from the nurse are able to clean their own perineal area with minimal assistance. The nurse may need to hand a moistened washcloth and soap to the client, rinse the washcloth, and provide a towel.

Because some clients are unfamiliar with terminology for the genitals and perineum, it may be difficult for nurses to explain what is expected. Most clients, however, understand what is meant if the nurse simply says, "I'll give you a washcloth to finish your bath." Older clients may be familiar with the term *private parts*. Whatever expression the nurse uses, it needs to be one that the client understands and one that is comfortable for the nurse to use.

The nurse needs to provide perineal care efficiently and matter-of-factly. Nurses should wear gloves while providing this care for the comfort of the client and to protect themselves from infection. Technique 10-2 explains how to provide perineal–genital care.

Nursing Process: Perineal–Genital Care

ASSESSMENT

Assess for the presence of:

- Irritation, excoriation, inflammation, swelling
- Excessive discharge
- Odor; pain or discomfort
- Urinary or fecal incontinence
- Recent rectal or perineal surgery
- Indwelling catheter

Determine:

- Perineal–genital hygiene practices
- Self-care abilities

PLANNING

Delegation

Perineal–genital care can be delegated to UAP. If the client has recently had perineal, rectal, or genital surgery, the nurse needs to assess if it is appropriate for the UAP to perform perineal–genital care.

IMPLEMENTATION:
TECHNIQUE 10-2 PROVIDING PERINEAL–GENITAL CARE

Equipment

Perineal–Genital Care Provided in Conjunction with the Bed Bath

- Bath towel
- Bath blanket
- Disposable gloves
- Bath basin with water at 43 to 46°C (110 to 115°F)
- Soap
- Washcloth

Special Perineal–Genital Care

- Bath towel
- Bath blanket
- Disposable gloves
- Cotton balls or swabs
- Solution bottle, pitcher, or container filled with warm water or a prescribed solution
- Bedpan to receive rinse water
- Moisture-resistant bag or receptacle for used cotton swabs
- Perineal pad

Preparation

- Determine whether the client is experiencing any discomfort in the perineal–genital area.
- Obtain and prepare the necessary equipment and supplies.

Performance

1. Explain to the client what you are going to do, why it is necessary, and how he or she can cooperate, being particularly sensitive to any embarrassment felt by the client.

2. Wash hands and observe other appropriate infection control procedures (e.g., disposable gloves).

3. Provide for client privacy.

4. Prepare the client
   - Fold the top bed linen to the foot of the bed and fold the gown up to expose the genital area.
   - Place a bath towel under the client's hips. *The bath towel prevents the bed from becoming soiled.*

5. Position and drape the client and clean the upper inner thighs.

For Females

- Position the female in a back-lying position with the knees flexed and spread well apart (abducted).
- Cover her body and legs with the bath blanket. Drape the legs by tucking the bottom corners of the bath blanket under the inner sides of the legs (Figure 10-4 ◆). *Minimum exposure lessens embarrassment and helps to provide warmth.* Bring the middle portion of the base of the blanket up over the pubic area.
- Put on gloves; wash and dry the upper inner thighs.

For Males

- Position the male client in a supine position with knees slightly flexed and hips slightly externally rotated.

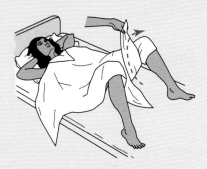

FIGURE 10-4 ◆ Draping the client for perineal–genital care.

- Put on gloves; wash and dry the upper inner thighs.

6. Inspect the perineal area.
   - Note particular areas of inflammation, excoriation, or swelling, especially between the labia in females and the scrotal folds in males.
   - Also note excessive discharge or secretions from the orifices and the presence of odors.

7. Wash and dry the perineal–genital area.

For Females

- Clean the labia majora. Then spread the labia to wash the folds between the labia majora and the labia minora (Figure 10-5 ◆). *Secretions that tend to collect around the labia minora facilitate bacterial growth.*
- Use separate quarters of the washcloth for each stroke, and wipe from the pubis to the rectum. For menstruating women and clients with indwelling catheters, use disposable wipes, cotton balls, or gauze. Take a clean ball for each stroke. *Using separate quarters of the washcloth or new cotton balls or gauzes prevents the transmission of microorganisms from one area to the other. Wipe from the area of least contamination (the pubis) to that of greatest (the rectum).*

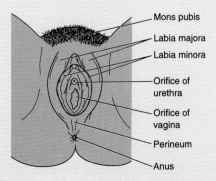

FIGURE 10-5 ◆ Female genitals.

Mons pubis
Labia majora
Labia minora
Orifice of urethra
Orifice of vagina
Perineum
Anus

- Rinse the area well. You may place the client on a bedpan and use a periwash or solution bottle to pour warm water over the area. Dry the perineum thoroughly, paying particular attention to the folds between the labia. *Moisture supports the growth of many microorganisms.*

For Males

- Wash and dry the penis, using firm strokes. *Handling the penis firmly may prevent an erection.*
- If the client is uncircumcised, retract the prepuce (foreskin) to expose the glans penis (the tip of the penis) for cleaning. Replace the foreskin after cleaning the glans penis (Figure 10-6 ◆). *Retracting the foreskin is necessary to remove the smegma that collects under the foreskin and facilitates bacterial growth. Replacing the foreskin prevents constriction of the penis, which may cause edema.*
- Wash and dry the scrotum. The posterior folds of the scrotum may need to be cleaned in step 9 with the buttocks. *The scrotum tends to be more soiled than the penis because of its proximity to the rectum; thus, it is usually cleaned after the penis.*

8. Inspect perineal orifices for intactness.
   - Inspect particularly around the urethra in clients with indwelling catheters. *A catheter may cause excoriation around the urethra.*

9. Clean between the buttocks.
   - Assist the client to turn onto the side facing away from you.
   - Pay particular attention to the anal area and posterior folds of the scrotum in males. Clean the anus with toilet tissue before washing it, if necessary.
   - Dry the area well.
   - For postdelivery or menstruating females, apply a perineal pad as needed from front to back. *This prevents contamination of the vagina and urethra from the anal area.*

 10. **Document** any unusual findings such as redness, excoriation, skin breakdown, discharge or drainage, and any localized areas of tenderness.

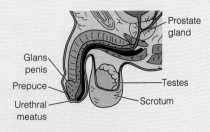

FIGURE 10-6 ◆ Male genitals.

Prostate gland
Glans penis
Prepuce
Urethral meatus
Testes
Scrotum

- Relate current assessments to previous assessments.
- Conduct appropriate follow-up such as prescribed ointment for excoriation.
- Report any deviation from normal to the physician.

Back Massage

Effleurage is a type of massage consisting of long, slow, gliding strokes (Labyak & Metzger, 1997). The back rub or back massage, terms referring to effleurage, is a technique traditionally used in nursing to promote rest and relaxation.

Research demonstrates that back massage has the ability to elicit a relaxation response (Gauthier, 1999). Other research findings (Labyak & Metzger, 1997) suggest that a simple 3-minute back rub can enhance client comfort and relaxation and have a positive effect on cardiovascular parameters such as blood pressure, heart rate, and respiratory rate (p. 62). Back massage improved the quality of sleep among critically ill clients (Richards, 1998). Rowe and Alfred (1999) found that slow-stroke massage could diffuse agitated behaviors in individuals with Alzheimer's disease. While not specifically back massage, research by Hayes and Cox (1999) indicated that a five-minute foot massage administered to critically ill clients in intensive care had the potential effect of increasing relaxation as evidenced by a decrease in heart rate, blood pressure, and respirations.

Ironically, nurses in acute care settings seldom use this basic nursing technique. The intensity of the acute care environment and the time demands of high-technology nursing may be contributing factors leading to the disappearance of the back rub (Labyak & Metzger, 1997). Nurses, however, need to reconsider this simple, effective, traditional technique when research indicates the positive client outcomes. Technique 10-9 provides guidelines for giving a back rub.

Nursing Process: Back Massage

ASSESSMENT

- Assess behaviors indicating potential need for a back massage, such as a complaint of stiffness, muscle tension in the back or shoulders, or difficulty sleeping related to tenseness or anxiety.
- Determine if the client is willing to have a massage, as some individuals may not enjoy a massage.
- Assess for contraindications of back massage (e.g., impaired skin integrity, back surgery, vertebral, rib fracture).

PLANNING

Delegation

The nurse can delegate this skill to UAP; however, the nurse should first assess for any contraindications and client willingness.

IMPLEMENTATION:
TECHNIQUE 10-3 PERFORMING A BACK MASSAGE

Equipment

- Lotion
- Towel for excess lotion

Preparation

Determine (1) previous assessments of the skin, (2) special lotions to be used, and (3) positions contraindicated for the client. Arrange for a quiet environment with no interruptions to promote maximum effect of the back massage.

Performance

1. Explain to the client what you are going to do, why it is necessary, and how he or she can cooperate. Encourage the client to give you feedback as to the amount of pressure you are using during the backrub.

2. Wash hands and observe other appropriate infection control procedures.

3. Provide for client privacy.

4. Prepare the client.
   - Assist the client to move to the near side of the bed within your reach and adjust the bed to a comfortable working height *to prevent back strain.*
   - Establish which position the client prefers. The prone position is recommended for a back rub. The side-lying position can be used if a client cannot assume the prone position.
   - Expose the back from the shoulders to the inferior sacral area. Cover the remainder of the body *to prevent chilling and minimize exposure.*

5. Massage the back.
   - Pour a small amount of lotion onto the palms of your hands and hold it for a minute. The lotion

bottle can also be placed in a bath basin filled with warm water. *Back rub preparations tend to feel uncomfortably cold to people. Warming the solution facilitates client comfort.*

- Using your palm, begin in the sacral area using smooth, circular strokes.
- Move your hands up the center of the back and then over both scapulae.
- Massage in a circular motion over the scapulae.
- Move your hands down the sides of the back.
- Massage the areas over the right and left iliac crests (Figure 10-7 ◆).
- Apply firm, continuous pressure without breaking contact with the client's skin.
- Repeat above for 3 to 5 minutes obtaining more lotion as necessary.
- While massaging the back, assess for skin redness and areas of decreased circulation.
- Pat dry any excess lotion with a towel.

 6. **Document** that a back rub was performed and the client's response. Record any unusual findings.

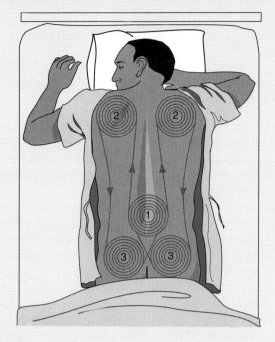

FIGURE 10-7 ◆ One suggested pattern for a back massage.

EVALUATION

Compare the client's current response to his or her previous response. Is there a positive client outcome such as increased relaxation and decrease in pain and anxiety as a result of the back massage?

Oral Hygiene

Good oral hygiene includes daily stimulation of the gums, mechanical brushing and flossing of the teeth, flushing of the mouth, and regular check-ups by a dentist. The nurse is often in a position to help people maintain oral hygiene by helping or teaching them to clean their teeth and oral cavity, by inspecting whether clients (especially children) have done so, or by actually providing mouth care to clients who are ill or incapacitated. The nurse can also be instrumental in identifying problems that require the intervention of a dentist or oral surgeon and arranging a referral.

Thorough brushing of the teeth is important in preventing tooth decay. The mechanical action of brushing removes food particles that can harbor and incubate bacteria. It also stimulates circulation in the gums, thus maintaining their healthy firmness. One of the techniques recommended for brushing teeth is called the **sulcular technique**, which removes plaque and cleans under the gingival margins. There are many toothpastes on the market. Fluoride toothpaste is often recommended because of its antibacterial protections. Technique 10-4 describes brushing and flossing teeth.

Some people have artificial teeth in the form of a plate—a complete set of teeth for one jaw. A person may have a lower plate, an upper plate, or both. When only a few artificial teeth are needed, the individual may have a bridge rather than a plate. A bridge may be fixed or removable.

Artificial dentures, like natural teeth, collect microorganisms and food. They need to be cleaned regularly, at least once a day. They can be removed from the mouth, scrubbed with a toothbrush, rinsed, and reinserted. Some people use a **dentifrice** (paste or powder used to clean or polish the teeth) for cleaning teeth and others use commercial cleaning compounds for plates.

Special Oral Hygiene

For the client who is debilitated or unconscious or who has excessive dryness, sores, or irritations of the mouth, it may be necessary to clean the oral mucosa and tongue in addition to the teeth. Agency practices differ in regard to special mouth care and the frequency with which it is provided. Depending on the health of the client's mouth, special care may be needed every 2 to 8 hours.

Mouth care for unconscious or debilitated people is important because their mouths tend to become dry and consequently predisposed to infections. Dryness occurs because the client cannot take fluids by mouth, is often breathing through the mouth, or may be receiving oxygen, which tends to dry the mucous membranes.

The nurse can use foam swabs to clean the mucous membranes. Long-term use of lemon–glycerine swabs can lead to further dryness of the mucosa and changes in tooth enamel. Mineral oil is contraindicated because aspiration of it can initiate an infection (lipid pneumonia). Hydrogen peroxide is not recommended for use in oral care because it irritates healthy oral mucosa and may alter the microflora of the mouth. Normal saline solution is recommended for oral hygiene for the dependent client who is not on a sodium restriction. Technique 10-5 focuses on oral care for the unconscious person but may be adapted for conscious persons who are seriously ill or have mouth problems.

Nursing Process: Oral Hygiene

ASSESSMENT

- Determine the extent of the client's self-care abilities.
- Assess the client's usual mouth care practices.
- Inspect lips, gums, oral mucosa, and tongue for deviations from normal.
- Identify presence of oral problems such as tooth caries, halitosis, gingivitis, or loose or broken teeth.
- Check if the client has bridgework or wears dentures. If the client has dentures, ask if any tenderness or soreness is present and, if so, the location of the area(s) for ongoing assessment.

PLANNING

Delegation

Oral care, brushing and flossing teeth, and denture care can be delegated to UAP. After performing the above assessment, the nurse should instruct the UAP as to the type of oral care and amount of assistance needed by the client. Remind the UAP to report changes in the client's oral mucosa.

IMPLEMENTATION:
TECHNIQUE 10-4 BRUSHING AND FLOSSING THE TEETH

Equipment

Brushing and Flossing
- Towel
- Disposable gloves
- Curved basin (emesis basin)
- Toothbrush
- Cup of tepid water
- Dentifrice (toothpaste)
- Mouthwash
- Dental floss, at least two pieces 20 cm (8 in) in length
- Floss holder (optional)

Cleaning Artificial Dentures
- Disposable gloves
- Tissue or piece of gauze
- Denture container
- Clean washcloth
- Toothbrush or stiff-bristled brush
- Dentifrice or denture cleaner
- Tepid water
- Container of mouthwash

- Curved basin (emesis basin)
- Towel

Preparation

Assemble all the necessary equipment.

Performance

1. Explain to the client what you are going to do, why it is necessary, and how he or she can cooperate.

2. Wash hands and observe other appropriate infection control procedures (e.g., disposable gloves). *Wearing gloves while providing mouth care prevents the nurse from acquiring infections. Gloves also prevent transmission of microorganisms to the client.*

3. Provide for client privacy.

4. Prepare the client.
   - Assist the client to a sitting position in bed, if health permits. If not, assist the client to a side-lying position with the head turned *so liquid may be prevented from draining down the client's throat.*

5. Prepare the equipment.
   - Place the towel under the client's chin.

- Put on gloves.
- Moisten the bristles of the toothbrush with tepid water and apply the dentrifice to the toothbrush.
- Use a soft toothbrush (a small one for a child) and the client's choice of dentrifice.
- For the client who must remain in bed, place or hold the curved basin under the client's chin, fitting the small curve around the chin or neck.
- Inspect the mouth and teeth.

6. Brush the teeth.
- Hand the toothbrush to the client, or brush the client's teeth as follows:
  a. Hold the brush against the teeth with the bristles at a 45-degree angle (Figure 10-8 ◆). The tips of the outer bristles should rest against and penetrate under the gingival sulcus (Figure 10-9 ◆). The brush will clean under the sulcus of two or three teeth at one time. *This sulcular technique removes plaque and cleans under the gingival margins.*
  b. Move the bristles back and forth using a vibrating or jiggling motion from the sulcus to the crowns of the teeth.
  c. Repeat until all outer and inner surfaces of the teeth and sulci of the gums are cleaned.
  d. Clean the biting surfaces by moving the brush back and forth over them in short strokes (Figure 10-10 ◆).
  e. If the tongue is coated, brush it gently with the toothbrush. *Brushing removes accumulated materials and coatings. A coated tongue may be caused by poor oral hygiene and low fluid intake. Brushing gently and carefully helps prevent gagging or vomiting.*

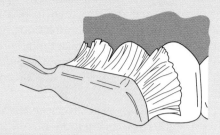

FIGURE 10-9 ◆ Directing the tips of the outer bristles under the gingival margins.

- Hand the client the water cup or mouthwash to rinse the mouth vigorously. Then ask the client to spit the water and excess dentifrice into the basin. Some agencies supply a standard mouthwash. Alternatively, a mouth rinse of normal saline can be an effective cleaner and moisturizer. *Vigorous rinsing loosens food particles and washes out already loosened particles.*
- Repeat the preceding steps until the mouth is free of dentifrice and food particles.
- Remove the curved basin and help the client wipe the mouth.

7. Floss the teeth.
- Assist the client to floss independently, or floss the teeth as follows. Waxed floss is less likely to fray than unwaxed floss; particles between the teeth attach more readily to unwaxed floss than to waxed floss. Some believe that waxed floss leaves a residue on the teeth and that plaque then adheres to the wax.
  a. Wrap one end of the floss around the third finger of each hand (Figure 10-11 ◆).
  b. To floss the upper teeth, use your thumb and index finger to stretch the floss (Figure 10-12 ◆). Move the floss up and down between the teeth from the tops of the crowns to the gum and along the gum lines as far as possible. Make a "C" with the floss around the tooth edge being flossed. Start at the back on the right side and work around to the back of the left side, or work from the center teeth to the back of the jaw on either side.

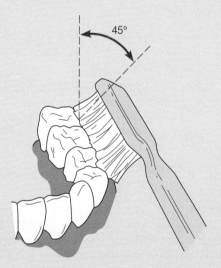

FIGURE 10-8 ◆ The sulcular technique: placing the bristles at a 45-degree angle against the teeth.

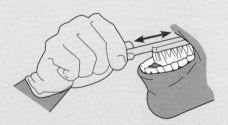

FIGURE 10-10 ◆ Brushing the biting surfaces.

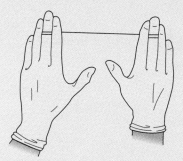

FIGURE 10-11 ◆ Stretching the floss between the third finger of each hand.

c. To floss the lower teeth, use your index fingers to stretch the floss (Figure 10-13 ◆).
- Give the client tepid water or mouthwash to rinse the mouth and a curved basin in which to spit the water.
- Assist the client in wiping the mouth.

8. Remove and dispose of equipment appropriately.
- Remove and clean the curved basin.
- Remove and discard the gloves.

9. **Document** assessment of the teeth, tongue, gums, and oral mucosa. Include any problems such as sores or inflammation and swelling of the gums. Brushing and flossing teeth are not usually recorded.

Variation: Artificial Dentures

1. Remove the dentures.
- Put on gloves. *Wearing gloves protects the nurse and client from infection.*
- If the client cannot remove the dentures, take the tissue or gauze, grasp the upper plate at the front teeth with your thumb and second finger, and move the denture up and down slightly (Figure 10-14 ◆). *The slight movement breaks the suction that holds the plate on the roof of the mouth.*
- Lower the upper plate, move it out of the mouth, and place it in the denture container.
- Lift the lower plate, turning it so that the left side, for example, is slightly lower than the right, to remove the plate from the mouth without stretching the lips. Place the lower plate in the denture container.

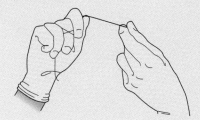

FIGURE 10-12 ◆ Flossing the upper teeth by using the thumbs and index fingers to stretch the floss.

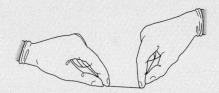

FIGURE 10-13 ◆ Flossing the lower teeth by using the index fingers to stretch the floss.

- Remove a partial denture by exerting equal pressure on the border of each side of the denture, not on the clasps, which can bend or break.

2. Clean the dentures.
- Take the denture container to a sink. Take care not to drop the dentures *as they may break.* Place a washcloth in the bowl of the sink *to prevent damage if the dentures are dropped.*
- Using a toothbrush or special stiff-bristled brush, scrub the dentures with the cleaning agent and tepid water. Hot water is not used *because heat will change the shape of some dentures.*
- Rinse the dentures with tepid running water. *Rinsing removes the cleaning agent and food particles.*
    a. If the dentures are stained, soak them in a commercial cleaner. Be sure to follow the manufacturer's directions. To prevent corrosion, dentures with metal parts should not be soaked overnight.

3. Inspect the dentures and the mouth.
- Observe the dentures for any rough, sharp, or worn areas that could irritate the tongue or mucous membranes of the mouth, lips, and gums.
- Inspect the mouth for any redness, irritated areas, or indications of infection.
- Assess the fit of the dentures. People who have them should see a dentist at least once a year to check the fit and the presence of any irritation to the soft tissues of the mouth. Clients who need repairs to their dentures or new dentures may need a referral for financial assistance.

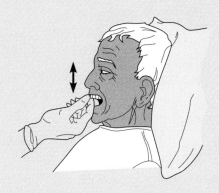

FIGURE 10-14 ◆ Removing the top dentures by first breaking the suction.

4. Return the dentures to the mouth.

  • Offer some mouthwash and a curved basin to rinse the mouth. If the client cannot insert the dentures independently, insert the plates one at a time. Hold each plate at a slight angle while inserting it, to avoid injuring the lips (Figure 10-15 ◆).

5. Assist the client as needed.

  • Wipe the client's hands and mouth with the towel.

  • If the client does not want to or cannot wear the dentures, store them in a denture container with water. Label the cup with the client's name and identification number.

6. Remove and discard gloves.

 7. **Document** all assessments and include any problems such as an irritated area on the mucous membrane.

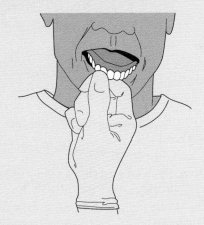

FIGURE 10-15 ◆ Inserting the dentures at a slight angle.

Equipment

• Towel

• Curved basin (emesis basin)

• Disposable gloves

• Bite-block to hold the mouth open and teeth apart (optional)

• Toothbrush

• Cup of tepid water

• Dentifrice or denture cleaner

• Tissue or piece of gauze to remove dentures (optional)

• Denture container as needed

• Mouthwash

• Rubber-tipped bulb syringe

• Suction catheter with suction apparatus (optional)

• Foam swabs and cleaning solution for cleaning the mucous membranes

• Petroleum jelly (Vaseline)

Performance

1. Explain to the client and the family what you are going to do and why it is necessary.

2. Wash hands and observe other appropriate infection control procedures (e.g., disposable gloves).

3. Provide for client privacy.

4. Prepare the client.

  • Position the unconscious client in a side-lying position, with the head of the bed lowered. *In this position, the saliva automatically runs out by gravity rather than being aspirated into the lungs.* This position is the one of choice for the unconscious client receiving mouth care. If the client's head cannot be lowered, turn it to one side. *The fluid will readily run out of the mouth or pool in the side of the mouth, where it can be suctioned.*

  • Place the towel under the client's chin.

  • Place the curved basin against the client's chin and lower cheek to receive the fluid from the mouth (Figure 10-16 ◆).

  • Put on gloves.

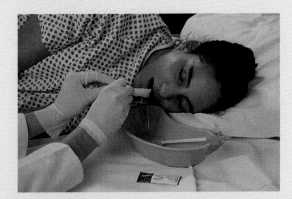

FIGURE 10-16 ◆ Position of client and placement of curved basin when providing special mouth care.

5. Clean the teeth and rinse the mouth.
   - If the person has natural teeth, brush the teeth as described in Technique 10-4. Brush gently and carefully to avoid injuring the gums. If the client has artificial teeth, clean them as described in the variation component of Technique 10-4.
   - Rinse the client's mouth by drawing about 10 mL of water or mouthwash into the syringe and injecting it gently into each side of the mouth. *If the solution is injected with force, some of it may flow down the client's throat and be aspirated into the lungs.*
   - Watch carefully to make sure that all the rinsing solution has run out of the mouth into the basin. If not, suction the fluid from the mouth. See the section on oropharyngeal suctioning in Chapter 21. *Fluid remaining in the mouth may be aspirated into the lungs.*
   - Repeat rinsing until the mouth is free of dentifrice, if used.

6. Inspect and clean the oral tissues.
   - If the tissues appear dry or unclean, clean them with the foam swabs or gauze and cleaning solution following agency policy.
   - Picking up a moistened foam swab, wipe the mucous membrane of one cheek. If no foam swabs are available, wrap a small gauze square around a tongue blade and moisten it. Discard the swab or tongue blade in a waste container, and with a fresh one clean the next area. *Using separate applicators for each area of the mouth prevents the transfer of microorganisms from one area to another.*
   - Clean all the mouth tissues in an orderly progression, using separate applicators: the cheeks, roof of the mouth, base of the mouth, and tongue.
   - Observe the tissues closely for inflammation and dryness.
   - Rinse the client's mouth as described in step 5.
   - Remove and discard gloves.

7. Ensure client comfort.
   - Remove the basin, and dry around the client's mouth with the towel. Replace artificial dentures, if indicated.
   - Lubricate the client's lips with petroleum jelly. *Lubrication prevents cracking and subsequent infection.*

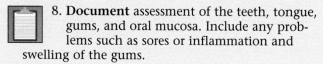 8. **Document** assessment of the teeth, tongue, gums, and oral mucosa. Include any problems such as sores or inflammation and swelling of the gums.

AMBULATORY AND COMMUNITY SETTINGS

Oral Hygiene

- Assess the oral hygiene practices and attitude toward oral hygiene of family members and the client.

- Clients with a nasogastric tube or who are receiving oxygen are likely to develop dry oral mucous membranes, especially if they breathe through their mouth. More frequent oral hygiene will be needed.

AGE-RELATED CONSIDERATIONS

Oral Hygiene

Infant

- Most dentists recommend that dental hygiene should begin when the first tooth erupts and be practiced after each feeding. Cleaning can be accomplished by using a wet washcloth or a cotton ball or small gauze moistened with water.

Child

- Beginning at about 18 months of age, brush the child's teeth with a soft toothbrush. Use only a toothbrush moistened with water. Introduce toothpaste later and use one that contains fluoride.

Elders

- Dryness of the oral mucosa is a common finding in older people because saliva production decreases with age.
- Promoting good oral hygiene can have a positive effect on the older adult's ability to eat.

EVALUATION

- Consider the client's medical diagnosis and treatment (e.g., chemotherapy, oxygen) and the necessary nursing interventions related to oral hygiene.

- Conduct an ongoing assessment, if appropriate, of the oral mucosa, gums, tongue, and lips.
- Report deviations from normal to the physician.
- Conduct appropriate follow-up such as a referral to a dentist for dental caries.

Hair Care

The appearance of the hair often reflects a person's feelings of self-concept and sociocultural well-being. Becoming familiar with hair care needs and practices that may be different than our own is an important aspect of providing competent nursing care to all clients. A person who feels ill may not groom their hair as before. Dirty scalp and hair is itchy, uncomfortable, and can have an odor. The hair may also reflect a state of health (e.g., excessive coarseness and dryness may be associated with endocrine disorders such as hypothyroidism). Box 10-2 lists common hair problems.

Long hair may present a problem for clients confined to bed as it may become matted. It should be combed and brushed at least once a day to prevent this. A brush with stiff bristles provides the best stimulation to blood circulation in the scalp. The bristles, however, should not be so sharp that they injure the client's scalp. A comb with dull, even teeth is advisable. A comb with sharp teeth might injure the scalp; combs that are too fine can pull and break the hair. Some clients are pleased to have their hair tied neatly in the back or braided until other assistance is available or until they feel better and can look after it themselves.

Shampooing the Hair

Hair should be washed as often as needed to keep it clean. There are several ways to shampoo clients' hair, depending on their health, strength, and age. The client who is well enough to take a shower can shampoo while in the shower. The client who is unable to shower may be given a shampoo while sitting on a chair in front of a sink. The back-lying client who can move to a stretcher can be given a shampoo on a stretcher wheeled to a sink. The client who must remain in bed can be given a shampoo with water brought to the bedside.

Shampoo basins to catch the water and direct it to the washbasin or other receptacle are usually made of plastic or metal. A pail or large washbasin can be used as a receptacle for the shampoo water. If possible, the receptacle should be large enough to hold all the shampoo water so that it does not have to be emptied during the shampoo (Figure 10-17 ◆).

Water used for the shampoo should be 40.5°C (105°F) for an adult or child to be comfortable and not injure the scalp. Usually, the client will supply a liquid or cream shampoo. If the shampoo is being given to destroy lice, a medicated shampoo should be used. Dry shampoos are also available. They will remove some of the dirt, odor, and oil. Their main disadvantage is that they dry the hair and scalp.

How often a person needs a shampoo is highly individual, depending to a large degree on the person's activities and the amount of sebum secreted by the scalp. Oily hair tends to look stringy and dirty, and it feels unclean to the person.

Beard and Mustache Care

Beards and mustaches also require daily care. The most important aspect of the care is to keep them clean. Food particles tend to collect in beards and mustaches and they need washing and combing periodically. Clients may also wish a beard or mustache trim to maintain a well-groomed appearance. A beard or mustache should not be shaved off without the client's

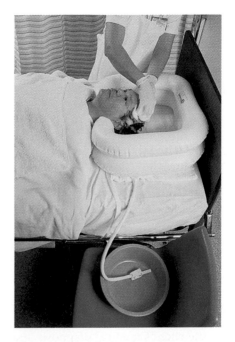

FIGURE 10-17 ◆ Shampooing the hair of a client confined to bed. Note the shampoo basin and the receptacle below.

Box 10-2 *Common Hair Problems*

- **Alopecia** (hair loss)—can be caused by chemotherapeutic agents and radiation of the head.
- **Dandruff**—a diffuse scaling of the scalp. Often accompanied by itching. Can usually be treated effectively with a commercial shampoo.
- **Pediculosis (lice)**—there are three common kinds:
  - *Head lice (Pediculus capitis):* Found on the scalp and tends to stay hidden in the hairs.
  - *Body lice (Pediculus corporis):* Tends to cling to clothing so that when a client undresses, the lice may not be in evidence on the body. These lice suck blood from the person and lay their eggs on the clothing.
  - *Crab lice (Pediculus pubis):* Stays hidden in pubic hair.
- **Hirsutism**—the growth of excessive body hair. The cause of excessive body hair is not always known.

Box 10-3 *Using a Safety Razor to Shave Facial Hair*

- Don gloves in case there are facial nicks and contact with blood.
- Apply shaving cream or soap and water to soften the bristles and make the skin more pliable.
- Hold the skin taut, particularly around creases, to prevent cutting the skin.
- Hold the razor so that the blade is at a 45-degree angle to the skin, and shave in short, firm strokes in the direction of hair growth.

- After shaving the entire area, wipe the client's face with a wet washcloth to remove any remaining shaving cream and hair.
- Dry the face well, then apply aftershave lotion or powder as the client prefers.
- To prevent irritating the skin, pat on the lotion with the fingers and avoid rubbing the face.

From *Fundamentals of nursing: Concepts, process, and practice,* 6th ed., by B. Kozier, G. Erb, A. Berman, & K. Burke, 2000, Upper Saddle River, NJ: Prentice Hall Health.

consent. Male clients often shave or are shaved after a bath. Frequently, clients supply their own electric or safety razors. See Box 10-3 for the steps involved in shaving facial hair with a safety razor.

African American Clients

Dark-skinned people often have thicker, drier, curlier hair than light-skinned people. Very curly hair may stand out from the scalp. Although the shafts of curly or kinky hair look strong and wiry, they have less strength than straight hair shafts and can break easily. Many African American people have hair that is naturally curly, and it can become matted and tangled in just an 8-hour period of time (Jackson, 1998). Cultural groups often have their own vocabulary for describing personal activities. Box 10-4 provides a list of words and hairstyles used by some African American clients to describe their hair.

Some African Americans have their hair straightened. Even if straightened, the hair tends to tangle and mat easily, especially at the back and the sides if

Box 10-4 *Terms Used by Some African American Clients to Describe Hair Condition and Hairstyle*

- *Nappy/kinky:* This means that the hair is very difficult to comb and is very curly, maybe even tangled at the root. The hair "draws" up and appears shorter than it really is because of this extreme curliness. It may have a rough, "steel wool" appearance.
- *Pressed:* The hair is straightened using a hot comb. However, if it gets wet, for example, sweating, high humidity, shampoo, or getting caught in the rain, it reverts back to being kinky.
- *Permanent:* This is a chemical means of straightening the hair. The hair will remain straight for 4 to 6 weeks, even if it gets wet. This is the major advantage of the permanent over using the hot comb.
- *Grease:* Clients may request some grease. They are not asking for vegetable shortening. This is a request to apply either lotion to the skin or hair oil to the scalp.
- *Braids/extensions:* Synthetic hair is braided into the person's real hair. The length is variable, usually shoulder length or longer. If the braids are left hanging, the ends are burned with a small lighter to keep them from unraveling and a small rubber band applied. The braids should be left intact, but care of the scalp is still very important. There are some special products

made especially for those with extensions that can be used to moisturize the hair and scalp. The hair can be shampooed with this style. Some place a stocking cap over the hair. Others just shampoo the hair gently, use a towel to press excess water from the hair, and keep it covered until the hair and scalp are completely dry. If there is a need to remove the synthetic braid extensions, care must be taken not to cut the client's real hair.

- *Dreadlocks:* Made popular by the Rastafarian religion, which reportedly originated in Jamaica. Not everyone who wears dreadlocks is a Rastafarian. Dreadlocks are worn by men, women, and children of all ages. The hair is not combed or picked—ever. Most people keep their locks extremely clean. The locks attract lint. Use tweezers to remove lint that's on top of the hair. With long dreadlocks, removing lint from inside the lock can destroy it. The lint acts as a bonding cement that holds the lock together. Since the hair is shampooed often, this lint is clean. Gently shampoo the hair, taking care not to destroy the locks. Some individuals use a stocking cap, others just gently shampoo the hair. Dreadlocks take a long time to dry when wet. Protect the client from drafts until the hair is dry.

From Jackson, F. (1998). The ABC's of black hair and skin care. *The ABNF Journal,* p. 101. Reprinted with permission.

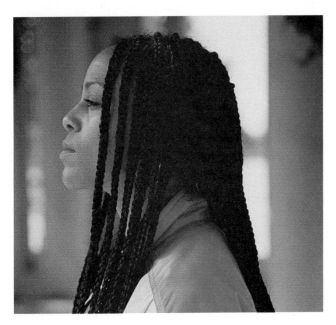

FIGURE 10-18 ◆ An African American's hair styled with braids.

the client is confined to bed. Other African Americans style their hair in small braids (Figure 10-18 ◆). These braids do not have to be unbraided for shampooing and washing. The nurse should obtain the client's permission before any such unbraiding. Some African American clients need to oil their hair daily because it tends to be dry. Oil also prevents the hair strands from breaking and the scalp from becoming too dry. Not all African American individuals have curly or kinky hair. Some have naturally straight hair. Keeping the scalp and hair clean and oiled remains important and necessary. Technique 10-6 describes how to provide hair care for clients.

Nursing Process: Hair Care

ASSESSMENT

Determine:

- History of the following conditions or therapies: recent chemotherapy, hypothyroidism, radiation of the head, unexplained hair loss, and growth of excessive body hair.
- Usual hair care practices and routinely used hair care products (e.g., hair spray, shampoo, conditioners, hair oil preparation, hair dye, curling or straightening preparations).
- Whether wetting the hair will make it difficult to comb. Kinky hair is easier to comb when wet; however, it is very difficult to comb when it dries (Jackson, 1998, p. 102).

Assess:

- Condition of the hair and scalp. Is the hair straight, curly, or kinky? Is the hair matted or tangled? Is the scalp dry?
- Evenness of hair growth over the scalp, in particular, any patchy loss of hair; hair texture, oiliness, thickness, or thinness; presence of lesions, infections, or infestations on the scalp; presence of hirsutism
- Self-care abilities (e.g., any problems managing hair care)

PLANNING

Delegation

Brushing and combing hair, shampooing hair, and shaving facial hair can be delegated to UAP unless the client has a condition in which the procedure would be contraindicated (e.g., cervical spinal injury or trauma). The nurse needs to assess the UAP's knowledge and experience of hair care for an African American client, if appropriate.

IMPLEMENTATION:
TECHNIQUE 10-6 PROVIDING HAIR CARE

Equipment

- Clean brush and comb
- A wide-toothed comb is usually used for many black-skinned people because finer combs pull the hair into knots and may also break the hair.
- Towel
- Hair oil preparation, if appropriate

Performance

1. Explain to the client what you are going to do, why it is necessary, and how he or she can cooperate.

2. Wash hands and observe other appropriate infection control procedures.

3. Provide for client privacy.

4. Position and prepare the client appropriately.

- Assist the client who can sit to move to a chair. *Hair is more easily brushed and combed when the client is in a sitting position.* If health permits, assist a client confined to a bed to a sitting position by raising the head of the bed. Otherwise, assist the client to alternate side-lying positions, and do one side of the head at a time.

- If the client remains in bed, place a clean towel over the pillow and the client's shoulders. Place it over the sitting client's shoulders. *The towel collects any removed hair, dirt, and scaly material.*
- Remove any pins or ribbons in the hair.

5. Remove any mats or tangles gradually.
- Mats can usually be pulled apart with fingers or worked out with repeated brushings.
- If the hair is very tangled, rub alcohol or an oil, such as mineral oil, on the strands to help loosen the tangles.
- Comb out tangles in a small section of hair toward the scalp. Stabilize the hair with one hand and comb towards the ends of the hair with the other hand. *This avoids scalp trauma. Note:* Excessive matting or tangled hair may be infested with lice.

6. Brush and comb the hair.
- For short hair, brush and comb one side at a time. Divide long hair into two sections by parting it down the middle from the front to the back. If the hair is very thick, divide each section into front and back subsections or into several layers.

7. Arrange the hair as neatly and attractively as possible, according to the individual's desires.
- Braiding long hair helps prevent tangles.

 8. **Document** assessments and special nursing interventions. Daily combing and brushing of the hair are not normally recorded.

Variation: Hair Care for African American Clients
- Position and prepare the client.
- Untangle the hair first, if appropriate.
  - Use fingers to reduce hair breakage and discomfort. Move fingers in a circular motion starting at the roots and gently moving up to the tip of the hair.
- Comb the hair.
  - Apply hair oil preparation as the client indicates.
  - Using a large and open-toothed comb, grasp a small section of hair and, holding the hair at the tip, start untangling at the tip and work down toward the scalp (Jackson, 1998, p. 102).

Oil Shampoo
An oil shampoo is composed of one part alcohol and four parts mineral oil. The alcohol is an antiseptic and both the alcohol and mineral oil are cleansing agents (Jackson, 1998, p. 102).
- Warm the mixture.
- Pour it into the hair and gently massage.
- Comb the hair.
- Remove excess oil with a towel.

Oiling the Hair
If a water-based shampoo was used, it may be necessary to oil and massage the scalp.
- Part the hair in sections.
- Place a small amount of hair oil on the scalp. *The hair is so dense that oiling the top of the hair will not help a dry scalp.*
- Ask the client if they would like their hair braided. *Braiding will decrease tangling; however, it is a client's preference.*

AGE-RELATED CONSIDERATIONS

Hair Care

Infant
- Some newborns have hair on their scalp and others are free of hair at birth but grow hair over the scalp during the first year of life.

Child
- In adolescence, the sebaceous glands increase in activity as a result of increased hormone levels. As a result, hair follicle openings enlarge to accommodate the increased amount of sebum, which can make the adolescent's hair more oily.

Elders
- The older person's hair tends to be drier than normal. With age, axillary and pubic hair becomes finer and scanter, in contrast to the eyebrows, which become bristly and coarse. Many women develop hair on their face, which may be a concern to them.

EVALUATION

- Conduct ongoing assessments for problems such as dandruff, alopecia, pediculosis, scalp lesions, or excessive dryness or matting.

- Evaluate effectiveness of medication (e.g. pediculosis), if appropriate.

Foot Care

Foot hygiene is particularly important for clients who have an infection or abrasion. Because of reduced peripheral circulation to the feet, clients with diabetes or peripheral vascular disease are particularly prone to infection if skin breakage occurs. Many foot problems can be prevented by teaching the client simple foot care guidelines (see Box 10-5).

Foot and nail care is often provided during the client's bath but may be provided at any time in the day to accommodate the client's preference or schedule. The frequency of foot care is determined by the nurse and the client and is based on objective assessment data and the client's specific problems. Technique 10-7 describes how to provide foot care.

Nursing Process: Foot Care

ASSESSMENT

Determine:

- History of any problems with foot odor; foot discomfort; foot mobility; circulatory problems (e.g., swelling, changes in skin color and/or temperature, and pain); structural problems (e.g., bunion, hammertoe, or overlapping digits).
- Usual foot care practices (e.g., frequency of washing feet and cutting nails, foot hygiene products used, how often socks are changed, whether the client ever goes barefoot).

Assess:

- Skin surfaces for cleanliness, odor, dryness, and intactness.
- Each foot and toe for shape, size, presence of lesions (e.g., corn, callus, wart, or rash), and areas of tenderness and ankle edema.
- Skin temperatures of the two feet to assess circulatory status and the dorsalis pedis pulses.
- Self-care abilities (e.g., any problems managing foot care).

PLANNING

Delegation

Foot care for the *nondiabetic* client can be delegated to UAP). Remind the UAP to notify the nurse of anything that looks out of the ordinary. Review with the UAP the agency policy about cutting or trimming nails.

BOX 10-5 *Foot Care Guidelines*

- Wash the feet daily, and dry them well, especially between the toes.
- When washing, inspect the skin of the feet for breaks or red or swollen areas. Use a mirror if needed to visualize all areas.
- To prevent burns, check the water temperature before immersing the feet.
- Use creams or lotions to moisten the skin, or soak the feet in warm water with Epsom salts to avoid excessive drying of the skin of the feet. Lotion will also soften calluses. A lotion that reduces dryness effectively is a mixture of lanolin and mineral oil.
- To prevent or control an unpleasant odor due to excessive foot perspiration, wash the feet frequently and change socks and shoes at least daily. Special deodorant sprays or absorbent foot powders are also helpful.
- File the toenails rather than cutting them to avoid skin injury. File the nails straight across the ends of the toes. If the nails are too thick or misshapen to file, consult a podiatrist.
- Wear clean stockings or socks daily. Avoid socks with holes or dams that can cause pressure areas.
- Wear correctly fitting shoes that neither restrict the foot nor rub on any area; rubbing can cause corns and calluses. Check worn shoes for rough spots in the lin-

ing. Break in new shoes gradually by increasing the wearing time 30 to 60 minutes each day.

- Avoid walking barefoot, because injury and infection may result. Wear slippers in public showers and in change areas to avoid contracting athlete's foot or other infections.
- Several times each day exercise the feet to promote circulation. Point the feet upward, point them downward, and move them in circles.
- Avoid wearing constricting garments such as knee-high elastic stockings and avoid sitting with the legs crossed at the knees, which may decrease circulation.
- When the feet are cold, use extra blankets and wear warm socks rather than using heating pads or hot water bottles, which may cause burns. Test bathwater before stepping into it.
- Wash any cut on the foot thoroughly, apply a mild antiseptic, and notify the physician.
- Avoid self-treatment for corns or calluses. Pumice stones and some callus and corn applications are injurious to the skin. Consult a podiatrist or physician first.
- Notify the physician if you notice abnormal sores or drainage, pain, or changes in temperature, color, and sensation of the foot.

From *Fundamentals of nursing: Concepts, process, and practice,* 6th ed., by B. Kozier, G. Erb, A. Berman, & K. Burke, 2000, Upper Saddle River, NJ: Prentice Hall Health.

Equipment

- Washbasin containing warm water
- Pillow
- Moisture-resistant disposable pad
- Towels
- Soap
- Washcloth
- Toenail cleaning and trimming equipment
- Lotion or foot powder

Performance

1. Explain to the client what you are going to do, why it is necessary, and how he or she can cooperate.

2. Wash hands and observe other appropriate infection control procedures.

3. Provide for client privacy.

4. Prepare the equipment and the client.

   - Fill the washbasin with warm water at about 40 to 43°C (105 to 110°F). *Warm water promotes circulation, comforts, and refreshes.*

   - Assist the ambulatory client to a sitting position in a chair, or the bed client to a supine or semi-Fowler's position.

   - Place a pillow under the bed client's knees. *This provides support and prevents muscle fatigue.*

   - Place the washbasin on the moisture-resistant pad at the foot of the bed for a bed client or on the floor in front of the chair for an ambulatory client.

   - For a bed client, pad the rim of the washbasin with a towel. *The towel prevents undue pressure on the skin.*

5. Wash the foot and soak it as required.

   - Place one of the client's feet in the basin and wash it with soap, paying particular attention to the interdigital areas. Prolonged soaking is generally not recommended for diabetic clients or individuals with peripheral vascular disease. *Prolonged soaking may remove natural skin oils, thus drying the skin and making it more susceptible to cracking and injury.*

- Rinse the foot well to remove soap. *Soap irritates the skin if not properly removed.*

- Rub callused areas of the foot with the washcloth. *This helps remove dead skin layers.*

- If the nails are brittle or thick and require trimming, replace the water and allow the foot to soak for 10 to 20 minutes. *Soaking softens the nails and loosens debris under them.*

- Clean the nails as required with an orange stick or the blunt end of a toothpick. *This removes excess debris that harbors microorganisms.*

- Remove the foot from the basin and place it on the towel.

6. Dry the foot thoroughly and apply lotion or foot powder.

   - Blot the foot gently with the towel to dry it thoroughly, particularly between the toes. *Harsh rubbing can damage the skin. Thorough drying reduces the risk of infection.*

   - Apply lotion or lanolin cream. *This lubricates dry skin.*

     or

   - Apply a foot powder containing a nonirritating deodorant if the feet tend to perspire excessively. *Foot powders have greater absorbent properties than regular bath powders; some also contain menthol, which makes the feet feel cool.*

7. If agency policy permits, trim the nails of the first foot while the second foot is soaking.

   - See Box 10-6 for information on the appropriate method to trim nails. Note that in many agencies, toenail trimming requires a physician's order or is contraindicated for clients with diabetes mellitus, toe infections, and peripheral vascular disease, unless performed by a podiatrist or general practice physician.

 8. **Document** any foot problems observed.

   - Foot care is not generally recorded unless problems are noted.

   - Record any signs of inflammation, infection, breaks in the skin, corns, troublesome calluses, bunions, and pressure areas. This is of particular importance for clients with peripheral vascular disease and diabetes.

AMBULATORY AND COMMUNITY SETTINGS

Home Care Assessment for Client Hygiene

- Determine whether caregiver individuals are available and able to assist with bathing, dressing, toileting, nail care, hair shampoo, shopping for hygienic or grooming aids, and so on.

- Assess whether the caregiver needs instruction in how to assist the client in and out of the tub, foot care, and so on.

Home Care Assessment for Client Hygiene (*continued*)

- Assess the effects of the client's illness on financial status, parenting, spousal roles, sexuality, and social roles.

- Explore resources that will provide assistance with bathing, laundry, and foot care (e.g., home health aid, podiatrist).

Box 10-6 *Nail Care*

- To provide nail care, the nurse needs a nail cutter or sharp scissors, a nail file, an orange stick to push back the cuticle, hand lotion or mineral oil to lubricate any dry tissue around the nails, and a basin of water to soak the nails if they are particularly thick or hard.

- One hand or foot is soaked, if needed, and dried. Then, the nail is cut or filed straight across beyond the end of the finger or toe. Avoid trimming or digging into nails at the lateral corners. *This predisposes the client to ingrown toenails.*

- Clients who have diabetes or circulatory problems should have their nails filed rather than cut. *Inadvertent injury to tissues can occur if scissors are used.*

- After the initial cut or filing, the nail is filed to round the corners and the nurse cleans under the nail.

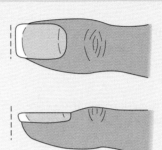

- Gently push back the cuticle, taking care not to injure it.
- The next finger or toe is cared for in the same manner.

EVALUATION

- Inspect nails and skin after the soak.
- Compare to prior assessment data.
- Report any abnormalities to the physician.

Ears

Normal ears require minimal hygiene. Clients who have excessive **cerumen** (earwax) and dependent clients who have **hearing aids** may require assistance from the nurse.

Cleaning the Ears

The auricles of the ear are cleaned during the bed bath. The nurse or client must remove excessive cerumen that is visible or that causes discomfort or hearing difficulty. Visible cerumen may be loosened and removed by retracting the auricle up and back. If this measure is ineffective, irrigation is necessary. Clients need to be advised never to use bobby pins, toothpicks, or cotton-tipped applicators to remove cerumen. Bobby pins and toothpicks can injure the ear canal and rupture the tympanic membrane. Cotton-tipped applicators can cause wax to become impacted within the canal.

Care of Hearing Aids

A hearing aid is a battery-powered, sound-amplifying device used by hearing-impaired persons. It consists of a microphone that picks up sound and converts it to electric energy, an amplifier that magnifies the electric energy electronically, a receiver that converts the amplified energy back to sound energy, and an **earmold** that directs the sound into the ear. See Box 10-7 for a description of several types of hearing aids.

For correct functioning, hearing aids require appropriate handling during insertion and removal, regular cleaning of the earmold, and replacement of dead batteries. With proper care, hearing aids generally last 5 to 10 years. Earmolds generally need readjustment every 2 to 3 years.

Technique 10-8 describes how to remove, clean, and insert a hearing aid.

Nursing Process: Ears

ASSESSMENT

Determine if the client has experienced any problems with the hearing aid and hearing aid practices. Assess for the presence of inflammation, excessive wax, drainage, or discomfort in the external ear.

Box 10-7 *Types of Hearing Aids*

- **Behind-the-ear (BTE or postaural) aid:** This is the most widely used type because it fits snugly behind the ear. The hearing aid case, which holds the microphone, amplifier, and receiver, is attached to the earmold by a plastic tube.
- **In-the-ear (ITE or intra-aural):** This one-piece aid has all its components housed in the earmold.
- **In-the-canal (ITC) aid:** This is the most compact and least visible aid, fitting completely inside the ear canal.

In addition to having cosmetic appeal, the ITC does not interfere with telephone use or the wearing of eyeglasses. However, it is not suitable for clients with progressive hearing loss; it requires adequate ear canal diameter and length for a good fit; and it tends to plug with cerumen more than other aids.

- **Eyeglasses aid:** This is similar to the behind-the-ear aid, but the components are housed in the temple of the eyeglasses. A hearing aid can be in one or both temples of the glasses.
- **Body hearing aid:** This pocket-sized aid, used for more severe hearing losses, clips onto an undergarment, shirt pocket, or harness carrier supplied by the manufacturer. The case, containing the microphone and amplifier, is connected by a cord to the receiver, which snaps into the earpiece.

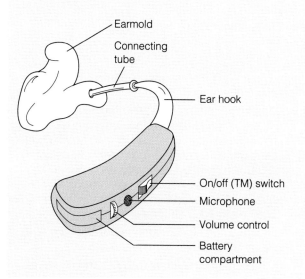

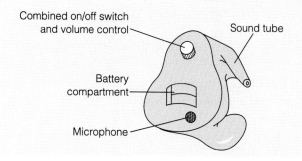

PLANNING

Delegation

A nurse can delegate the task of caring for a hearing aid to UAP. It is important, however, for the nurse to first determine that the UAP knows the correct way to care for a hearing aid. Inform the UAP to report the presence of ear inflammation, discomfort, excess wax, or drainage to the registered nurse.

IMPLEMENTATION:
TECHNIQUE 10-8 REMOVING, CLEANING, AND INSERTING A HEARING AID

Equipment

- Client's hearing aid
- Soap, water, and towels or a damp cloth
- Pipe cleaner or toothpick (optional)
- New battery (if needed)

Performance

1. Explain to the client what you are going to do, why it is necessary, and how he or she can cooperate.

2. Wash hands and observe other appropriate infection control procedures.

3. Provide for client privacy.

4. Remove the hearing aid.
   - Turn the hearing aid off and lower the volume. The on/off switch may be labeled "O" (off), "M" (microphone), "T" (telephone), or "TM" (telephone/microphone). *The batteries continue to run if the hearing aid is not turned off.*
   - Remove the earmold by rotating it slightly forward and pulling it outward.
   - If the hearing aid is not to be used for several days, remove the battery. *Removal prevents corrosion of the hearing aid from battery leakage.*
   - Store the hearing aid in a safe place. Avoid exposure to heat and moisture. *Proper storage prevents loss or damage.*

5. Clean the earmold.

- Detach the earmold if possible. Disconnect the earmold from the receiver of a body hearing aid or from the hearing aid case of behind-the-ear and eyeglasses hearing aids where the tubing meets the hook of the case. Do not remove the earmold if it is glued or secured by a small metal ring. *Removal facilitates cleaning and prevents inadvertent damage to the other parts.*

- If the earmold is detachable, soak it in a mild soapy solution. Rinse and dry it well. Do not use isopropyl alcohol. *Alcohol can damage the hearing aid.*

- If the earmold is not detachable or is for an in-the-ear aid, wipe the earmold with a damp cloth.

- Check that the earmold opening is patent. Blow any excess moisture through the opening or remove debris (e.g., earwax) with a pipe cleaner or toothpick.

- Reattach the earmold if it was detached from the rest of the hearing aid.

6. Insert the hearing aid.

- Determine from the client if the earmold is for the left or the right ear.

- Check that the battery is inserted in the hearing aid. Turn off the hearing aid, and make sure the volume is turned all the way down. *A volume that is too loud is distressing.*

- Inspect the earmold to identify the ear canal portion. Some earmolds are fitted for only the ear canal and concha; others are fitted for all the contours of the ear. The canal portion, common to all, can be used as a guide for correct insertion.

- Line up the parts of the earmold with the corresponding parts of the client's ear.

- Rotate the earmold slightly forward, and insert the ear canal portion.

- Gently press the earmold into the ear while rotating it backward.

- Check that the earmold fits snugly by asking the client if it feels secure and comfortable.

- Adjust the other components of a behind-the-ear or body hearing aid.

- Turn the hearing aid on, and adjust the volume according to the client's needs.

7. Correct problems associated with improper functioning.

- If the sound is weak or there is no sound:

  a. Ensure that the volume is turned high enough.

  b. Ensure that the earmold opening is not clogged.

  c. Check the battery by turning the hearing aid on, turning up the volume, cupping your hand over the earmold, and listening. A constant whistling sound indicates the battery is functioning. If necessary, replace the battery. Be sure that the negative (–) and positive (+) signs on the battery match those where indicated on the hearing aid.

  d. Ensure that the ear canal is not blocked with wax, which can obstruct sound waves.

- If the client reports a whistling sound or squeal after insertion:

  a. Turn the volume down.

  b. Ensure that the earmold is properly attached to the receiver.

  c. Reinsert the earmold.

 8. **Document** pertinent data.

  - The removal and the insertion of a hearing aid are not normally recorded.

- Report and record any problems the client has with the hearing aid.

AMBULATORY AND COMMUNITY SETTINGS

Hearing Aids

- People who need a hearing aid may not wear one because they view the hearing aid as a stigma of old age.

- It is important for the client who just purchased a hearing aid to know that it often takes weeks or even months to adjust to the hearing aid. At first, the sounds will seem shrill as they start hearing high-frequency sounds that had been forgotten. Remind them that it is a hearing aid, not a hearing cure. Encourage them to not give up.

- The client needs to adjust to the hearing aid gradually by increasing the amount of time each day until the aid can be worn for a full day (Anderson, 1998).

- Encourage clients to purchase their hearing aid from a company that has a minimum warranty of a 30-day return policy.

- Emphasize the importance for maintenance of the hearing aid—having it cleaned and checked regularly.

- Speak to the client in a normal conversational tone and observe client behaviors.

- Compare the client's hearing ability to previous assessments.

- Report to the physician any deviations from normal for the client.

Chapter Summary

TERMINOLOGY

afternoon care	early morning care	pediculosis (lice)
alopecia	earmold	peri-care
as-needed (prn) care	effleurage	perineal care
bag bath	hearing aid	self-help bed bath
cerumen	hirsutism	shower
cleaning baths	hour of sleep (HS) care	sulcular technique
complete bed bath	hygiene	therapeutic baths
dandruff	morning care	towel bath
dentifrice	partial (abbreviated) bath	tub bath

FORMING CLINICAL JUDGMENTS

Consider This:

1. An unlicensed assistive person comes to you and informs you that a client "refuses her bath." The UAP tells you that the client has an unpleasant body odor and her hair is oily and matted. What will you do?

2. A client complains of not being able to hear after the cleaning of his hearing aid. What will you do?

RELATED RESEARCH

Blood, I. M. (1997). The hearing aid effect: Challenges for counseling. *The Journal of Rehabilitation, 63*(10), 59–62.

Gauthier, D. M. (1999). The healing potential of back massage. *Online Journal of Knowledge Synthesis for Nursing, 6*(5).

Norwood-Chapman, L., & Burchfield, S. B. (1999). Nursing home personnel knowledge and attitudes about hearing loss and hearing aids. *Gerontology and Geriatrics Education, 20*(2), 37–47.

REFERENCES

Anderson, E. G. (1998). Deafness is a scourge (and you can say that again). *Geriatrics, 53*(8), 65–69.

Dempster, J. (1999). The advantages of the bag bath in resident hygiene care. *Canadian Nursing Home, 10*(2), 15–17.

Feldman, C. B. (1998). Caring for feet: Patients and nurse practitioners working together. *Nurse Practitioner Forum, 9*(2), 87–93.

Foss-Durant, A. M., & McAfee, A. (1997). A comparison of three oral care products commonly used in practice. *Clinical Nursing Research, 6*(1), 90–104.

Freeman, E. M. (1997). International perspectives on bathing. *Journal of Gerontological Nursing, 23*(5), 40–44.

Gauthier, D. M. (1999). The healing potential of back massage. *Online Journal of Knowledge Synthesis for Nursing, 6*(5).

Hayes, J., & Cox, C. (1999). Immediate effects of a five-minute foot massage on patients in critical care. *Intensive and Critical Care Nursing, 15*(2), 77–82.

Hektor, L. M., & Touhy, T. A. (1997). The history of the bath: From art to task? *Journal of Gerontological Nursing, 23*(5), 7–15.

Hoeffer, B, Rader, J., McKenzie, D., Lavelle, M., & Stewart, B. (1997).

References (continued)

Reducing aggressive behavior during bathing cognitively impaired nursing home residents. *Journal of Gerontological Nursing, 23*(5), 16–23.

Jackson, F. (1998). The ABC's of black hair and skin care. *The ABNF Journal, 9*(5), 100–104.

Labyak, S. E., & Metzger, B. L. (1997). The effects of effleurage backrub on the physiological components of relaxation: A meta-analysis. *Nursing Research, 46*(1), 59–62.

McConnell, E. A. (1998). Clinical do's & don'ts. Teaching a patient with diabetes how to protect her feet. *Nursing, 28*(12), 32.

Miller, M. F. (1997). Physically aggressive resident behavior during hygienic care. *Journal of Gerontological Nursing, 23*(5), 24–39.

Nursing Procedures (3rd ed.). (2000). Springhouse, PA: Springhouse Corporation.

Rader, J., Lavelle, M., Hoeffer, B., & McKenzie, D. (1996). Maintaining cleanliness: An individualized approach. *Journal of Gerontological Nursing, 22*(3), 32–38.

Richards, K. C. (1998). Effect of a back massage and relaxation intervention on sleep in critically ill patients. *American Journal of Critical Care, 7*(4), 288–299.

Rowe, M., & Alfred, D. (1999). The effectiveness of slow-stroke massage in diffusing agitated behaviors in individuals with Alzheimer's disease. *Journal of Gerontological Nursing, 25*(6), 22–34.

Skewes, S. (1997). Bathing: It's a tough job! *Journal of Gerontological Nursing, 23*(5), 45–49.

Chapter 11

Bedmaking

Techniques

OBJECTIVES

- Identify safety and comfort measures underlying bedmaking techniques.
- Make a closed and open unoccupied bed, surgical bed, and occupied bed effectively.

Because people are usually confined to bed when ill, often for long periods, the bed becomes an important element in the client's life. A place that is clean, safe, and comfortable contributes to the client's ability to rest and sleep and to a sense of well-being. Basic furniture in a health care facility includes the bed, bedside table, overbed table, one or more chairs, and a storage space for clothing. Most bed units also have a call light, light fixtures, electric outlets, and hygienic equipment in the bedside table.

Hospital Beds

The frame of a hospital bed is divided into three sections. This permits the head and the foot to be elevated separately. Most hospital beds have electric motors to operate the movable joints. The motor is activated by pressing a button or moving a small lever, located either at the side of the bed or on a small panel separate from the bed but attached to it by a cable, which the client can readily use. Common bed positions are shown in Table 11-1.

Hospital beds are usually 66 cm (26 in) high and 0.9 m (3 ft) wide, narrower than the usual bed, so that the nurse can reach the client from either side of the bed without undue stretching. The length is usually 1.9 m (6.5 ft). Some beds can be extended in length to accommodate very tall clients. Long-term facilities for ambulatory clients usually have low beds to facilitate movement in and out of bed. Most hospital beds have "high" and "low" positions that can be adjusted either mechanically or electrically by a button or lever. The high position permits the nurse to reach the client without undue stretching or stooping. The low position allows the client to step easily from the bed to the floor.

Mattresses

Mattresses are usually covered with a water-repellent material that resists soiling and can be cleaned easily. Most mattresses have handles on the sides called lugs by which the mattress can be moved.

Many special mattresses are also used in hospitals to relieve pressure on the body's bony prominences, such as the heels. They are particularly helpful for clients confined to bed for a long time.

Side Rails

Side rails, or safety sides, are used on both hospital beds and stretchers. They are of various shapes and sizes and are usually made of metal. Devices to raise and lower them differ. Often, one or two knobs are pulled to release the side and permit it to be moved. When side rails are being used, it is important that the nurse *never* leave the bedside while the rail is lowered. Some side rails have two positions: up and down. Others have three: high, intermediate, and low. The

down and low positions are employed when a side rail is not needed. With some models, the bed foundations (the mattress and frame supporting it) must be raised before the side rail can be put in the low position; otherwise, the side rail might hit the floor and be damaged. The intermediate position is used when the bed is in the low position and the nurse is present. The up or high side rail position is used when a client is in bed and requires protection from falling. Some agencies have a release form that the client can sign if the use of side rails is refused.

Footboard

A footboard is used to support the immobilized client's foot in a normal right angle to the legs to prevent plantar flexion contractures.

Bed Cradles

A bed cradle, sometimes called an *Anderson frame,* is a device designed to keep the top bedclothes off the feet, legs, and even abdomen of a client. The bedclothes are arranged over the device and may be pinned in place. There are several types of bed cradles. One of the most common is a curved metal rod that fits over the bed. Part of the cradle fits under the mattress and small metal brackets press down on each side of the mattress to keep the cradle in place. The frame of some cradles extends over half of the width of the bed, above one leg.

Intravenous Rods

Intravenous rods (poles, stands, standards), usually made of metal, support intravenous (IV) infusion containers while fluid is being administered to a client. These rods can be freestanding on the floor beside the bed or attached to the hospital bed. Some hospital units have overhead hanging rods on a track for IVs.

Making Beds

Nurses need to be able to prepare hospital beds in different ways for specific purposes. In most instances, beds are made after the client receives certain care and when beds are unoccupied. At times, however, nurses need to make an occupied bed or prepare a bed for a client who is having surgery (an anesthetic, postoperative, or surgical bed). Regardless of what type of bed equipment is available, whether the bed is occupied, or the purpose for which the bed is being prepared, certain guidelines pertain to all bed-making. These are summarized in Box 11-1.

Unoccupied Bed

An **unoccupied bed** can be either closed or open. Generally, the top covers of an **open bed** are folded back (thus the term open bed) to make it easier for a

TABLE 11-1	COMMONLY USED BED POSITIONS	
Postion	**Description**	**Indications for Use**
Flat Foot of bed / Head of bed	Mattress is completely horizontal.	Client sleeping in a variety of bed positions, such as back-lying, side-lying, and prone (face down) To maintain spinal alignment for clients with spinal injuries To assist clients to move and turn in bed Bedmaking by nurse
Fowler's position	Semisitting position in which head of bed is raised to angle of at least 45°. Knees may be flexed or horizontal.	Convenient for eating, reading, visiting, watching TV Relief from lying positions To promote lung expansion for client with respiratory problem To assist a client to a sitting position on the edge of the bed
Semi-Fowler's position	Head of bed is raised only to 30° angle.	Relief from lying position To promote lung expansion
Trendelenburg's position	Head of bed is lowered and the foot raised in a straight incline.	To promote venous circulation in certain clients To provide postural drainage of basal lung lobes
Reverse Trendelenburg's position	Head of bed raised and the foot lowered. Straight tilt in direction opposite to Trendelenburg's position.	To promote stomach emptying and prevent esophageal reflex in client with hiatal hernia

From *Fundamentals of nursing: Concepts, process, and practice*, 6th ed., by B. Kozier, G. Erb, A. Berman, & K. Burke, 2000, Upper Saddle River, NJ: Prentice Hall Health.

client to get in. Open and closed beds are made the same way, except that the top sheet, blanket, and bedspread of a **closed bed** are drawn up to the top of the bed and under the pillows.

Beds are often changed after bed baths. The linen can be collected before the bath. The linen is not usually changed unless it is soiled. Check the policy at each clinical agency. Unfitted sheets, blankets, and

Box 11-1 *Bedmaking Guidelines*

- Wash hands thoroughly after handling a client's bed linen. Linens and equipment that have been soiled with secretions and excretions harbor microorganisms that can be transmitted to others directly or by the nurse's hands or uniform.
- Hold soiled linen away from uniform.
- Linen for one client is *never* (even momentarily) placed on another client's bed.
- Place soiled linen directly in a portable linen hamper or tucked into a pillow case at the end of the bed before it is gathered up for disposal.

- Do not shake soiled linen in the air because shaking can disseminate secretions and excretions and the microorganisms they contain.
- When stripping and making a bed, conserve time and energy by stripping and making up one side as much as possible before working on the other side.
- To avoid unnecessary trips to the linen supply area, gather all linen before starting to strip a bed.

From *Fundamentals of nursing: Concepts, process, and practice*, 6th ed., by B. Kozier, G. Erb, A. Berman, & K. Burke, 2000, Upper Saddle River, NJ: Prentice Hall Health.

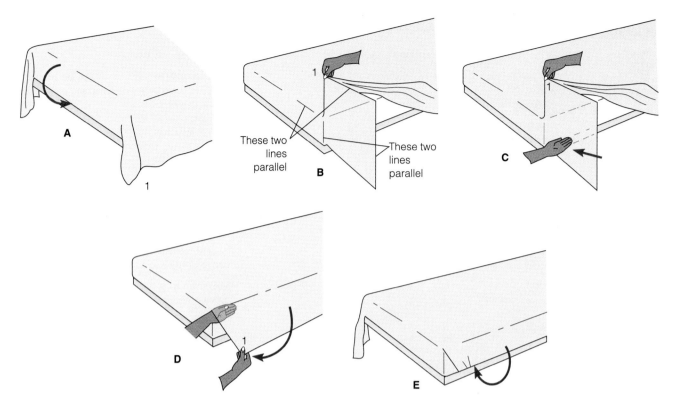

FIGURE 11-1 ◆ Mitering the corner of a bed: (A) Tuck in the bedcover (sheet, blanket, and/or spread) firmly under the mattress at the bottom or top of the bed. (B) Lift the bedcover at point 1 so that it forms a triangle with the side edge of the bed and the edge of the bedcover is parallel to the end of the bed. (C) Tuck the part of the cover that hangs below the mattress under the mattress while holding the cover at point 1 against the mattress. (D) Bring point 1 down toward the floor while the other hand holds the fold of the cover against the side of the mattress. (E) Remove the hand and tuck the remainder of the cover under the mattress, if appropriate. The sides of the top sheet, blanket, and bedspread may be left hanging freely rather than tucked in. The bedspread is mitered separately and left hanging freely if the top sheet and blanket are tucked in.

bedspreads are mitered at the corners of the bed. The purpose of mitering is to secure the bedclothes while the bed is occupied. Figure 11-1 ◆ shows how to miter the corner of a bed. Technique 11-1 explains how to change an unoccupied bed.

Nursing Process: Making Beds

ASSESSMENT

- Assess the client's health status to determine that the person can safely get out of bed. In some hospitals, it is necessary to have a written order if the client has been in bed continuously.

- Assess the client's pulse and respirations if indicated.

- Note all the tubes and equipment connected to the client *as this may influence the need for additional linens or waterproof pads.*

PLANNING

Delegation

Bedmaking is usually delegated to unlicensed assistive personnel (UAP). If appropriate, inform the UAP of the proper disposal method of linens that contain drainage. Ask the UAP to inform you immediately if any tubes or dressings become dislodged or removed. Stress the importance of the call light's being readily available while the client is out of bed.

IMPLEMENTATION:
TECHNIQUE 11-1 CHANGING AN UNOCCUPIED BED

Equipment
- Two flat sheets or one fitted and one flat sheet

- Cloth drawsheet (optional)
- One blanket

- One bedspread
- Waterproof drawsheet or waterproof pads (optional)
- Pillowcase(s) for the head pillow(s)
- Plastic laundry bag or portable linen hamper, if available

Preparation

Determine what linens the client may already have in the room *to avoid a stockpiling of unnecessary extra linens.*

Performance

1. Explain to the client what you are going to do, why it is necessary, and how he or she can cooperate.

2. Wash hands and observe other appropriate infection control procedures.

3. Provide for client privacy.

4. Place the fresh linen on the client's chair or overbed table; do not use another client's bed. *This prevents* **cross-contamination** *(the movement of microorganisms from one client to another) via soiled linen.*

5. Assess and assist the client out of bed.
   - Make sure that this is an appropriate and convenient time for the client to be out of bed.
   - Assist the client to a comfortable chair.

6. Strip the bed.
   - Check bed linens for any items belonging to the client, and detach the call bell or any drainage tubes from the bed linen.
   - Loosen all bedding systematically, starting at the head of the bed on the far side and moving around the bed up to the head of the bed on the near side. *Moving around the bed systematically prevents stretching and reaching and possible muscle strain.*
   - Remove the pillowcases, if soiled, and place the pillows on the bedside chair near the foot of the bed.
   - Fold reusable linens, such as the bedspread and top sheet on the bed, into fourths. First, fold the linen in half by bringing the top edge even with the bottom edge, and then grasp it at the center of the middle fold and bottom edges (Figure 11-2 ◆). *Folding linens saves time and energy when reapplying the linens on the bed.*
   - Remove the waterproof pad and discard it if soiled.
   - Roll all soiled linen inside the bottom sheet, hold it away from your uniform, and place it directly in the linen hamper. *These actions are essential to prevent the transmission of microorganisms to the nurse and others.*
   - Grasp the mattress securely, using the lugs if

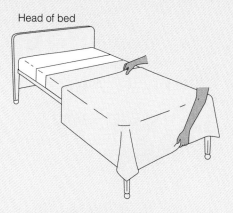

Head of bed

FIGURE 11-2 ◆ **Folding reusable linens.**

present, and move the mattress up to the head of the bed.

7. Apply the bottom sheet and drawsheet.
   - Place the folded bottom sheet with its center fold on the center of the bed. Make sure the sheet is hem side down for a smooth foundation. Spread the sheet out over the mattress, and allow a sufficient amount of sheet at the top to tuck under the mattress. *The top of the sheet needs to be well tucked under to remain securely in place, especially when the head of the bed is elevated.* Place the sheet along the edge of the mattress at the foot of the bed and do not tuck it in (unless it is a contour or fitted sheet).
   - Miter the sheet at the top corner on the near side (see Figure 11-1) and tuck the sheet under the mattress, working from the head of the bed to the foot.
   - If a waterproof drawsheet is used, place it over the bottom sheet so that the center fold is at the center line of the bed and the top and bottom edges extend from the middle of the client's back to the area of the midthigh or knee. Fanfold the uppermost half of the folded drawsheet at the center or far edge of the bed and tuck in the near edge.
   - Lay the cloth drawsheet over the waterproof sheet in the same manner.
   - *Optional:* Before moving to the other side of the bed, place the top linens on the bed hem side up, unfold them, tuck them in, and **miter** the bottom corners. *Completing the entire side of the bed saves time and energy.*

8. Move to the other side and secure the bottom linens.
   - Tuck in the bottom sheet under the head of the mattress, pull the sheet firmly, and miter the corner of the sheet.
   - Pull the remainder of the sheet firmly so that there are no wrinkles. *Wrinkles can cause discomfort for the client. Tuck the sheet in at the side.*
   - Complete this same process for the drawsheet(s).

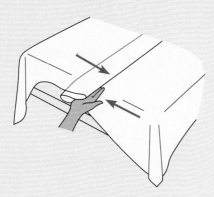

FIGURE 11-3 ◆ A vertical toe pleat.

9. Apply or complete the top sheet, blanket, and spread.

- Place the top sheet, hem side up, on the bed so that its center fold is at the center of the bed and the top edge is even with the top edge of the mattress.
- Unfold the sheet over the bed.
- *Optional:* Make a vertical or a horizontal **toe pleat** in the sheet to provide additional room for the client's feet.
  - a. *Vertical toe pleat:* Make a fold in the sheet 5 to 10 cm (2 to 4 in) perpendicular to the foot of the bed (Figure 11-3 ◆).
  - b. *Horizontal toe pleat:* Make a fold in the sheet 5 to 10 cm (2 to 4 in) across the bed near the foot (Figure 11-4 ◆). Loosening the top covers around the feet after the client is in bed is another way to provide additional space.
- Follow the same procedure for the blanket and the spread, but place the top edges about 15 cm (6 in) from the head of the bed to allow a cuff of sheet to be folded over them.
- Tuck in the sheet, blanket, and spread at the foot of the bed, and miter the corner, using all three layers of linen. Leave the sides of the top

sheet, blanket, and spread hanging freely unless toe pleats were provided.
- Fold the top of the top sheet down over the spread, providing a cuff. *The cuff of sheet makes it easier for the client to pull the covers up.*
- Move to the other side of the bed and secure the top bedding in the same manner.

10. Put clean pillowcases on the pillows as required.

- Grasp the closed end of the pillowcase at the center with one hand.
- Gather up the sides of the pillowcase and place them over the hand grasping the case. Then grasp the center of one short side of the pillow through the pillowcase (Figure 11-5 ◆).
- With the free hand, pull the pillowcase over the pillow.
- Adjust the pillowcase so that the pillow fits into the corners of the case and the seams are straight. *A smoothly fitting pillowcase is more comfortable than a wrinkled one.*
- Place the pillows appropriately at the head of the bed.

11. Provide for client comfort and safety.

- Attach the signal cord so that the client can conveniently use it. Some cords have clamps that attach to the sheet or pillowcase. Others are attached by a safety pin.
- If the bed is currently being used by a client, either fold back the top covers at one side or fanfold them down to the center of the bed. *This makes it easier for the client to get into the bed.*
- Place the bedside table and the overbed table so that they are available to the client.
- Leave the bed in the high position if the client is returning by stretcher, or place in the low position if the client is returning to bed after being up.

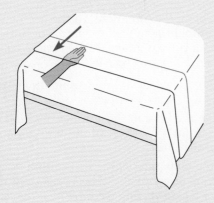

FIGURE 11-4 ◆ A horizontal toe pleat.

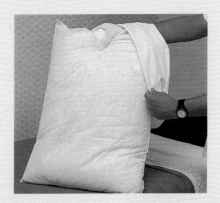

FIGURE 11-5 ◆ Method for putting a clean pillowcase on a pillow.

12. **Document** and report pertinent data.
   - Bedmaking is not normally recorded.
   - Record any nursing assessments, such as the client's physical status and pulse and respiratory rates before and after being out of bed, as indicated.

Variation: Surgical Bed

While the client is in the operating room, the client's bed is prepared for the postoperative phase. In some agencies, the client is brought back to the unit on a stretcher and transferred to the bed in the room. In other agencies, the client's bed is brought to the surgery suite and the client is transferred there. In the latter situation, the bed needs to be made with clean linens as soon as the client goes to surgery so that it can be taken to the operating room when needed.

- Strip the bed.
- Place and leave the pillows on the bedside chair. *Pillows are left on a chair to facilitate transferring the client into the bed.*
- Apply the bottom linens as for an unoccupied bed. Place a bath blanket on the foundation of the bed

if this is agency practice. *A flannel bath blanket provides additional warmth.*

- Place the top covers (sheet, blanket, and bedspread) on the bed as you would for an unoccupied bed. Do not tuck them in, miter the corners, or make a toe pleat.
- Make a cuff at the top of the bed as you would for an unoccupied bed. Fold the top linens up from the bottom.
- On the side of the bed where the client will be transferred, fold up the two outer corners of the top linens so they meet in the middle of the bed, forming a triangle (Figure 11-6 ◆).
- Pick up the apex of the triangle and fanfold the top linens lengthwise to the other side of the bed *to facilitate the client's transfer into the bed* (Figure 11-7 ◆).
- Leave the bed in high position with the side rails down. *The high position facilitates the transfer of the client.*
- Lock the wheels of the bed if the bed is not to be moved. *Locking the wheels keeps the bed from rolling when the client is transferred from the stretcher to the bed.*

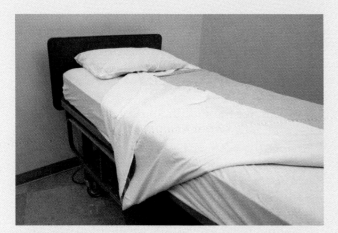

FIGURE 11-6 ◆ Fold up the two outer corners of the top linens forming a triangle.

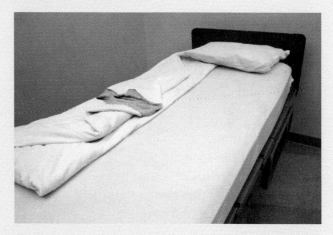

FIGURE 11-7 ◆ Surgical bed. The linens are horizontally fanfolded to the other side of the bed to facilitate transfer of the client into the bed.

EVALUATION

- Make sure the call light is accessible to the client.
- Relate client parameters of activity (e.g., pulse and respirations) to previous assessment data particularly if the client has been on bedrest for an extended period of time or it is the first time that the client is getting out of bed after surgery.

Occupied Bed

Some clients may be too weak to get out of bed. Either the nature of their illness may contraindicate their sitting out of bed or they may be restricted in bed by the

presence of traction or other therapies. When changing an **occupied bed**, the nurse works quickly and disturbs the client as little as possible to conserve the client's energy. See Box 11-2 for guidelines.

Nursing Process: Occupied Beds

ASSESSMENT

- Note specific orders or precautions for moving and positioning the client.
- Determine presence of incontinence or excessive drainage from other sources indicating the need for protective waterproof pads.

BOX 11-2 *Guidelines for Changing an Occupied Bed*

- Maintain the client in good body alignment. Never move or position a client in a manner that is contraindicated by the client's health. Obtain help if necessary to ensure safety.
- Move the client gently and smoothly. Rough handling can cause the client discomfort and abrade the skin.

- Explain what you plan to do throughout the procedure before you do it. Use terms that the client can understand.
- Use the bedmaking time, like the bed bath time, to assess and meet the client's needs.

- Assess skin condition and need for special mattress (e.g., egg crate), footboard, or heel protectors.

PLANNING

Delegation

Bedmaking is usually delegated to UAP. Inform the UAP to what extent the client can assist or if another person will be needed to assist the UAP. Instruct the UAP about the handling of any dressings and/or tubes of the client and also the need for special equipment (e.g., footboard, heel protectors), if appropriate.

IMPLEMENTATION:
TECHNIQUE 11-2 CHANGING AN OCCUPIED BED

Equipment

- Two flat sheets or one fitted and one flat sheet
- Cloth drawsheet (optional)
- One blanket
- One bedspread
- Waterproof drawsheet or waterproof pads (optional)
- Pillowcase(s) for the head pillow(s)
- Plastic laundry bag or portable linen hamper, if available

Performance

1. Explain to the client what you are going to do, why it is necessary, and how he or she can cooperate.

2. Wash hands and observe other appropriate infection control procedures. Put on disposable gloves if linen is soiled with body fluids.

3. Provide for client privacy.

4. Remove the top bedding.
   - Remove any equipment attached to the bed linen, such as a signal light.
   - Loosen all the top linen at the foot of the bed, and remove the spread and the blanket.
   - Leave the top sheet over the client (the top sheet can remain over the client if it is being changed and if it will provide sufficient warmth), or replace it with a bath blanket as follows:
     a. Spread the bath blanket over the top sheet.
     b. Ask the client to hold the top edge of the blanket.
     c. Reaching under the blanket from the side, grasp the top edge of the sheet and draw it down to the foot of the bed, leaving the blanket in place.
     d. Remove the sheet from the bed and place it in the soiled linen hamper.

5. Change the bottom sheet and drawsheet.
   - Assist the client to turn on the side facing away from the side where the clean linen is.
   - Raise the side rail nearest the client. *This protects the client from falling.* If there is no side rail, have another nurse support the client at the edge of the bed.
   - Loosen the foundation of the linen on the side of the bed near the linen supply.
   - Fanfold the drawsheet and the bottom sheet at the center of the bed (Figure 11-8 ◆), as close to the client as possible. *Doing this leaves the near half of the bed free to be changed.*
   - Place the new bottom sheet on the bed, and vertically fanfold the half to be used on the far side of the bed as close to the client as possible. Tuck the sheet under the near half of the bed and miter the corner if a contour sheet is not being used.
   - Place the clean drawsheet on the bed with the center fold at the center of the bed. Fanfold the uppermost half vertically at the center of the bed and tuck the near side edge under the side of the mattress.
   - Assist the client to roll over toward you onto the clean side of the bed. The client rolls over the fanfolded linen at the center of the bed.

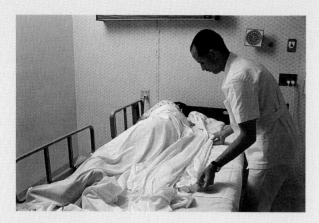

FIGURE 11-8 ◆ Fanfold soiled linen as close to the client as possible.

- Move the pillows to the clean side for the client's use. Raise the side rail before leaving the side of the bed.
- Move to the other side of the bed and lower the side rail.
- Remove the used linen and place it in the portable hamper.
- Unfold the fanfolded bottom sheet from the center of the bed.
- Facing the side of the bed, use both hands to pull the bottom sheet so that it is smooth and tuck the excess under the side of the mattress.
- Unfold the drawsheet fanfolded at the center of the bed and pull it tightly with both hands. Pull the sheet in three sections: (1) face the side of the bed to pull the middle section; (2) face the far top corner to pull the bottom section; and (3) face the far bottom corner to pull the top section.
- Tuck the excess drawsheet under the side of the mattress.

6. Reposition the client in the center of the bed.
- Reposition the pillows at the center of the bed.
- Assist the client to the center of the bed. Determine what position the client requires or prefers and assist the client to that position.

7. Apply or complete the top bedding.
- Spread the top sheet over the client and either ask the client to hold the top edge of the sheet or tuck it under the shoulders. The sheet should remain over the client when the bath blanket or used sheet is removed.
- Complete the top of the bed.

8. Ensure continued safety of the client.
- Raise the side rails. Place the bed in the low position before leaving the bedside.
- Attach the signal cord to the bed linen within the client's reach.
- Put items used by the client within easy reach.

 9. Bedmaking is not normally recorded.

AMBULATORY AND COMMUNITY SETTINGS

Bedmaking

- If the client needs to remain in bed, determine the caregiver's knowledge and experience with making an occupied bed. The nurse may need to demonstrate how to change the linen. Emphasize safety for the client and use of correct body mechanics for the caregiver.
- Assess and discuss with the caregiver the following: need for linens (e.g., incontinence, drainage), available linen supply, and laundry accommodations.

AGE-RELATED CONSIDERATIONS

Bedmaking
Child

- Check if the child has a favorite blanket and if it was brought from home. If so, make sure to replace it on the bed after changing the bed linens.

Elders

- Because of the older adult's thin, tender, and fragile skin, be sure to check that the linens are dry and free of wrinkles and be especially careful when pulling linens underneath the older client.

EVALUATION

Conduct appropriate follow-up, such as determining client's comfort and safety, patency of all drainage tubes and client's access to call light to summon help when needed.

Chapter Summary

TERMINOLOGY

closed bed

cross-contamination

Fowler's position

miter

occupied bed

open bed

reverse Trendelenburg's position

semi-Fowler's position

surgical bed

toe pleat

Trendelenburg's position

unoccupied bed

FORMING CLINICAL JUDGMENTS

Consider This:

1. What should you do if the UAP complains of back discomfort during or after making a bed?

REFERENCES

Elkin, M. K., Perry, A. G., & Potter, P. A. (2000). *Nursing Interventions & Clinical Skills* (2nd ed.). St. Louis: Mosby.

Nursing Procedures (3rd ed.). (2000). Springhouse, PA: Springhouse Corp.

Smith, S. F., Duell, D. J., & Martin, B. C. (2000). *Clinical Nursing Skills Basic to Advanced Skills.* New Jersey: Prentice Hall Health.

Chapter 12

Infection Control

Techniques

OBJECTIVES

- Describe six links in the chain of infection.
- Establish and maintain a sterile field.
- Apply and remove sterile gloves.
- Compare and contrast category-specific, disease-specific, universal, standard, transmission-based, and body substance isolation precaution systems.
- Correctly implement practices appropriate for caring for a client with an infection, including bagging articles and managing equipment used for isolation clients.

Chain of Infection

Six links make up the chain of infection: the **etiologic agent**, or microorganism; the place where the organism naturally resides (**reservoir**); a **portal of exit** from the reservoir; a method (**mode**) of transmission; a **portal of entry** into a host; and the susceptibility of the host (see Figure 12-1 ◆). The goal of infection control measures is to break the chain whenever and wherever possible so that disease is not transmitted from one person to another.

Method of Transmission

After a microorganism leaves its source or reservoir (see Table 12-1), it requires a means of transmission to reach another person or host through a receptive portal of entry. There are three mechanisms:

1. **Direct transmission.** Direct transmission involves immediate and direct transfer of microorganisms from person to person through touching, biting, kissing, or sexual intercourse. Droplet spread is also a form of direct contact but can occur only if the persons are within 3 feet of each other. Sneezing, coughing, spitting, singing, or talking can project droplet spray into the conjunctiva or onto the mucous membranes of the eye, nose, or mouth of another person.

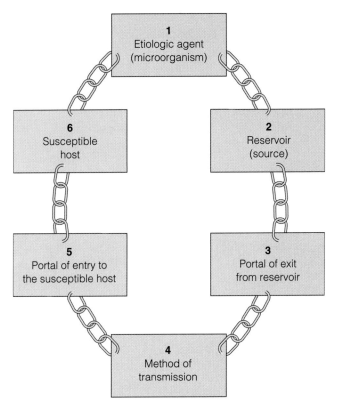

FIGURE 12-1 ◆ The chain of infection.

TABLE 12-1	HUMAN RESERVOIRS, COMMON INFECTIOUS ORGANISMS, AND PORTALS OF EXIT	
Body Area (Source)	**Common Infectious Organisms**	**Portals of Exit**
Respiratory tract	Parainfluenza virus Mycobacterium tuberculosis Staphylococcus aureus	Nose or mouth through sneezing, coughing, breathing, or talking; endotracheal tubes or tracheostomies
Gastrointestinal tract	Hepatitis A virus Salmonella species	Mouth: saliva, vomitus; anus: feces; ostomies; drainage tubes (e.g., nasogastric or T-tubes)
Urinary tract	Escherichia coli enterococci Pseudomonas aeruginosa	Urethral meatus and urinary diversion ostomies
Reproductive tract (including genitals)	Neisseria gonorrhoeae Treponema pallidum Herpes simplex virus type 2 Hepatitis B virus	Vagina: vaginal discharge; urinary meatus: semen, urine
Blood	Hepatitis B virus Human immunodeficiency virus (HIV) Staphylococcus aureus Staphylococcus epidermidis	Open wound, needle puncture site, any disruption of intact skin or mucous membrane surfaces
Tissue	Staphylococcus aureus Escherichia coli Proteus species Streptococcus beta-hemolytic A or B	Drainage from cut or wound

From *Fundamentals of nursing: Concepts, process, and practice,* 6th ed., by B. Kozier, G. Erb, A. Berman, & K. Burke, 2000, Upper Saddle River, NJ: Prentice Hall Health.

2. **Indirect transmission.** Indirect transmission may be either vehicle-borne or vector-borne.

    a. **Vehicle-borne transmission.** A vehicle is any substance that serves as an intermediate means to transport and introduce an infectious agent into a susceptible host through a suitable portal of entry. **Fomites** (inanimate materials or objects), such as handkerchiefs, toys, soiled clothes, cooking or eating utensils, and surgical instruments or dressings, can act as vehicles. For example, an intravenous needle can be a vehicle for transmission of microorganisms from the reservoir to the host. Water, food, milk, blood, serum, and plasma are other vehicles. For example, a food handler who transports the hepatitis A virus may contaminate food or water. A susceptible host then ingests the food.

    b. **Vector-borne transmission.** A vector is an animal or flying or crawling insect that serves as an intermediate means of transporting the infectious agent. Transmission may occur by injecting salivary fluid during biting or by depositing feces or other materials on the skin through the bite wound or a traumatized skin area.

3. **Airborne transmission.** Airborne transmission occurs when droplet nuclei (residue of evaporated droplets that may remain in the air for long periods of time) emitted by an infected host (e.g., one with tuberculosis) or dust particles containing the infectious agent (e.g., *Clostridium difficile* spores from the soil) are transmitted by air currents to a suitable portal of entry, usually the respiratory tract, of another person.

Breaking the Chain of Infection

Various practices break the chain of infection or interrupt the infectious disease process (see Table 12-2). For example, the etiologic agent is interrupted by the use of **antiseptics** (agents that inhibit the growth of some microorganisms) and **disinfectants** (agents that destroy microorganisms other than **spores**), and by sterilization. The aim of most hospital precautions is breaking the chain during the mode of transmission phase of the cycle.

Reducing Risks for Infection

Planned nursing strategies to reduce the risk of transmission of organisms from one person to another

TABLE 12-2	NURSING INTERVENTIONS THAT BREAK THE CHAIN OF INFECTION	
Link	**Interventions**	**Rationale**
Etiologic agent (microorganism)	Ensure that articles are correctly cleaned and disinfected or sterilized before use.	Correct cleaning, disinfecting, and sterilizing reduce or eliminate microorganisms.
	Educate clients and support persons about appropriate methods to clean, disinfect, and sterilize articles.	Knowledge of ways to reduce or eliminate microorganisms reduces the numbers of microorganisms present and the likelihood of transmission.
Reservoir (source)	Change dressings and bandages when they are soiled or wet.	Moist dressings are ideal environments for microorganisms to grow and multiply.
	Assist clients to carry out appropriate skin and oral hygiene.	Hygienic measures reduce the numbers of resident and transient microorganisms and the likelihood of infection.
	Dispose of damp, soiled linens appropriately.	Damp, soiled linens harbor more microorganisms than dry linens.
	Dispose of feces and urine in appropriate receptacles.	Urine and feces in particular contain many microorganisms. Feces may also be the source of certain microorganisms, such as the hepatitis A virus in asymptomatic carriers.
	Ensure that all fluid containers, such as bedside water jugs and suction and drainage bottles, are covered or capped.	Prolonged exposure increases the risk of contamination and promotes microbial growth.
	Empty suction and drainage bottles at the end of each shift or before they become full, or according to agency policy.	Drainage harbors microorganisms, that, if left for long periods, proliferate and can be transmitted to others.
Portal of exit from the reservoir	Avoid talking, coughing, or sneezing over open wounds or sterile fields, and cover the mouth and nose when coughing and sneezing.	These measures limit the number of microorganisms that escape from the respiratory tract.

TABLE 12-2

NURSING INTERVENTIONS THAT BREAK THE CHAIN OF INFECTION (continued)

Link	Interventions	Rationale
Method of transmission	Wash hands between client contacts, after touching body substances, and before performing invasive procedures or touching open wounds. Instruct clients and support persons to wash hands before handling food or eating, after eliminating, and after touching infectious material.	Handwashing is an important means of controlling and preventing the transmission of microorganisms.
	Place discarded soiled materials in moistureproof refuse bags.	Moistureproof bags prevent the spread of microorganisms to others.
	Hold used bedpans steadily to prevent spillage, and dispose of urine and feces in appropriate receptacles.	Feces in particular contain many microorganisms.
	Initiate and implement aseptic precautions for all clients.	All clients may harbor potentially infectious microorganisms that can be transmitted to others.
	Wear masks and eye protection when in close contact with clients who have infections transmitted by droplets from the respiratory tract.	Masks and eyewear reduce the spread of droplet-transmitted microorganisms.
	Wear gloves when handling secretions and excretions. Wear gowns if there is danger of soiling clothing with body substances.	Gloves and gowns prevent soiling of the hands and clothing.
	Wear masks and eye protection when sprays of body fluid are possible (e.g., during irrigation procedures).	Masks and eye protection provide protection from microorganisms in clients' body substances.
Portal of entry to the susceptible host	Use sterile technique (see pp. 303–307) for invasive procedures (e.g., injections, catheterizations).	Invasive procedures penetrate the body's natural protective barriers to microorganisms.
	Use sterile technique when exposing open wounds or handling dressings.	Open wounds are vulnerable to microbial infection.
	Place used disposable needles and syringes in puncture-resistant containers for disposal.	Injuries from needles contaminated by blood or body fluids from an infected client or carrier are a primary cause of hepatitis B virus (HBV) and human immunodeficiency virus (HIV) transmission to health care workers.
Susceptible host	Provide all clients with their own personal care items.	People have less resistance to another person's microorganisms than to their own.
	Maintain the integrity of the client's skin and mucous membranes.	Intact skin and mucous membranes protect against invasion by microorganisms.
	Ensure that the client receives a balanced diet.	A balanced diet supplies proteins and vitamins necessary to build or maintain body tissues.
	Educate the public about the importance of immunizations.	Immunizations protect people against virulent infectious diseases.

From *Fundamentals of nursing: Concepts, process, and practice*, 6th ed., by B. Kozier, G. Erb, A. Berman, & K. Burke, 2000, Upper Saddle River, NJ: Prentice Hall Health.

include the use of meticulous asepsis. **Asepsis** is the freedom from infection or infectious material. There are two basic types of asepsis: medical and surgical. **Medical asepsis** includes all practices intended to confine a specific microorganism to a specific area, limiting the number, growth, and spread of microorganisms. **Surgical asepsis**, or sterile technique, refers to those practices that keep an area or objects free of all microorganisms; it includes practices that destroy all microorganisms.

Maintaining Surgical Asepsis

An object is sterile only when it is free of all microorganisms. It is well known that surgical asepsis is practiced in operating rooms and special diagnostic areas. Surgical asepsis is also employed for many procedures in general care areas (such as administering injections, changing wound dressings, performing urinary catheterizations, and administering intravenous therapy). In these situations, all of the principles of surgical asepsis are applied as in the operating or delivery room; however, not all of the sterile techniques that follow are always required. For example, before an operating room procedure, the nurse generally puts on a mask and cap, performs a surgical hand scrub, and then dons a sterile gown and gloves. In a general care area, the nurse may only perform a handwash and don sterile gloves. The nine basic principles of surgical asepsis and practices that relate to each principle appear in Table 12-3.

TABLE 12-3	PRINCIPLES AND PRACTICES OF SURGICAL ASEPSIS
Principles	**Practices**
All objects used in a sterile field must be sterile.	All articles are sterilized appropriately by dry or moist heat, chemicals, or radiation before use.
	Sterile articles can be stored for only a prescribed time; after that, they are considered unsterile.
	Always check a package containing a sterile object for intactness, dryness, and expiration date. Any package that appears already open, torn, punctured, or wet is considered unsterile. Never assume an item is sterile.
	Storage areas should be clean, dry, off the floor, and away from sinks.
	Always check the sterilization dates and periods on the labels of wrapped items before use.
	Always check chemical indicators of sterilization before using a package. The indicator is often a tape used to fasten the package or contained inside the package. The indicator changes color during sterilization, indicating that the contents have undergone a sterilization procedure. If the color change is not evident, the package is considered unsterile. Commercially prepared sterile packages may not have indicators but are marked with the word *sterile*.
Sterile objects become unsterile when touched by unsterile objects.	Handle sterile objects that will touch open wounds or enter body cavities only with sterile forceps or sterile gloved hands.
	Discard or resterilize objects that come into contact with unsterile objects.
	Whenever the sterility of an object is questionable, assume the article is unsterile.
Sterile items that are out of vision or below the waist level of the nurse are considered unsterile.	Once left unattended, a sterile field is considered unsterile.
	Sterile objects are always kept in view. Nurses do not turn their backs on a sterile field.
	Only the front part of a sterile gown (from the waist to the shoulder) and 2 inches above the elbows to the cuff of the sleeves are considered sterile.
	Always keep sterile gloved hands in sight and above waist level; touch only objects that are sterile.
	Sterile draped tables in the operating room or elsewhere are considered sterile only at surface level.
	Once a sterile field becomes unsterile, it must be set up again before proceeding.
Sterile objects can become unsterile by prolonged exposure to airborne microorganisms.	Keep doors closed and traffic to a minimum in areas where a sterile procedure is being performed, because moving air can carry dust and microorganisms.
	Keep areas in which sterile procedures are carried out as clean as possible by frequent damp cleaning with detergent germicides to minimize contaminants in the area.
	Keep hair clean and short or enclose it in a net to prevent hair from falling on sterile objects. Microorganisms on the hair can make a sterile field unsterile.
	Wear surgical caps in operating rooms, delivery rooms, and burn units.
	Refrain from sneezing or coughing over a sterile field. This can make it unsterile because droplets containing microorganisms from the respiratory tract can travel 1 m (3 ft). Some nurses recommend that masks covering the mouth and the nose should be worn by anyone working over a sterile field or an open wound.
	Nurses with mild upper respiratory tract infections refrain from carrying out sterile procedures or wear masks.

TABLE 12-3   PRINCIPLES AND PRACTICES OF SURGICAL ASEPSIS (continued)

Principles	Practices
	When working over a sterile field, keep talking to a minimum. Avert the head from the field if talking is necessary.
	To prevent microorganisms from falling over a sterile field, refrain from reaching over a sterile field unless sterile gloves are worn and refrain from moving unsterile objects over a sterile field.
Fluids flow in the direction of gravity.	Unless gloves are worn, always hold wet forceps with the tips below the handles. When the tips are held higher than the handles, fluid can flow onto the handle and become contaminated by the hands. When the forceps are again pointed downward, the fluid flows back down and contaminates the tips.
	During a surgical handwash, hold the hands higher than the elbows to prevent contaminants from the forearms from reaching the hands.
Moisture that passes through a sterile object draws microorganisms from unsterile surfaces above or below to the sterile surface by capillary action.	Sterile moistureproof barriers are used beneath sterile objects. Liquids (sterile saline or antiseptics) are frequently poured into containers on a sterile field. If they are spilled onto the sterile field, the barrier keeps the liquid from seeping beneath it.
	Keep the sterile covers on sterile equipment dry. Damp surfaces can attract microorganisms in the air.
	Replace sterile drapes that do not have a sterile barrier underneath when they become moist.
The edges of a sterile field are considered unsterile.	A 2.5-cm (1-in) margin at each edge of an opened drape is considered unsterile because the edges are in contact with unsterile surfaces.
	Place all sterile objects more than 2.5 cm (1 in) inside the edges of a sterile field.
	Any article that falls outside the edges of a sterile field is considered unsterile.
The skin cannot be sterilized and is unsterile.	Use sterile gloves or sterile forceps to handle sterile items.
	Prior to a surgical aseptic procedure, wash the hands to reduce the number of microorganisms on them.
Conscientiousness, alertness, and honesty are essential qualities in maintaining surgical asepsis.	When a sterile object becomes unsterile, it does not necessarily change in appearance.
	The person who sees a sterile object become contaiminated must correct or report the situation.
	Do not set up a sterile field ahead of time for future use.

From *Fundamentals of nursing: Concepts, process, and practice*, 6th ed., by B. Kozier, G. Erb, A. Berman, & K. Burke, 2000, Upper Saddle River, NJ: Prentice Hall Health.

Sterile Field

A **sterile field** is a microorganism-free area. Nurses often establish a sterile field by using the innermost side of a sterile wrapper or by using a sterile drape. When the field is established, sterile supplies and sterile solutions can be placed on it. Sterile forceps are used in many instances to handle and transfer the sterile supplies.

So that its sterility can be maintained, equipment is wrapped in a variety of materials. Commercially prepared items are frequently wrapped in plastic, paper, or glass. Commercially prepared sterile liquids for both internal and external use are often supplied in plastic or glass containers. Sterile liquids (e.g., sterile water for irrigations) are preferably packaged in amounts adequate for one use only.

Nursing Process: Maintaining Surgical Asepsis

ASSESSMENT

Review the client's record or discuss with the client exactly what procedure will be performed that requires a sterile field. Assess the client for presence of or excessive risk for infection and the client's ability to cooperate with the procedure.

PLANNING

Determine, if possible, what supplies and techniques have been used in the past to perform these procedures for this client. Also attempt to determine if the procedures will performed again in the future so that you can conduct appropriate client teaching and have adequate supplies available. Schedule the procedure at a time consistent with the physician's order, the need for the procedure, and the client's other activities.

Delegation

Sterile procedures are not delegated to unlicensed assistive personnel (UAP).

Equipment

- Package containing a sterile drape
- Sterile equipment as needed (e.g., wrapped sterile gauze, wrapped sterile bowl, antiseptic solution, sterile forceps)

Preparation

1. Confirm the sterility of the package.
   - Ensure that the package is clean and dry; if moisture is noted on the inside of a plastic-wrapped package or the outside of a cloth-wrapped package, it is considered contaminated and must be discarded.
   - Check the sterilization expiration dates on the package, and look for any indications that it has been previously opened.
   - Follow agency practice about the disposal of possibly contaminated packages.

Performance

1. Explain to the client what you are going to do, why it is necessary, and how he or she can cooperate. Discuss how the results will be used in planning further care or treatments.

2. Observe other appropriate infection control procedures (see Techniques 1-1, 1-2, 1-3, and 12-3).

3. Provide for client privacy.

4. Open the package. If the package is inside a plastic cover, remove the cover.

Opening a Wrapped Package on a Surface

- Place the package in the center of the work area so that the top flap of the wrapper opens away from you. *This position prevents you from subsequently reaching directly over the exposed sterile contents, which could contaminate them.*
- Reaching around the package (not over it), pinch the first flap on the outside of the wrapper between the thumb and index finger (Figure 12-2 ◆). *Touching only the outside of the wrapper maintains the sterility of the inside of the wrapper.* Pull the flap open, laying it flat on the far surface.
- Repeat for the side flaps, opening the top one first. Use the right hand for the right flap, and the left hand for the left flap (Figure 12-3 ◆). *By using both hands, you avoid reaching over the sterile contents.*
- Pull the fourth flap toward you by grasping the corner that is turned down (Figure 12-4 ◆). Make sure that the flap does not touch any object. *If the inner surface touches any unsterile article, it is contaminated.*

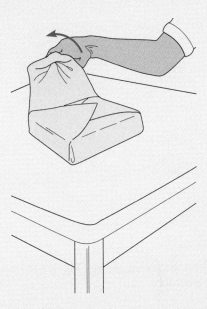

FIGURE 12-2 ◆ Opening the first flap of a sterile wrapped package.

Variation: Opening a Wrapped Package While Holding It

- Hold the package in one hand with the top flap opening away from you.
- Using the other hand, open the package as described above, pulling the corners of the flaps well back (Figure 12-5 ◆). *The hands are considered contaminated, and at no time should they touch the contents of the package.*

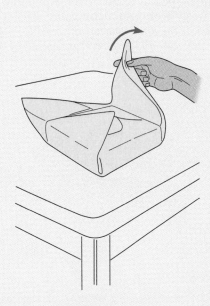

FIGURE 12-3 ◆ Opening the second flap to the side.

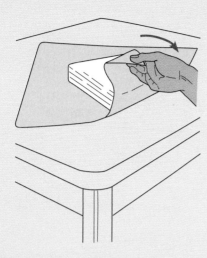

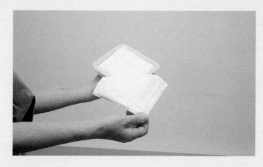

FIGURE 12-6 ◆ Opening a sterile package that has an unsealed corner.

FIGURE 12-4 ◆ Pulling the last flap toward oneself by grasping the corner.

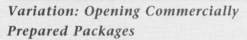

Variation: Opening Commercially Prepared Packages

- If the flap of the package has an unsealed corner, hold the container in one hand, and pull back on the flap with the other hand (Figure 12-6 ◆).

- If the package has a partially sealed edge, grasp both sides of the edge, one with each hand, and pull apart gently (Figure 12-7 ◆).

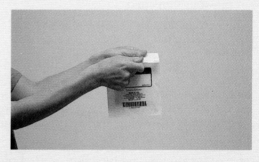

FIGURE 12-7 ◆ Opening a sterile package that has a partially sealed edge.

5. Establish a sterile field by using a drape.

- Open the package containing the drape as described above.

- With one hand, pluck the corner of the drape that is folded back on the top.

- Lift the drape out of the cover, and allow it to open freely without touching any articles (Figure 12-8 ◆). *If the drape touches the outside of the package or any unsterile surface, it is considered contaminated.*

- Discard the cover.

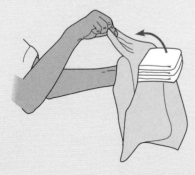

FIGURE 12-5 ◆ Opening a wrapped package while holding it.

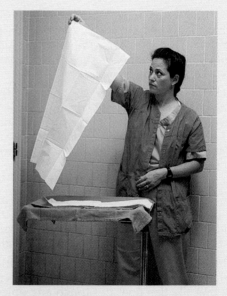

FIGURE 12-8 ◆ Allowing a drape to open freely without touching any objects.

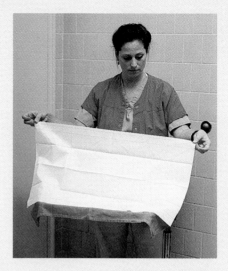

FIGURE 12-9 ◆ Placing a drape on a surface.

- With the other hand, carefully pick up another corner of the drape, holding it well away from you.
- Lay the drape on a clean and dry surface, placing the bottom (i.e., the freely hanging side) farthest from you (Figure 12-9 ◆). *By placing the lowermost side farthest away, you avoid leaning over the sterile field and contaminating it.*

6. Add necessary sterile supplies.

Adding Wrapped Supplies to a Sterile Field

- Open each wrapped package as described in the preceding steps.
- With the free hand, grasp the corners of the wrapper, and hold them against the wrist of the

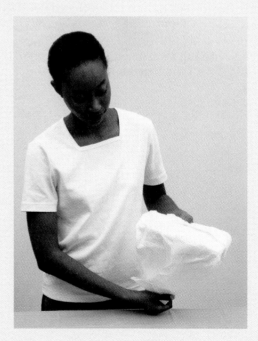

FIGURE 12-10 ◆ Adding wrapped sterile supplies to a sterile field.

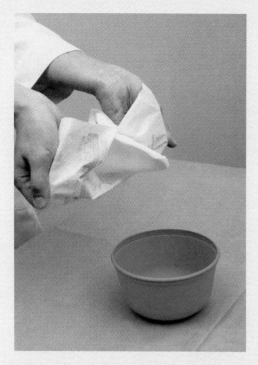

FIGURE 12-11 ◆ Adding commercially packaged gauze to a sterile field.

other hand (Figure 12-10 ◆). *The sterile wrapper now covers the unsterile hand.*

- Place the sterile bowl, drape, or other supply on the sterile field by approaching from an angle rather than holding the arm over the field.
- Discard the wrapper.

Variation: Adding Commercially Packaged Supplies to a Sterile Field

- Open each package as previously described.
- Hold the package 15 cm (6 in) above the field, and allow the contents to drop on the field (Figure 12-11 ◆). Keep in mind that 2.5 cm (1 in) around the edge of the field is considered contaminated. *At a height of 15 cm (6 in), the outside of the package is not likely to touch and contaminate the sterile field.*

Adding Solution to a Sterile Bowl

Liquids (e.g., normal saline) may need to be poured into containers within a sterile field. Unwrapped bottles or flasks that contain sterile solution are considered sterile on the inside and contaminated on the outside because the bottle may have been handled. Bottles used in an operating room may be sterilized on the outside as well as the inside, however, and these are handled with sterile gloves.

- Before pouring any liquid, read the label three times to make sure you have the correct solution and concentration (strength).
- Obtain the exact amount of solution, if possible. *Once a sterile container has been opened, its sterility*

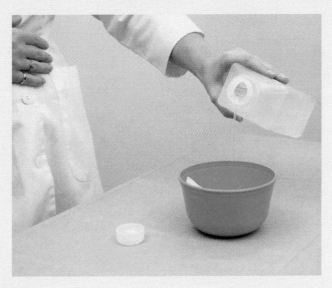

FIGURE 12-12 ◆ Adding a liquid to a sterile bowl.

cannot be ensured for future use. Follow agency policy for reuse of open sterile solutions.

• Remove the lid or cap from the bottle and invert the lid before placing it on a surface that is not sterile. *Inverting the lid maintains the sterility of the inside surface because it is not allowed to touch an unsterile surface.*

• Hold the bottle at a slight angle so that the label is uppermost (Figure 12-12 ◆). *Any solution that flows down the outside of the bottle during pouring will not damage or obliterate the label.*

• Hold the bottle of fluid at a height of 10 to 15 cm (4 to 6 in) over the bowl and to the side of the sterile field so that as little of the bottle as possible is over the field. *At this height, there is less likelihood of contaminating the sterile field by touching the field or by reaching an arm over it.*

• Pour the solution gently to avoid splashing the liquid. *If a barrier drape (one that has a water-resistant layer) is not used and the drape is on an unsterile surface, moisture will contaminate the field by wicking microorganisms through the drape.*

• If the bottle will be used again, replace the lid securely and write on the label the date and time of opening. *Replacing the lid immediately maintains the sterility of the inner aspect of the lid and the solution.* Depending on agency policy, a sterile container of solution that is opened may be used only once and then discarded or kept up to 24 hours.

7. Use sterile forceps to handle sterile supplies.

• Forceps are usually used to move a sterile article from one place to another, for example, transferring sterile gauze from its package to a sterile dressing tray. Forceps may be disposable or resterilized after use. Commonly used forceps include

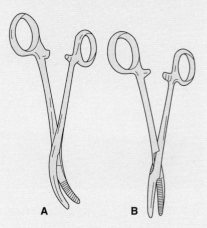

FIGURE 12-13 ◆ Hemostats: (A) curved; (B) straight.

hemostats (Figure 12-13 ◆) and tissue forceps (Figure 12-14 ◆).

• Keep the tips of wet forceps lower than the wrist at all times, unless you are wearing sterile gloves (Figure 12-15 ◆). *Gravity prevents liquids on the tips of the forceps from flowing to the unsterile handles and later back to the tips.*

• Hold sterile forceps above waist level. *Items held below waist level are considered contaminated.*

• Hold sterile forceps within sight. *While out of sight, forceps may, unknown to the user, become unsterile. Any forceps that go out of sight should be considered unsterile.*

• When using forceps to lift sterile supplies, be sure that the forceps do not touch the edges or outside of the wrapper. *The edges and outside of the sterile field are considered unsterile.*

• When placing forceps whose handles were in contact with the bare hand, position the handles

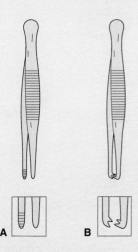

FIGURE 12-14 ◆ Tissue forceps: (A) plain; (B) toothed.

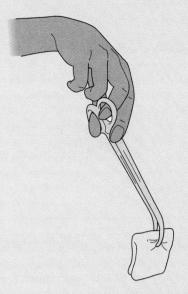

outside the sterile area. *The handles of these forceps harbor microorganisms from the bare hand.*

- Deposit a sterile item on a sterile field without permitting moist forceps to touch the sterile field when the surface under the absorbent sterile field is unsterile and a barrier drape is not used.

 8. **Document** that sterile technique was used in the performance of the procedure.

FIGURE 12-15 ◆ Holding forceps with an ungloved hand, keeping the tips lower than the wrist.

EVALUATION

Conduct any follow-up indicated during your care of the client. Ensure that adequate numbers and types of sterile supplies are available for the next health care provider.

Sterile Gloves

Sterile gloves may be donned by the open method or the closed method. The open method is most frequently used outside the operating room, since the closed method requires that the nurse wear a sterile gown. Gloves are worn during many procedures to enable the nurse to handle sterile objects freely and to prevent clients at risk (e.g., those with open wounds) from becoming infected by microorganisms on the nurse's hands.

Sterile gloves are packaged with a cuff and with the palms facing upward when the package is opened. The package usually indicates the size of the glove (e.g., size 7½ or size medium). Latex and vinyl gloves are available to protect the nurse from contact with blood and body fluids. Latex is more flexible than vinyl, molds to the wearer's hands, allows freedom of movement, and has the added feature of resealing tiny punctures automatically. However, increasing num-

bers of health care providers and clients are developing latex allergies. Therefore, nonlatex gloves that have similar characteristics must be available. Vinyl gloves should be chosen for tasks unlikely to stress the glove material, requiring minimal precision, and with minimal risk of exposure to pathogens.

Nursing Process: Establishing and Maintaining a Sterile Field

ASSESSMENT

Review the client's record and orders to determine exactly what procedure will be performed that requires sterile gloves. Check the client record and ask about latex allergies.

PLANNING

Think through the procedure, planning which steps need to be completed before the gloves can be applied. Determine what additional supplies are needed to perform the procedure for this client. Always have an extra pair of sterile gloves available.

Delegation

Sterile procedures are not delegated to UAP.

IMPLEMENTATION:
TECHNIQUE 12-2 DONNING AND REMOVING STERILE GLOVES (OPEN METHOD)

Equipment

- Packages of sterile gloves

Performance

1. Explain to the client what you are going to do, why it is necessary, and how he or she can cooper-

ate. Discuss how the results will be used in planning further care or treatments.

2. Observe appropriate infection control procedures (see Techniques 1-1, 1-2, 1-3, and 12-3).

3. Provide for client privacy.

4. Open the package of sterile gloves.

- Place the package of gloves on a clean dry surface. *Any moisture on the surface could contaminate the gloves.*

- Some gloves are packed in an inner as well as an outer package. Open the outer package without contaminating the gloves or the inner package. See Procedure 12-1.

- Remove the inner package from the outer package.

- Open the inner package as in step 4 of Procedure 12-1 or according to the manufacturer's directions. Some manufacturers provide a numbered sequence for opening the flaps and folded tabs to grasp for opening the flaps. If no tabs are provided, pluck the flap so that the fingers do not touch the inner surfaces. *The inner surfaces, which are next to the sterile gloves, will remain sterile.*

5. Put the first glove on the dominant hand.

- If the gloves are packaged so that they lie side by side, grasp the glove for the dominant hand by its folded cuff edge (on the palmar side) with the thumb and first finger of the nondominant hand. Touch only the inside of the cuff (Figure 12-16 ◆). *The hands are not sterile. By touching only the inside of the glove, the nurse avoids contaminating the outside.*

  or

- If the gloves are packaged one on top of the other, grasp the cuff of the top glove as above, using the opposite hand.

- Insert the dominant hand into the glove and pull the glove on. Keep the thumb of the inserted hand against the palm of the hand during inser-

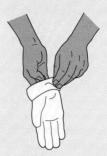

FIGURE 12-17 ◆ Putting on the first sterile glove.

tion (Figure 12-17 ◆). *If the thumb is kept against the palm, it is less likely to contaminate the outside of the glove.*

- Leave the cuff turned down.

6. Put the second glove on the nondominant hand.

- Pick up the other glove with the sterile gloved hand, inserting the gloved fingers under the cuff and holding the gloved thumb close to the gloved palm (Figure 12-18 ◆). *This helps prevent accidental contamination of the glove by the bare hand.*

- Pull on the second glove carefully. Hold the thumb of the gloved first hand as far as possible from the palm (Figure 12-19 ◆). *In this position, the thumb is less likely to touch the arm and become contaminated.*

- Adjust each glove so that it fits smoothly, and carefully pull the cuffs up by sliding the fingers under the cuffs.

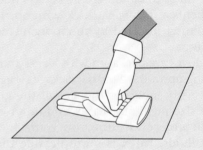

FIGURE 12-18 ◆ Picking up the second sterile glove.

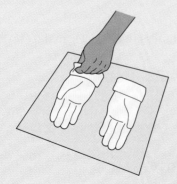

FIGURE 12-16 ◆ Picking up the first sterile glove.

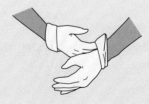

FIGURE 12-19 ◆ Putting on the second sterile glove.

7. Remove and dispose of used gloves.
   - There is no special technique for removing sterile gloves. If they are soiled with secretions, remove them by turning them inside out. See removal of disposable gloves on page 8.

8. **Document** that sterile technique was used in the performance of the procedure.

Establishing and Maintaining a Sterile Field

- Clean and dry a flat surface for the sterile field.
- Keep pets out of the area when setting up for and performing sterile procedures.
- Dispose of all soiled materials in a waterproof bag. Check with the agency as to how to dispose of medical refuse.

- Remove all instruments from the home or other setting where others might accidentally find them. New or used instruments can be sharp or capable of causing injury. Used instruments may transmit infection. Check with the agency for instructions on cleansing of reusable supplies and disposal of single use instruments.
- If appropriate, teach the client and family members the principles of using a sterile field.

EVALUATION

Conduct any follow up indicated during your care of the client. Ensure that adequate numbers and types of sterile supplies are available for the next health care provider.

Caring for Clients with Known or Suspected Infections

As discussed in Chapter 1, nurses care for all clients using **Standard Precautions** (see Technique 1-2). That is, the risk of caregiver exposure to client body tissues and fluids rather than the suspected presence or absence of infectious organisms determines the use of clean gloves, gowns, masks, and eye protection. Isolation refers to measures designed to prevent the spread of infection or potentially infectious material.

In the past, the Centers for Disease Control and Prevention (CDC) recommended that hospitals choose one of the following alternative systems for isolation or design their own system.

- **Category-specific isolation system** based on seven categories: strict isolation, contact isolation, respiratory isolation, tuberculosis isolation, enteric precautions, drainage/secretions precautions, and blood/body fluid precautions.

- **Disease-specific isolation precautions** that delineated use of private rooms, special ventilation, and use of gowns to care for clients with particular diseases or microorganisms.

- A third system, **body substance isolation (BSI)** is based on three premises (Jackson & Lynch, 1991):

1. All people have an increased risk for infection from microorganisms placed on their mucous membranes and nonintact skin.
2. All people are likely to have potentially infectious microorganisms in all of their moist body sites and substances.
3. An unknown portion of clients and health care workers will always be colonized or infected with potentially infectious microorganisms in their blood and other moist body sites and substances.

The CDC's **Universal Precautions**, issued in 1987 and used with all clients to prevent transmission of bloodborne pathogens, was designed to be used with one of the above systems. In 1996, the CDC published revised recommendations for isolation precautions in hospitals:

Tier 1: Standard Precautions (see Chapter 1)

Tier 2: **Transmission-based precautions** (see Technique 12-3)

- Airborne (e.g., measles [rubeola], varicella, tuberculosis)
- Droplet (e.g., pertussis, mumps, pneumonia)
- Contact (e.g., *Clostridium difficile,* drug-resistant bacteria, hepatitis A, herpes simplex, scabies)

Nursing Process: Caring for Clients with Known or Suspected Infection

ASSESSMENT

If precautions have not already been ordered or specified, determine needed Tier 2 precautions based on the client's history and current signs and symptoms. Consult with appropriate infection control personnel as needed. In most cases, the strictest precautions indicated should always be used until a definitive diagnosis has been made.

PLANNING

Notify all agency departments as specified by policy. These may include placing biohazard or isolation labels on equipment, rooms, or charts and notifying the dietary, housekeeping, laboratory, and other relevant departments of the precautions being implemented.

Delegation

Care of clients requiring transmission-based precautions may be delegated to UAP. However, the nurse is responsible for ensuring that all personnel are aware of the specific isolation procedures required for the individual client and can implement them.

IMPLEMENTATION:
TECHNIQUE 12-3 IMPLEMENTING TRANSMISSION-BASED PRECAUTIONS

Equipment

As indicated by the specific precautions:

- Clean gloves
- Gown
- Mask or respirator
- Protective eyewear
- A private room or specialized isolation room

Performance

1. Explain to the client what you are going to do, why it is necessary, and how he or she can cooperate. It is extremely important that clients and family members understand the rationale for use of barriers to infection transmission. They must be given the opportunity to ask questions and express feelings. Hospitalized clients are already socially isolated from others and use of additional barriers can initiate negative feelings such as depression and withdrawal.

2. Use Tier 1: Standard Precautions (Technique 1-2).

3. Implement indicated Tier 2 precautions

Airborne Precautions

1. Place the client in a private room that has negative air pressure, 6 to 12 air changes per hour, and either discharge of air to the outside or a filtration system for the room air. Keep the room door closed.

2. If a private room is not available, place the client with another client who is infected with the same organism.

3. Wear a respiratory device (N95 respirator) when entering the room of a client who is known or suspected of having pulmonary tuberculosis.

4. Susceptible persons should not enter the room of a client who has rubella (measles) or varicella (chickenpox). If they must enter, they should wear a respirator mask.

5. Limit movement of client outside the room to essential purposes. Place a surgical mask on the client while outside of the room.

Droplet Precautions

1. Place the client in a private room.

2. If a private room is not available, place the client with another client who is infected with the same organism.

3. Wear a mask when working within 3 feet of the client.

4. Limit movement of client outside the room to essential purposes. Place a surgical mask on the client while outside of the room.

Contact Precautions

1. Place the client in a private room.

2. If a private room is not available, place the client with another client who is infected with the same organism.

3. Wear gowns and gloves as described in Standard Precautions (see Technique 1-2)

   a. Change gowns and gloves after contact with infectious material.

   b. Remove gowns and gloves before leaving the client's room.

   c. Wash hands immediately after removing gloves.

4. Bag contaminated articles.

   - Identify and separate items that are disposable from those that are reusable.

   - Place garbage and disposable items such as dressings or single-use equipment in the plastic bags that line the wastebasket and tie the bag. If the bag is sturdy and impermeable to microorganisms (waterproof or solid enough to prevent organisms from moving through it even when wet), a single bag is adequate. If not, place the first bag inside another impermeable bag. Some agencies have a particular location where such garbage is to be placed and some use bags of a particular color (e.g., red) to indicate potentially infective waste.

   - Place used disposable sharps (e.g., needles, scalpels, syringes) directly into designated sharps containers. Do not disassemble or recap sharps *since this increases the chances of sustaining a puncture injury.*

- Place contaminated reusable items in an impermeable bag and send to the proper area for decontamination. In some agencies, glass and metal are separated from plastic and rubber equipment since they require different methods of decontamination.
- Place soiled linen directly in the linen hamper. Close the bag and send to the laundry as specified by policy. In some agencies, a bag that dissolves in hot water (melt-away) is used as the first bag and then the entire bundle is placed in a cloth or plastic bag. *In this way, laundry workers need never actually touch soiled linens.* In other

agencies, all contaminated linen is double bagged.

- Specimens to be sent to the laboratory must be placed in an impermeable container with a secure lid. If the outside of the container is contaminated, place the container in a sealable plastic bag.
- Food dishes and silverware require no special handling. Some agencies use disposable dishes for convenience.

 5. **Document** observance of infection control procedures in the client record using forms or checklists supplemented by narrative notes when appropriate.

AMBULATORY AND COMMUNITY SETTINGS

Infection Control

- Teach handwashing and related hygienic measures to all family members (see Technique 12-1).
- Discuss use of antimicrobial soaps and disinfectants.
- Ensure access to and proper use of gloves and other barriers as indicated by the type of infection or risk.
- Teach signs and symptoms of infection, and when to contact a health care provider.
- Teach how to avoid infections:

- When to wash hands
- Not to share personal care items such as toothbrushes
- Wash raw fruits and vegetables
- Cleanse and disinfect used equipment
- Properly dispose of contaminated items such as dressings
- Properly dispose of used sharps such as needles and syringes
- Emphasize the importance of proper immunizations for all members of the household.

EVALUATION

Report any concerns regarding breaks in isolation technique to the appropriate persons (often the infection control nurse). An infection control committee monitors unusual occurrences of infections.

Chapter Summary

TERMINOLOGY

airborne transmission
antiseptics
asepsis
body substance isolation (BSI)
category-specific isolation system
contact precautions
direct transmission
disease-specific isolation
  precautions

disinfectants
etiologic agent
fomite
indirect transmission
medical asepsis
mode of transmission
portal of entry
portal of exit
reservoir

spore
Standard Precautions
sterile field
surgical asepsis
transmission-based precautions
Universal Precautions
vehicle-borne transmission
vector-borne transmission

Forming Clinical Judgments

Consider This:

1. While dropping commercially packaged sterile gauze onto an already established sterile field, the gauze lands with one corner almost off the edge of the field. Does this present any concerns regarding its sterility? If so, how would you handle the situation?

2. After establishing a sterile field and applying sterile gloves, you realize that you have forgotten to open the bottle of saline that needs to be poured into a bowl on the field. The bottle is not sterile on the outside. What are two ways you could solve this dilemma?

3. A client is being admitted to the hospital with a diagnosis of severe diarrhea, unknown origin. What infection control precautions would be appropriate at this time?

4. You are assigned to care for a client with disseminated herpes zoster infections (shingles). In reviewing the agency infection control manual, you learn that persons who have not had chickenpox should not enter this client's room. Persons who have had chickenpox or a blood titer indicating immunity to chickenpox may interact with the client. Explain why this is the case.

Related Research

Kretzer, E. K., & Larson, E. L. (1998). Behavioral interventions to improve infection control practices. *American Journal of Infection Control, 26,* 245–253.

References

Beaumont, E. (1997). Technology scorecard: Focus on infection. *American Journal of Nursing, 98*(12), 51–54.

Garner, J. S., & Hospital Infection Control Practices Advisory Committee. (1996). Guideline for isolation precautions in hospitals. Part I. Evolution of isolation practices. *American Journal of Infection Control, 24,* 24–31.

Jackson, M. M., & Lynch, P. (1991). An attempt to make an issue less murky: A comparison of four systems for infection precautions. *Infection Control and Hospital Epidemiology, 12,* 448–450.

Jones, L., & Hannum, D. (1998). Playing it safe with a particulate respirator. *Nursing 98, 28*(1), 50–51.

Larson, E. L. (1995). APIC guideline for handwashing and hand antisepsis in health care settings. *American Journal of Infection Control, 23,* 251–269.

Rosenheimer, L. (1999). Establishing an effective infection control and surveillance program in the home care setting. *Home HealthCare Consultant, 6*(12), 38–42.

U. S. Department of Health and Human Services. (1996). Guideline for isolation precautions in hospitals. Part II. Recommendations for isolation precautions in hospitals. *American Journal of Infection Control, 24,* 32–52.

U. S. Department of Health and Human Services. Centers for Disease Control and Prevention. (1997). Draft guideline for infection control in health care personnel, 1997. *Federal Register, 62*(173).

Xavier, G. (1999). Asepsis. *Nursing Standard, 13*(36), 49–53, 56.

Chapter 13

Heat and Cold Measures

Techniques

OBJECTIVES

- Identify reasons for administering hot and cold applications.
- Identify essential guidelines for applying heat and cold.
- Describe methods of applying dry and moist heat.
- Describe methods of applying dry and moist cold.

Heat and Cold Therapy

H eat and cold are applied to the body to promote the repair and healing of tissues. The form of **thermal** applications generally depends on their purpose. Cold applied to a body part draws heat from the area; heat, of course, warms the area. The application of heat or cold produces physiologic changes in the temperature of the tissues, size of the blood vessels, capillary blood pressure, capillary surface area for exchange of fluids and electrolytes, and tissue metabolism. The duration of the application also affects the response. See Table 13-1 for a summary of the physiologic effects of heat and cold.

Heat and cold can be applied to the body in both dry and moist forms. Dry heat is applied locally, for heat conduction, by means of a hot water bottle, electric pad, **aquathermia pad**, or disposable heat pack. Moist heat can be provided, through **conduction**, by compress, hot pack, soak, or bath. Dry cold is administered for local effect by the use of ice bags, **ice collars**, ice gloves, and disposable cold packs. Cold **moist compresses** are administered to body parts for a local effect; tepid sponge baths are given for a systemic cooling effect. Cold is often applied to the body to decrease bleeding by constricting blood vessels; to decrease inflammation by causing vasoconstriction; and to decrease pain by slowing nerve conduction

TABLE 13-1	PHYSIOLOGIC EFFECTS OF HEAT AND COLD

Heat	Cold
Vasodilation	Vasoconstriction
Increases capillary permeability	Decreases capillary permeability
Increases cellular metabolism	Decreases cellular metabolism
Relaxes muscles	Relaxes muscles
Increases inflammation; increases blood flow to an area	Slows bacterial growth, decreases inflammation
Decreases pain by relaxing muscles	Decreases pain by numbing the area, slowing the flow of pain impulses, and by increasing the pain threshold
Sedative effect	Local anesthetic effect
Reduces joint stiffness by decreasing viscosity of synovial fluids	Decreases bleeding

From *Fundamentals of nursing: Concepts, process, and practice,* 6th ed., by B. Kozier, G. Erb, A. Berman, & K. Burke, 2000, Upper Saddle River, NJ: Prentice Hall Health.

rate, producing numbness, and acting as a counterirritant. Selected indications for the use of heat and cold are found in Box 13-1.

Guidelines for Applying Heat and Cold

An understanding of the adaptive response of thermal receptors, the rebound phenomenon, systemic effects, tolerance to heat and cold, and contraindications is essential when administering hot and cold applications.

Adaptation of Thermal Receptors

Thermal receptors adapt to temperature changes. When a cold receptor is subjected to an abrupt fall in temperature or when a warmth receptor is subjected to an abrupt rise in temperature, the receptor is strongly stimulated initially. This strong stimulation declines rapidly during the first few seconds and then more slowly during the next half hour or more as the receptor adapts to the new temperature.

Nurses need to understand this adaptive response when applying heat and cold. Clients may be tempted to change the temperature of a thermal application because of the change in thermal sensation following adaptation. Increasing the temperature of a hot application after adaptation has occurred can result in serious burns. Decreasing the temperature of a cold application can result in pain and serious impairment of circulation to the body part. See Table 13-2 for recommended temperatures of hot and cold applications.

Rebound Phenomenon

The **rebound phenomenon** occurs at the time the maximum therapeutic effect of the hot or cold application is achieved and the opposite effect begins. For example, heat produces maximum vasodilation in 20 to 30 minutes; continuation of the application beyond 30 to 45 minutes brings tissue congestion, and the blood vessels then *constrict* for reasons unknown. If the heat application is continued further, the client is at risk for burns, since the constricted blood vessels are unable to dissipate the heat adequately via the blood circulation.

With cold applications, maximum vasoconstriction occurs when the involved skin reaches a temperature of 15°C (60°F). Below 15°C, vasodilation begins. This mechanism is protective: It helps to prevent freezing of body tissues normally exposed to cold, such as the nose and ears. It also explains the ruddiness of the skin of a person who has been walking in cold weather.

An understanding of the rebound phenomenon is essential for the nurse. Thermal applications must be halted *before* the rebound phenomenon begins.

Box 13-1 *Selected Indications of Heat and Cold*

Indication	Effect of Heat	Effect of Cold
Muscle spasm	Relaxes muscles and increases their contractility	Relaxes muscles and decreases their contractility
Inflammation	Increases blood flow, softens exudates	Vasoconstriction decreases capillary permeability, decreases blood flow, slows cellular metabolism
Pain	Relieves pain, possibly by promoting muscle relaxation, increasing circulation, promoting psychological relaxation and a feeling of comfort; acts as a counterirritant	Decreases pain by slowing nerve conduction rate and blocking nerve impulses, produces numbness, acts as a counterirritant, increases pain threshold
Contracture	Reduces contracture and increases joint range of motion by allowing greater distention of muscles and connective tissue	
Joint stiffness	Reduces joint stiffness by decreasing viscosity of synovial fluid and increasing tissue distensibility	
Traumatic injury		Decreases bleeding by constricting blood vessels, decreases edema by reducing capillary permeability

Systemic Effects

Heat applied to a localized body area, particularly a large body area, may increase cardiac output and pulmonary ventilation. These increases are a result of excessive peripheral vasodilation, which diverts large supplies of blood from the internal organs and produces a drop in blood pressure. A significant drop in blood pressure can cause fainting. Clients who have heart or pulmonary disease and who have circulatory disturbances such as arteriosclerosis are more prone to this effect than healthy persons.

With extensive cold applications (such as when a client is placed on a cooling blanket) and vasoconstriction, a client's blood pressure can increase, because blood is shunted from the cutaneous circula-tion to the internal blood vessels. This shunting of blood, a normal protective response to prolonged cold, is the body's attempt to maintain its core temperature. Shivering, another generalized effect of prolonged cold, is a normal response as the body attempts to warm itself.

Tolerance and Contraindications

Various parts of the body differ in tolerance to heat and cold. The physiologic tolerance of individuals also varies. See Box 13-2.

Specific conditions contraindicate the use of hot or cold applications. In addition, certain conditions call for precautions in administering heat and cold therapy. See Box 13-3.

TABLE 13-2	RECOMMENDED TEMPERATURES FOR HOT AND COLD APPLICATIONS	
Description	**Temperature**	**Application**
Very cold	Below 15°C (59°F)	Ice bags
Cold	15–18°C (59–65°F)	Cold pack
Cool	18–27°C (65–80°F)	Cold compresses
Tepid	27–37°C (80–98°F)	Alcohol sponge bath
Warm	37–40°C (98–105°F)	Warm bath, aquathermia pads
Hot	40–46°C (105–115°F)	Hot soak, irrigations, hot compresses
Very hot	Above 46°C (above 115°F)	Hot water bags for adults

From *Fundamentals of nursing: Concepts, process, and practice,* 6th ed., by B. Kozier, G. Erb, A. Berman, & K. Burke, 2000, Upper Saddle River, NJ: Prentice Hall Health.

Box 13-2 *Variables Affecting Physiologic Tolerance to Heat and Cold*

• *Body part.* The back of the hand and foot are not very temperature sensitive. In contrast, the inner aspect of the wrist and forearm, the neck, and the perineal area are temperature sensitive.

• *Size of the exposed body part.* The larger the area exposed to heat and cold, the lower the tolerance.

• *Individual tolerance.* The very young and the very old generally have the lowest tolerance. Persons who have

neurosensory impairments may have a high tolerance, but the risk of injury is greater.

• *Length of exposure.* People feel hot and cold applications most while the temperature is changing. After a period of time, tolerance increases.

• *Intactness of skin.* Injured skin areas are more sensitive to temperature variations.

From *Fundamentals of nursing: Concepts, process, and practice,* 6th ed., by B. Kozier, G. Erb, A. Berman, & K. Burke, 2000, Upper Saddle River, NJ: Prentice Hall Health.

Nursing Process: Applying Heat or Cold

ASSESSMENT

Assess:

1. The capacity of the client to recognize when the heat is injurious. *Establish whether the client is aware of heat and cold and can discern a temperature that is too hot or too cold for the tissues.*

2. The client's degree of consciousness and general physical condition. *Very young, very old, unconscious, or debilitated clients do not tolerate heat well.*

3. The area to be treated for:
   • Alterations in skin integrity, such as the presence of edema, bruises, redness, open lesions, discharge, and bleeding
   • Circulatory status (color, temperature, and sensation). *Tissues that feel cold, have a pale or bluish hue, and lack sensation or feel numb indicate circulatory impairment.*
   • Level of discomfort and range of motion if muscle spasm or pain is being treated.

4. Pulse, respirations, and blood pressure. *Assessing these factors is particularly important before hot or cold is applied to large body areas.*

Box 13-3 *Contraindications to the Use of Heat and Cold*

Determine the presence of any conditions contraindicating the use of heat:

• *The first 24 hours after traumatic injury.* Heat increases bleeding and swelling.

• *Active hemorrhage.* Heat causes vasodilation and increases bleeding.

• *Noninflammatory edema.* Heat increases capillary permeability and edema.

• *Localized malignant tumor.* Because heat accelerates cell metabolism and cell growth and increases circulation, it may accelerate metastases (secondary tumors).

• *Skin disorder that causes redness or blisters.* Heat can burn or cause further damage to the skin.

Determine the presence of any conditions contraindicating the use of cold:

• *Open wounds.* Cold can increase tissue damage by decreasing blood flow to an open wound.

• *Impaired circulation.* Cold can further impair nourishment of the tissues and cause tissue damage. In clients with Raynaud's disease, cold increases arterial spasm.

• *Allergy or hypersensitivity to cold.* Some clients have an allergy to cold that may be manifested by an inflammatory response (e.g., erythema, hives, swelling, joint

pain, and occasional muscle spasm). Some react with a sudden increase in blood pressure, which can be hazardous if the person is hypersensitive.

Determine the presence of any conditions indicating the need for special precautions during heat and cold therapy:

• *Neurosensory impairment.* Persons with sensory impairments are unable to perceive that heat is damaging the tissues and are at risk for burns, or they are unable to perceive discomfort from cold and are unable to prevent tissue injury.

• *Impaired mental status.* Persons who are confused or have an altered level of consciousness need monitoring and supervision during applications to ensure safe therapy.

• *Impaired circulation.* Persons with peripheral vascular disease, diabetes, or congestive heart failure lack the normal ability to dissipate heat via the blood circulation, which puts them at risk for tissue damage with heat applications. Cold applications are contraindicated for these people.

• *Open wounds.* Tissues around an open wound are more sensitive to heat and cold.

PLANNING

Before applying heat or cold, determine:

- Whether the client is required to sign a release for the application (if a release is required, check the client's chart for the signed release)
- Type of heat or cold to be used, the temperature, and the duration and frequency of the application (check the order if necessary)
- Agency protocol about the type of equipment used, the temperature recommended, and the length of applications
- At what time the treatment should be applied

Delegation

Application of certain heat and cold measures may be delegated to unlicensed assistive personnel (UAP) (e.g., sitz baths, cooling baths) if they meet the general criteria for delegation (see Chapter 1). However, in all cases, assessment of the client and the determination that the measure is safe to employ is the responsibility of the nurse. UAP may observe the area being treated during usual care and must report abnormal findings to the nurse. Abnormal findings must be validated and interpreted by the nurse.

IMPLEMENTATION:

TECHNIQUE 13-1 APPLYING DRY HEAT MEASURES: HOT WATER BOTTLE, ELECTRIC HEATING PAD, AQUATHERMIA PAD, DISPOSABLE HOT PACK

Equipment

- Hot water bottle (bag)
  - Hot water bottle with a stopper
  - Cover
  - Hot water and a thermometer
- Electric heating pad
  - Electric pad and control
  - Cover (waterproof if there will be moisture under the pad when it is applied)
  - Gauze ties (optional)
- Aquathermia pad
  - Pad
  - Distilled water
  - Control unit
  - Cover
  - Gauze ties or tape (optional)
- Disposable hot pack
  - One or two commercially prepared disposable hot packs

Performance

1. Explain to the client what you are going to do, why it is necessary, and how he or she can cooperate. Discuss how the results will be used in planning further care or treatments.
2. Wash hands and observe appropriate infection control procedures.
3. Provide for client privacy.
4. Apply the heat

Variation: Hot Water Bottle

- Measure the temperature of the water. Follow agency practice for the appropriate temperature.

Temperatures commonly used are

a. 46 to 52°C (125°F) for a normal adult.

b. 40.5 to 46°C (105 to 115°F) for a debilitated or unconscious adult.

- Fill the hot water bottle about two-thirds full.
- Expel the air from the bottle. *Air remaining in the bottle prevents it from molding to the body part being treated.*
- Secure the stopper tightly.
- Hold the bottle upside down, and check for leaks.
- Dry the bottle.
- Wrap the bottle in a towel or hot water bottle cover.
- Apply the pad to the body part using pillows to support it if necessary.

Variation: Electric Heating Pad

- Ensure that the body area is dry. *Electricity in the presence of moisture can conduct a shock.*
- Check that the electric pad is functioning and in good repair. The cord should be free from cracks, wires should be intact, heating components should not be exposed, and temperature distribution over the pad should be even.
- Place the cover on the pad. Some models have waterproof covers to be used when the pad is placed over a moist dressing. *Moisture could cause the pad to short circuit and burn or shock the client.*
- Plug the pad into the electric socket.
- Set the control dial for the correct temperature.
- After the pad has heated, place the pad over the body part to which heat is being applied.
- Use gauze ties instead of safety pins to hold the pad in place, if needed. *A pin might strike a wire, damaging the pad and giving an electric shock to the client.*

IMPLEMENTATION:

TECHNIQUE 13-1 APPLYING DRY HEAT MEASURES: HOT WATER BOTTLE, ELECTRIC HEATING PAD, AQUATHERMIA PAD, DISPOSABLE HOT PACK (*continued*)

Variation: Aquathermia Pad, also Referred to as a K-pad (Figure 13-1 ◆)

- Fill the unit with distilled water until it is two-thirds full. The unit will warm the water, which circulates through the pad.
- Remove air bubbles, and secure the top.
- Regulate the temperature with the key if it has not been preset. Normal temperature is 40.5°C (105°F). Check the manufacturer's instructions.
- Cover the pad with a towel or pillowcase.
- Plug in the unit.
- Check for any leak or malfunctions of the pad before use.
- Use tape or gauze ties to hold the pad in place. Never use safety pins. They can cause leakage.
- If unusual redness or pain occurs, discontinue the treatment, and report the client's reaction.

Variation: Disposable Hot Pack (Figure 13-2 ◆)

- Microwave, strike, squeeze, or knead the pack according to the manufacturer's directions.

- Note the manufacturer's instructions about the length of time that heat is produced.

5. Give the client the following instructions:
   - Do not insert any sharp, pointed object (e.g., a pin) into the bottle or pad.
   - Do not lie directly on the bottle or pad. *The surface below the object promotes heat absorption instead of normal heat dissipation.*
   - To prevent injury, avoid adjusting the heat higher than specified. *The degree of heat felt shortly after application will decrease, because the body's temperature receptors quickly adapt to the temperature. This adaptive mechanism can lead to tissue injury if the temperature is adjusted higher.*
   - Call the nurse if any discomfort is felt.

6. Leave the heat in place for only the designated period of time to avoid the rebound phenomenon. For a hot water bottle, this is 30 to 45 minutes; for an electric pad, 10 to 15 minutes.

 7. **Document** the application of the heat and the client's response in the client record using forms or checklists supplemented by narrative notes when appropriate.

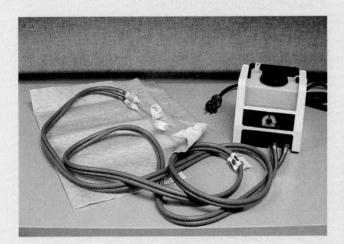

FIGURE 13-1 ◆ An aquathermia heating unit.

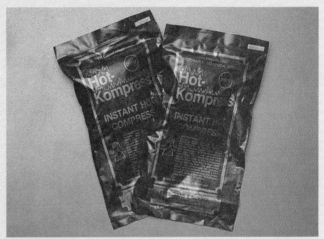

FIGURE 13-2 ◆ Commercially prepared disposable hot packs.

AGE-RELATED CONSIDERATIONS

Applying Heat Measures

Infant/Child

- The temperature of water in a hot water bottle should be 40.5 to 46°C (105 to 115°F) for a child under 2 years of age.

Elders

- Use special care in assessing the area to be treated and in evaluating the effects of the treatment since elders have many of the conditions predisposing to injury with heat measures.

EVALUATION

- Perform a follow-up examination of the client to determine the effectiveness of the therapy and assess for any complications. Relate findings to previous assessment data if available.

- Report significant deviations from normal to the physician.

IMPLEMENTATION:

TECHNIQUE 13-2 APPLYING DRY COLD MEASURES: ICE BAG, ICE COLLAR, ICE GLOVE, DISPOSABLE COLD PACK

Equipment

- Ice bag, collar, glove, or cold pack
- Ice chips
- Protective covering
- Roller gauze, a binder or a towel, and tape

Performance

1. Explain to the client what you are going to do, why it is necessary, and how he or she can cooperate. Discuss how the results will be used in planning further care or treatments.

2. Wash hands and observe appropriate infection control procedures.

3. Provide for client privacy. Expose only the area to be treated, and provide warmth to avoid chilling.

4. Prepare the client.
   - Assist the client to a comfortable position, and support the body part requiring the application.

5. Apply the cold measure.

Variation: Ice Bag, Collar, or Glove

- Fill the device one-half to two-thirds full of crushed ice. *Partial filling makes the device more pliable so that it can be molded to a body part.*

- Remove excess air by bending or twisting the device. *Air inflates the device so that it cannot be molded to the body part.*

- Insert the stopper securely into an ice bag or collar, or tie a knot at the open end of a glove. *This prevents leakage of fluid when the ice melts.*

- Hold the device upside down, and check it for leaks.

- Cover the device with a soft cloth cover, if it is not already equipped with one. *The cover absorbs moisture that condenses on the outside of the device. It is also more comfortable for the client.*

- Hold the device in place with roller gauze, a binder, or a towel. Secure with tape as necessary.

Variation: Disposable Cold Pack

- Strike, squeeze, or knead the cold pack according to the manufacturer's instructions. *The action activates the chemical reaction that produces the cold.*

- Cover with a soft cloth cover, if the pack does not have a cover. Most commercially prepared cold packs have soft outer coverings to permit application directly to the body part.

6. Instruct the client as follows:
   - Remain in position for the duration of the treatment.
   - Call the nurse if discomfort is felt.

7. Monitor the client during the application.
   - Assess the client in terms of comfort and skin reaction (e.g., pallor, mottled appearance) as frequently as necessary for the client's safety (e.g., every 5 to 10 minutes). Factors such as previous responses to applications and the client's ability to report any problems need to be considered.
   - Report untoward reactions and remove the application.

8. Leave the heat in place for only the designated period of time to *avoid the rebound phenomenon and the harmful effects of prolonged cold.*

 9. **Document** the application of the cold and the client's response in the client record using forms or checklists supplemented by narrative notes when appropriate.

EVALUATION

- Perform a follow-up examination of the client to determine the effectiveness of the therapy and assess for any complications. Relate findings to previous assessment data if available.

- Report significant deviations from normal to the physician.

Compresses and Moist Packs

Compresses and moist packs can be either hot or cold. A compress is a moist gauze dressing, applied frequently to an open wound. When hot compresses are ordered, the solution is heated to the temperature indicated by the physician, for example, 40.5°C (105°F). When there is a break in the skin or when the body part (e.g., an eye) is vulnerable to microbial invasion, sterile technique is necessary; therefore, sterile gloves or sterile forceps are needed to apply the compress, and all materials (solution, container, thermometer, towels, gauze squares, and petroleum jelly) must be sterile.

A **hot or cold pack** is a hot or cold moist cloth applied to an area of the body. Packs are usually unsterile; after application, they are covered with a water-resistant material (e.g., plastic wrap) to contain the moisture and prevent the transfer of airborne microorganisms to the area.

IMPLEMENTATION:
TECHNIQUE 13-3 APPLYING COMPRESSES AND MOIST PACKS

Equipment

Use sterile equipment and supplies for an open wound.

Compress

- Disposable gloves or sterile gloves (for an open wound)
- Container for the solution
- Solution at the strength and temperature specified by the physician or the agency
- Thermometer
- Gauze squares
- Sterile gloves, forceps, and cotton applicator sticks (if compress must be sterile)
- Petroleum jelly
- Insulating towel
- Plastic
- Ties (e.g., roller gauze or masking tape)
- Hot water bottle or aquathermia pad (optional)

  or
- Ice bag (optional)
- Sterile dressing, if required

Moist Pack

- Disposable gloves
- Flannel pieces or towel packs
- Hot-pack machine for heating the packs

  or
- Basin of water with some ice chips
- Thermometer if a specific temperature is ordered for the pack
- Sterile gloves, forceps, and cotton applicator sticks (if sterility must be maintained)
- Petroleum jelly
- Insulating material (e.g., flannel or towels)
- Plastic
- Hot water bottle (optional)

or
- Ice bag (optional)
- Sterile dressing, if required

Performance

1. Explain to the client what you are going to do, why it is necessary, and how he or she can cooperate. Discuss how the results will be used in planning further care or treatments.

2. Wash hands and observe appropriate infection control procedures.

3. Provide for client privacy.

4. Prepare the client.
   - Assist the client to a comfortable position.
   - Expose the area for the compress or pack.
   - Provide support for the body part requiring the compress or pack.
   - Don disposable gloves, and remove the wound dressing, if present. A dry, sterile dressing is often placed over open wounds between applications of moist heat or cold.

5. Moisten the compress or the pack.
   - Place the gauze in the solution.

     or
   - Heat the flannel or towel in a steamer, or chill it in the basin of water and ice chips.

6. Protect the surrounding skin as indicated.
   - With a cotton swab or an applicator stick, apply petroleum jelly to the skin surrounding the wound, not on the wound or open areas of the skin. *Jelly protects the skin from possible burns, maceration, and the irritating effects of some solutions.*

7. Apply the moist compress or pack.
   - Wring out the gauze compress so that the solution does not drip from it. For a sterile compress, use sterile forceps or sterile gloves to wring out the gauze.

- Apply the gauze lightly and gradually to the designated area and, if tolerated by the client, mold the compress close to the body. Pack the gauze snugly against all wound surfaces. *Air is a poor conductor of cold or heat, and molding excludes air.*

  or

- Wring out the flannel (for a sterile pack, use sterile gloves).
- Apply the flannel to the body area, molding it closely to the body part.

8. Immediately insulate and secure the application.

- Cover the gauze or flannel quickly with a dry towel and a piece of plastic. *This step helps maintain the temperature of the application and thus its effectiveness.*
- Secure the compress or pack in place with gauze ties or tape.
- *Optional:* Apply a hot water bottle or aquathermia pad or ice bag over the plastic to maintain the heat or cold.

9. Monitor the client.

- Assess the client for discomfort at 5- to 10-minute intervals. If the client feels any discomfort, assess the area for erythema, numbness, maceration, or blistering.
- For applications to large areas of the body, note any change in the pulse, respirations, and blood pressure.
- In the event of unexpected reactions, terminate the treatment and report to the nurse in charge.

10. Remove the compress or pack at the specified time.

- Compresses and packs with external heat or cold may remain in place 1 to 2 hours. Without external heat or cold, they need to be changed every few minutes.
- Apply a sterile dressing if one is required.

11. **Document** the application of the compress or pack and the client's response in the client record using forms or checklists supplemented by narrative notes when appropriate.

EVALUATION

- Perform a follow-up examination of the client to determine the effectiveness of the therapy and assess for any complications. Relate findings to previous assessment data if available.
- Report significant deviations from normal to the physician.

Chapter Summary

TERMINOLOGY

aquathermia pad	K-pad	rebound phenomenon
conduction	ice collar	thermal
hot/cold pack	moist compress	

FORMING CLINICAL JUDGMENTS

Consider This:

1. The client reports that she has been using a heating pad at home for low back pain. She says it "used to help" but now, even on the highest setting, it doesn't feel very warm to her. What are three possible explanations for her experience?

2. A friend tells you that she has injured her ankle and wants to know whether ice or heat should be applied. Based on your understanding of the effects of heat and cold on various tissues, how would you respond?

3. The physician has ordered "cooling baths for temperature greater than 104°F." You observe the nursing assistant using cool tap water and rubbing the client's legs. The client is shivering. Which of these observations require you to intervene?

RELATED RESEARCH

Myrer, J. W., Measom, G., Durrant, E., & Fellingham, G. W. (1997). Cold- and hot-pack contrast therapy: Subcutaneous temperature change. *Journal of Athletic Training, 32,* 238–241.

REFERENCES

McConnell, E. A. (1997). Clinical do's and don'ts: Using dry heat to promote healing. *Nursing, 27*(5), 22.

McConnell, E. A. (1998). Clinical do's and don'ts: Using cold treatment. *Nursing, 28*(6), 26.

Todd, J. F. (1997). Heating devices: How to avoid burns. *Nursing, 27*(10), 83.

Chapter 14

Pain Management

Techniques

OBJECTIVES

- Describe the nature of pain, including the types of pain.
- Identify barriers to effective pain management.
- Identify subjective and objective data to collect and analyze when assessing pain.
- Assess the client in pain effectively.
- Describe nonpharmacologic pain control interventions.

The Nature of Pain

Pain is a highly unpleasant and very personal sensation that cannot be shared with others. It can occupy all a person's thinking, direct all activities, and change a person's life. Yet, pain is a difficult concept for a client to communicate. A nurse can neither feel nor see a client's pain.

No two people experience pain in exactly the same way. In addition, the differences in individual pain perception and reaction, as well as the many causes of pain, present the nurse with a complex situation when developing a plan to relieve pain and provide comfort. Effective pain management is an important aspect of nursing care.

Although pain is a universal experience, its exact nature remains a mystery. It is known that pain is highly subjective and individual and that it is one of the body's defense mechanisms indicating that there is a problem. Unrelieved pain presents both physiologic and psychological dangers to health and recovery. McCaffery defines *pain* as "whatever the experiencing person says it is, existing whenever he (or she) says it does" (McCaffery & Pasero, 1999, p. 5). Basic to this definition is the care provider's willingness to believe that the client is experiencing pain and that the client is the real authority on that pain.

Types of Pain

Pain may be described in terms of the duration, location, or etiology. When pain lasts only through the expected recovery period, it is described as **acute pain** whether it has a sudden or slow onset and regardless of the intensity. **Chronic pain**, on the other hand, is prolonged, usually recurring or persisting over six months or longer, and interferes with functioning. Chronic pain can be further classified as chronic malignant pain when associated with cancer or other life-threatening conditions or as chronic nonmalignant pain when the etiology is a nonprogressive disorder. Acute and chronic pain result in different physiologic and behavioral responses as shown in Table 14-1.

Pain can be categorized according to its origin. **Cutaneous pain** originates in the skin or subcutaneous tissue. A paper cut causing a sharp pain with some burning is an example of cutaneous pain. **Deep somatic pain** arises from ligaments, tendons, bones, blood vessels, and nerves. It is diffuse and tends to last longer than cutaneous pain. An ankle sprain is an example of deep somatic pain. **Visceral pain** results from stimulation of pain receptors in the abdominal cavity, cranium, and thorax. Visceral pain tends to appear diffuse and often feels like deep somatic pain, that is, burning, aching, or a feeling of pressure. Visceral pain is frequently caused by stretching of the tissues, ischemia, or muscle spasms. For example, an obstructed bowel will result in visceral pain.

Pain may also be described according to where it is experienced in the body. **Radiating pain** is perceived at the source of the pain and extends to nearby tissues. For example, cardiac pain may be felt not only in the chest but also along the left shoulder and down the arm. **Referred pain** is pain felt in a part of the body that is considerably removed from the tissues causing the pain. For example, pain from one part of the abdominal viscera may be perceived in an area of the skin remote from the organ causing the pain (see Figure 14-1 ◆).

TABLE 14-1	COMPARISON OF ACUTE AND CHRONIC PAIN
Acute Pain	**Chronic Pain**
Mild to severe	Mild to severe
Sympathetic nervous system responses:	Parasympathetic nervous system responses:
Increased pulse rate	Vital signs normal
Increased respiratory rate	Dry, warm skin
Elevated blood pressure	Pupils normal or dilated
Diaphoresis	
Dilated pupils	
Related to tissue injury; resolves with healing	Continues beyond healing
Client appears restless and anxious	Client appears depressed and withdrawn
Client reports pain	Client often does not mention pain unless asked
Client exhibits behavior indicative of pain: crying, rubbing area, holding area	Pain behavior often absent

From *Fundamentals of nursing: Concepts, process, and practice*, 6th ed., by B. Kozier, G. Erb, A. Berman, & K. Burke, 2000, Upper Saddle River, NJ: Prentice Hall Health.

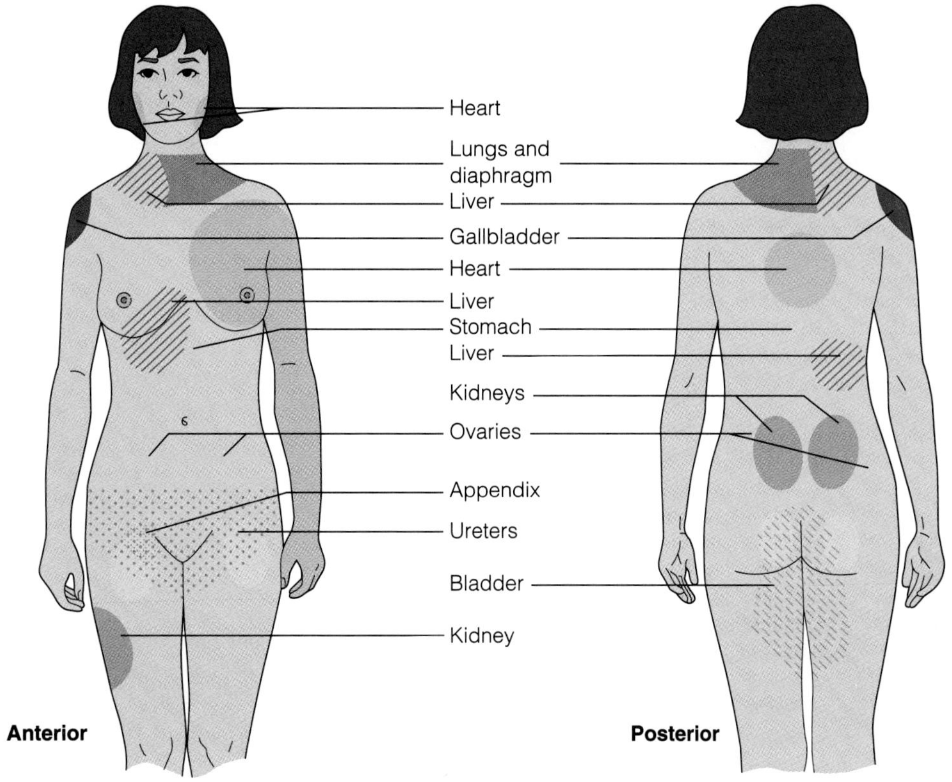
Heart
Lungs and diaphragm
Liver
Gallbladder
Heart
Liver
Stomach
Liver
Kidneys
Ovaries
Appendix
Ureters
Bladder
Kidney
Anterior
Posterior

FIGURE 14-1 ◆ Common sites of referred pain from various body organs.

Intractable pain is pain that is highly resistant to relief. One example is the pain from an advanced malignancy. Often, nurses are challenged to use a number of methods, such as imagery and **patient-controlled analgesia (PCA)** to provide a client with pain relief.

Neuropathic pain is the result of current or past damage to the peripheral or central nervous system and may not have a stimulus, such as tissue or nerve damage, for the pain. Neuropathic pain is long lasting, unpleasant, and can be described as burning, dull, and aching; episodes of sharp, shooting pain can also be experienced (Hawthorn & Redmond, 1998).

Phantom pain, which is a painful sensation perceived in a body part that is missing (e.g., an amputated leg) or paralyzed by a spinal cord injury, is also an example of neuropathic pain. This can be distinguished from phantom sensation, that is, the feeling that the missing body part is still present.

Concepts Associated with Pain

When an individual perceives pain from injured tissue, the pain threshold is reached. An individual's **pain threshold** is the amount of pain stimulation a person requires in order to feel pain. People's pain threshold is generally fairly uniform; however, it can change. For example, the same stimuli that once produced mild pain can at another time produce intense pain. Excessive sensitivity to pain is called **hyperalgesia.**

Pain sensation can be considered the same as pain threshold; **pain reaction** includes the autonomic nervous system and behavioral responses to pain. The autonomic nervous system response is the automatic reaction of the body that often protects the individual from further harm, for example, the automatic withdrawal of the hand from a hot stove. The behavioral response is a learned response used as a method of coping with the pain.

Pain tolerance is the maximum amount and duration of pain that an individual is willing to endure. Some clients are unable to tolerate even the slightest pain, whereas others are willing to endure severe pain rather than be treated for it. Thus, pain tolerance varies greatly among people and is widely influenced by psychological and sociocultural factors. Pain tolerance appears to increase with age.

Factors Affecting the Pain Experience

Numerous factors can affect a person's perception of and reaction to pain.

Ethnic and Cultural Values

Ethnic background and cultural heritage has long been recognized as a factor that influences both a person's reaction to pain and the expression of pain. Behavior related to pain is a part of the socialization process.

Although there appears to be little variation in pain threshold, cultural background can affect the level of pain that an individual is willing to tolerate. In some Middle Eastern and African cultures, self-infliction of pain is a sign of mourning or grief. In other groups, pain may be anticipated as part of the ritualistic practices and therefore tolerance of pain signifies strength and endurance. Additionally, there are significant variations in the expression of pain. Studies have shown that individuals of northern European descent tend to be more stoic and less expressive of their pain than individuals from southern European backgrounds. One study showed that even the descriptors of pain used varied by cultural group (Andrews & Boyle, 1995).

Developmental Stage

The age and developmental stage of a client is an important variable that will influence both the reaction to and the expression of pain. Age variations are presented in Table 14-2.

TABLE 14-2	AGE VARIATIONS IN THE PAIN EXPERIENCE
Age Group	**Pain Perception and Behavior**
Infant	• Perceives pain. • Responds to pain with increased sensitivity. • Older infant tries to avoid pain; for example, turns away and physically resists.
Toddler and preschooler	• Develops the ability to describe pain and its intensity and location. • Often responds with crying and anger because child perceives pain as a threat to security. • Reasoning with child at this stage is not always successful. • May consider pain as punishment. • Feels sad. • May learn there are gender differences in pain expression. • Tends to hold someone accountable for the pain.
School-aged child	• Tries to be brave when facing pain. • Rationalizes in an attempt to explain the pain. • Responsive to explanations. • Can usually identify the location and describe the pain. • With persistent pain, may regress to an earlier stage of development.
Adolescent	• May be slow to acknowledge pain. • Recognizing pain or "giving in" may be considered weakness. • Wants to appear brave in front of peers and not report pain.
Adult	• Behaviors exhibited when experiencing pain may be gender-based behaviors learned as a child. • May ignore pain because to admit it is perceived as a sign of weakness or failure. • May use pain for secondary gain, for example, to get attention. • Fear of what pain means may prevent some adults from taking action.
Older adult	• May perceive pain as part of the aging process. • May have decreased sensations or perceptions of the pain. • Lethargy, anorexia, and fatigue may be indicators of pain. • May withhold complaints of pain because of fear of the treatment, of any lifestyle changes that may be involved, or of becoming dependent. • May describe pain differently, that is, as *ache*, *hurt*, or *discomfort*. • May consider it unacceptable to admit or show pain.

Environment and Support People

A strange environment such as a hospital, with its noises, lights, and activity, can compound pain. In addition, the lonely person who is without a support network may perceive pain as severe, whereas the person who has supportive people around may perceive less pain. Some people prefer to withdraw when they are in pain, whereas others prefer the distraction of people and activity around them. Family caregivers can be a significant support for a person in pain. With the increase in outpatient and home care, families are assuming an increased responsibility for the management of pain.

Past Pain Experiences

Previous pain experiences alter a client's sensitivity to pain. People who have personally experienced pain or who have been exposed to the suffering of someone close are often more threatened by anticipated pain than people without a pain experience. In addition, the success or lack of success of pain relief measures influences a person's expectations for relief. For example, a person who has tried several pain relief measures without success may have little hope about the helpfulness of nursing interventions.

Meaning of Pain

Some clients may accept pain more readily than others depending on the circumstances and the client's interpretation of its significance. A client who associates the pain with a positive outcome may withstand the pain amazingly well. For example, a woman giving birth to a child or an athlete undergoing knee surgery to prolong his career may tolerate pain better because of the benefit associated with it. These clients may view the pain as a temporary inconvenience rather than a potential threat or disruption to daily life.

By contrast, clients with unrelenting chronic pain may suffer more intensely. They may respond with despair, anxiety, and depression because they cannot attach a positive significance or purpose to the pain. In this situation, the pain may be looked upon as a threat to body image or lifestyle and as a sign of possible impending death.

Anxiety and Stress

Anxiety often accompanies pain. Threat of the unknown and the inability to control the pain or the events surrounding it often augment the pain perception. Fatigue also reduces a person's ability to cope, thereby increasing pain perception. When pain interferes with sleep, fatigue and muscle tension often result and increase the pain; thus, a cycle of pain, fatigue, and pain develops. People in pain who believe that they have control of their pain have decreased fear and anxiety that decreases their pain perception. A perception of lacking control or a sense of helplessness tends to increase pain perception.

Barriers to Pain Management

Misconceptions and biases can affect pain management. Some of these involve attitudes of the nurse or the client as well as knowledge deficits. Clients respond to pain experiences based on their culture, personal experiences, and the meaning the pain has for them. For many people, pain is expected and accepted as a normal aspect of illness. Clients and families may lack knowledge of the adverse effects of pain and may have misinformation regarding the use of analgesics. Other common misconceptions are shown in Table 14-3.

TABLE 14-3	COMMON MISCONCEPTIONS ABOUT PAIN
Misconception	**Correction**
Clients experience severe pain only when they have had major surgery.	Even after minor surgery, clients can experience intense pain.
The nurse or other health care professionals are the authorities about a client's pain.	The person who experiences the pain is the only authority about its existence and nature.
Administering analgesics regularly for pain will lead to addiction.	Clients are unlikely to become addicted to an analgesic provided to treat pain.
The amount of tissue damage is directly related to the amount of pain.	Pain is a subjective experience, and the intensity and duration of pain vary considerably among individuals.
Visible physiologic or behavioral signs accompany pain and can be used to verify its existence.	Even with severe pain, periods of physiologic and behavioral adaptation can occur.

From *Fundamentals of nursing: Concepts, process, and practice*, 6th ed., by B. Kozier, G. Erb, A. Berman, & K. Burke, 2000, Upper Saddle River, NJ: Prentice Hall Health.

Key Factors in Pain Management

Acknowledging and Accepting

Basic to all strategies for reducing pain is that nurses convey to clients that they believe the client is having pain. Good communication and interaction that conveys respect and belief is vital to effective pain management.

Assisting Support Persons

Support persons often need assistance to respond positively to the client experiencing pain. Nurses can help by giving them accurate information about the pain and providing opportunities for them to discuss their emotional reactions that may include anger, fear, frustration, and feelings of inadequacy. Enlisting the aid of support persons in the provision of pain relief to the client, such as massaging the client's back, may diminish their feelings of helplessness and foster a more positive attitude toward the client's pain experience.

Reducing Misconceptions About Pain

Reducing a client's misconceptions about the pain and its treatment will often avoid intensifying the pain. The nurse should explain to the client that pain is a highly individual experience and that it is only the client who really experiences the pain, although others can understand and empathize.

Reducing Fear and Anxiety

It is important to help relieve the emotional component, that is, anxiety or fear associated with the pain. When clients have no opportunity to talk about their pain and associated fears, their perceptions and reactions to the pain can be intensified. The client may become angry or complain about the nurse's care when the problem really is a belief that the pain is not being attended to. If the nurse is honest and sincere and promptly attends to the client's needs, the client is much more likely to know that the nurse does believe the client is in pain.

By providing accurate information, the nurse can also reduce many of the client's fears, such as fear of addiction or a fear that the pain will always be present. It also helps many clients to have privacy when they are experiencing pain.

Preventing Pain

A preventive approach to pain management involves the provision of measures to treat the pain before it occurs or before it is severe. **Preemptive analgesia** is the administration of analgesics prior to an invasive or operative procedure. Painful procedures can be yet another physical insult to clients who may already be compromised. Pasero (1998) recommends that if there is any question about whether a procedure is painful, the clinicians must assume that it is and provide analgesia. Another example of a preemptive approach to pain management is when nurses provide analgesics around the clock (ATC) rather than as needed (PRN).

Pain Assessment

Accurate pain assessment is essential for effective pain management. Because pain is subjective and experienced uniquely by each individual, nurses need to assess all factors affecting the pain experience—physiological, psychologic, behavioral, emotional, and sociocultural.

The extent and frequency of the pain assessment varies according to the situation. For clients experiencing acute or severe pain, the nurse may focus only on location, quality, severity, and early intervention. Clients with less severe or chronic pain can usually provide a more detailed description of the experience. Frequency of pain assessment usually depends on the pain control measures being used and the clinical circumstances. For example, in the initial postoperative period, pain is often assessed whenever vital signs are taken, which may be as often as every 15 minutes and then extended to every 2 to 4 hours.

Because it has been found that many people will not voice their pain unless asked about it, the nurse *must* initiate pain assessments. Some of the many reasons clients may be reluctant to report pain are listed in Box 14-1.

Pain assessments consist of two major components: (1) a pain history to obtain facts from the client and (2) direct observation of behavioral and physiologic responses of the client. The goal of assessment is to gain an objective understanding of a subjective experience.

Pain History

While taking pain histories, the nurse must provide an opportunity for clients to express in their own words how they view the pain and the situation. This will help the nurse understand what the pain means to the client and how the client is coping with the pain. Remember that each person's pain experience is unique and that the client is the best interpreter of the pain experience. This history should be geared to the specific client: for example, questions asked of an accident victim would be different from those asked of a postoperative client or one suffering from chronic pain. The initial pain assessment for someone in severe acute pain may consist of only a few questions before intervention occurs. In contrast, for the person with chronic pain, the nurse may ask more questions focusing on the client's coping mechanisms, effective-

Box 14-1 *Why Clients May Be Reluctant to Report Pain*

- Unwillingness to trouble staff who are perceived as busy
- Fear of the injectable route of analgesic administration—children in particular
- Belief that pain is to be expected as part of the recovery process
- Belief that pain is a normal part of aging or a necessary part of life—older adults in particular
- Difficulty expressing personal discomfort

- Concern about risks associated with opioid drugs (e.g., addiction)
- Fear about the cause of pain or that reporting pain will lead to further tests and expenses
- Concern about unwanted side effects, especially of opioid drugs
- Concern that use of drugs now will render the drug inefficient if or when the pain becomes worse

From *Fundamentals of nursing: Concepts, process, and practice,* 6th ed., by B. Kozier, G. Erb, A. Berman, & K. Burke, 2000, Upper Saddle River, NJ: Prentice Hall Health.

ness of current pain management, and ways in which the pain has affected activities of daily living (ADL).

Data that should be obtained in a comprehensive pain history include pain location, intensity, quality, patterns, precipitating factors, alleviating factors, associated symptoms, effect on ADL, past pain experiences, meaning of the pain to the person, coping resources, and affective responses.

Location

To ascertain the specific location of the pain, ask the individual to point to the site of the discomfort. A chart consisting of drawings of the body can assist in identifying pain locations. The client marks the location of pain on the chart. This tool can be especially effective with clients who have more than one source of pain.

Pain Intensity or Rating Scales

The single most important indicator of the intensity of pain is the *client's* report of pain. Studies have shown that health care providers may underrate or overrate the client's pain intensity. The inaccuracy of the nurse's rating of a client's pain tends to be even greater when the pain is severe (Pasero, 1996). In contrast, the use of pain intensity scales is an easy and reliable method of determining the client's pain intensity. Such scales provide consistency for nurses to communicate with the client and other health care providers. Most scales use either a 0 to 5 or 0 to 10 range with 0 indicating "no pain" and the highest number indicating the "worst pain possible" for that individual. A 10-point rating scale is shown in Figure 14-2 ◆. The inclusion of word modifiers on the scale can assist some clients who find it difficult to apply a number level to their pain. The client is asked to indicate the scale point that best represents the pain intensity. The American Pain Society suggests that pain become the fifth vital sign, that is, the nurse make pain intensity rating a part of the assessment and documentation of the client's vital signs (McCaffery & Pasero, 1999).

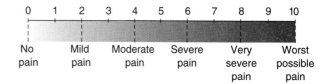

FIGURE 14-2 ◆ A 10-point pain intensity scale with word modifiers.

Not all clients can understand or relate to numerical pain intensity scales. These include children who are unable to communicate discomfort verbally, elderly clients with impairments in cognition or communication, and people who do not speak English. For these clients, the Wong-Baker FACES Pain Rating Scale (Figure 14-3 ◆) may be easier to use (Pasero, 1997b). The face scale includes a number scale in relation to each expression so that the pain intensity can be documented. When it is not possible to use any kind of rating scale with a client, the nurse must rely on observation of behavior and any physiologic signs. The input of the client's significant others, such as parents or caregivers, can assist the nurse in interpreting the observations.

For effective use of pain rating scales, clients need to not only understand the use of the scale but also be educated about how the information will be used to determine changes in their condition and the effectiveness of pain management interventions. This will ensure that adequate pain management is achieved (Pasero, 1997a).

Pain Quality

Descriptive adjectives help people communicate the quality of pain. Some of the terms commonly used to describe pain are listed in Table 14-4. Nurses need to record the *exact* words clients use to describe pain. A client's words are more accurate and descriptive than an interpretation in the nurse's words.

Pattern

The pattern of pain includes time of onset, duration, and recurrence or intervals without pain. The nurse

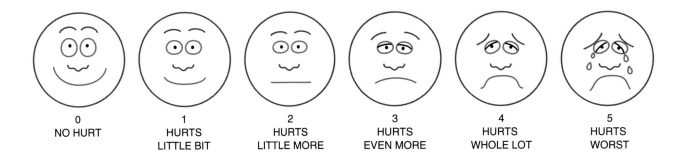

	0	1	2	3	4	5
	NO HURT	HURTS LITTLE BIT	HURTS LITTLE MORE	HURTS EVEN MORE	HURTS WHOLE LOT	HURTS WORST

Explain to the person that each face is for a person who feels happy because he has no pain (hurt) or sad because he has some or a lot of pain. Face 0 is very happy because he doesn't hurt at all. Face 1 hurts just a little bit. Face 2 hurts a little more. Face 3 hurts even more. Face 4 hurts a whole lot. Face 5 hurts as much as you can imagine, although you don't have to be crying to feel this bad. Ask the person to choose the face that best describes how he is feeling.

Rating scale is recommended for persons age 3 years and older.

Brief word instructions: Point to each face using the words to describe the pain intensity. Ask the child to choose face that best describes own pain and record the appropriate number.

FIGURE 14-3 ◆ The Wong-Baker FACES Rating Scale

From Wong DL, Hockenberry-Eaton M, Wilson D, Winkelstein ML, Schwartz P: *Wong's Essentials of Pediatric Nursing, 6/e*, St. Louis, 2001, P. 1301. Copyrighted by Mosby, Inc. Reprinted by permission.

TABLE 14-4	COMMONLY USED PAIN DESCRIPTORS	
Term	**Sensory Words**	**Affective Words**
Pain	searing	unbearable
	scalding	killing
	sharp	intense
	piercing	torturing
	drilling	agonizing
	wrenching	terrifying
	shooting	exhausting
	burning	suffocating
	crushing	frightful
	penetrating	punishing
		miserable
Hurt	hurting	
	pricking	heavy
	pressing	throbbing
	tender	
Ache	numb	annoying
	cold	nagging
	flickering	tiring
	radiating	troublesome
	dull	gnawing
	sore	uncomfortable
	aching	sickening
	cramping	tender

therefore determines when the pain began, how long the pain lasts, whether it recurs and, if so, the length of the interval without pain and when the pain last occurred.

Precipitating Factors

Certain activities sometimes precede pain. For example, physical exertion may precede chest pain or abdominal pain may occur after eating. Environmental factors such as extreme cold or heat and extremes of humidity can affect some types of pain. Physical and emotional stressors can also precipitate pain.

Alleviating Factors

Nurses must ask clients to describe anything that they have done to help alleviate the pain (e.g., home remedies, rest, over-the-counter medications, heat, cold, prayer, or distractions like TV). It is important to explore the effect any of these measures had on the pain, whether relief was obtained or whether the pain became worse.

Associated Symptoms

Also included in the clinical appraisal of pain are other associated symptoms, such as nausea, vomiting, dizziness, and diarrhea. These symptoms may relate to the onset of the pain or they may result from the presence of the pain.

Behavioral and Physiologic Responses

There are wide variations in nonverbal responses to pain (see Box 14-2). For clients who are very young, aphasic, confused, or disoriented, nonverbal expres-

- Clenched teeth
- Tightly shut eyes
- Biting of lower lip
- Facial grimaces
- Moaning, groaning
- Whimpering
- Crying
- Screaming
- Immobilization of body
- Guarding a part of the body
- Restlessness, tossing, turning
- Rhythmic body movements
- Rubbing a part of the body
- Supporting the affected part

sions may be the only means of communicating pain. Facial expression is often the first indication of pain, and it may be the only one. It is important to note that behavioral responses can be controlled and so may not be very revealing. When pain is chronic, there are rarely overt behavioral responses as the individual develops personal coping styles for dealing with pain, discomfort, or suffering.

Physiologic responses vary with the origin and duration of the pain. Early in the onset of acute pain the sympathetic nervous system is stimulated resulting in increased blood pressure, pulse rate, respiratory rate, pallor, diaphoresis, and pupil dilation. The body does not sustain the increased sympathetic function over a prolonged period of time and, therefore, the sympathetic nervous system adapts making the physiologic responses less evident or even absent. Physiologic responses are most likely to be absent in people with chronic pain because of central nervous system (CNS) adaptation. Thus, it is important that the nurse assess more than only physiologic responses, as they may be poor indicators of pain.

Affective Responses

Affective responses vary according to the situation, the degree and duration of pain, the interpretation of it, and many other factors. The nurse needs to explore the client's feelings, for example, anxiety, fear, exhaustion, depression, or a sense of failure. Because many people with chronic pain become depressed and potentially suicidal, it may also be necessary to assess the client's suicide risk.

Effect on Activities of Daily Living

Knowing how ADL are affected by chronic pain helps the nurse understand the client's perspective on the pain's severity. The nurse asks the client to describe how the pain has affected the following aspects of life: sleep, appetite, concentration, work/school, interpersonal relationships, marital relationship/sex, home activities, driving/walking, leisure activities, and emotional status.

Coping Resources

Each individual will exhibit personal ways of coping with pain. Strategies may relate to past pain experiences or the specific meaning of the pain; some may reflect religious or cultural influences. Nurses can encourage and support the client's use of methods known to have helped in modifying pain. Strategies may include use of distraction, prayer or other religious practices, and support from significant others.

PLANNING

Delegation

The nurse is responsible for the initial and regular reassessment of pain. After the assessment and in collaboration with the client, the nurse can discuss and delegate the performance of appropriate comfort measures to the unlicensed assistive personnel (UAP). For example, the UAP may reposition the client at regular intervals, give the client a back massage, or provide rest periods. Emphasize the importance of the UAP's reporting any changes in the client's pain to the nurse.

IMPLEMENTATION:
TECHNIQUE 14-1 ASSESSING THE CLIENT IN PAIN

Equipment

- Pain Assessment Flow Sheet (Figure 14-4 ◆)
- Pain Rating Scale

Preparation

Identify those factors that may cause the client to be in pain. For example, does the client have a prior his-

tory of low back pain or diabetic neuropathy? Has the client had a major surgical procedure? Has the client experienced recent trauma? Note the client's baseline vital signs.

Performance

1. Explain to the client what you are going to do, why it is necessary, and how he or she can cooper-

Sunshine Hospital and Medical Center & Sunrise Children's Hospital
Pain Management Flow Sheet

SR-1420 (6/00)

* **Monitoring Guidelines outlined on back of form**

Patient's stated pain level goal: _____

Mode of Administration

A - PO opioid and nonopioid medications
B - PCA Infuser Basal with Patient Control
C - Continuous Infusion
D - Epidural Infuser Continuous Basal Only
E - Epidural Infuser Basal & Patient Control
F - Intermittent IV/IM Injection
G - Transdermal opioids
H - On-Q Pump
I - Per Rectum

Level of Pain Assessment Scales

Faces Pain Rating Scale

0 .... 2 .... 4 .... 6 .... 8 10

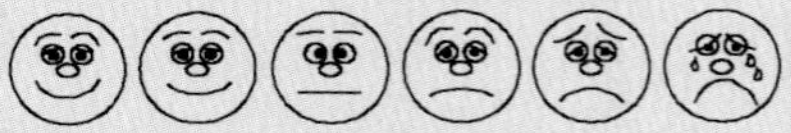

1 - 10 Pain Scale

0 ----------------- 10

No pain or pain relieved   Worst pain imaginable

0 - 10 Sum Scale

A. Vocal   C. Facial
0 = Positive/ETT   0 = Smiling
1 = Whimpers   1 = Neutral
2 = Crying   2 = Frown/grimace
3 = Screaming   3 = Clenched teeth

B. Body Movement   D. Touching (localizing)
0 = Moves easily   0 = No touching
1 = Neutral shifting   1 = Reaching/patting
2 = Tense/flailing limbs   2 = Grabbing

Location of Pain:

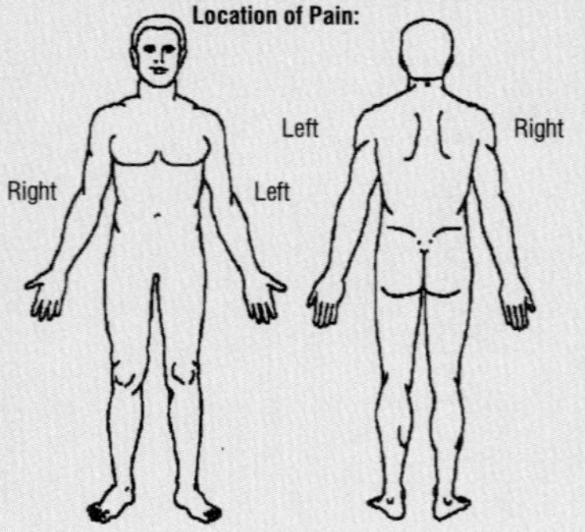

Right   Left   Left   Right

A = No pain
B-Z = Use letters to mark location of pain on graph

Frequency of Pain:
0 = Occasional   F = Frequent   C = Constant

Type of Pain:
A = Burning   D = Sharp   G = Isolated
B = Stabbing   E = Shooting   H = Other
C = Radiating   F = Dull

Arousal Score:
0 = Alert   1 = Medically sedated / ETT
2 = Drowsy   3 = Somnolent
                   4 = Asleep

Non-Pharmacologic Interventionsl
C = Cold   P = Pacifier
D = Distraction   PO = Positioning
H = Heat   R = Relaxation
HO = Holding   RO = Rocking
I = Imagery   S = Security Object
M = Massage   T = Tens Unit
MU = Music   O = Other

Analgesia Order:
1 = Increase in dosage/rate
2 = Decrease in doseage/rate
3 = Extra bolus
4 = PRN medication for break-through pain
5 = Discontinue

Reason for Analgesia Order:
1 = Unrelieved pain
2 = Decreased arousal/neuro score
3 = Side effects (See below)
4 = Discontinue therapy/change to oral route
5 = Adverse drug reactions
(Document all adverse drug reactions in Nsg
notes and complete an ADR report)

Side Effects: 0 = None
A = Anxiety   N = Nausea
C = Confused   R = Respiratory Depression
Co = Constipation   U = Urinary Retention
I = Itching   V = Vomiting

Sensory Function   Epidural Only
0 = Moves all extremities well
1 = Unable to move all extremities well

Motor Function   Epidural Only
0 = Able to feel tactile pressure
1 = Unable to feel tactile pressure

Neuro Score: Epidural Only
0 = No numbness, no weakness
1 = Medically sedated / ETT
2 = Numbness without weakness
3 = Numbness and weakness

Catheter Site: Epidural Only
1 = No redness, drainage, inflammation or swelling
2 = Red, inflamed
3 = Visable clear drainage
4 = Visable purulent drainage
5 = Visable serosanguinous/sanguinous drainage
6 = Swelling

Catheter Integrity Upon Removal: Epidural Only
1 = Catheter tip visually intact
2 = Catheter NOT visually intact - See Nsg Notes

Date
Time
Initials
Mode of Admin
Level of Pain
Location of Pain
Frequency of Pain
Type of Pain
Arousal Score
Non-Pharm. Intervent.
Analgesia Order
Reason for Order
Side Effects
Adverse Effects (Y/N)
Sensory Function   Epidural Only
Motor Function   Epidural Only
Neuro Score   Epidural Only
Catheter Site   Epidural Only
Cath Integrity   Epidural Only
O2 Saturation
Respirations
Pulse
Blood Pressure
See Nursing Notes   (Y / N)

Initials   Signature

Patient Identification Label

FIGURE 14-4 ◆ Pain Management Flow Sheet.

ate. Discuss how the results will be used in planning further care or treatments.

2. Wash hands and observe other appropriate infection control procedures.

3. Provide for client privacy.

4. Assess client's perception of pain. For clients experiencing acute or severe pain, the nurse may focus on the first three assessments and follow with an intervention. Clients with less severe or chronic pain can usually provide a more detailed description and the nurse can obtain a comprehensive pain assessment.

   - *Location.* Ask the client to place a mark on the figure on the form, if appropriate. If there is more than one area of pain, use letters (e.g., A, B, C) to differentiate between the various sites. If the client is unable or unwilling to mark the figure, ask the client to tell you where the pain is located. Follow up by asking the client to point to the painful site with one finger. *This will help verify if the verbal description and the location are the same.*

   - *Intensity.* Ask the client to rate the pain using the appropriate scale per agency policy.

   - *Quality.* Ask the client, "What words would you use to describe your pain?" *Although this question may be difficult for the client to answer, the assessment is most accurate when the client provides the description.*

   - *Onset, duration, and recurrence.* This assessment can include such questions as, "How long have you been having pain?" "Have you noticed any activity (e.g., swallowing, eating, stress, urinating, exertion) that causes the pain or increases the pain?" "How long does the pain last?" "How often does the pain occur?" "Is the pain better or worse at certain times of the day or night?"

   - *Manner of expressing pain.* Observe for behavioral cues such as grimacing, crying, or a change in body posture. *Learning how a client expresses pain is particularly important for the client who cannot communicate or is very young or unable to hear.*

   - *Precipitating factors.* Ask what causes or increases the pain. *Knowledge of those activities can both help prevent the pain from occurring and, sometimes, help determine the cause.*

   - *Alleviating factors.* Ask questions such as: "What makes the pain go away or lessen?" "What methods of relief have you tried?" "How long did you use them?" "How effective were they?" *Asking these questions can assist the nurse and the client to determine if some of the methods (such as listening to music or relaxation) can continue while at the health care facility.*

   - *Associated symptoms.* Ask if there are any other symptoms (e.g., nausea, vomiting, dizziness) that occur prior to, with, or after the pain. *These symptoms may relate to the onset of the pain or may result from the presence of the pain.*

   - *Effects of pain.* Explore the client's feelings and the effect the pain has on his or her life. This is particularly important for the client with chronic pain. *Assessing the areas of sleep, appetite, physical activity, relationships, emotions, and concentration provides the nurse with information about the level of the client's functioning on a daily basis.*

   - *Other comments.* Ask if there is any other information that would be helpful for the doctors and nurses to know. Emphasize that you want to work with the client and family to get the best control of the pain.

5. Assess physiological response to pain. Note blood pressure, pulse rate, respiratory rate, skin color, and presence of diaphoresis. *Signs of sympathetic nervous system stimulation (flight or fight) may be present with acute pain, however, clients with chronic pain may not have physical signs because of CNS adaptation.*

6. Assess affected body part, if appropriate. *Additional assessment may provide additional information about the pain and possible intervention.*

 7. **Document** findings of the pain assessment and include the intervention(s) and the client's response to the interventions. *Thorough assessment and documentation assists the nurse to gain insights into the nature and pattern of the client's pain and ensures continuity of care.*

Variation: Daily Pain Diary

For clients who experience chronic pain, a daily diary may help the client and nurse identify pain patterns and factors that exacerbate or mediate the pain experience. In home care, the family or other caregiver can be taught to complete the diary. The record can include:

- Time or onset of pain
- Activity before pain
- Pain-related positions or behaviors
- Pain intensity level
- Use of analgesics or other relief measures
- Duration of pain
- Time spent in relief activities

Recorded data can provide the basis for developing or modifying the plan of care.

AMBULATORY AND COMMUNITY SETTINGS

Pain Assessment

Home Care Assessment includes the following:

Client

- *Level of knowledge:* Pharmacologic and nonpharmacologic pain relief measures selected; adverse effects and measures to counteract these effects; warning signs to report to health care provider.
- *Self-care abilities for analgesic administration:* Ability to use analgesics appropriately; physical dexterity to take pills or to administer intravenous medications and to store medications safely; and ability to obtain prescriptions or over-the-counter medications at the pharmacy.

Family

- *Caregiver availability, skills, and willingness:* Primary and secondary persons able and willing to assist

with pain management; shopping if the client has restricted activity; ability to comprehend selected therapies (e.g., infusion pumps, imagery, massage, positioning, and relaxation techniques) and perform them or assist the client with them as needed.
- *Family role changes and coping:* Effect on financial status, parenting and spousal roles, sexuality, social roles.

Community

- *Resources:* Availability of and familiarity with resources such as supplies, home health aid, or financial assistance.

EVALUATION

- Conduct appropriate follow-up assessments to determine the effectiveness of the pain management intervention. Include the response of the client, the changes in the pain, and the client's perceptions of the effectiveness of the therapy.
- Relate findings to previous assessment data if available.
- Report significant deviations from normal to the physician.

Pain Management

Pain management is the alleviation of pain or a reduction in pain to a level of comfort that is acceptable to the client. It includes two basic types of nursing interventions: pharmacologic and nonpharmacologic interventions. Nursing management of pain consists of both independent and collaborative nursing actions. In general, noninvasive measures may be performed as an independent nursing function and administration of analgesic medications requires a physician's order. The decision, however, to administer the prescribed medication is frequently the nurse's and often requires judgment as to the dose to be given and the time of administration.

Generally speaking, a combination of strategies is best for the client in pain. Sometimes, strategies need to be tried and changed until the client obtains effective pain relief.

Pharmacologic Pain Management

Pharmacologic pain management involves the use of opioids (narcotics), nonopioids/NSAIDs (nonsteroidal anti-inflammatory drugs), and adjuvants or coanalgesic drugs.

Opioid analgesics include opium derivatives such as morphine and codeine. **Narcotics** relieve pain and provide a sense of euphoria. When administering any analgesic, the nurse must review side effects. All opioids result in some initial drowsiness when first administered, but with regular administration, this side effect tends to decrease. Opioids also may cause nausea, vomiting, constipation, and respiratory depression and must be used cautiously in clients with respiratory problems. Opioids can be administered by a variety of routes as shown in Box 14-3.

Nonopioids (nonnarcotic analgesics) include **nonsteroidal anti-inflammatory drugs (NSAIDs)** such as aspirin and ibuprofen. They relieve pain by acting on peripheral nerve endings at the injury site and decreasing the level of inflammatory mediators generated at the site of injury. Pharmacologic management of mild to moderate pain should begin with NSAIDs, unless there is a specific contraindication (U.S. Department of Health and Human Services, 1992a, p. 16). For example, NSAIDs are contraindicated in clients with impaired blood clotting and gastrointestinal bleeding or ulcer risk.

Adjuvant analgesics are medications that were developed for uses other than analgesia but have been found to reduce certain types of chronic pain in addi-

Box 14-3 *Routes for Opioid Delivery*

- *Oral:* Preferred because of ease of administration. Duration of action is approximately 4 hours. Long-acting forms with duration of 8 or more hours are also available. Another method of oral opiate delivery is high-concentration liquid morphine that allows clients who can swallow only small amounts to continue taking the drug orally.
- *Nasal:* Has the advantage of rapid action of the medication because of direct absorption through the vascular nasal mucosa.
- *Transdermal:* Delivers a relatively stable plasma drug level and is noninvasive. Can provide drug delivery for up to 72 hours.

- *Rectal:* This route is useful for clients who have difficulty swallowing or nausea and vomiting.
- *Subcutaneous:* A traditional route.
- *Intramuscular:* The least desirable route because of variable absorption, pain involved with administration, and the need to repeat administration every 3 to 4 hours.
- *Intravenous:* Provides rapid and effective pain relief with few side effects. Can be administered by IV bolus or by continuous infusion controlled by the client using a PCA machine at the bedside (see Chapter 28).
- *Intraspinal:* Infusion of opiates into the epidural or intrathecal (subarachnoid) space (see Chapter 28).

tion to their primary action. Mild sedatives or tranquilizers, for example, may help reduce painful muscle spasms as well as reduce anxiety, stress, and tension so that the client can obtain a good night's sleep. Antidepressants are used to treat underlying depression or mood disorders but may also enhance other pain strategies.

Nonpharmacologic Pain Management

Physical Pain Management Strategies

Nonpharmacologic pain management consists of a variety of physical and cognitive–behavioral pain management strategies. Physical interventions include cutaneous stimulation, immobilization, **transcutaneous electrical nerve stimulation (TENS)**, and acupuncture.

See Table 14-5 for additional information regarding nonpharmacologic physical interventions. Technique 14-2 describes how to manage a TENS unit.

Transcutaneous Electrical Nerve Stimulation (TENS)

TENS is a method of applying low-voltage electrical stimulation directly over identified pain areas, at an acupressure point, along peripheral nerve areas that innervate the pain area, or along the spinal column. The TENS unit consists of a portable, battery-operated device with lead wire and electrode pads that are applied to the chosen area of skin (see Figure 14-5 ◆). The purposes of using a TENS unit include: (1) reducing chronic and acute pain, (2) decreasing opioid requirements and reducing the chances of depressed

TABLE 14-5	NONPHARMACOLOGIC PHYSICAL INTERVENTIONS
Physical Intervention	**Comments**
Cutaneous stimulation techniques:	Can provide effective temporary pain relief. It distracts the client and focuses attention on the tactile stimuli, away from the painful sensations, thus reducing pain perception.
• Massage	A comfort measure that can aid relaxation, decrease muscle tension, and may ease anxiety.
• Heat and cold applications	A warm bath, heating pads, ice bags, ice massage, hot or cold compresses, and warm or cold sitz baths in general relieve pain and promote healing of injured tissues.
• Acupressure	A form of healing in which the therapist exerts finger pressure on specific sites. Six hundred fifty-seven designated points can be massaged according to the theory underlying acupressure. These points are similar to those used in acupuncture and shiatsu massage.
• Contralateral stimulation	Stimulating the skin in an area opposite to the painful area (e.g., stimulating the left knee if the pain is in the right knee). The contralateral area may be scratched for itching, massaged for cramps or treated with cold packs or analgesic ointments. This method is useful when the painful area cannot be touched because it is hypersensitive, inaccessible by a cast or bandages, or when the pain is felt in a missing part (phantom pain).
Immobilization	Immobilizing or restricting the movement of a painful body part may help to manage episodes of acute pain. Splints or supportive devices should hold joints in the position of optimal function and should be removed regularly to provide range-of-motion exercises.

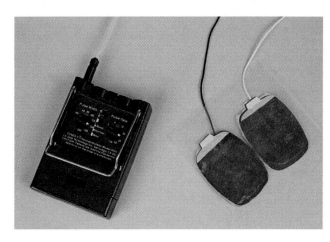

FIGURE 14-5 ◆ A transcutaneous electric nerve stimulator (TENS).

respiratory function from narcotic usage, and (3) facilitating client involvement in managing pain control.

Nursing Process: Transcutaneous Electric Nerve Stimulation (TENS)

ASSESSMENT

Assess the following:

- Client's mental status and ability to follow instructions in using the TENS unit

- Intactness of skin and absence of signs of infection and irritation
- Appearance of incisional area of postoperative client
- Characteristics of pain (intensity, location, associated factors, precipitating factors, and alleviating factors)
- Amount of pain medication required before and during treatment

PLANNING

Before applying a TENS unit, determine the presence of factors contraindicating usage, such as the presence of a cardiac pacemaker, history of dysrhythmias, myocardial ischemia, myocardial infarction, first-trimester pregnancy, confusion, or history of peripheral vascular problems altering neurosensory perception.

Delegation

The assessment for and application of a TENS unit requires specialized knowledge and problem solving. It is important that the nurse understand how this method of pain management works. In an acute care health setting, the nurse would not delegate the skill of managing a TENS unit to UAP. A TENS unit is often ordered for home use and the nurse is responsible for teaching the client or caregiver.

IMPLEMENTATION:

TECHNIQUE 14-2 MANAGING A TRANSCUTANEOUS ELECTRICAL NERVE STIMULATION (TENS) UNIT

Equipment

- TENS Unit
- Bath basin with warm water
- Soap
- Washcloth
- Towel
- Conduction cream, gel, or water (see manufacturer's instructions)
- Hypoallergenic tape

Performance

1. Explain the purpose and application procedure to the client and family. Explain that the TENS unit may not completely eliminate pain but should reduce pain to a level that allows the client to rest more comfortably and/or carry out everyday activities.

2. Wash hands and observe other appropriate infection control procedures.

3. Provide for client privacy.

4. Prepare the equipment.
   - Insert the battery into the TENS unit to test its functioning.
   - With the TENS unit off, plug the lead wires into the battery-operated unit at one end, leaving the electrodes at the other end.

5. Clean the application area.
   - Wash, rinse, and dry the designated area with soap and water. *This reduces skin irritation and facilitates adhesion of the electrodes to the skin for a longer period of time.*

6. Apply the electrodes to the client.
   - If the electrodes are not pregelled, moisten them with a small amount of water or apply conducting gel. (Consult the manufacturer's instructions). *This facilitates electrical conduction.*
   - Place the electrodes on a clean, unbroken skin area. Choose the area according to the location, nature, and origin of the pain.

- Ensure that the electrodes make full surface contact with the skin. Tape all sides evenly with hypoallergenic tape. *This prevents an inadvertent burn.*

7. Turn the unit on.
   - Ascertain that the amplitude control is set at level 0.
   - Slowly increase the intensity of the stimulus (amplitude) until the client notes a slight increase in discomfort.
   - When the client notes discomfort, slowly decrease the amplitude until the client notes a pleasant sensation. Once this has been achieved, keep the TENS unit set at this level to maintain blockage of the pain sensation. Most clients select frequencies between 60 and 100 Hertz.

8. Monitor the client.
   - If the client complains of itching, pricking, or burning, explore the following options:
     a. Turn the pulse-width dial down.
     b. Check that the entire electrode surface is in contact with the skin.
     c. Increase the distance between the electrodes.
     d. Select another type of electrode suitable for the model of TENS unit in use.
     e. Discontinue the TENS and consider the possibility of another brand of TENS.
   - If the sensation of the stimulus is unpleasant, too intense, or distracting, turn down both the amplitude and pulse-width dial.
   - If the client complains of headache or nausea during application or use, turn down both the amplitude and the pulse-width dial.

Repositioning of the electrodes may also be helpful.
   - If further troubleshooting is not effective, discontinue the use of the TENS unit and notify the physician.

9. After the treatment:
   - Turn off the controls and unplug the lead wires from the control box.
   - Clean the electrodes according to the manufacturer's instructions. Clean the client's skin with soap and water.
   - Replace the used battery pack with a charged battery. Begin recharging the used battery.
   - If continuous therapy is used, remove the electrode patches and inspect the skin at least once daily.

10. Provide client teaching.
    - Review instructions for use with the client and verify that the client understands.
    - Have the client demonstrate the use of the TENS unit and verbalize ways to troubleshoot if headache, nausea, or unpleasant sensations occur.
    - Instruct the client not to submerge the unit in water but instead to remove and reapply it after bathing.

11. **Document** all relevant information.
    - Record the date and time TENS therapy was initiated, the location of electrode placement and status of skin in that area, the character and quality of the pain, settings of TENS unit used, and side effects experienced and the client's response.

TENS Unit

TENS units are frequently ordered for home use to relieve chronic pain. Instruct the client or caregiver:
- How to use and care for the TENS equipment.
- How to troubleshoot if side effects or problems occur and who to call if the equipment malfunctions.

- Where and how to obtain supplies needed for the TENS unit.
- To remove the electrodes daily and check for skin breakdown at the electrode sites.

EVALUATION

- Perform a follow-up assessment of the client to determine pain relief or side effects experiences.
- Relate findings to previous assessment data if available.
- Report significant deviations from normal to the physician.

Cognitive–Behavioral Pain Management Strategies

Mind–body (cognitive–behavioral) interventions include distraction activities, relaxation techniques, imagery, meditation, biofeedback, hypnosis, and therapeutic touch. Different types of distractions are shown in Box 14-4. Additionally, Techniques 14-3

Box 14-4 *Types of Distraction*

Visual Distraction
- Reading or watching TV
- Watching a baseball game
- Guided imagery

Tactile Distraction
- Slow, rhythmic breathing
- Massage
- Holding or stroking a pet or toy

Auditory Distraction
- Humor
- Listening to music

Intellectual Distraction
- Crossword puzzles
- Card games (e.g., bridge)
- Hobbies (e.g., stamp collecting, writing a story)

From *Fundamentals of nursing: Concepts, process, and practice*, 6th ed., by B. Kozier, G. Erb, A. Berman, & K. Burke, 2000, Upper Saddle River, NJ: Prentice Hall Health.

(Teaching Progressive Relaxation) and 14-4 (Assisting with Guided Imagery) provide examples of mind–body interventions.

Nursing Process: Cognitive–Behavioral Pain Management Strategies

ASSESSMENT

- Assess the client's willingness to participate in the relaxation or imagery exercises. Note the nature and location of any pain.

- Check the client's vital signs, if appropriate.
- Note any signs of stress being exhibited by the client.

PLANNING

Delegation

Noninvasive pain management techniques can be delegated to UAP if they feel comfortable and/or have experience using the technique. The nurse is responsible for assessing the client's willingness to participate in the relaxation or imagery exercise. The UAP is instructed to report the client's response to the nurse.

IMPLEMENTATION:
TECHNIQUE 14-3 TEACHING PROGRESSIVE RELAXATION

Equipment

- A printed relaxation script that an individual can read until the client learns the technique.
- Tape recorder and tape (optional). The tape recorder could be used to provide the script for the exercise or for the playing of background music.

Preparation

Ensure that the environment is quiet, peaceful, and at a temperature that promotes comfort to the client. *Interruptions or distractions and a room that is too cool interfere with the client's ability to achieve full relaxation.*

Performance

1. Tell the client how **progressive relaxation** works.
   - Provide a rationale for the procedure. *This enables the client to understand how stress affects the body.*
   - Ask the client to identify the stressors operating in the client's life and the reactions to these stressors.

   - Demonstrate the method of tensing and relaxing the muscles. *Demonstration enables the client to understand the complete relaxation procedure clearly.*

2. Wash hands and observe other appropriate infection control procedures.

3. Provide for client privacy.

4. Assist the client to a comfortable position.
   - Ensure that all body parts are supported and the joints slightly flexed with no strain or pull on the muscles (e.g., arms and legs should not be crossed). *Assuming a position of comfort facilitates relaxation.*

5. Encourage the client to rest the mind.
   - Ask the client to gaze slowly around the room (e.g., across the ceiling, down the wall, along a window curtain, around the fabric pattern and back up the wall). *This exercise focuses the mind outside the body and creates a second center of concentration facilitating relaxation.*

6. Instruct the client to tense and then relax each muscle group.
   - Progress through each muscle group in the following order starting with the dominant side:
     a. Hand and forearm
     b. Upper arm
     c. Forehead
     d. Central face
     e. Lower face and jaw
     f. Neck
     g. Chest, shoulders, and upper back
     h. Abdomen
     i. Thigh
     j. Calf muscles
     k. Foot
   - Encourage the client to breathe slowly and deeply during the entire procedure. *Slow, deep breathing facilitates relaxation.*
   - Encourage the client to focus on each muscle group being tensed and relaxed.
   - Speak in a soothing voice that encourages a relaxation and coach the client to focus on each muscle group (e.g., "Make a tight fist," "Clench your fist tightly," "Hold the tension for 5 to 7 seconds," "Let all the tension go," and "Enjoy the feelings as your muscles become relaxed and loose.").

7. Ask the client to state whether any tension remains after all muscle groups have been tensed and relaxed.
   - Repeat the procedure for muscle groups that are not relaxed.

8. Terminate the relaxation exercise slowly by counting backward from 4 to 1.
   - Ask the client to move the body slowly: first the hands and feet, then arms and legs, and finally the head and neck.

 9. **Document** the client's response to the exercise.

Preparation

Provide a comfortable, quiet environment free of distractions. *An environment free of distractions is necessary for the client to focus on the selected image.*

Performance

1. Explain the rationale and benefits of imagery. *The client is an active participant in an imagery exercise and must understand completely what to do and the expected outcomes.*

2. Wash hands and observe other appropriate infection control procedures.

3. Provide for client privacy.

4. Assist the client to a comfortable position.
   - Assist the client to a reclining position and ask the client to close their eyes. *A position of comfort can enhance the client's focus during the imagery exercise.*
   - Use touch only if this does not threaten the client. For some clients, physical touch may be disturbing because of cultural or religious beliefs.

5. Implement actions to induce relaxation.
   - Use the client's preferred name. *During imagery exercise, the client is more likely to respond to the preferred name.*
   - Speak clearly in a calming and neutral tone of voice. *Positive voice coaching can enhance the effect of imagery. A shrill or loud voice can distract the client from the image.*
   - Ask the client to take slow, deep breaths and to relax all muscles.
   - Use progressive relaxation exercises as needed to assist the client to achieve total relaxation (see Technique 14-3).
   - For pain or stress management, encourage the client to "go to a place where you have previously felt very peaceful." For internal imagery, encourage the client to focus on a meaningful image of power and to use it to control the specific problem.

6. Assist the client to elaborate on the description of the image.
   - Ask the client to use all the senses in describing the image and the environment of the image. Sometimes, clients will think only of visual images. *Using all the senses enhances the client's benefit from imagery.*

7. Ask the client to describe the physical and emotional feelings elicited by the image.
   - Direct the client to explore the response to the image as this enables the client to modify the image. Negative responses can be redirected by the nurse to provide a more positive outcome. Positive responses can be enhanced by describing them in detail.

8. Provide the client with continuous feedback.
   - Comment on signs of relaxation and peacefulness.

9. Take the client out of the image.

- Slowly count backward from 5 to 1. Tell the client that they will feel rested when the eyes are opened.
- Remain until the client is alert.

10. Following the experience, discuss the client's feelings about the experience.
    - Identify anything that could enhance the experience.

11. Encourage the client to practice the imagery technique
    - Imagery is a technique that can be done independently by the client once one knows how.

 12. **Document** the client's response to the exercise.

AMBULATORY AND COMMUNITY SETTINGS

Pain Management

- Teach client to keep a pain diary to monitor pain onset, activity before pain, pain intensity, use of analgesics or other relief measures, and so on.
- Instruct client to contact a health care professional if planned pain control measures are ineffective.
- Teach the use of preferred and selected nonpharmacologic techniques such as relaxation, guided imagery, distraction, music therapy, massage, and so on.
- Instruct the client to use pain control measures before the pain becomes severe.
- Inform the client of the effects of untreated pain.
- Provide appropriate information about how to access community resources, home care agencies, and associations that offer self-help groups and educational materials.

AGE-RELATED CONSIDERATIONS

Pain Management

Infant

- Giving an infant, particularly a very-low-birth-weight infant, a water and sucrose solution administered through a pacifier is effective in reducing pain during procedures that may be painful.

Child

- Distract the child with toys, books, or pictures.
- Hold the child to provide comfort.
- Explore misconceptions about pain.
- Children can use their imagination during **guided imagery.** To use the "pain switch," ask the child to imagine a pain switch (even give it a color) and tell them to visualize turning the switch off in the area where there is pain. A "magic glove" or "magic blanket" is an imaginary object that the child applies on areas of the body (e.g., hand, thigh, back, hip) to lessen discomfort.

Elders

- Focus on the client's control in dealing with the pain.
- Spend time with the client and listen carefully.
- Clarify misconceptions. Encourage independence whenever possible.

EVALUATION

- Conduct a follow-up assessment of the client for signs of relaxation and/or decreased pain (e.g., decreased muscle tension; slow, restful breathing; and peaceful affect).
- Determine the client's feelings regarding success or problems with the relaxation technique or the effectiveness of the image selected.
- Relate findings to previous assessment data if available.

Chapter Summary

TERMINOLOGY

acupressure

acute pain

adjuvants

chronic pain

contralateral stimulation

cutaneous pain

cutaneous stimulation

deep somatic pain

epidural

guided imagery

hyperalgesia

intractable pain

intraspinal

narcotics

neuropathic pain

nonopioids

nonsteroidal anti-inflammatory
    drugs (NSAIDs)

opioids

pain reaction

pain sensation

pain threshold

pain tolerance

patient-controlled analgesia (PCA)

phantom pain

preemptive analgesia

progressive relaxation

radiating pain

referred pain

transcutaneous electrical nerve
    stimulation (TENS)

visceral pain

FORMING CLINICAL JUDGMENTS

Consider This:

1. You are caring for two clients, both with the diagnosis of low back pain. One client's low back pain resulted from an on-the-job injury yesterday. He lifted a heavy object without using proper body mechanics. The other client's pain has been bothering him for over 8 months, and there is no known cause despite many medical tests. Describe the differences in your nursing assessment, goals, and nursing interventions.

2. You are a home health nurse visiting a client recently diagnosed with cancer. The client has had a great deal of pain lately. You notice that he yawns a lot during your visit and also that his wife is listless and doesn't follow the conversation that you are having with her husband. What assessments would you include for this family?

3. Describe how you would assess pain intensity for each of the following clients who are experiencing pain:
   • 4-year-old child
   • Teenager
   • 30 year old
   • 82 year old with impaired hearing

4. Some clients grew up hearing the slogan, "Just Say No to Drugs." What are the implications, if any, of this statement on effective pain management?

RELATED RESEARCH

Bergh, I., & Sjostrom, B. (1999). A comparative study of nurses' and elderly patients' ratings of pain and pain tolerance. *Journal of Gerontological Nursing, 25*(5), 30–36.

Coyne, M. L., Reinert, B., Cater, K., Dubuisson, W., Smith, J. F. H., Parker, M. M., & Cantham, C. (1999). Nurses' knowledge of pain assessment, pharmacologic and nonpharmacologic interventions. *Clinical Nursing Research, 8*(2), 153–165.

Jacob, E., & Puntillo, K. A. (1999). A survey of nursing practice in the assessment and management of pain in children. *Pediatric Nursing, 25*(3), 278–286.

Kleiber, C., & Harper, D. C. (1999). Effects of distraction on children's pain and distress during medical procedures: A meta-analysis. *Nursing Research, 48*(1), 44–49.

Stevens, B., Johnston, C., Franck, L., Petryshen, P., Jack, A., & Foster, G. (1999). The efficacy of developmentally sensitive interventions and sucrose for relieving procedural pain in very low birth weight neonates. *Nursing Research, 48*(1), 35–43.

REFERENCES

Andrews, M. M., & Boyle, J. S. (1995). *Transcultural Concepts in Nursing Care* (2nd ed.). Philadelphia: Lippincott.

Chapman, G. F. (1999). Charting tips: Documenting a pain assessment. *Nursing, 29*(11), 25.

Faries, J. (1998). Making a smooth switch from IV analgesia. *Nursing, 28*(7), 26.

Galloway, S., & Turner, L. (1999). Pain assessment in older adults who are cognitively impaired. *Journal of Gerontological Nursing, 25*(7), 34–39.

Hawthorn, J., & Redmond, K. (1998). *Pain Causes and Management.* Oxford: Blackwell Science Ltd.

Kedziera, P. (1998). The two faces of pain. *RN, 61*(2), 45–46.

McCaffery, M. (1999). Understanding your patient's pain tolerance. *Nursing, 29*(12), 17.

McCaffery, M. (1997). Pain management handbook. *Nursing, 27*(4), 42–45.

McCaffery, M., & Ferrell, B. R. (1999). Opioids and pain management: What do nurses know? *Nursing, 29*(3), 48–52.

McCaffery, M., & Pasero, C. (1999). *Pain Clinical Manual* (2nd ed.). St. Louis: Mosby.

Music shown to decrease infant pain. (2000). *Sigma Theta Tau Excellence in Clinical Practice, 1*(3), 2.

Newshan, G. (2000). Pain management in the addicted patient: Practical considerations. *Nursing Outlook, 48*(2), 81–85.

Pasero, C. L. (1999). Teaching patients to use a numerical pain-rating scale. *American Journal of Nursing, 99*(12), 22.

Pasero, C. L. (1998). Talking with patients and families about addiction. *American Journal of Nursing, 98*(3), 18–21.

Pasero, C. L. (1998). Procedural pain management. *American Journal of Nursing, 98*(7), 18–20.

Pasero, C. L. (1997a). Pain ratings: The fifth vital sign. *American Journal of Nursing, 97*(2), 15–16.

Pasero, C. L. (1997b). Using the Faces Scale to assess pain. *American Journal of Nursing, 97*(7), 19–20.

Pasero, C. L. (1996). Mismatch: When nurses rate patients' pain. *American Journal of Nursing, 96*(5), 21.

Strevy, S. R. (1998). Myths and facts about pain. *RN, 61*(2), 42–44.

U.S. Department of Health and Human Services (1992a). *Clinical Practice Guidelines: Acute Pain Management in Adults: Operative Procedures: Quick Reference Guide for Clinicians.* Rockville, MD: Public Health Service Agency for Health Care Policy and Research, Pub. No. 92-0019.

U.S. Department of Health and Human Services (1992b). *Clinical Practice Guidelines: Acute Pain Management in Infants, Children and Adolescents: Operative and Medical Procedures: Quick Reference Guide for Clinicians.* Rockville, MD: Public Health Service Agency for Health Care Policy and Research, Pub. No. 92-0020.

Young, D. M. (1999). Acute pain management protocol. *Journal of Gerontological Nursing, 25*(6), 10–21.

Chapter 15

Feeding Clients

Techniques

OBJECTIVES

- Describe nutrition and malnutrition.
- Identify factors influencing nutrition.
- State types of and reasons for modified diets.
- Describe essential steps involved in assisting clients with meals.
- Describe some aids that enable self-feeding.
- Safely insert and remove a nasogastric tube.
- Administer a nasogastric, gastrostomy, or jejunostomy feeding effectively.
- Obtain essential assessment data before administering tube feedings.

Nutrition

Nutrition is the sum of all the interactions between an organism and the food it consumes. In other words, nutrition is what a person eats and how the body uses it. **Nutrients** are organic, inorganic, and energy-producing substances found in foods and required for body functioning. People require the essential nutrients in foods for the growth and maintenance of all body tissues and the normal functioning of all body processes.

An adequate food intake consists of a balance of essential nutrients: water, carbohydrates, proteins, fats, vitamins, and minerals. Nutrients have three major functions: providing energy for body processes and movement, providing structural material for body tissues, and regulating body processes.

The body's most basic nutrient need is water.

Because every cell requires a continuous supply of fuel, the most urgent nutritional need, after water, is for nutrients that provide fuel or energy. The energy-providing nutrients are carbohydrates, fats, and proteins. Hunger impels people to eat enough energy-providing nutrients to satisfy their energy needs but no clear-cut body signal leads a person to ingest certain vitamins or minerals.

Although the nutritional content of food is an important consideration when planning a diet, an individual's food preferences and habits are often a major factor affecting actual food intake. Habits about eating are influenced by many factors, as described in Table 15-1.

Altered Nutrition

Malnutrition is commonly defined as the lack of necessary or appropriate food substances but in practice

TABLE 15-1	FACTORS AFFECTING NUTRITION
Factor	**Comments**
Development	People in rapid periods of growth (i.e., infancy and adolescence) have increased needs for nutrients.
Gender	Nutrient requirements are different for men and women because of body composition and reproductive functions. The larger muscle mass of men means a greater need for calories and proteins. Because of menstruation, women require more iron then men.
Ethnicity and culture	Ethnicity often determines food preferences. Traditional foods (e.g., rice for Asians, pasta for Italians, curry for Indians) are eaten long after other customs are abandoned. Food preference, however, probably differs as much among individuals of the same cultural background as they do generally between cultures.
Beliefs about food	Beliefs about effects of foods on health and well-being can affect food choices. Many people acquire their beliefs about food from television, magazines, and other media.
Personal preferences	Some adults are very adventuresome and eager to try new foods. Others prefer to eat the same foods over and over again. Preferences in the tastes, smells, flavors (blends of taste and smell), temperatures, colors, shapes, and sizes of food influence a person's food choices.
Religious practices	Some Roman Catholics avoid meat on certain days and some Protestant faiths prohibit meat, tea, coffee, or alcohol. Both Orthodox Judaism and Islam prohibit pork. Orthodox Jews observe kosher customs, eating certain foods only if they are inspected by a rabbi and prepared according to dietary laws.
Lifestyle	Certain lifestyles are linked to food-related behaviors. People who are always in a hurry probably buy convenience grocery items or eat restaurant meals. Individual differences also influence lifestyle patterns (e.g., cooking skills, concern about health).
Medications and therapy	The effects of drugs on nutrition vary considerably. They may alter appetite, disturb taste perception, or interfere with nutrient absorption or excretion.
Health	An individual's health status greatly affects eating habits and nutritional status. The lack of teeth, ill-fitting teeth, or a sore mouth makes chewing food difficult. Difficulty swallowing (dysphagia) due to a painfully inflamed throat or a stricture of the esophagus can prevent a person from obtaining adequate nourishment. Disease processes and surgery of the gastrointestinal tract can affect digestion, absorption, metabolism, and excretion of essential nutrients.
Alcohol abuse	Excessive alcohol use contributes to nutritional deficiencies in a number of ways. Alcohol may replace food in a person's diet, and it can also depress the appetite.
Advertising	Food producers try to persuade people to change from the product they currently use to the brand of the producer.
Psychological factors	Although some people overeat when stressed, depressed, or lonely, others eat very little under the same conditions. Anorexia and weight loss can indicate severe stress or depression.

includes both undernutrition and overnutrition (obesity). **Overnutrition** refers to a caloric intake in excess of daily energy requirements, resulting in storage of energy in the form of increased adipose tissue.

Undernutrition refers to an intake of nutrients insufficient to meet daily energy requirements as a result of inadequate food intake or improper digestion and absorption of food. An inadequate food intake may be caused by the inability to acquire and prepare food, inadequate knowledge about essential nutrients and a balanced diet, discomfort during or after eating, **dysphagia** (difficulty swallowing), **anorexia** (loss of appetite), nausea or vomiting, and so on. Improper digestion and absorption of nutrients may be caused by an adequate production of hormones or enzymes or by medical conditions resulting in inflammation or obstruction of the gastrointestinal tract.

Malnutrition is a major risk for morbidity and mortality among elderly hospital and nursing home clients (Morrisson, 1997, p. 792). More than 50 percent of elderly clients admitted to hospitals and nursing facilities suffer from or are in danger of malnutrition (Holzapfel et al., 1996). Examples of individuals at greater risk include the elderly client who is cognitively impaired or the client with significant dementia who exhibits agitated behaviors at mealtime because of the overwhelming stimuli. Many clients in skilled nursing facilities are dependent on staff assistance for feeding, ranging from verbal direction to total assistance. The role of nutrition cannot be underestimated in its importance to not only optimal physical and cognitive function of clients but also to quality of life. Therefore, assessing and promoting adequate nutrition for clients is an important and vital aspect of nursing care.

Diet Modification

Nursing interventions to promote optimal nutrition for hospitalized clients are often provided in collaboration with the physician, who writes the diet orders, and the dietitian, who informs clients about special diets. The nurse reinforces this instruction and, in addition, creates an atmosphere that encourages eating, provides assistance with eating, monitors the client's appetite and food intake, administers enteral and parenteral feedings, and consults with the physician and dietitian about nutritional problems that arise.

Clients who do not have special needs eat the regular (standard or house) diet, a balanced diet that supplies the metabolic requirements of a sedentary person (about 2,000 kcal). A variation of the regular diet is the **light diet**, designed for postoperative and other clients who are not ready for the regular diet. Foods in the light diet are cooked plainly and fat is usually omitted, as are bran and foods containing a great deal of fiber. Not all agencies provide a light diet.

Diets that are modified in consistency are often given to clients before and after surgery or to promote healing in clients with gastrointestinal distress. See Table 15-2 for a description of these diets.

Many special diets may be prescribed to meet requirements for disease processes or altered metabolism. For example, a client with diabetes mellitus may need a diabetic diet recommended by the National Diabetic Association, an obese client may need a calorie-restricted diet, a cardiac client may need sodium and cholesterol restrictions, and a client with allergies will need a nonallergic diet.

Physical illness, unfamiliar or unpalatable food, environmental and psychological factors, and physi-

TABLE 15-2	TEMPORARY CONSISTENCY DIETS
Diet	**Description**
NPO	Food and fluid are prohibited, for example, before anesthesia to prevent aspiration of stomach contents or after surgery until bowel sounds return.
Clear liquid	Limited to water, tea, coffee, clear broths, ginger ale or other carbonated beverages, strained and clear juices, and plain gelatin. It is a short-term diet (24 to 36 hours) provided for clients after certain surgery or in the acute stages of infection, particularly of the gastrointestinal tract.
Full liquid	Contains only liquids or foods that turn to liquid at body temperature such as ice cream. Clients who have gastrointestinal disturbances or are otherwise unable to tolerate solid or semisolid foods often eat full liquid diets to tolerate solid or semisolid foods.
Soft	Because this diet is easily chewed and digested, it is often ordered for clients who have difficulty chewing and swallowing. The **pureed diet** is a modification of the soft diet in which liquid may be added to the food, which is then blended to a semisolid consistency.
Diet as tolerated (DAT)	This diet is ordered when the client's appetite, ability to eat, and tolerance for certain foods may change. For example, on the first postoperative day a client may be given a clear liquid diet. If no nausea occurs, normal intestinal motility has returned and the client feels like eating, the diet may be advanced to a full liquid, light, or **regular diet.**

• Relieve illness symptoms that depress appetite prior to mealtime; for example, give an analgesic for pain or an antipyretic for a fever or allow rest for fatigue.

• Provide familiar food that the person likes. Often, the relatives of clients are pleased to bring food from home but may need some guidance about special diet requirements.

• Select small portions so as not to discourage the anorexic client.

• Avoid unpleasant or uncomfortable treatments immediately before or after a meal.

• Provide a tidy, clean environment that is free of unpleasant sights and odors. A soiled dressing, a used bedpan, an uncovered irrigation set, or even used dishes can negatively affect the appetite.

• Encourage or provide oral hygiene before mealtime. This improves the client's ability to taste.

• Reduce psychologic stress. A lack of understanding of therapy, the anticipation of an operation, and fear of the unknown can cause anorexia. Often, the nurse can help by discussing feelings with the client, giving information and assistance, and allaying fears.

From *Fundamentals of nursing: Concepts, process, and practice*, 6th ed., by B. Kozier, G. Erb, A. Berman, & K. Burke, 2000, Upper Saddle River, NJ: Prentice Hall Health.

cal discomfort or pain may depress the appetites of many clients. A short-term decrease in food intake usually is not a problem for adults. Over time, however, it leads to weight loss, decreased strength and stamina, and other nutritional problems. Stimulating a person's appetite requires the nurse to determine the reason for the lack of appetite and then deal with the problem. See Box 15-1 for interventions to improve a client's appetite.

Assisting Clients with Meals

Because clients in health care agencies are frequently confined to their beds, meals are often brought to the client. The client receives a tray that has been assembled in a central kitchen. Nursing personnel may be responsible for giving out and collecting the trays. In most settings, however, special dietary personnel do this. Long-term facilities and some hospitals serve meals to ambulatory clients in a special dining area.

Four groups of people frequently require help with their meals: older adults who are weakened; the handicapped, such as blind clients; those who must remain in a back-lying position; or those who cannot use their hands. The client's nursing care plan will indicate that assistance is required with meals.

The nurse must be sensitive to clients' feelings of embarrassment, resentment, and loss of autonomy. Whenever possible, the nurse should help incapacitated clients feed themselves rather than feed them. Some clients become depressed because they require help and because they believe they are burdensome to busy nursing personnel. Although feeding a client is time consuming, nurses should try to appear unhurried and convey that they have ample time. Sitting at the bedside, preferably at eye level, is one way to convey this impression.

Although normal utensils should be used whenever possible, special utensils may be needed to assist a client to eat. Many adaptive feeding aids are available to help clients maintain independence. A standard eating utensil with a built-up or widened handle helps clients who cannot grasp objects easily. Collars or bands that prevent the utensil from being dropped can be attached to the end of the handle and fit over the client's hand. Plates with rims and plastic or metal plate guards enable the client to pick up the food by first pushing it against this raised edge. A suction cup or damp sponge or cloth may be placed under the dish to keep it from moving while the client is eating. No-spill mugs and two-handled drinking cups are especially useful for persons with impaired hand coordination. Figures 15-1 ◆ and 15-2 ◆ show some of these aids. Technique 15-1 explains the steps involved in assisting adult clients to eat.

Special mealtime care is required for clients with dementia, cognitive impairment, or medical disorders that put them at risk for aspiration. Often, feeding a client is delegated to unlicensed assistive personnel (UAP). If possible, assigning the same person to feed an individual client can be beneficial in a number of

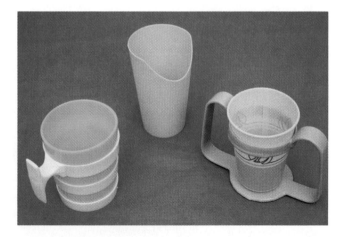

FIGURE 15-1 ◆ Left to right: glass holder, cup with hole for hose, two-handled cup holder.

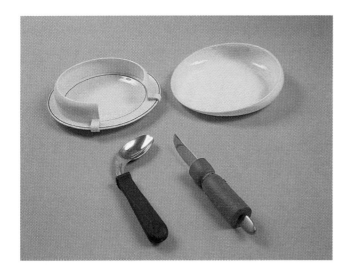

FIGURE 15-2 ◆ Dinner plate with guard attached and lipped plate facilitates scooping; spoon and knife facilitate grip.

ways. The UAP develops a rapport and relationship with the client that may promote better eating through cuing and guidance. The UAP, by knowing the client, would be able to determine if any changes are occurring such as improved appetite, changes in mental status, or signs of swallowing problems such as coughing and choking. For cognitively impaired clients, a helpful strategy is to provide one course at a time and give only those eating utensils that the person can use. By reducing the distractions, the client can focus on eating the meal. Denney (1997) found that playing quiet classical music during mealtime significantly decreased the incidence of agitated behaviors of clients with dementia.

Nursing Process: Assisting Clients with Meals

ASSESSMENT

Assess the client's:

- Self-care abilities for eating and assistance required (note hand coordination, level of consciousness, and visual acuity)
- Appetite for and tolerance of food and fluid
- Need for a special diet
- Food allergies and food likes and dislikes

PLANNING

Confirm the client's diet order.

- Check the client's chart or plan of care for the diet order and to determine whether the client is fasting for laboratory tests or surgery or whether the physician has ordered nothing by mouth (NPO). For clients who are fasting or NPO, ensure that the appropriate signs are placed on either the room door or the client's bed, according to agency practice.
- If there is a change in the type of food the client is to receive, notify the dietary staff.

Delegation

Assisting or feeding a client is often delegated to a UAP. It is, however, the responsibility of the nurse to assess the client's ability to eat and to identify actual or potential risk factors that may impact the client's nutritional status. The nurse must instruct the UAP about strategies that promote the client's nutritional health as well as the importance of the UAP's reporting any unusual or different client behaviors to the nurse.

IMPLEMENTATION:
TECHNIQUE 15-1 ASSISTING AN ADULT TO EAT

Equipment

- Meal tray with the correct food and fluids
- Extra napkin or small towel
- Straw, special drinking cup, weighted glass, or other adaptive feeding aid as required

Preparation

Prepare the client and overbed table.

- Assist the client to the bathroom or onto a bedpan or commode if the client needs to urinate.
- Offer the client assistance in washing the hands prior to a meal. If the client has problems with oral hygiene, brushing the teeth or using a mouthwash

can improve the taste in the mouth and hence the appetite.

- Clear the overbed table so that there is space for the tray. If the client must remain in a lying position in bed, arrange the overbed table close to the bedside so that the client can see the food.

Performance

1. Explain to the client what you are going to do, why it is necessary, and how they can cooperate.

2. Wash hands and observe other appropriate infection control procedures.

3. Provide for client privacy.

4. Position the client and yourself appropriately.

- Assist the client to a comfortable position for eating. Most people sit during a meal; if it is permitted, assist the client to sit in bed (Figure 15-3 ◆) or in a chair.

- If the client is unable to sit, assist the client to a lateral position. *People will swallow more easily in these positions than in a back-lying position.*

- If the client requires assistance with feeding, assume a sitting position, if possible, beside the client. *This conveys a more relaxed presence and encourages the client to eat an adequate meal.*

5. Assist the client as required.

- Check each tray for the client's name, the type of diet, and completeness. If the diet does not seem to be correct, check it against the client's chart. Confirm the client's name by checking the wristband before leaving the tray. Do *not* leave an incorrect diet for a client to eat.

- Encourage the client to eat independently, assisting as needed. Do not take over the feeding process. *Participation by the client enhances feelings of independence.*

- Remove the food covers, butter the bread, pour the drink, and cut the meat, if needed.

- For a blind person, identify the placement of the food as you would describe the time on a clock. For instance, say "The potatoes are at 8 o'clock; the chicken at 12 o'clock and the green beans at 4 o'clock" (Figure 15-4 ◆).

- If the client needs assistance with feeding:

a. Ask in which order the client desires to eat the food.

b. Use normal utensils whenever possible. *Using ordinary utensils enhances self-esteem.*

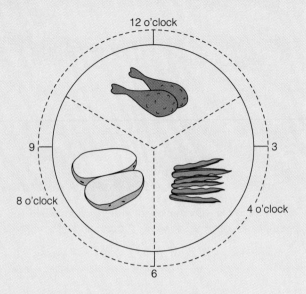

FIGURE 15-4 ◆ The clock system used to describe the location of food on the plate for a blind client.

c. If the client cannot see, tell which food you are giving.

d. Warn the client if the food is hot or cold.

e. Allow ample time for the client to chew and swallow the food before offering more.

f. Provide fluids as requested, or, if the client is unable to tell you, offer fluids after every three or four mouthfuls of solid food.

g. Use a straw or special drinking cup for fluids that would spill from normal containers.

h. Make the time a pleasant one, choosing topics of conversation that are of interest to the client, if the person wants to talk.

6. After the meal, ensure client comfort.

- Assist the client to clean the mouth and hands.

- Reposition the client.

- Replace the food covers and remove the food tray from the bedside.

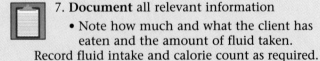

7. **Document** all relevant information

- Note how much and what the client has eaten and the amount of fluid taken. Record fluid intake and calorie count as required.

- If the client is on a special diet or is having problems eating, record the amount of food eaten and any pain, fatigue, or nausea experienced.

- If the client is not eating, notify the nurse in charge so that the diet can be changed or other nursing measures can be taken (e.g., rescheduling the meals, providing small, more frequent meals, or obtaining special self-feeding aids).

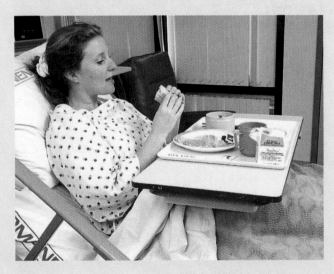

FIGURE 15-3 ◆ A supported sitting position contributes to a client's comfort while eating.

Assisting an Adult to Eat

- Assess the home for adequate facilities to prepare and store food such as a working refrigerator and stove.
- Assess the client's and caregiver's ability to obtain food and prepare meals.
- Evaluate problems that can interfere with eating such as ill-fitting dentures, sore gums, constipation, diarrhea, or a special diet.

- Instruct the caregiver about the importance of regular, nutritious meals and allowing the client to remain independent when possible.
- Provide written guidelines for the client's diet and any special feeding techniques.

Assisting an Adult to Eat

Elders

- Offer fluids frequently to prevent dry mouth. Initially avoid dry foods such as crackers and sticky foods such as bananas. *Saliva production decreases with age.*
- Allow the older client time to eat and offer to rewarm the food if needed. *Hand tremors and arthritic joint changes may slow the eating process for older clients.*

- Observe for dysphagia (difficulty swallowing) and adapt the older client's diet accordingly. *Esophageal nerve degeneration, which often occurs with aging, can affect the ability to swallow.*
- Older clients may need extra seasoning on food. *Aging decreases the ability to taste, especially sweet and salty foods.*

EVALUATION

- Note the client's appetite, tolerance of food and fluids taken, amount of fluid intake, calorie count, if required, any chewing or swallowing difficulties, and the need for any adjustments in food consistency (e.g., minced or pureed foods, need for special feeding aids).
- Relate these findings to previous assessment data if available.
- Report significant deviations from normal to the physician.

Enteral Nutrition

Alternative feeding methods to ensure adequate nutrition include both **enteral** (through the gastrointestinal system) and **parenteral** (intravenous) methods. **Enteral nutrition (EN)**, also referred to as **total enteral nutrition (TEN)**, is provided when the client is unable to ingest foods or the upper gastrointestinal tract is impaired and the transport of food to the small intestine is interrupted. Enteral feedings are administered through nasogastric and small-bore feeding tubes or through gastrostomy or jejunostomy tubes.

Enteral Access Devices

Enteral access is achieved by means of nasogastric or nasoenteric tubes or gastrostomy or jejunostomy tubes.

A **nasogastric tube** is inserted through one of the nostrils, down the nasopharynx, and into the alimentary tract. In some instances, the tube is passed through the mouth and pharynx, although this route may be more uncomfortable for the adult client and cause gagging. This approach is often used for infants, who are obligatory nose breathers (must breathe through the nose), and premature infants, who have no gag reflex.

Traditional firm, **large-bore tubes**, those larger than 12 French (Fr) in diameter, are placed in the stomach. Examples are the Levin tube, a flexible rubber or plastic single-lumen tube with holes near the tip, and the Salem sump tube with a double lumen. The larger tube of the Salem sump tube drains gastric contents; the smaller tube allows for an inflow of atmospheric air, which prevents a vacuum if the gastric tube adheres to the wall of the stomach. Irritation of the gastric mucosa is thereby avoided.

Nasogastric tubes may be inserted for reasons other than providing a route for feeding the client, including: (1) to remove stomach contents for laboratory analysis, (2) to lavage (wash) the stomach in cases of poisoning or overdose of medications, and (3) to prevent nausea, vomiting, and gastric distention following surgery and, in this case, the tube is attached to a suction source.

Nasogastric tubes are used for clients who have intact gag and cough reflexes, who have adequate gastric emptying, and who require short-term feedings. Technique 15-2 provides guidelines for inserting a

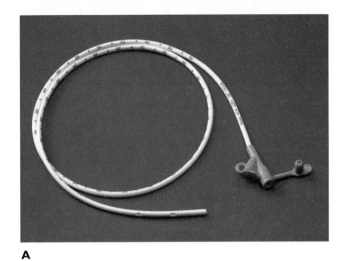

A

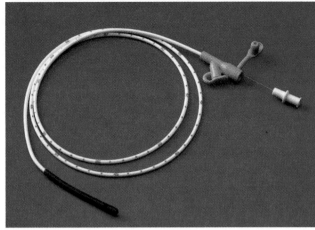

B

FIGURE 15-5 ◆ Nasoenteric feeding tubes. (A) 12F, 36"; (B) 8F, opaque, 45", stylet, weighted tip. Note that both have a Y-port connector to permit irrigation and medication administration without disconnecting feeding device.

nasogastric tube and Technique 15-3 outlines the steps for removing a nasogastric tube.

Nasoenteric tubes are the most common type of enteral device inserted. Softer, more flexible, and less irritating **small-bore tubes**, ranging from 5 to 12 Fr in diameter, are frequently used (Figure 15-5 ◆). Tube lengths vary from 22 to 60 inches. The longer tube length (at least 40 inches for an adult) is needed for passage into the upper small intestine. The tip of the feeding tube may be blunt or tapered and the tube may or may not have a weighted tip. Research varies as to whether the weighted tips facilitate passage into the small bowel and keep the tube in place longer (Lord, 1997). Some tubes may have medication ports in order to administer medications and water flushes without disconnecting the formula from the feeding device. Bedside placement for small bowel feeding tube placement requires specially trained nurses or physicians and a variety of approaches can be used. Nasoenteric tubes are used for clients who are at risk for aspiration.

Gastrostomy and jejunostomy devices are used for long-term nutritional support, generally more than 6 to 8 weeks. Conventional tubes are placed surgically or by laparoscopy through the abdominal wall into the stomach (gastrostomy) or into the jejunum (jejunostomy). See Figure 15-6 ◆ for the various placements for enteral access.

The surgical opening is sutured tightly around the tube or catheter to prevent leakage. Care of this opening before it heals requires surgical asepsis. When the incision heals (10 to 14 days), a low-profile gastrostomy device may be used (Figure 15-7 ◆). This device is flush with the skin and requires an extension tube to connect it to the feeding tubing. After the feeding, the extension tubing is removed and the device is capped off. A one-way valve prevents leakage between the feedings (Lord, 1997, p. 695).

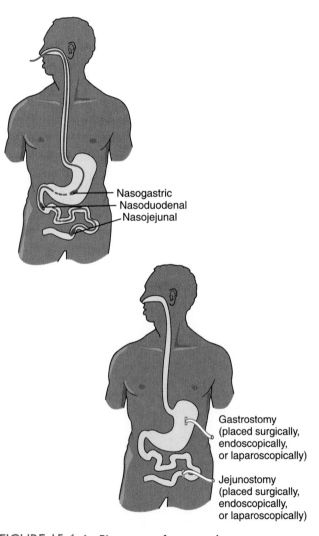

Nasogastric
Nasoduodenal
Nasojejunal

Gastrostomy
(placed surgically,
endoscopically,
or laparoscopically)

Jejunostomy
(placed surgically,
endoscopically,
or laparoscopically)

FIGURE 15-6 ◆ Placements for enteral access.

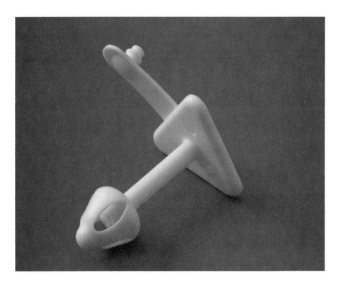

FIGURE 15-7 ◆ Low-profile gastrostomy device.

Increasingly, **percutaneous endoscopic gastrostomy (PEG)** and **percutaneous endoscopic jejunostomy (PEJ)** are being used (see Figures 15-8 ◆ and 15-9 ◆). These procedures do not require general anes-

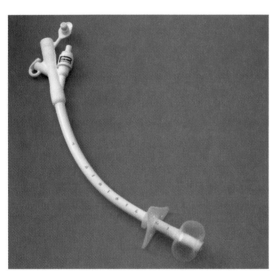

A

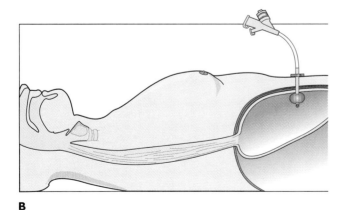

B

FIGURE 15-8 ◆ Percutaneous endoscopic gastrostomy (PEG) tube.

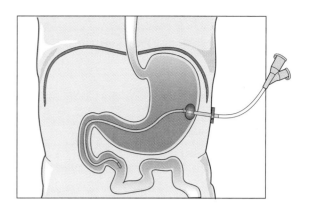

FIGURE 15-9 ◆ Percutaneous endoscopic jejunostomy (PEJ) tube.

thesia or the use of an operating room. PEG or PEJ is usually performed in the endoscopy suite but may also be done in the client's room. Using an endoscope to visualize the inside of the stomach, the physician makes a puncture through the skin and subcutaneous tissues of the abdomen into the stomach and inserts the PEG or PEJ catheter through the puncture. The catheter has internal and external bumpers and an inflatable retention balloon to maintain placement. Once the opening has healed, replacement tubes can be inserted without the use of endoscopy.

Nursing Process: Enteral Nutrition

ASSESSMENT

- Check patency of nares and intactness of nasal tissues. Check for history of nasal surgery or deviated septum.
- Determine presence of gag reflex.
- Assess mental status or ability to cooperate with procedure.

PLANNING

Before inserting a nasogastric tube, determine the size of tube to be inserted and whether or not the tube is to be attached to suction.

Delegation

Insertion of a nasogastric tube is an invasive procedure requiring application of knowledge (e.g., anatomy and physiology, risk factors, etc.) and problem solving. Delegation of this skill to UAP is not appropriate. The UAP, however, can assist with the oral hygiene needs of a client with a nasogastric tube.

Equipment

- Large- or small-bore tube
- Guidewire or stylet for small-bore tube
- Solution basin filled with warm water (if a plastic tube is being used) or ice (if a rubber tube is being used)
- Nonallergenic adhesive tape, 2.5 cm (1 in) wide
- Disposable gloves
- Water-soluble lubricant
- Facial tissues
- Glass of water and drinking straw
- 20- to 50-mL syringe with an adapter
- Basin
- pH test strip or meter
- Stethoscope
- Disposable pad or towel
- Clamp or plug (optional)
- Suction apparatus if required
- Gauze square or plastic specimen bag and elastic band
- Safety pin and elastic band

Preparation

- Assist the client to a high-Fowler's position if his or her health condition permits, and support the head on a pillow. *It is often easier to swallow in this position and gravity helps the passage of the tube.*
- Place a towel or disposable pad across the chest.

Performance

1. Explain to the client what you plan to do. The passage of a gastric tube is not painful, but it is unpleasant because the gag reflex is activated during insertion.

2. Wash hands and observe other appropriate infection control procedures (e.g., disposable gloves).

3. Provide for client privacy.

4. Assess the client's nares.
   - Ask the client to hyperextend the head, and, using a flashlight, observe the intactness of the tissues of the nostrils, including any irritations or abrasions.
   - Examine the nares for any obstructions or deformities by asking the client to breathe through one nostril while occluding the other.
   - Select the nostril that has the greater airflow.

5. Prepare the tube.
   - If a rubber tube is being used, place it on ice for 5 to 10 minutes. *This stiffens the tube, facilitating insertion.* If a plastic tube is being used, place it in warm water until the tube is softer and more flexible. *This facilitates insertion.*
   - If a small-bore tube is being used, insert stylet or guidewire into the tube making sure that it is secured in position. *An improperly positioned stylet or guidewire can traumatize the nasopharynx, esophagus, and stomach.*

6. Determine how far to insert the tube.
   - Use the tube to mark off the distance from the tip of the client's nose to the tip of the earlobe and then from the tip of the earlobe to the tip of the sternum (Figure 15-10 ◆). *This length approximates the distance from the nares to the stomach. This distance varies among individuals.*
   - Mark this length with adhesive tape if the tube does not have markings.

7. Insert the tube.
   - Put on gloves.
   - Lubricate the tip of the tube well with water-soluble lubricant or water to ease insertion. *A water-soluble lubricant dissolves if the tube accidentally enters the lungs. An oil-based lubricant, such as petroleum jelly, will not dissolve and could cause respiratory complications if it enters the lungs.*

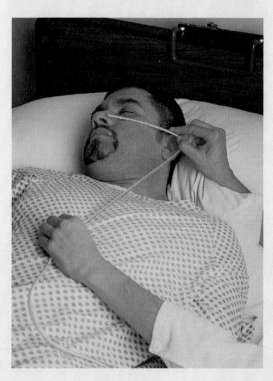

FIGURE 15-10 ◆ Measuring the appropriate length to insert a nasogastric tube.

- Insert the tube, with its natural curve toward the client, into the selected nostril. Ask the client to hyperextend the neck, and gently advance the tube toward the nasopharynx. *Hyperextension of the neck reduces the curvature of the nasopharyngeal junction.*

- Direct the tube along the floor of the nostril and toward the ear on that side. *Directing the tube along the floor avoids the projections (turbinates) along the lateral wall.*

- Slight pressure is sometimes required to pass the tube into the nasopharynx, and some clients' eyes may water at this point. *Tears are a natural body response.* Provide the client with tissues as needed.

- If the tube meets resistance, withdraw it, relubricate it, and insert it in the other nostril. *The tube should never be forced against resistance because of the danger of injury.*

- Once the tube reaches the oropharynx (throat) the client will feel the tube in the throat and may gag and retch. Ask the client to tilt the head forward, and encourage the client to drink and swallow. *Tilting the head forward facilitates passage of the tube into the posterior pharynx and esophagus rather than into the larynx; swallowing moves the epiglottis over the opening to the larynx* (Figure 15-11 ◆).

- If the client gags, stop passing the tube momentarily. Have the client rest, take a few breaths, and take sips of water to calm the gag reflex.

- In cooperation with the client, pass the tube 5 to 10 cm (2 to 4 in) with each swallow, until the indicated length is inserted.

- If the client continues to gag and the tube does not advance with each swallow, withdraw it

slightly, and inspect the throat by looking through the mouth. *The tube may be coiled in the throat.* If so, withdraw it until it is straight, and try again to insert it.

8. Ascertain correct placement of the tube.

- Aspirate stomach contents, and check the pH. *Research indicates that testing pH is a more reliable way to determine location of a feeding tube.*

- Auscultate air insufflation by placing a stethoscope over the client's epigastrium and injecting 10 to 30 mL of air into the tube while listening for a "whooshing" sound. Do not use this method as the primary method for determining placement of the feeding tube *as it is often unreliable.*

- If the signs do not indicate placement in the stomach, advance the tube 5 cm (2 in), and repeat the tests.

- If a small-bore tube is used, leave the stylet or guidewire in place until correct position is verified by x-ray.

9. Secure the tube by taping it to the bridge of the client's nose.

- If the client has oily skin, wipe the nose first with alcohol.

- Cut 7.5 cm (3 in) of tape, and split it lengthwise at one end, leaving a 2.5-cm (1-in) tab at the end.

- Place the tape over the bridge of the client's nose, and bring the split ends either under and around the tubing or, under the tubing and back up over the nose (Figure 15-12 ◆). *Taping in this manner prevents the tube from pressing against and irritating the edge of the nostril.*

10. Attach the tube to a suction source or feeding apparatus as ordered, or clamp the end of the tubing.

- The tube, if inserted preoperatively, is usually clamped or plugged; or it may be covered with a gauze square or plastic specimen bag and an elastic band.

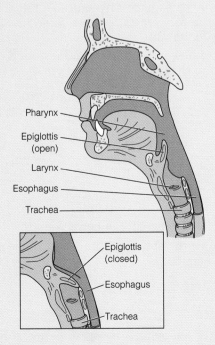

Pharynx

Epiglottis (open)

Larynx

Esophagus

Trachea

Epiglottis (closed)

Esophagus

Trachea

FIGURE 15-11 ◆ Swallowing closes the epiglottis.

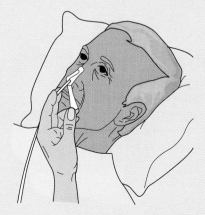

FIGURE 15-12 ◆ Taping a nasogastric tube to the bridge of the nose.

11. Secure the tube to the client's gown.
   - Loop an elastic band around the end of the tubing, and attach the elastic band to the gown with a safety pin.

      or

   - Attach a piece of adhesive tape to the tube, and pin the tape to the gown. *The tube is attached to prevent it from dangling and pulling.*

 12. **Document** relevant information.
   - Document the insertion of the tube, the means by which correct placement was determined, and client responses (e.g., discomfort or abdominal distention).

13. Establish a plan for providing daily nasogastric tube care.
   - Inspect the nostril for discharge and irritation.
   - Clean the nostril and tube with moistened, cotton-tipped applicators.
   - Apply water-soluble lubricant to the nostril if it appears dry or encrusted.

   - Change the adhesive tape as required.
   - Give frequent mouth care. The client may breathe through the mouth and cannot drink.

14 If suction is applied, ensure that the patency of both the nasogastric and suction tubes is maintained.
   - Irrigations of the tube with 30 mL of normal saline may be required at regular intervals. In some agencies, irrigations must be ordered by the physician. Managing gastrointestinal suction and irrigating a nasogastric tube are discussed in Chapter 32.
   - Keep accurate records of the client's fluid intake and output, and record the amount and characteristics of the drainage.
   - Document the type of tube inserted, date and time of tube insertion, type of suction used, color and amount of gastric contents, and the client's tolerance of the procedure.

AGE-RELATED CONSIDERATIONS

Inserting a Nasogastric Tube

Infants and Young Children

- Restraints may be necessary during tube insertion and throughout therapy. *Restraints will prevent accidental dislodging of the tube.*
- Place the infant in an infant seat or position the infant with a rolled towel or pillow under the head and shoulders.
- When assessing the nares, obstruct one of the infant's nares and feel for air passage from the other. If the nasal passageway is very small or is obstructed, an orogastric tube may be more appropriate.

- Measure appropriate nasogastric tube length from the nose to the tip of the earlobe and then to the point midway between the umbilicus and the xiphoid process.
- If an orogastric tube is used, measure from the tip of the earlobe to the corner of the mouth to the xiphoid process.
- Do not hyperextend or hyperflex an infant's neck. *Hyperextension or hyperflexion of the neck could occlude the airway.*
- Tape the tube to the area between the end of the nares and the upper lip as well as to the cheek.

EVALUATION

Conduct appropriate follow-up, such as degree of client comfort, client tolerance of the nasogastric tube, correct placement of nasogastric tube in stomach, client understanding of restrictions, color and amount of gastric contents if attached to suction, or stomach contents aspirated.

Removing a Nasogastric Tube

ASSESSMENT

- Check for the presence of bowel sounds.
- Determine the absence of nausea or vomiting when tube is clamped.

PLANNING

Delegation

The skill of removing a nasogastric tube is not delegated to a UAP.

Equipment

- Disposable pad
- Tissues
- Disposable gloves
- 50-mL syringe (optional)
- Plastic disposable bag

Preparation

- Confirm the physician's order to remove the tube.
- Assist the client to a sitting position if health permits.
- Place the disposable pad across the client's chest to collect any spillage of mucous and gastric secretions from the tube.
- Provide tissues to the client to wipe the nose and mouth after tube removal.

Performance

1. Explain to the client what you are going to do, why it is necessary, and how he or she can cooperate. Explain that the procedure will cause no discomfort.

2. Wash hands and observe other appropriate infection control procedures (e.g., disposable gloves).

3. Provide for client privacy.

4. Detach the tube.
   - Disconnect the nasogastric tube from the suction apparatus, if present.
   - Unpin the tube from the client's gown.
   - Remove the adhesive tape securing the tube to the nose.

5. Remove the nasogastric tube.
   - Put on disposable gloves.

- (Optional) Instill 50 mL of air into the tube. *This clears the tube of any contents such as feeding or gastric drainage.*
- Ask the client to take a deep breath and to hold it. *This closes the glottis, thereby preventing accidental aspiration of any gastric contents.*
- Pinch the tube with the gloved hand. *Pinching the tube prevents any contents inside the tube from draining into the client's throat.*
- Quickly and smoothly withdraw the tube.
- Place the tube in the plastic bag. *Placing the tube immediately into the bag prevents the transference of microorganisms from the tube to other articles or people.*
- Observe the intactness of the tube.

6. Ensure client comfort.
   - Provide mouth care if desired.
   - Assist the client as required to blow the nose. *Excessive secretions may have accumulated in the nasal passages.*

7. Dispose of the equipment appropriately.
   - Place the pad, bag with tube, and gloves in the receptacle designated by the agency. *Correct disposal prevents the transmission of microorganisms.*

8. Assess the nasogastric drainage if suction was used.
   - Measure the amount of gastric drainage and record it on the client's fluid output record.
   - Inspect the drainage for appearance and consistency.

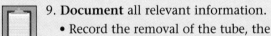 9. **Document** all relevant information.
   - Record the removal of the tube, the amount and appearance of any drainage if connected to suction, and any relevant assessments of the client.

EVALUATION

- Perform a follow-up examination, such as presence of bowel sounds, absence of nausea or vomiting when tube is removed, and intactness of tissues of the nares.
- Relate findings to previous assessment data if available.
- Report significant deviations from normal to the physician.

Testing Feeding Tube Placement

Before feedings are introduced, tube placement is confirmed by radiography, particularly when a small-bore tube has been inserted or when the client is at risk for aspiration. After placement is confirmed, the nurse marks the tube with indelible ink or tape at its exit point from the nose and documents the length of visible tubing for baseline data. The nurse is responsible, however, for verifying tube placement (i.e., gastrointestinal placement versus respiratory placement) before each intermittent feeding and at regular intervals (e.g., at least once per shift) when continuous feedings are being administered.

Methods nurses use to check tube placement include the following:

1. *Aspirate 20 to 30 mL of gastrointestinal secretions.* Small-bore tubes offer more resistance during aspi-

rations than large-bore tubes and are more likely to collapse when negative pressure is applied. An effective method for aspirating fluid from small-bore tubes is outlined in Box 15-2. Gastric secretions tend to be a grassy-green, off-white, or tan color; intestinal fluid is stained with bile and has a golden yellow or brownish-green color.

2. *Measure the pH of aspirated fluid.* This is the recommended method to determine tube placement. Testing the pH of aspirates can help distinguish gastric from respiratory and intestinal placement (Metheny, Wehrle, Wiersema, & Clark, 1998a; Metheny, Smith, Wehrle, Wiersema, & Clark, 1998b; Lord, 1997) as follows:

   • Gastric aspirates tend to be acidic and have a pH of 1 to 4 but may be as high as 6 if the client is receiving medications that control gastric acid.

   • Small intestine aspirates generally have a pH equal to or higher than 6.

   • Respiratory secretions are more alkaline with values of 7 or higher. However, there is a slight possibility of respiratory placement when the pH reading is as low as 6.

   Therefore, when pH readings are 6 or higher, radiographic confirmation of tube location needs to be considered, especially in clients with diminished cough and gag reflexes (Metheny et al., 1998a). Metheny (1998a) cautions nurses to not use test strips designed for testing urine pH as they have a narrower pH range and are not suitable for testing feeding tube placement.

3. *Auscultate the epigastrium while injecting 5 to 20 mL of air.* Air injected into the stomach produces whooshing, gurgling, or bubbling sounds over the epigastrium and the upper left quadrant. Accuracy of this method in predicting placement is less reliable than pH testing and should not be the primary method of determining tube placement (Metheny et al., 1998a; 1998b; Lord, 1997).

   Currently, the most effective method appears to be radiographic verification of tube placement.

Repeated x-ray studies, however, are not feasible in terms of cost and radiation risk. More research is required to devise effective alternatives, especially for placement of small-bore tubes. In the meantime, nurses should (1) ensure initial radiographic verification of small-bore tubes, (2) aspirate contents when possible and check their acidity, (3) closely observe the client for signs of obvious distress, and (4) suspect tube dislodgement after episodes of coughing, sneezing, and vomiting.

Enteral Feeding

The frequency of feedings and amounts to be administered are ordered by the physician. Liquid feeding mixtures are available commercially. Enteral feedings can be given intermittently or continuously. **Intermittent feedings** are the administration of 300 to 500 mL of enteral formula several times per day. The stomach is the preferred site for these feedings, which are usually administered over at least 30 minutes. **Bolus intermittent feedings** are those that use a syringe to deliver the formula into the stomach. Because the formula is delivered rapidly by this method, it is not usually recommended but may be used in long-term situations if the client tolerates them. These feedings must be given only into the stomach and the client must be monitored closely for distention and aspiration.

Continuous feedings are generally administered over a 24-hour period using an infusion pump that guarantees a constant flow rate (Figure 15-13 ◆). Continuous feedings are essential when feedings are administered in the small bowel. They are also used when smaller-bore gastric tubes are in place or when gravity flow is insufficient to instill the feeding.

Cyclic feedings are continuous feedings that are administered in less than 24 hours (e.g., 12 to 16 hours). These feedings, often administered at night and referred to as *nocturnal feedings,* allow the client to attempt to eat regular meals through the day.

Box 15-2 *Aspirating Gastrointestinal Secretions from Small-Bore Tubes*

• Using a 30- to 60-mL syringe, inject 20 mL of air into the tube. This clears the tube of fluid and residual feeding, and moves the tip of the tube away from the mucosal lining.

• Aspirate the air and gastrointestinal fluid. Removing the air prevents gastric distention. Avoid exerting excessive negative pressure when aspirating to prevent tube collapse.

• If fluid *is* aspirated, measure its volume, test its pH, and flush the tube with water to maintain its patency.

• If fluid *is not* aspirated, inject another 20 mL of air and replace the larger syringe with a smaller syringe (e.g.,

10 mL) before attempting to aspirate. The smaller syringe may create less negative pressure and decrease the possibility of tube collapse.

• If still unsuccessful, repeat the above step using the larger syringe to instill air and then attaching the smaller syringe, except this time leave the smaller syringe attached to the tube for 15 minutes before aspirating air and fluid. This allows time for fluid to accumulate.

• Change the client's position from side to side or raise or lower the head of the bed. These actions may make the tube move to an area where fluid has collected.

From *Fundamentals of nursing: Concepts, process, and practice,* 6th ed., by B. Kozier, G. Erb, A. Berman, & K. Burke, 2000, Upper Saddle River, NJ: Prentice Hall Health.

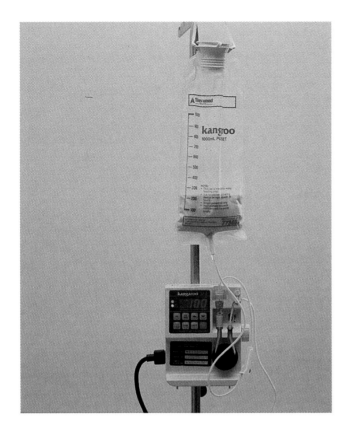

FIGURE 15-13 ◆ An enteric feeding pump.

Enteral feedings are administered to clients through open or closed systems. **Open systems** use an open-top container or a syringe for administration. Enteral feedings for use with open systems are provided in flip-top cans or powdered formulas that are reconstituted with sterile water. Sterile water, rather than tap water, is used to reduce the risk of microbial contamination. **Closed systems** consist of a prefilled container that is spiked with enteral tubing and attached to the enteral access device. Prefilled containers generally have one liter of formula and can hang safely for 24 to 36 hours if sterile technique is used (Lord et al., 1997, p. 407).

Technique 15-4 provides the essential steps involved in administering a tube feeding, and Technique 15-5 indicates the steps involved in administering a gastrostomy or jejunostomy tube feeding.

ASSESSMENT

- Assess for any clinical signs of malnutrition or dehydration.
- Check for allergies to any food in the feeding.
- Assess for the presence of bowel sounds.
- Note any problems that suggest lack of tolerance of previous feedings (e.g., delayed gastric emptying, abdominal distention, dumping syndrome, constipation, or dehydration).

PLANNING

Before commencing a nasogastric or orogastric feeding, determine the type, amount, and frequency of feedings and tolerance of previous feedings.

Delegation

Administering a tube feeding requires application of knowledge and problem solving and it is not usually delegated to UAP. Some agencies, however, may allow a trained UAP to administer a feeding. In this case, it is the responsibility of the nurse to assess tube placement and determine that the tube is patent. The nurse should reinforce major points, such as making sure the client is sitting upright, and instruct the UAP to report any difficulty administering the feeding or any complaints voiced by the client.

IMPLEMENTATION:
TECHNIQUE 15-4 ADMINISTERING A TUBE FEEDING

Equipment

- Correct amount of feeding solution
- 20- to 50-mL syringe with an adapter
- Emesis basin
- Disposable gloves
- Large syringe with plunger or calibrated plastic feeding bag with tubing that can be attached to the feeding tube or prefilled bottle with a drip chamber, tubing, and a flow-regulator clamp
- pH test strip or meter
- Measuring container from which to pour the feeding (if using open system)
- Water (60 mL unless otherwise specified) at room temperature
- Feeding pump as required

Preparation

- Assist the client to a Fowler's position in bed or a sitting position in a chair, the normal position for eating. If a sitting position is contraindicated, a slightly elevated right side-lying position is acceptable. *These positions enhance the gravitational flow of the solution and prevent aspiration of fluid into the lungs.*

Performance

1. Explain to the client what you are going to do, why it is necessary, and how he or she can cooperate. Inform the client that the feeding should not cause any discomfort but may cause a feeling of fullness. For an adult, the usual intermittent feeding will take about 30 minutes; the exact length of time depends largely on the volume of the feeding.

2. Wash hands and observe appropriate infection control procedures (e.g., disposable gloves).

3. Provide privacy for this procedure if the client desires it. Nasogastric or nasoenteric feedings are embarrassing to some people.

4. Assess tube placement.
   - Attach the syringe to the open end of the tube and aspirate alimentary secretions. Check the pH. McConnell (1997b, p. 26) advises (1) allowing 1 hour to elapse before testing the pH if the client has received a medication and (2) using a pH meter rather than pH paper if the client is receiving a continuous feeding or if food coloring has been added to the formula.

5. Assess residual feeding contents.
   - Aspirate all the stomach contents, and measure the amount prior to administering the feeding. *This is done to evaluate absorption of the last feeding, that is, whether undigested formula from a previous feeding remains.*
   - If 100 mL (or more than half the last feeding) is withdrawn, check with the nurse in charge or refer to agency policy before proceeding. The precise amount is usually determined by the physician's order or by agency policy. *At some agencies, a feeding is withheld when the specified amount or more of formula remains in the stomach. In other agencies, the amount withdrawn is subtracted from the total feeding and that volume (less the undigested portion) is administered slowly.*

   or

   - Reinstill the gastric contents into the stomach if this is the agency policy or physician's order. Remove the syringe bulb or plunger, and pour the gastric contents via the syringe into the nasogastric tube. *Removal of the contents could disturb the client's electrolyte balance.*
   - If the client is on a continuous feeding, check the gastric residual every 4 to 6 hours or according to agency protocol.

6. Administer the feeding.
   - Before administering feeding:
   a. Check the expiration date of the feeding.

   b. Warm the feeding to room temperature. *An excessively cold feeding may cause cramps.*
   - When an open system is used, clean the top of the feeding container with alcohol before opening it. *This minimizes the risk of contaminants entering the feeding syringe or feeding bag.*

Feeding Bag (Open System)

- Hang the bag from an infusion pole about 30 cm (12 in) above the tube's point of insertion into the client.
- Clamp the tubing and add the formula to the bag.
- Open the clamp, run the formula through the tubing, and reclamp the tube. *The formula will displace the air in the tubing, thus preventing the instillation of excess air into the client's stomach or intestine.*
- Attach the bag to the nasogastric/nasoenteric tube (Figure 15-14 ◆), and regulate the drip by adjusting the clamp to the drop factor on the bag (e.g., 20 drops/mL).

Syringe (Open System)

- Remove the plunger from the syringe and connect the syringe to a pinched or clamped nasogastric tube. *Pinching or clamping the tube prevents excess air from entering the stomach and causing distention.*
- Add the feeding to the syringe barrel (Figure 15-15 ◆).
- Permit the feeding to flow in slowly at the prescribed rate. Raise or lower the syringe to adjust

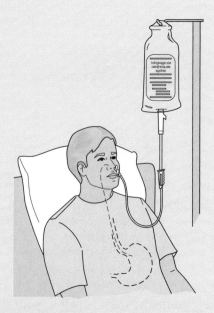

FIGURE 15-14 ◆ Using a calibrated plastic bag to administer a tube feeding.

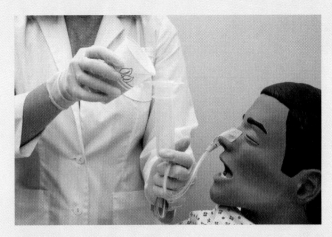

FIGURE 15-15 ◆ Using the barrel of a syringe to administer a tube feeding.

the flow as needed. Pinch or clamp the tubing to stop the flow for a minute if the client experiences discomfort. *Quickly administered feedings can cause flatus, cramps, and/or reflux vomiting.*

Prefilled Bottle with Drip Chamber (Closed System)

- Remove the screw-on cap from the container and attach the administration set with the drip chamber and tubing.
- Close the clamp on the tubing.
- Hang the container on an intravenous pole about 30 cm (12 in) above the tube's insertion point into the client. *At this height, the formula should run at a safe rate into the stomach or intestine.*
- Squeeze the drip chamber to fill it to one-third to one-half of its capacity.
- Open the tubing clamp, run the formula through the tubing, and reclamp the tube. *The formula will displace the air in the tubing, thus preventing the instillation of excess air.*
- Attach the feeding set tubing to the feeding tube, and regulate the drip rate to deliver the feeding over the desired length of time. Prefilled tube-feeding sets can be attached to a feeding pump to regulate the flow.

7. Rinse the feeding tube immediately before all of the formula has run through the tubing.
- Instill 50 to 100 mL of water through the feeding tube. *Water flushes the lumen of the tube, preventing future blockage by sticky formula.*
- Be sure to add the water before the feeding solution has drained from the neck of a syringe or from the tubing of an administration set. Before adding water to a feeding bag or prefilled tubing set, first clamp and disconnect both feeding and administration tubes. *Adding the water before the syringe or tubing is empty prevents the instillation of air into the stomach or intestine and thus prevents unnecessary distention.*

8. Clamp and cover the feeding tube.
- Clamp the feeding tube before all of the water is instilled. *Clamping prevents leakage and air from entering the tube if done before water is instilled.*
- Cover the end of the feeding tube with gauze held by an elastic band. *Covering the tube end prevents leakage from it.*

9. Ensure client comfort and safety.
- Pin the tubing to the client's gown. *This minimizes pulling of the tube, thus preventing discomfort and dislodgement.*
- Ask the client to remain sitting upright in Fowler's position or in a slightly elevated right lateral position for at least 30 minutes. *These positions facilitate digestion and movement of the feeding from the stomach along the alimentary tract, and prevent the potential aspiration of the feeding into the lungs.*
- Check the agency's policy on the frequency of changing the nasogastric tube and the use of smaller-lumen tubes if a large-bore tube is in place. *These measures prevent irritation and erosion of the pharyngeal and esophageal mucous membranes.*

10. Dispose of equipment appropriately.
- If the equipment is to be reused, wash it thoroughly with soap and water so that it is ready for reuse.
- Change the equipment every 24 hours or according to agency policy.

11. **Document** all relevant information.
- Document the feeding, including amount and kind of solution taken, duration of the feeding, and assessments of the client.
- Record the volume of the feeding and water administered on the client's intake and output record.

12. Monitor the client for possible problems.
- Carefully assess clients receiving tube feedings for problems.
- To prevent dehydration, give the client supplemental water in addition to the prescribed tube feeding as ordered.

Variation: Continuous-Drip Feeding
- If the feeding is a continuous-drip tube feeding, place a label on the container.
- Clamp the tubing at least every 4 to 6 hours or as indicated by agency protocol or the manufacturer, and aspirate and measure the gastric contents. Then flush the tubing with 30 to 50 mL of water. *This determines adequate absorption and verifies correct placement of the tube. If placement of a small-bore tube is questionable, a repeat x-ray should be done.*
- Determine agency protocol regarding withholding a feeding. Many agencies withhold the feed-

ing if more than 75 to 100 mL of feeding is aspirated.

• To prevent spoilage or bacterial contamination, do not allow the feeding solution to hang longer than 4 to 8 hours. *Check agency policy or manufacturer's recommendations regarding time limits.*

• Follow agency policy regarding how frequently to change the feeding bag and tubing. *Changing the feeding bag and tubing every 24 hours reduces the risk of contamination.*

AMBULATORY AND COMMUNITY SETTINGS

Administering a Tube Feeding

• Teach the client or caregiver how to assess for tube placement using pH measurement before administering the feeding.

• Provide instructions for care of the tube and insertion site.

• Teach signs and symptoms to report to the doctor or home health nurse.

AGE-RELATED CONSIDERATIONS

Administering a Tube Feeding

Infant

• Feeding tubes may be reinserted at each feeding to prevent irritation of the mucous membrane, nasal airway obstruction, and stomach perforation that may occur if the tube is left in place continuously. Check agency practice.

Child

• Position a small child or infant in your lap, provide a pacifier, and hold and cuddle the child during feedings. This promotes comfort, supports the normal sucking instinct of the infant, and facilitates digestion.

Elders

• Physiologic changes associated with changing may make the older adult more vulnerable to complications associated with enteral feedings. Decreased gastric emptying may necessitate checking frequently for gastric residual. Diarrhea from administering the feeding too fast or too high concentration of the feeding may cause dehydration in the older adult. If the feeding has a high concentration of glucose, assess for hyperglycemia as with aging there is a decreased ability to handle increased glucose levels.

EVALUATION

• Perform a follow-up examination of the following:
  • Tolerance of feeding
  • Regurgitation and feelings of fullness after feedings
  • Weight gain or loss
  • Fecal elimination pattern (e.g., diarrhea, flatulence, constipation)
  • Skin turgor
  • Urine output
  • Glucose and acetone in urine
• Relate findings to previous assessment data if available. Report significant deviations from normal to the physician.

Nursing Process: Gastrostomy or Jejunostomy Feeding

ASSESSMENT

See Technique 15-4.

PLANNING

Before commencing a gastrostomy or jejunostomy feeding, determine the type and amount of feeding to be instilled, frequency of feedings, and any pertinent information about previous feedings (e.g., the positioning which the client best tolerates the feeding).

Delegation

See Technique 15-4.

Equipment

- Correct amount of feeding solution
- Graduated container to hold the feeding
- Large bulb syringe
- Graduated container with 60 mL of water to flush the tubing
- Graduated container to measure residual formula

For a Tube Sutured in Place

- 4" × 4" gauze squares to cover the end of the tube
- Elastic band

For Tube Insertion

- Clean disposable gloves
- Moistureproof bag
- Water-soluble lubricant
- 18 Fr whistle-tip catheter or other feeding tube
- Tubing clamp

For Cleaning the Peristomal Skin and Dressing the Stoma

- Mild soap and water
- Petrolatum, zinc oxide ointment, or other skin protectant
- Precut 4" × 4" gauze squares
- Uncut 4" × 4" gauze squares
- Abdominal pads
- Abdominal binder or Montgomery straps

Performance

1. Explain to the client what you are going to do, why it is necessary, and how he or she can cooperate.

2. Wash hands and observe other appropriate infection control procedures.

3. Provide for client privacy.

4. Assess and prepare the client.
   - See Technique 15-4.

5. Insert a feeding tube, if one is not already in place.
   - Wearing gloves, remove the ostomy dressing. Then discard the dressing and gloves in the moistureproof bag.
   - Lubricate the end of the tube, and insert it into the ostomy opening 10 to 15 cm (4 to 6 in).

6. Check the patency of a tube that is sutured or secured in place.
   - Determine correct placement of the tube by aspirating secretions and checking the pH.
   - Pour 15 to 30 mL of water into the syringe, remove the tube clamp, and allow the water to flow into the tube. This determines the patency of the tube. If water flows freely, the tube is patent.
   - If the water does not flow freely, notify the nurse in charge and/or physician.

7. Check for residual formula.
   - Attach the bulb to the syringe, and compress the bulb. *Compressing the bulb before the syringe is attached to the feeding tube prevents the instillation of air into the stomach or jejunum.*
   - Attach the syringe to the end of the feeding tube, and withdraw and measure the stomach or jejunal contents.
   - Follow agency practice if there is no more than 50 mL of undigested formula. Hold the feeding if there is more than 150 mL, and recheck in 3 to 4 hours or according to agency policy. Notify the physician if a large residual still remains.
   - For continuous feedings, check the residual every 4 to 6 hours, and hold feedings according to agency policy. The physician should be notified if a large residual persists.

8. Administer the feeding.
   - Hold the barrel of the syringe 7 to 15 cm (3 to 6 in) above the ostomy opening.
   - Slowly pour the solution into the syringe, and allow it to flow through the tube by gravity.
   - Just before all the formula has run through and the syringe is empty, add 30 mL of water. Water flushes the tube and preserves its patency.
   - If the tube is sutured in place, hold it upright, remove the syringe, and then clamp or plug the tube to prevent leakage. Cover the end of the tube with a 4" × 4" gauze, and secure the gauze with a rubber band.
   - If a catheter was inserted for the feeding, remove it.

9. Ensure client comfort and safety.
   - After the feeding, ask the client to remain in the sitting position or a slightly elevated right lateral position for at least 30 minutes. *This minimizes the risk of aspiration.*
   - Assess status of peristomal skin. *Gastric or jejunal drainage contains digestive enzymes that can irritate the skin.* Document any redness and broken skin areas.
   - Check orders about cleaning the peristomal skin, applying a skin protectant, and applying appropriate dressings. Generally, the peristomal skin is washed with mild soap and water at least once daily. Petrolatum, zinc oxide ointment, or other skin protectant may be applied around the stoma, and precut 4" × 4" gauze squares may be

placed around the tube. The precut squares are then covered with regular 4″ × 4″ gauze squares, and the tube is coiled over them. The coiled tube is covered with abdominal pads and secured with either an abdominal binder or Montgomery straps.

- Observe for common complications of enteral feedings: aspiration, hyperglycemia, abdominal distention, diarrhea, and fecal impaction. Report findings to physician. Often, a change in formula or rate of administration can correct problems.

- When appropriate, teach the client how to administer feedings and when to notify the health care provider concerning problems.

Variation: Percutaneous Endoscopic Gastrostomy (PEG)

- A PEG is kept in place with a short crosspiece or bolster near the skin level at the stoma.

- Clean the stoma daily with soap and water using a cotton swab or small piece of gauze in a circular motion.

- Rotate the bolster and clean the skin under it.

- Rotate the tube in a full circle between the thumb and forefinger daily.

- After cleaning, allow the skin to air dry.

- Report any signs of redness, pain, soreness, swelling, or drainage to the health care provider.

- Do not apply a dressing over the PEG. *A dressing and tape may result in skin excoriation and breakdown.*

 10. **Document** all assessments and interventions.

EVALUATION

See Technique 15-4.

Maintaining Feeding Tube Patency

All enteral feeding devices require periodic flushing to maintain patency and water continues to be the best flushing solution. Enteral devices in adults should be flushed with at least 20 to 30 mL of warm water every 4 hours during continuous feedings and before and after intermittent feedings and medications (Lord, 1997).

Tube clogging can occur with any enteral device, but smaller diameters and longer lengths of nasoenteric and jejunostomy tubes predispose them to a higher incidence of clogging. Most tube clogging is caused by viscous enteral feeding (e.g., those that contain fiber) or medications. Contamination of the formula can lead to coagulation, causing clogging. Prevention is facilitated by frequent flushing of the tube, using a pump if the infusion rate is slow, and prompt attention to pump alarms.

When administering medications through enteral devices, the following actions suggested by Lord (1997) will help prevent clogging:

- Crush a tablet into a fine powder and dilute with enough water to dissolve it. Enteric coated or sustained release medications should not be crushed or given through enteral devices.

- Give liquid forms of medications whenever possible.

- Check compatibility of medications with formula *to avoid formation of a precipitate.*

- Flush before and after medication administration.

- Give medications separately and flush with 15 mL of warm water between each medication. *This avoids medication interactions.*

Chapter Summary

TERMINOLOGY

anorexia

bolus intermittent feedings

clear liquid diet

closed systems

continuous feedings

cyclic feedings

diet as tolerated (DAT)

dysphagia

enteral

enteral nutrition (EN)

full liquid diet

intermittent feedings

large-bore tube

light diet

malnutrition

nasoenteric tube

nasogastric tube

nothing by mouth (NPO)

nutrients

nutrition

open systems

overnutrition

parenteral

percutaneous endoscopic gastrostomy (PEG)

percutaneous endoscopic jejunostomy (PEJ)

pureed diet

regular diet

small-bore tube

soft diet

total enteral nutrition (TEN)

undernutrition

FORMING CLINICAL JUDGMENTS

Consider This:

1. A 75-year-old female client has recently been diagnosed with chronic lung cancer that has left her susceptible to pneumonia. As a result, her physician has ordered three different oral medications that have resulted in her losing her appetite and a 22-pound weight loss. Once overweight, the client is now within the weight parameters for her height and age. The client tells her home health nurse that "nothing sounds good and nothing tastes good." The client lives alone and is responsible for her own meal preparation.

   a. Do you have any concerns regarding this client's nutritional needs?

   b. What information would be helpful to you as the nurse in order to meet or maintain the client's nutritional needs?

   c. What suggestions do you have for ways to enhance the client's intake during this period of decreased appetite?

   d. Do you think the client is a good candidate for a feeding tube? Why or why not?

2. It is time for the next tube feeding. You have just checked feeding tube placement and obtained the pH of the aspirated fluid for the following three clients. What actions would you take for each client?

   Client A: pH = 3

   Client B: pH = 6

   Client C: pH = 7

3. Contaminated enteral feeding formula can put the client at risk for many problems. How can you minimize or avoid the risk of contamination for both the open and closed feedings systems?

RELATED RESEARCH

Holzapfel, S. K., Ramirez, R. F., Layton, M. S., Smith, I. W., Sagl-Massey, K., & DuBose, J. Z. (1996). Feeder position and food and fluid consumed by nursing home residents. *Journal of Gerontological Nursing, 22*(4), 6–12.

McHale, J. M., Phipps, M. A., Horvath, K., & Schmelz, J. (1998). Expert nursing knowledge in the care of patients at risk of impaired swallowing. *Image: Journal of Nursing Scholarship, 30*(2), 137–141.

REFERENCES

Denney, A. (1997). Quiet music: An intervention for mealtime agitation? *Journal of Gerontological Nursing, 23*(7), 16–23.

Evans-Stoner, N. (1997). Guidelines for care of the patient on home nutrition support. *Nursing Clinics of North America, 32*(4), 769–775.

Hall, J. C. (1997). Learning about low-profile gastrostomy devices. *Nursing, 27*(6), 62–64.

Kayser-Jones, J., & Schell, E. (1997). The mealtime experience of a cognitively impaired elder: Ineffective and effective strategies. *Journal of Gerontological Nursing, 23*(7), 33–39.

Kohn-Keeth, C. (2000). How to keep feeding tubes flowing freely. *Nursing, 30*(3), 58–59.

Loan, T., Magnuson, B., & Williams, S. (1998). Debunking six myths about enteral feeding. *Nursing, 28*(8), 43–48.

Lord, L. M. (1997). Enteral access devices. *Nursing Clinics of North America, 32*(4), 685–703.

McConnell, E. A. (1996). Maintaining a feeding tube exit site. *Nursing, 26*(12), 61.

McConnell, E. A. (1997a). Clinical do's & don'ts. Inserting a nasogastric tube. *Nursing, 27*(1), 72.

McConnell, E. A. (1997b). Clinical do's & don'ts. How to determine gastric pH. *Nursing, 27*(8), 26.

Metheny, N., Wehrle, M. A., Wiersema, L, & Clark, J. (1998a). Testing feeding tube placement: Auscultation vs. pH method. *American Journal of Nursing, 98*(5), 37–42.

Metheny, N., Smith, L., Wehrle, M. A., Wiersema, L., & Clark, J. (1998b). pH, color, and feeding tubes. *RN, 61*(1), 25–27.

Miceli, B. V. (1999). Nursing unit meal management maintenance program: Continuation of safe swallowing and feeding beyond skilled therapeutic intervention. *Journal of Gerontological Nursing, 25*(8), 22–36.

Morrisson, S. G. (1997). Feeding the elderly population. *Nursing Clinics of North America, 32*(4), 791–812.

Chapter 16

Assisting with Fecal Elimination

Techniques

OBJECTIVES

- Describe essential aspects of defecation.
- Describe common fecal elimination problems and factors contributing to them.
- Describe the use of various types of bedpans.
- Identify the steps in the administration of selected types of enemas.
- Discuss methods of removing a fecal impaction.
- Discuss selected nursing interventions appropriate for caring for clients with bowel diversion ostomies.
- Identify the steps in irrigating a colostomy.

Defecation

The pattern of **defecation** is highly individual, varying from several times per day to two or three times per week. The amount defecated also varies from person to person. Repeated inhibition of the urge to defecate can result in expansion of the rectum to accommodate accumulated feces and eventual loss of sensitivity to the need to defecate. Constipation can be the ultimate result.

Normal **feces** are made of about 75 percent water and 25 percent solid materials. They are soft but formed. Feces are normally brown, chiefly due to the presence of stercobilin and urobilin, which are derived from bilirubin. Another factor that affects fecal color is the action of bacteria such as *Escherichia coli*, which are normally present in the large intestine. An adult usually forms 7 to 10 liters of flatus (air or gas) in the large intestine every 24 hours. The gases include carbon dioxide, methane, hydrogen, oxygen, and nitrogen. Some are swallowed with food and fluids taken by mouth, and others are formed through the action of bacteria. The action of microorganisms is responsible for the odor of feces and flatus. See Table 16-1 for characteristics of normal and abnormal feces.

TABLE 16-1 CHARACTERISTICS OF NORMAL AND ABNORMAL FECES

Characteristic	Normal	Abnormal	Possible Cause
Color	Adult: brown Infant: yellow	Clay or white	Absence of bile pigment (bile obstruction): diagnostic study using barium
		Black or tarry	Drug (e.g., iron); bleeding from upper gastrointestinal tract (e.g., stomach, small intestine); diet high in red meat and dark green vegetables (e.g., spinach)
		Red	Bleeding from lower gastrointestinal tract (e.g., rectum); some foods (e.g., beets)
		Pale	Malabsorption of fats; diet high in milk and milk products and low in meat
		Orange or green	Intestinal infection
Consistency	Formed, soft, semisolid, moist	Hard, dry	Dehydration; decreased intestinal motility resulting from lack of fiber in diet, lack of exercise, emotional upset, laxative abuse
		Diarrhea	Increased intestinal motility (e.g., due to irritation of the colon by bacteria)
Shape	Cylindrical (contour of rectum) about 2.5 cm (1 in) in diameter in adults	Narrow, pencil-shaped, or stringlike stool	Obstructive condition of the rectum
Amount	Varies with diet (about 100–400 g/day)		
Odor	Aromatic: affected by ingested food and person's own bacterial flora	Pungent	Infection, blood
Constituents	Small amounts of undigested roughage, sloughed dead bacteria and epithelial cells, fat, protein, dried constituents of digestive juices (e.g., bile pigments), inorganic matter (calcium, phosphates)	Pus Mucus Parasites Blood Large quantities of fat Foreign objects	Bacterial infection Inflammatory condition Gastrointestinal bleeding Malabsorption Accidental ingestion

From *Fundamentals of nursing: Concepts, process, and practice*, 6th ed., by B. Kozier, G. Erb, A. Berman, & K. Burke, 2000, Upper Saddle River, NJ: Prentice Hall Health.

Factors That Affect Defecation

Patterns of defecation vary during different stages of life. Following are factors affecting adults.

Diet

Sufficient bulk (cellulose, fiber) in the diet is necessary to provide fecal volume. Individuals who eat at the same times every day have a regularly timed, physiologic response to the food intake and a regular pattern of peristaltic activity in the colon. Spicy foods can produce diarrhea and flatus in some individuals.

Fluid

Healthy fecal elimination usually requires a daily fluid intake of 2,000 to 3,000 mL. When fluid intake is inadequate or output (urine or vomitus, for example) is excessive, the body continues to reabsorb fluid from the **chyme** (contents of the colon). This can result in hard stools and slowed elimination. If peristalsis is speeded up, there may be inadequate time for fluid to be absorbed into the blood, and the feces are soft or even watery.

Activity

Activity stimulates peristalsis, thus facilitating the movement of chyme along the colon. Weak abdominal and pelvic muscles are often ineffective in increasing the intra-abdominal pressure during defecation or in controlling defecation.

Psychological Factors

Certain diseases that involve severe diarrhea, such as ulcerative colitis, may have a psychological component. Some people who are anxious or angry experience increased peristaltic activity and subsequent diarrhea. People who are depressed may experience slower intestinal motility, resulting in constipation.

Medications

Some drugs have side effects that can interfere with normal elimination. Some cause diarrhea; others, such as morphine and codeine, cause constipation. Some medications directly affect elimination. Laxatives are medications that stimulate bowel activity and so assist fecal elimination. There are medications that soften stool, facilitating defecation. Certain medications suppress peristaltic activity and sometimes are used to treat diarrhea. Several drugs cause a change in the color of the stool, from black (iron), to green (antibiotics), to white (antacids).

Anesthesia and Surgery

General anesthetics cause the normal colonic movements to cease or slow down by blocking parasympathetic stimulation to the muscles of the colon. Clients who have regional or spinal anesthesia are less likely to experience this problem. Surgery that involves direct handling of the intestines can cause temporary cessation of intestinal movement. This is called **paralytic ileus**, a condition that usually lasts 24 to 48 hours.

Pathologic Conditions

Spinal cord injuries and head injuries, for example, can decrease the sensory stimulation for defecation. Impaired mobility may limit the client's ability to respond to the urge to defecate when the client is unable to reach a toilet or summon assistance. As a result, the client may experience constipation. Or a client may experience fecal **incontinence** because of poorly functioning anal sphincters.

Positioning

Normal defecation is facilitated by (1) thigh flexion, which increases the pressure within the abdomen, and (2) a sitting or squatting position, which increases the downward pressure on the rectum. Clients restricted to bed may have to use a bedpan rather than the toilet.

Bedpans

There are two main types of bedpans: the regular, or high-back, pan and the slipper, or fracture, pan (Figure 16-1 ◆). The slipper pan has a low back and is used for people who are unable to elevate their buttocks because of physical problems or therapy that contraindicates such movement. Many people confined to bed are able to use a bedpan independently, provided the equipment is placed within safe and easy reach. Some, however, require varying degrees of assistance from a nurse. The nurse has to determine the individual's needs and provide the appropriate assistance. Using a bedpan can be embarrassing to many people. For the elderly, physically impaired, or critically ill people, it can also be a tiring procedure.

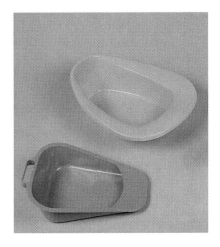

FIGURE 16-1 ◆ Two types of bedpans: high-back, or regular, pan; the slipper, or fracture, pan.

Guidelines for the Care of Bedpans

The care of bedpans relates largely to preventing the transmission of microorganisms and to the feelings people attach to elimination.

- To maintain medical asepsis, each client in a hospital is provided with a separate bedpan.

- Bedpans are stored in an appropriate place out of sight. Bedside units are often designed to provide a specific place for bedpans that is not visible to others and is separate from the client's personal possessions. It is usually also separated from other equipment used for hygienic care. Medical aseptic practice prohibits the placing of a bedpan on the floor under the bed or on overbed tables.

- A clean bedpan cover is placed over the bedpan after use and for transporting it to and from the bedside.

- Bedpans should always be handled from the outside. Slipper (fracture) pans have handles that the nurse can use to carry them. The high-back bedpan needs to be supported with both hands on its base for transport.

- Elimination equipment is thoroughly cleaned and dried after use. Disposable equipment is discarded. Rinsing devices, cleaning brushes, and disinfectant solutions are generally located in the bathrooms or unit dirty utility rooms. Bedpans periodically need to be recycled through a central supply area for comprehensive cleaning, which includes resterilization.

Nursing Process: Bedpans

ASSESSMENT

Following are key assessments for any client related to fecal elimination. The nurse selects those items most pertinent to the interaction with the client at a particular time.

Determine:

- *Defecation pattern:* The frequency and time of day of the client's defecation. Has this pattern changed recently? Does it ever change? If so, does the client know what factors affect it?

- *Behavioral patterns:* The use of enemas, laxatives, fluids, and other methods to maintain normal defecation. What routines does the client follow to maintain the usual defecation pattern (e.g., a glass of hot lemon juice with breakfast or a long walk before breakfast)?

- *Diet:* What foods does the client believe affect defecation? Are meals taken at a regular time?

- *Fluid intake:* What amount and kind of fluid does the client take each day (e.g., six glasses of water, five cups of coffee)?

- *Exercise:* What is the client's usual daily exercise pattern? Obtain specifics about exercise rather than asking whether it is sufficient or not, since people have different ideas of what is sufficient.

- *Medications:* Has the client taken any medications that could affect the gastrointestinal tract (e.g., iron, antacids, narcotic analgesics)?

- *Pertinent illness or surgery:* Has the client had any surgery or illness that affects the intestinal tract? The presence of any ostomies must be explored (e.g., a colostomy or ileostomy).

Assess:

- *Abdominal distention:* Distention will appear as an overall outward protuberance of the abdomen, with the skin appearing tight and tense. When palpated, the abdomen feels firm.

- *Bowel sounds:* Auscultate all four abdominal quadrants for 5 to 15 seconds to determine the degree of activity or frequency of sounds. See Technique 3-15 Assessing the Abdomen.

- *Consistency and color of feces.*

- *Perianal region and anus:* Inspect these areas for discolorations, inflammations, scars, lesions, fissures, fistulas, or hemorrhoids.

- *Presence of abdominal or rectal pain.*

Clients at risk for developing fecal elimination problems are those who:

- Have insufficient fluid or roughage in the diet
- Do not exercise sufficiently
- Use constipating medications
- Ingest excessive gas-forming foods

PLANNING

Inquire whether the client has used a bedpan previously. If so, determine if the client has any unique needs related to the use of the bedpan. Locate the client's bedpan.

Delegation

Unlicensed assistive personnel (UAP) commonly assist clients with bedpans. The nurse must determine if the specific client has unique needs that would require special training of the UAP in the use of the bedpan. Ensure that personnel are aware of any specimens that need to be collected. Abnormal findings must be validated and interpreted by the nurse.

Equipment

- Clean bedpan and cover
- Toilet tissue
- Basin of water, soap, washcloth, and towel
- Aerosol freshener (optional)
- Equipment for a specimen as required (see Technique 4-3)
- Disposable gloves
- Disposable linen-saver pad

Preparation

- If the bedpan is metal, warm it by rinsing it with warm water. Dry the outside of the pan, and place it on the foot of the bed or on an adjacent chair. *A cold bedpan may make a person tense and thus hinder elimination. When warming a metal pan, which retains heat, take care not to burn the client.*
- Adjust the bed to a height appropriate *to prevent straining your back.*
- Elevate the rail on the opposite side of the bed *to prevent the client from falling and to provide a hand grasp for the client if needed.*

Performance

1. Explain to the client what you are going to do, why it is necessary, and how he or she can cooperate. Discuss how the results will be used in planning further care or treatments.

2. Wash hands, apply clean gloves, and observe appropriate infection control procedures.

3. Provide for client privacy.

4. Prepare the client.
   - For clients who can assist by raising their buttocks, fold down the top bed linen on the near side to expose the hip, and adjust the gown so that it will not fall into the bedpan. *A pie fold of the top bedclothes exposes the client minimally and facilitates placement of the bedpan.*
   - For clients who cannot raise their buttocks onto and off a bedpan, fold the top bedclothes down to the hips.

5. Give the bedpan.
   - For clients who can lift their buttocks:
   a. Ask the client to flex the knees, rest the weight on the back and the heels, and then raise the buttocks. The client can use a trapeze, if present, or grasp the side rail for support. Assist the client to lift the buttocks by placing the hand nearest the person's head palm up under the lower back, resting the elbow on the mattress,

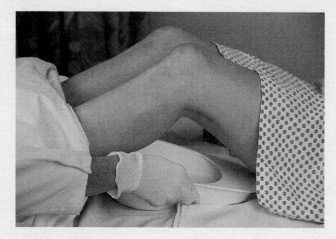

FIGURE 16-2 ◆ Placing a fracture bedpan under the client's buttocks.

and using the forearm as a lever. *Use of appropriate body mechanics by both client and nurse prevents unnecessary muscle strain and exertion.*

   b. Place the linen-saver pad on the bed where the bedpan will be located. Position a regular bedpan under the buttocks with the narrow end toward the foot of the bed and the buttocks resting on the smooth, rounded rim. Place a slipper (fracture) pan with the flat end under the client's buttocks (Figure 16-2 ◆). *Improper placement of the bedpan can cause skin abrasion to the sacral area and spillage of the bedpan's contents.*

   - For clients who cannot lift their buttocks:
   a. Assist the client to a side-lying position.
   b. Place the bedpan against the buttocks with the open rim toward the foot of the bed.
   c. Smoothly roll the client onto the bedpan while holding the bedpan against the buttocks (Figure 16-3 ◆).

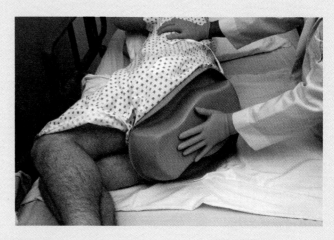

FIGURE 16-3 ◆ Placing a regular bedpan against the client's buttocks.

6. Elevate the head of the bed to a semi-Fowler's position. *This position relieves strain on the client's back and permits a more normal position for elimination.*

   • If the person is unable to assume a semi-Fowler's position, place a small pillow under the back, or help the client to another comfortable position.

7. Replace the top bed linen.

8. Provide the client with toilet tissue, raise the side rail, lower the bed height, and ensure that the call light is readily accessible. Ask the client to signal when finished. Leave only when, in your judgment, it is safe to do so. *Having necessary items within reach prevents falls.*

Removing a Bedpan

9. Reposition the bed and client to that used when giving the bedpan.

   • Remove the bedpan in the same manner it was placed, holding the pan with one hand to ensure the contents are not spilled.

   • Cover the bedpan, and place it on an adjacent chair. *Covering the bedpan reduces offensive odors and reduces the client's embarrassment.*

10. Assist the client with any needed hygienic measures.

   • Wrap toilet tissue several times around the gloved hand, and wipe the person from the pubic area to the anal area, using one stroke for each piece of tissue. *Cleaning in this direction— from the less soiled area to the more soiled area— helps prevent the spread of microorganisms.*

• Place the soiled tissue in the bedpan.

• Wash the anal area with soap and water as indicated, and thoroughly dry the area. *Adequate washing and drying prevents skin abrasion and excessive accumulation of microorganisms.*

• Remove the linen-saver pad or replace the drawsheet if it is soiled.

• Offer the client materials to wash and dry the hands. *Handwashing following elimination is a practice that helps prevent the spread of microorganisms.*

11. Attend to any unpleasant odors in the environment.

   • Spray the air with an air freshener unless contraindicated because of respiratory problems, allergies, or because it is offensive. *Elimination odor can be embarrassing to clients and visitors alike. However, sprays may be harmful to people with respiratory problems, and some perfume sprays are offensive to some people.*

12. Attend to the used bedpan.

   • Acquire a specimen if required. Place it in the appropriately labeled container.

   • Empty and clean the bedpan. Provide a clean bedpan cover, if necessary, before returning it to the client's unit.

13. **Document** findings in the client record using forms or checklists supplemented by narrative notes when appropriate.

AGE-RELATED CONSIDERATIONS

Factors Affecting Defecation

Infant

• **Meconium**, a black, tarry, sticky, odorless stool is passed for the first 24 hours after birth.

• Loose transitional stools, greenish yellow, with mucus, are passed for about 1 week following meconium.

• Soft or liquid stools are common, especially after eating.

• Breast-fed infants' stool is yellow while milk/formula fed infants stool is dark yellow or tan.

Child

• Bowel control begins at about age 18 months.

Elders

• Constipation is common.

• A change in bowel elimination patterns can be a sign of disease.

EVALUATION

• Perform follow-up treatment or client teaching based on findings that deviated from expected or normal for the client. Relate findings to previous data if available.

• Report significant deviations from normal to the physician.

Enemas

An **enema** is used most often as a treatment for constipation. **Constipation** refers to the passage of small, dry, hard stool or the passage of no stool for a period of time. It is important to define constipation in relation to the person's regular elimination pattern but may be defined as fewer than three bowel movements per week (Vickery, 1997). It occurs when the movement of feces through the large intestine is slow, thus allowing time for additional reabsorption of fluid from the large intestine.

An enema is a solution introduced into the rectum and sigmoid colon. Its function is to remove feces and/or flatus. Enemas are classified into five groups, according to their action: cleansing, carminative, retention, return flow, or therapeutic. A **cleansing enema** stimulates peristalsis by irritating the colon and rectum and/or by distending the intestine with the volume of fluid introduced.

A **carminative enema** is given primarily to expel flatus. The solution instilled into the rectum releases gas, which in turn distends the rectum and the colon, thus stimulating peristalsis.

A **retention enema** introduces oil into the rectum and sigmoid colon. It acts to soften the feces and to lubricate the rectum and anal canal, thus facilitating passage of the feces.

A **return flow enema**, sometimes referred to as the **Harris flush** or **colonic irrigation**, is used to expel flatus. Alternating flow of fluid into and out of the large intestine stimulates peristalsis.

Therapeutic enemas deliver nutrients or medication. Corticosteroid, antibiotic, and kayexalate (a resin used to remove excess potassium) are examples of medicated enemas.

Various solutions are used for enemas. The specific solution may be ordered by the physician or indicated by agency protocol. Table 16-2 describes some of these solutions.

An enema is a relatively safe procedure for the client. The chief dangers are irritation of the rectal mucosa by too much soap or an irritating soap and negative effects of a hypertonic solution or hypotonic solution on the shifting of body fluid and electrolytes.

The repeated administration of hypotonic solutions, such as tap water enemas, can result in absorption of the water from the colon into the bloodstream. This increases the blood volume and can produce water intoxication. For this reason, some health agencies limit to three the number of tap water enemas given consecutively. This is of particular concern when the order is "enemas until returns are clear"—for example, prior to a visual examination of the large intestine.

Guidelines for Administering Enemas

- Before administering an enema, determine whether a physician's order is required. At some agencies, a physician must order the kind of enema and the time to give it, for example, the morning of an examination. When the client has rectal disease, the physician may also specify the size of the rectal tube to use. At other agencies, enemas are given at the nurses' discretion (i.e., as necessary on a PRN order).

- Enemas for adults are usually given at 40 to 43°C (105 to 110°F); unless otherwise specified. High temperatures can be injurious to the bowel mucosa; cold temperatures are uncomfortable for the client and may trigger a spasm of the sphincter muscles.

- The force of flow of the solution is governed by the (1) height of the solution container, (2) size of the tubing, (3) viscosity of the fluid, and (4) resistance

TABLE 16-2	COMMONLY USED ENEMA SOLUTIONS			
Solution	Constituents	Action	Time to Take Effect	Adverse Effects
Hypertonic	90–120 mL of solution (e.g., sodium phosphate)	Draws water into the colon	5–10 min	Retention of sodium
Hypotonic	500–1,000 mL of tap water	Distends colon, stimulates peristalsis, and softens feces	15–20 min	Fluid and electrolyte imbalance; water intoxication
Isotonic	500–1,000 mL of normal saline (9 mL NaCl to 1,000 mL water)	Distends colon, stimulates peristalsis, and softens feces	15–20 min	Possible sodium retention
Soapsuds	500–1,000 mL (3–5 mL soap to 1,000 mL water)	Irritates mucosa, distends colon	10–15 min	Irritates and may damage mucosa
Oil (mineral, olive, cottonseed)	90–120 mL	Lubricates the feces and the colonic mucosa	30–60 min	

From *Fundamentals of nursing: Concepts, process, and practice*, 6th ed., by B. Kozier, G. Erb, A. Berman, & K. Burke, 2000, Upper Saddle River, NJ: Prentice Hall Health.

of the rectum. The higher the solution container is held above the rectum, the faster the flow and the greater the force (pressure) in the rectum.

- The time it takes to administer an enema largely depends on the amount of fluid to be instilled and the client's tolerance. Large volumes, such as 1,000 mL, may take 10 to 15 minutes to instill; small volumes require less time.

- The amount of time the client retains the enema solution depends on the purpose of the enema and the client's ability to contract the external sphincter to retain the solution. Oil retention enemas are usually retained 2 to 3 hours. Other enemas are normally retained 5 to 10 minutes.

Nursing Process: Enemas

ASSESSMENT

Determine when the client last had a bowel movement and the amount, color, and consistency of the feces; presence of abdominal distention (the distended abdomen appears swollen and feels firm rather than soft when palpated); whether the client has sphincter control; and whether the client can use a toilet or commode or must remain in bed and use a bedpan.

PLANNING

Delegation

Administration of enemas may be delegated to UAP. However, the nurse must ensure that personnel are competent in the use of Standard Precautions. Abnormal findings such as inability to insert the rectal tip, client inability to retain the solution, or unusual return from the enema must be validated and interpreted by the nurse.

IMPLEMENTATION:
TECHNIQUE 16-2 ADMINISTERING ENEMAS

Equipment

- Disposable linen-saver pad
- Bath blanket
- Bedpan or commode
- Disposable gloves
- Water-soluble lubricant if tubing not prelubricated
- Paper towel

Large-Volume Enema

- Solution container with tubing of correct size and tubing clamp
- Correct solution, amount, and temperature
- IV pole

Small-Volume Enema

- Prepackaged container of enema solution with lubricated tip

Preparation

- Lubricate about 5 cm (2 in) of the rectal tube (some commercially prepared enema sets have prelubricated nozzles). Lubrication facilitates insertion through the sphincters and minimizes trauma.

- Run some solution through the connecting tubing of a large volume enema set and the rectal tube to expel any air in the tubing; then close the clamp. *Air instilled into the rectum, although not harmful, causes unnecessary distention.*

Performance

1. Explain to the client what you are going to do, why it is necessary, and how he or she can cooperate. Discuss how the results will be used in planning further care or treatments. Indicate that the client may experience a feeling of fullness while the solution is being administered.

2. Wash hands, apply clean gloves, and observe appropriate infection control procedures.

3. Provide for client privacy.

4. Assist the adult client to a left lateral position, with the right leg as acutely flexed as possible (Figure 16-4 ◆) and the linen-saver pad under the buttocks. *This position facilitates the flow of solution by gravity into the sigmoid and descending colon, which are on the left side. Having the right leg acutely flexed provides for adequate exposure of the anus.*

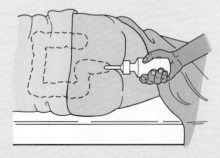

FIGURE 16-4 ◆ Assuming a left lateral position for an enema.

5. Insert the rectal tube.
- For clients in the left lateral position, lift the upper buttock *to ensure good visualization of the anus.*
- Insert the tube smoothly and slowly into the rectum, directing it toward the umbilicus (Figure 16-5 ◆). *The angle follows the normal contour of the rectum. Slow insertion prevents spasm of the sphincter.*
- Insert the tube 7 to 10 cm (3 to 4 in). *Because the anal canal is about 2.5 to 5 cm (1 to 2 in) long in the adult, insertion to this point places the tip of the tube beyond the anal sphincter into the rectum.*
- If resistance is encountered at the internal sphincter, ask the client to take a deep breath, then run a small amount of solution through the tube *to relax the internal anal sphincter.*
- Never force tube entry. If resistance persists, withdraw the tube, and report the resistance to the nurse in charge.
6. Slowly administer the enema solution.
- Raise the solution container, and open the clamp to allow fluid flow.
  or
- Compress a pliable container by hand.
- During most low enemas, hold or hang the solution container no higher than 30 cm (12 in) above the rectum. *The higher the solution container is held above the rectum, the faster the flow and the greater the force (pressure) in the rectum.* During a high enema, hang the solution container about 45 cm (18 in). *The fluid must be instilled farther to clean the entire bowel.* Follow agency protocol.
- Administer the fluid slowly. If the client complains of fullness or pain, use the clamp to stop the flow for 30 seconds, and then restart the flow at a slower rate. *Administering the enema slowly and stopping the flow momentarily decrease the likelihood of intestinal spasm and premature ejection of the solution.*
- If you are using a plastic commercial container, roll it up as the fluid is instilled. This prevents subsequent suctioning of the solution (see Figure 16-6 ◆).
- After all the solution has been instilled or when

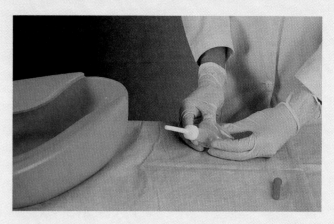

FIGURE 16-6 ◆ Rolling up a commercial enema container.

the client cannot hold any more and feels the desire to defecate (the urge to defecate usually indicates that sufficient fluid has been administered), close the clamp, and remove the rectal tube from the anus.
- Place the rectal tube in a disposable towel as you withdraw it.
7. Encourage the client to retain the enema.
- Ask the client to remain lying down. *It is easier for the client to retain the enema when lying down than when sitting or standing, because gravity promotes drainage and peristalsis.*
- Request that the client retain the solution for the appropriate amount of time, for example, 5 to 10 minutes for a cleansing enema or at least 30 minutes for a retention enema.
8. Assist the client to defecate.
- Assist the client to a sitting position on the bedpan, commode, or toilet. A sitting position facilitates the act of defecation.
- Ask the client who is using the toilet not to flush it. The nurse needs to observe the feces.
- If a specimen of feces is required, ask the client to use a bedpan or commode.

Variation: Administering an Enema to an Incontinent Client

Occasionally, a nurse needs to administer an enema to a client who is unable to control the external sphincter muscle and thus cannot retain the enema solution for even a few minutes. In that case, after the rectal tube is inserted, the client assumes a supine position on a bedpan. The head of the bed can be elevated slightly, to 30 degrees if necessary for easier breathing, and pillows support the client's head and back.

Variation: Administering a Return-Flow Enema

For a return-flow enema, the solution (100 to 200 mL for an adult) is instilled into the client's rectum and

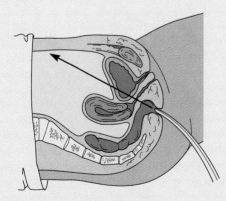

FIGURE 16-5 ◆ Inserting the rectal tube following the direction of the rectum.

sigmoid colon. Then the solution container is lowered so that the fluid flows back out through the rectal tube into the container, pulling the flatus with it. The inflow–outflow process is repeated five or six times (to stimulate peristalsis and the expulsion of flatus), and the solution is replaced several times during the procedure if it becomes thick with feces.

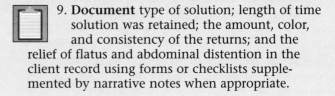 9. **Document** type of solution; length of time solution was retained; the amount, color, and consistency of the returns; and the relief of flatus and abdominal distention in the client record using forms or checklists supplemented by narrative notes when appropriate.

AMBULATORY AND COMMUNITY SETTINGS

Enemas

Teach the caregiver or client the following:

- To make saline solution, mix 1 teaspoon of table salt to 500 mL of tap water.

- Use enemas only as directed. Do not rely on them for regular bowel evacuation.

- Prior to administration, make sure a bedpan, commode, or toilet is nearby.

AGE-RELATED CONSIDERATIONS

Enemas

Infant/child

- Children may require an enema prior to undergoing procedures. The enema solution should be isotonic (usually normal saline). Some hypertonic commercial solutions (e.g., Fleet enema) can lead to hypovolemia and electrolyte imbalances. In addition, the osmotic effect of the Fleet enema may produce diarrhea and subsequent metabolic acidosis.

- Infants and small children do not exhibit sphincter control and need to be assisted in retaining the enema. The nurse administers the enema while the infant or child is lying with the buttocks over the bedpan and the nurse firmly presses the buttocks together to prevent the immediate expulsion of the solution. Older children can usually hold the solution if they understand what to do and are not required to hold it for too long a period. It may be necessary to ensure that the bathroom is available for an ambulatory child before starting the procedure or to have a bedpan ready.

- Enema temperature should be 37.7°C (100°F) unless otherwise ordered

- Large-volume enemas consist of 50 to 200 mL in children less than 18 months old; 200 to 300 mL in children 18 months to 5 years; 300 to 500 mL in children 5 years to 12 years old.

- Careful explanation is especially important for the preschool child. An enema is an intrusive procedure and therefore threatening.

- For infants and small children, the dorsal recumbent position is frequently used. Position them on a small padded bedpan with support for the back and head. Secure the legs by placing a diaper under the bedpan and then over and around the thighs (Figure 16-7 ◆). Place the underpad under the client's buttocks to protect the bed linen, and drape the client with the bath blanket.

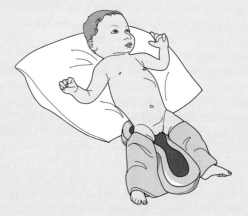

FIGURE 16-7 ◆ Immobilizing an infant's legs for an enema by placing a diaper under the bedpan and then over and around the thighs.

- Insert the tube 5 to 7.5 cm (2 to 3 in) in the child and only 2.5 to 3.75 cm (1 to 1.5 in) in the infant.

- For children, lower the height of the solution container appropriately for the age of the child. Follow agency protocol.

- To assist a small child in retaining the solution, apply firm pressure over the anus with tissue wipes, or firmly press the buttocks together.

Elders

- Elders may fatigue easily.

- Elders may be more susceptible to fluid and electrolyte imbalances. Use tap water enemas with great caution.

- Monitor the client's tolerance during the procedure, watching for vagal episodes and dysrhythmias.

- Protect older adults' skin from prolonged exposure to moisture.

- Assist older clients with perineal care as indicated.

EVALUATION

Perform a detailed follow-up based on findings that deviated from expected or normal for the client. Relate findings to previous assessment data if available. Report significant deviations from expected to the physician.

Fecal Impaction

Fecal **impaction** is a mass or collection of hardened feces in the rectum. Impaction results from prolonged retention and accumulation of fecal material. Fecal impaction is recognized by the passage of liquid fecal seepage (diarrhea) and no normal stool. The liquid portion of the feces seeps out around the impacted mass (Figure 16-8 ◆). Although fecal impaction can generally be prevented, digital removal of impacted feces is sometimes necessary. When fecal impaction is suspected, the client is often given an oil retention enema, a cleansing enema 2 to 4 hours later, and daily additional cleansing enemas (see Technique 16-2), suppositories, or stool softeners. If these measures fail, manual removal is often necessary.

Removing a Fecal Impaction Digitally

Digital removal involves breaking up the fecal mass using a finger and removing it in portions. Because the bowel mucosa can be injured during this procedure, some agencies restrict and specify the personnel permitted to conduct digital disimpactions. Rectal stimulation is also contraindicated for some people because it may cause an excessive vagal response resulting in cardiac arrhythmia. Prior to disimpaction, an oil retention enema, held for 30 minutes, is recommended to help soften the stool. After a disimpaction, the nurse can use various interventions to remove remaining feces (e.g., a cleansing enema or the insertion of a suppository).

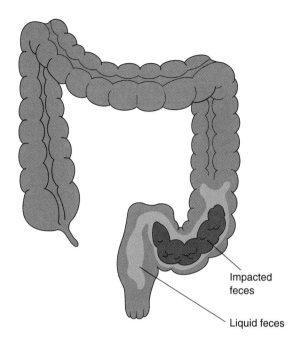

FIGURE 16-8 ◆ Fecal impaction with liquid feces leaking around the impaction.

Nursing Process: Fecal Impaction

ASSESSMENT

Confirm the presence of an impaction by digital examination; presence of nausea, headache, abdominal pain, malaise, or abdominal distention.

PLANNING

Delegation

Due to the potential results of stimulation of the vagus nerve during the procedure, digital removal of an impaction is generally not delegated to UAP.

IMPLEMENTATION:
TECHNIQUE 16-3 REMOVING A FECAL IMPACTION

Equipment

- Bath blanket
- Disposable linen-saver pad
- Bedpan and cover
- Toilet tissue
- Disposable gloves
- Lubricant
- Soap, water, and towel
- Topical lidocaine (if agency permits)

Preparation

If the agency permits the use of the topical anesthetic, lidocaine, 1 to 2 mL, should be inserted into the anal canal 5 minutes prior to the procedure. *This will numb the anal and rectal areas, reducing the pain of the procedure.*

Performance

1. Explain to the client what you are going to do, why it is necessary, and how he or she can cooperate. Discuss how the results will be used in planning further care or treatments. This procedure is

distressing, tiring, and uncomfortable, so the person may desire the presence of another nurse or support person.

2. Wash hands, apply clean gloves, and observe appropriate infection control procedures.

3. Provide for client privacy.

4. Assist the client to a right or left lateral or Sims' position with the back toward you. *When the person lies on the right side, the sigmoid colon is uppermost; thus, gravity can aid removal of the feces. Positioning on the left side allows easier access to the sigmoid colon.*

5. Place the linen-saver pad under the client's hips, and arrange the top bedclothing so that it falls obliquely over the hips, exposing only the buttocks.

6. Place the bedpan and toilet tissue nearby on the bed or a bedside chair.

7. Lubricate the gloved index finger. *Lubricant reduces resistance by the anal sphincter as the finger is inserted.*

8. Remove the impaction. Have the client take slow, deep breaths during the procedure.
   - Gently insert the index finger into the rectum, moving toward the umbilicus.
   - Gently massage around the stool. *Gentle action prevents damage to the rectal mucosa. A circular motion around the rectum dislodges the stool, stimulates peristalsis, and relaxes the anal sphincter.*
   - Work the finger into the hardened mass of stool to break it up (Figure 16-9 ◆). If you cannot break up the impaction with one finger, insert

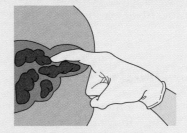

FIGURE 16-9 ◆ Digital removal of fecal impaction.

two fingers and try to break up the impaction scissor style.
   - Work the stool down to the anus, remove it in small pieces, and place them in the bedpan.
   - Carefully continue to remove as much fecal material as possible; at the same time, assess for bleeding or signs of pallor, feelings of faintness, shortness of breath, perspiration, or changes in pulse rate. Terminate the procedure if these occur. *Manual stimulation could result in mucosal damage, excessive vagal nerve stimulation, and subsequent cardiac arrhythmia.*
   - Assist the client to a position on a clean bedpan, commode, or toilet. *Digital stimulation of the rectum may induce the urge to defecate.*

9. Assist the client with hygienic measures as needed.
   - Wash the rectal area with soap and water and dry gently.

 10. **Document** the results of the procedure in the client record using forms or checklists supplemented by narrative notes when appropriate.

EVALUATION
- Perform a detailed follow-up based on findings that deviated from expected or normal for the client.
- Report significant deviations from normal (such as extensive bleeding) to the physician.
- Perform client teaching indicated to help prevent the formation of an impaction in the future.

Bowel Diversion Ostomies

An **ostomy** is an opening on the abdominal wall for the elimination of feces or urine. A **colostomy** is an opening into the colon (large bowel). An ascending colostomy empties from the ascending colon. A transverse colostomy empties from the transverse colon. A descending colostomy empties from the descending colon. A sigmoidostomy empties from the sigmoid

colon (Figure 16-10 ◆). The location of the ostomy influences the character and management of the fecal drainage.

- An **ileostomy** produces constant liquid fecal drainage and cannot be regulated. Ileostomy clients must take special precautions to prevent skin breakdown because ileostomy drainage contains digestive enzymes, which are damaging to the skin. Odor is minimal because few bacteria are present.
- An ascending colostomy is similar to an ileostomy in that the drainage is liquid and cannot be regulated, and digestive enzymes are present. Odor, however, is a problem requiring control (e.g., a deodorant inside the appliance).
- A transverse colostomy produces a malodorous, mushy drainage because some of the liquid has been reabsorbed. There is usually no control.

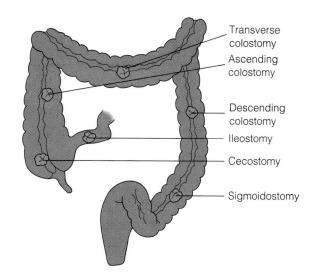

FIGURE 16-10 ◆ The location of bowel diversion ostomies.

- A descending colostomy produces increasingly solid fecal drainage. Stools are of normal or formed consistency, and the frequency of discharge can be regulated. Odors can usually be controlled.

There are four major types of **stoma** constructions: the single, loop, double-barreled, and divided colostomies.

- A **single (end) colostomy** has only one stoma (Figure 16-11 ◆), which arises from the end of the proximal portion of the bowel.
- For a **loop colostomy** (Figure 16-12 ◆), a loop of bowel is brought out onto the abdomen, supported by a plastic rod. If two openings are made, the proximal (or functioning) opening discharges fecal material and the distal or nonfunctioning end discharges only mucus. The loop colostomy is relatively large and cumbersome.

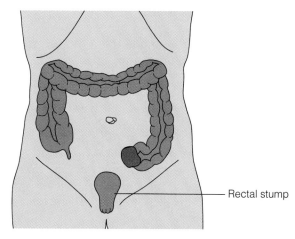

FIGURE 16-11 ◆ End colostomy with the disease portion of bowel removed and a rectal stump remaining.

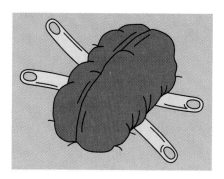

FIGURE 16-12 ◆ Loop colostomy using plastic rods to support the bowel on the abdomen.

- In the **double-barreled colostomy** (Figure 16-13 ◆), two separate stomas are constructed. One is the proximal, or functioning, stoma, and the other is the distal, or resting, stoma. The stomas are generally adjacent to one another—one above the other or side by side.
- A **divided colostomy** (Figure 16-14 ◆) has two stomas, separated on the abdominal wall.

Stoma and Skin Care

Enterostomal therapists or wound–ostomy–continence nurses are specially trained to assist the physician and client with all aspects of ostomy management. The equipment (appliance) used by a particular client is selected by the ostomy team and should not be modified without their advice. However, all nurses should be familiar with the basic aspects of caring for a fecal stoma.

The **ostomy appliance** consists of the skin barrier, flange or wafer, and the **ostomy pouch** (collection bag or reservoir) (Figure 16-15 ◆). The barrier has a pectin or synthetic faceplate with a skin adhesive that protects the skin surrounding the stoma. Pouches may be disposable or reusable, and either one-piece or two-piece systems. Temporary, disposable pouches are made of transparent plastic and have a hole into which the size of the stoma is cut. They are closed ended and, therefore, are removed and discarded rather than emptied. Permanent pouches may be clear or opaque, rubber or

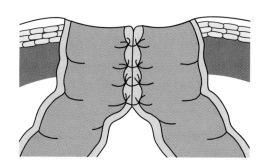

FIGURE 16-13 ◆ Double-barreled colostomy.

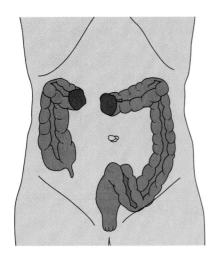

FIGURE 16-14 ◆ Divided colostomy: two separated stomas.

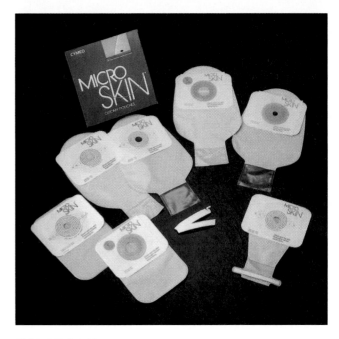

FIGURE 16-15 ◆ Ostomy appliances.

vinyl, and have a solid ring faceplate that fits around the stoma. They are drainable through removal of a clip at the bottom. One-piece systems have the pouch integrated with the barrier, whereas with two-piece systems the pouch attaches to a separate barrier with a ring.

Nursing Process: Bowel Diversion Ostomies

ASSESSMENT

Determine:

- The kind of ostomy and its placement on the abdomen. Surgeons often draw diagrams when there are two stomas. If there is more than one stoma, it is important to confirm which is the functioning stoma.
- The type and size of appliance currently used and the special barrier substance applied to the skin, according to the nursing care plan.
- Tape allergy.

Assess:

- *Stoma color:* The stoma should appear red, similar in color to the mucosal lining of the inner cheek. Very pale or darker-colored stomas with a bluish or purplish hue indicate impaired blood circulation to the area.
- *Stoma size and shape:* Most stomas protrude slightly from the abdomen. New stomas normally appear swollen, but swelling generally decreases over 2 or 3 weeks or for as long as 6 weeks. Failure of swelling to recede may indicate a problem (e.g., blockage).
- *Stomal bleeding:* Slight bleeding initially when the stoma is touched is normal, but other bleeding should be reported.

- *Status of peristomal skin:* Any redness and irritation of the peristomal skin—the 5 to 13 cm (2 to 5 in) of skin surrounding the stoma—should be noted. Transient redness after removal of adhesive is normal.
- *Amount and type of feces:* For ileal effluent and feces (colostomy effluent), assess the amount, color, odor, and consistency. Inspect for abnormalities, such as pus or blood.
- *Complaints:* Complaints of burning sensation under the faceplate may indicate skin breakdown. The presence of abdominal discomfort and/or distention also needs to be determined.
- The client's and family members' learning needs regarding the ostomy and self-care.
- The client's emotional status, especially strategies used to cope with the ostomy.

PLANNING

Review features of the appliance to ensure that all parts are present and function correctly.

Delegation

Due to the need for careful assessment and teaching, care of a new ostomy is not delegated to UAP. However, aspects of ostomy function are observed during usual care and may be recorded by persons other than the nurse. Abnormal findings must be validated and interpreted by the nurse. In some agencies, UAP may remove and replace well-established ostomy appliances.

Equipment

- Disposable gloves
- Electric or safety razor
- Bedpan
- Solvent (presaturated sponges or liquid)
- Moistureproof bag (for disposable pouches)
- Cleaning materials, including tissues, warm water, mild soap (optional), washcloth or cotton balls, towel
- Tissue or gauze pad
- Skin barrier (paste, powder and water, or liquid skin sealant)
- Stoma measuring guide
- Pen or pencil and scissors
- Clean ostomy appliance, with optional belt
- Tail closure clamp
- Special adhesive, if needed
- Stoma guidestrip, if needed
- Deodorant (liquid or tablet) for a nonodorproof colostomy bag

Preparation

1. Determine the need for an appliance change.
   - Assess the used appliance for leakage of effluent. *Effluent can irritate the peristomal skin.*
   - Ask the client about any discomfort at or around the stoma. *A burning sensation may indicate breakdown beneath the faceplate of the pouch.*
   - Assess the fullness of the pouch. Pouches need to be emptied when they are one-third to one-half full. *The weight of an overly full bag may loosen the faceplate and separate it from the skin, causing the effluent to leak and irritate the peristomal skin.*

2. If there is pouch leakage or discomfort at or around the stoma, change the appliance.

3. Select an appropriate time to change the appliance.
   - Avoid times close to meal or visiting hours. *Ostomy odor and effluent may reduce appetite or embarrass the client.*
   - Avoid times immediately after meals or the administration of any medications that may stimulate bowel evacuation. *It is best to change the pouch when drainage is least likely to occur.*

Performance

1. Explain to the client what you are going to do, why it is necessary, and how he or she can cooperate. Discuss how the results will be used in planning further care or treatments. Changing an ostomy appliance should not cause discomfort, but it may be distasteful to the client. Communicate acceptance and support to the client. It is important to change the appliance competently and quickly. Include support persons as appropriate.

2. Wash hands, apply clean gloves, and observe appropriate infection control procedures.

3. Provide for client privacy preferably in the bathroom, where clients can learn to deal with the ostomy as they would at home.

4. Assist the client to a comfortable sitting or lying position in bed or preferably a sitting or standing position in the bathroom. *Lying or standing positions may facilitate smoother pouch application, that is, avoid wrinkles.*

5. Unfasten the belt if the client is wearing one.

6. Shave the peristomal skin of well-established ostomies as needed.
   - Use an electric or safety razor on a regular basis to remove excessive hair. *Hair follicles can become irritated or infected by repeated pulling out of hairs during removal of the appliance and skin barrier. Excessive hair can interfere with adhesive action.*

7. Empty and remove the ostomy appliance.
   - Empty the contents of the pouch through the bottom opening into a bedpan. *Emptying before removing the pouch prevents spillage of effluent onto the client's skin.*
   - Assess the consistency and the amount of effluent.
   - Peel the bag off slowly while holding the client's skin taut. *Holding the skin taut minimizes client discomfort and prevents abrasion of the skin.*
   - If the appliance is disposable, discard it in a moistureproof bag.

8. Clean and dry the peristomal skin and stoma (Figure 16-16 ◆).
   - Use toilet tissue to remove excess stool.
   - Use warm water, mild soap (optional), and cotton balls or a washcloth and towel to clean the skin and stoma. Check agency practice on the use of soap. *Soap is sometimes not advised because it can be irritating to the skin.*
   - Use a special skin cleanser to remove dried, hard stool. *This emulsifies the stool, making removal less damaging to the skin.*
   - Dry the area thoroughly by patting with a towel or cotton balls. *Excess rubbing can abrade the skin.*

9. Assess the stoma and peristomal skin.

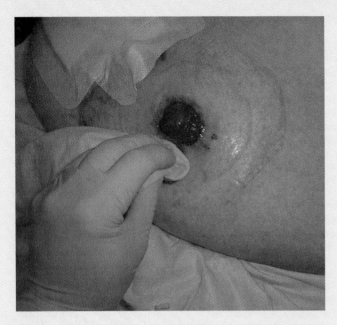

FIGURE 16-16 ◆ Cleaning the skin.

- Inspect the stoma for color, size, shape, and bleeding.
- Inspect the peristomal skin for any redness, ulceration, or irritation. Transient redness after the removal of adhesive is normal.
- Place a piece of tissue or gauze pad over the stoma, and change it as needed. This absorbs any seepage from the stoma.

10. Apply paste-type skin barrier if needed.
    - Fill in abdominal creases or dimples with paste. *This establishes a smooth surface for application of the skin barrier and pouch.*
    - Allow the paste to dry for 1 to 2 minutes or as recommended by the manufacturer.

11. Prepare and apply the skin barrier (peristomal seal).

For a Solid Wafer or Disc Skin Barrier

- Use the guide (Figure 16-17 ◆) to measure the size of the stoma.
- On the backing of the skin barrier, trace a circle the same size as the stomal opening.
- Cut out the traced stoma pattern to make an opening in the skin barrier. Make the opening no more than 0.3 to 0.4 cm (⅛ to ⅙ in) larger than the stoma. *This minimizes the risk of effluent contacting peristomal skin.*
- Remove the backing to expose the sticky adhesive side.
- Center the skin barrier over the stoma, and gently press it onto the client's skin, smoothing out any wrinkles or bubbles (Figure 16-18 ◆).

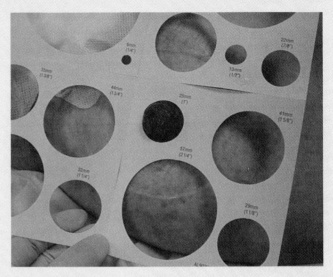

FIGURE 16-17 ◆ A guide for measuring the stoma.

For Liquid Skin Sealant

- Cover the stoma with a gauze pad. *This prevents contact with the skin sealant.*
- Either wipe or apply the product evenly around the peristomal skin to form a thin layer of the liquid plastic coating to the same area.
- Allow the skin sealant to dry until it no longer feels tacky.

12. Fill in any exposed skin around an irregularly shaped stoma.
    - Apply paste to any exposed skin areas. Use a non–alcohol-based product if the skin is excoriated. *Alcohol may cause stinging and burning.*

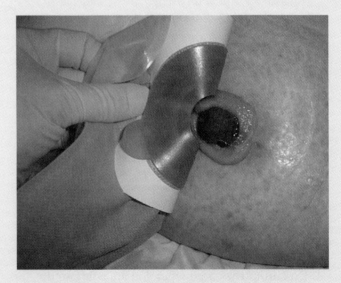

FIGURE 16-18 ◆ Centering the skin barrier over the stoma.

or

- Sprinkle peristomal powder on the skin, wipe off the excess, and dab the powder with a slightly moist gauze or an applicator moistened with a liquid skin barrier. *This creates a barrier or seal.*

13. Prepare and apply the clean appliance.

- Remove the tissue over the stoma before applying the pouch.

For a Disposable Pouch with Adhesive Square

- If the appliance does not have a precut opening, trace a circle 0.3 to 0.4 cm (⅛ to ⅙ in) larger than the stoma size on the appliance's adhesive square. *The opening is made slightly larger than the stoma to prevent rubbing, cutting, or trauma to the stoma.*
- Cut out a circle in the adhesive (Figure 16-19 ◆). Take care not to cut any portion of the pouch.

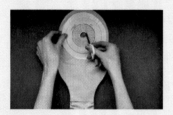

FIGURE 16-19 ◆ Cutting the wafer.

- Peel off the backing from the adhesive seal.
- Center the opening of the pouch over the client's stoma, and apply it directly onto the skin barrier (Figure 16-20 ◆).
- Gently press the adhesive backing onto the skin and smooth out any wrinkles, working from the stoma outward. *Wrinkles allow seepage of effluent, which can irritate the skin or soil clothing.*
- Remove the air from the pouch. *Removing the air helps the pouch lie flat against the abdomen.*
- Place a deodorant on the pouch (optional).
- Close the pouch by turning up the bottom a few times, fanfolding its end lengthwise, and securing it with a tail closure clamp.

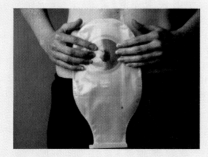

FIGURE 16-20 ◆ Applying the disposable pouch.

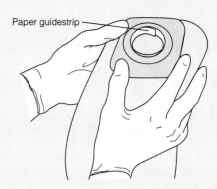

FIGURE 16-21 ◆ The coiled paper guidestrip in the faceplate opening.

For a Reusable Pouch with Faceplate Attached

- Apply either adhesive cement or a double-faced adhesive disc to the faceplate of the appliance, depending on the type of appliance being used. Follow the manufacturer's directions.
- Insert a coiled paper guidestrip (15-cm [6-in] strip of 1.3-cm [½-in] wide paper) into the faceplate opening (Figure 16-21 ◆). The strip should protrude slightly from the opening and expand to fit it. *The guidestrip helps the nurse center the appliance over the stoma and prevents pressure or irritation to the stoma due to an ill-fitting appliance.*
- Using the guidestrip, center the faceplate over the stoma.
- Firmly press the adhesive seal to the peristomal skin. The guidestrip will fall into the pouch; commercially prepared guidestrips will dissolve in the pouch.
- Place a deodorant in the bag if the bag is not odorproof. Most pouches are odorproof.
- Close the end of the pouch with the designated clamp.
- Attach the pouch belt, and fasten it around the client's waist (optional).

Variation: Applying a Reusable Pouch with Detachable Faceplate

- Some nurses recommend applying a skin sealant (e.g., Skin Prep) to the faceplate before attaching the adhesive disc. *This makes it easier to remove the adhesive disc from the faceplate.*
- Remove the protective paper strip from one side of the double-faced adhesive disc.
- Apply the sticky side to the back of the faceplate.
- Remove the remaining protective paper strip from the other side of the adhesive disc.
- Center the faceplate over the stoma and skin barrier, then press and hold the faceplate against the client's skin for a few minutes to secure the seal.
- Press the adhesive around the circumference of the adhesive disc.

• Tape the faceplate to the client's abdomen using four or eight 7.5-cm (3-in) strips of hypoallergenic tape. Place the strips around the faceplate in a "picture-framing" manner, one strip down each side, one across the top, and one across the bottom (Figure 16-22 ◆). The additional four strips can be placed diagonally over the other tapes to secure the seal.

• Stretch the opening on the back of the pouch, and position it over the base of the faceplate. Ease it over the faceplate flange.

• Place the lock ring between the pouch and the faceplate flange (Figure 16-23 ◆) to seal the pouch against the faceplate.

• Close the base of the pouch with the appropriate clamp.

• Attach the pouch belt, and fasten it around the client's waist (optional).

14. Dispose of equipment, or clean reusable equipment.

• Discard a disposable bag in a moistureproof bag before placing in the waste container.

• If feces are liquid, measure the volume. Note the feces' character, consistency, and color before emptying the feces into a toilet or hopper.

• Wash reusable bags with cool water and mild soap, rinse, and dry.

• Wash a soiled belt with warm water and mild soap, rinse, and dry.

• Remove and discard gloves.

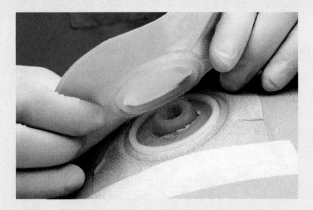

FIGURE 16-23 ◆ Sealing the pouch against the faceplate.

Variation: Applying the Skin Barrier and Appliance as One Unit

If a disc- or wafer-type skin barrier is used, the skin barrier and appliance can be applied as one unit. Applying the skin barrier and the appliance together not only is quicker but also is thought to reduce the chance of wrinkles. It also is easier for the client to apply without help.

• Prepare the skin barrier by measuring the size of the stoma, tracing a circle on the backing of the skin barrier, and cutting out the traced stoma pattern to make an opening in the skin barrier.

• Prepare the appliance by cutting an opening 0.3 to 0.4 cm (⅛ to ⅙ in) larger than the stoma size (if not already present) and peeling off the backing from the adhesive seal.

• Center the opening of the pouch over the skin barrier.

• Remove the skin barrier backing to expose the sticky adhesive side.

• Center the skin barrier and appliance over the stoma, and press it onto the client's skin.

15. **Document** the technique in the client record using forms or checklists supplemented by narrative notes when appropriate. Report and record pertinent assessments and interventions. Report any increase in stoma size, change in color indicative of circulatory impairment, and presence of skin irritation or erosion. Record on the client's chart discoloration of the stoma, the appearance of the peristomal skin, the amount and type of drainage, the client's experience with the ostomy, and skills learned by the client.

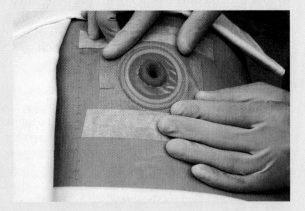

FIGURE 16-22 ◆ Taping the faceplate to the client's abdomen.

Changing an Ostomy Appliance

- Provide the client with the names and phone numbers of an enterostomal therapist, supply vendor, and other resource people to contact when needed.
- Inform the client of signs to report to a health care provider (e.g., peristomal redness, skin breakdown, and changes in stomal color).
- Provide client and family education regarding care of the ostomy and appliance when traveling.

- Educate the client and family regarding infection control precautions, including proper disposal of used pouches since these cannot be flushed down a toilet.
- Younger clients may have special concerns about odor and appearance. Provide information about ostomy care and community support groups. A visit from someone who has had an ostomy under similar circumstances may be helpful.

EVALUATION

- Relate findings to previous data if available. Adjust the teaching plan and nursing care plan as needed. Include on the teaching plan the equipment and procedure used. *Client learning is facilitated by consistent nursing interventions.*
- Perform detailed follow-up based on findings that deviated from expected or normal for the client.
- Report significant deviations from normal to the physician.

Colostomy Irrigation

A colostomy irrigation, similar to an enema, is a form of stoma management used for clients who have a sigmoid or descending colostomy. The purpose of irrigation is to distend the bowel sufficiently to stimulate peristalsis, which promotes evacuation. Clients who achieve a regular evacuation pattern usually need not wear a colostomy pouch.

Whether to perform routine daily irrigations to control the time of elimination is ultimately the client's decision. Some clients prefer to control the time of elimination through rigid dietary regulation, thus avoiding irrigations, which can take up to an hour to complete. Clients who elect to perform irrigations should perform them at the same time each day. Control by irrigations also necessitates some control of the diet. For example, clients need to avoid laxative foods that might cause an unexpected evacuation.

Nursing Process: Colostomy Irrigation

ASSESSMENT

Before commencing a colostomy irrigation, determine (1) whether the stoma needs to be dilated; (2) which is the distal stoma and which is the proximal stoma, if the colostomy is not an end colostomy, and which stoma is to be irrigated (usually the proximal stoma is irrigated, to stimulate evacuation of the bowel; however, it may be necessary to irrigate the distal stoma in preparation for diagnostic procedures); and (3) why the irrigation is being performed.

PLANNING

Determine if the client has had an irrigation previously. If so, gather history data regarding the purpose, equipment used, results, and client feelings about the procedure. If the client has had a colostomy for a long time, the irrigation needs to be given at the time the client has established, or the pattern of regularity will be disrupted. For a newly established colostomy, select a time based on the client's previous bowel habits and one that will allow the client to participate in usual daily activities. Encourage the client to select the time and to maintain it.

Delegation

Irrigation of a new colostomy is not delegated to UAP. However, they may perform irrigations of well-established ostomies if there are no complications anticipated. The nurse should reinforce use of standard precautions and what findings must be reported to the nurse. Abnormal findings must be validated and interpreted by the nurse.

IMPLEMENTATION:
TECHNIQUE 16-5 IRRIGATING A COLOSTOMY

Equipment

- Disposable linen-saver pad and a bedpan, if the client is to remain in bed

- Bath blanket
- Irrigation equipment (Figures 16-24 ◆ and 16-25 ◆)
  - A bag to hold the solution

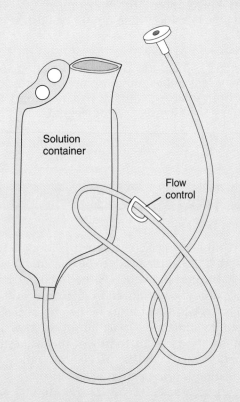

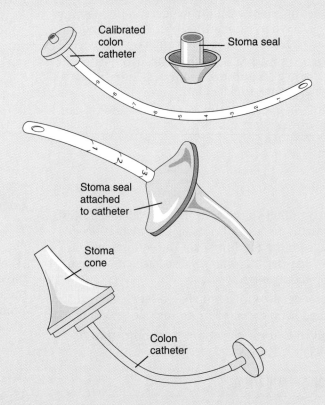

FIGURE 16-24 ◆ Colostomy irrigation equipment.

- Tubing attached to the bag
- Tubing clamp or flow regulator
- #28 rubber colon catheter, calibrated in either centimeters or inches, with a stoma cone or seal
- Disposable stoma irrigation drainage sleeve with belt to direct the fecal contents into the toilet or bedpan
- IV pole
- Moisture-resistant bag
- Clean gloves
- Lubricant

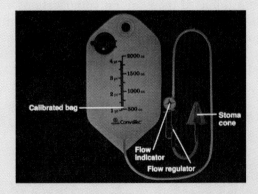

FIGURE 16-25 ◆ A commercially prepared colostomy irrigation set.

- Clean colostomy appliance or dressings
- Washcloth and towel

Preparation

- Fill the solution bag with 500 mL of warm (body temperature) tap water, or other solution as ordered.
- Hang the solution bag on an IV pole so that the bottom of the container is at the level of the client's shoulder, or 30 to 45 cm (12 to 18 in) above the stoma. *This height provides a pressure gradient that allows fluid to flow into the colon.*
- Attach the colon catheter securely to the tubing.
- Open the regulator clamp, and run fluid through the tubing to expel all air from it. Close the clamp until ready for the irrigation. *Air should not be introduced into the bowel because it distends the bowel and can cause cramps.*

Performance

1. Explain to the client what you are going to do, why it is necessary, and how he or she can cooperate. Discuss how the results will be used in planning further care or treatments.

2. Wash hands, apply clean gloves, and observe appropriate infection control procedures.

3. Provide for client privacy.

4. Assist the client who must remain in bed to a side-lying position. Place a disposable pad on the bed in front of the client, and place the bedpan on top of the disposable pad, beneath the stoma.

   or

   Assist an ambulatory client to sit on the toilet or on a commode in the bathroom. Ensure that the client's gown or pajamas are moved out of the way to prevent soiling, and cover the client appropriately with the bath blanket to prevent undue exposure.

   Throughout the technique, provide explanations, and encourage the client to participate.

5. Remove the colostomy bag and then position the irrigation drainage sleeve.

   • Remove the soiled colostomy bag, and place it in the moisture-resistant bag. *Placing the colostomy bag in this container prevents the transmission of microorganisms and helps reduce odor.*

   • Center the irrigation drainage sleeve over the stoma, and attach it snugly. *This prevents seepage of the fluid onto the skin.*

   • Direct the lower, open end of the drainage sleeve into the bedpan or between the client's legs into the toilet.

6. If ordered by the physician, dilate the stoma.

   • Lubricate the tip of the gloved little finger.

   • Gently insert the finger into the stoma, using a massaging motion (Figure 16-26 ◆). *A massaging motion relaxes the intestinal muscles.*

   • Repeat the previous two steps, using progressively larger fingers, until maximum dilation is achieved. *Stoma dilation is performed to stretch and relax the stomal sphincter and to assess the direction of the proximal colon prior to an irrigation.*

7. Insert the stoma cone or colon catheter.

   • Lubricate the tip of the stoma cone or colon catheter. *Lubricating the tip of the cone or catheter eases insertion and prevents injury to the stoma.*

   • Using a rotating motion, insert the catheter or stoma cone through the opening in the top of the irrigation drainage sleeve and gently

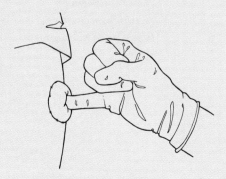

FIGURE 16-26 ◆ Dilating a colostomy stoma.

through the stoma. *A rotating motion on insertion helps to open the stoma.*

• Insert a catheter only 7 cm (3 in); insert a stoma cone just until it fits snugly. Many practitioners prefer using a cone to avoid the risk of perforating the bowel.

• If you have difficulty inserting the catheter or cone, do not apply force. *Forcing the cone or catheter may traumatize or perforate the bowel.*

8. Irrigate the colon.

   • Open the tubing clamp, and allow the fluid to flow into the bowel. If cramping occurs, stop the flow until the cramps subside and then resume the flow. *Fluid that is too cold or administered too quickly may cause cramps.*

   • If the fluid flows out as fast as you put it in, press the stoma cone or seal more firmly against the stoma to occlude it. If a stoma cone or seal is not available, press around the stoma with your fingers to close the stoma against the catheter.

   • After all the fluid is instilled, remove the catheter or cone and allow the colon to empty. Although not always indicated, you may ask the client to gently massage the abdomen and sit quietly for 10 to 15 minutes until initial emptying has occurred. *Massaging the abdomen encourages initial emptying.* In some agencies, the stoma cone is left in place for 10 to 15 minutes before it is removed.

9. Seal the drainage sleeve and allow complete emptying of the colon.

   • Clean the base of the irrigation drainage sleeve, and seal the bottom with a drainage clamp, following the manufacturer's instructions.

   • Encourage an ambulatory client to move around for about 30 minutes. *Complete emptying of the colon often takes up to half an hour. Moving around promotes peristalsis.*

10. Empty and remove the irrigation sleeve.

11. Ensure client comfort.

    • Clean the area around the stoma, and dry it thoroughly.

    • Put a colostomy appliance on the client as needed (see Technique 16-4).

12. **Document** findings in the client record using forms or checklists supplemented by narrative notes when appropriate.

    • Document all assessments and interventions. Include the time of the irrigation, the type and amount of fluid instilled, the returns, any problems experienced, and the client's response.

    • Promptly report to the nurse in charge any problems, such as no fluid or stool returns, difficulties inserting the tube, peristomal skin redness or irritation, and stomal discoloration.

AMBULATORY AND COMMUNITY SETTINGS

Irrigating an Ostomy

- Perform the procedure in an area where privacy can be maintained.
- Educate client and family about the importance of maintaining a regular irrigation schedule.
- If possible, teach a family member how to perform or assist with the irrigation.
- Discuss alternatives to the use of an IV pole based on the client's home setting (such as the hook on the back of the bathroom door). The bag should hang at about head height when the client is sitting.
- Provide information about how to modify the techniques when traveling. Teach the client that if the water is unsafe to drink, bottled water should be used for the irrigation.
- Ensure that the client is familiar with community resources and has means for obtaining supplies.

AGE-RELATED CONSIDERATIONS

Irrigating an Ostomy

Elders

- Older clients may need assistance with the procedure due to arthritic joints, hand tremors, or poor eyesight. Offer to assist only as needed, so the client can remain independent.

EVALUATION

- Perform detailed follow-up based on findings that deviated from expected or normal for the client. Relate findings to previous assessment data if available.
- Report significant deviations from normal to the physician.

Chapter Summary

TERMINOLOGY

carminative enema	enema	ostomy appliance
chyme	feces	ostomy pouch
cleansing enema	Harris flush	paralytic ileus
colonic irrigation	ileostomy	retention enema
colostomy	impaction	return flow enema
constipation	incontinence	single (end) colostomy
defecation	loop colostomy	stoma
divided colostomy	meconium	
double-barreled colostomy	ostomy	

Forming Clinical Judgments

Consider This:

1. An extremely heavy male client has requested the bedpan for a bowel movement. How would you assist him in getting onto the bedpan?

2. After you have administered about 150 mL of a soapsuds enema to the client, fluid begins to leak back out the anus and the client complains of rectal discomfort. What would you do?

3. During a home visit, a young client shares that her grandmother taught her to use digital stimulation to remove hard stool every week or so. What advice would you provide to this client?

4. When beginning to assist a client in changing a colostomy bag, you notice that the client is not using a skin barrier. When you ask about this, the client states that the barriers are too expensive since the bag is changed every day. The client's skin around the stoma appears in good condition. How would you respond?

5. You are teaching a client with a new colostomy about irrigation. The client expresses concern that the irrigation takes so long and may cause the client to be late to work. What suggestions might you make?

Related Research

Piwonka, M. A., & Merino, J. M. (1999). A muiltidimensional modeling of predictors influencing the adjustment to a colostomy. *Journal of Wound, Ostomy, Continence Nursing, 26,* 298–305.

References

Addison, R., Ness, W., Abulafi, M., & Swift, I. (2000). How to administer enemas and suppositories. *Nursing Times, 96*(6), 3–4.

Borwell, B. (1996). Colostomies and their management. *Nursing Standard, 11*(8), 49–55.

Fries, C. F. (1999). Wound care: Managing an ostomy. *Nursing, 29*(8), 26.

Lovell, J. (1997). About ostomy care. *Nursing, 27*(7), 25.

Moppett, S. (1999). Practical procedures for nurses: Administration of an enema. *Nursing Times, 95*(22), 2p.

O'Brien, B. K. (1999). Coming of age with an ostomy: Life with a stoma may be especially difficult for teens. *American Journal of Nursing, 99*(8), 71–74, 76.

(2000). Quick reference guide 13: Protocols for stoma care. *Nursing Standard, 14*(20), 2p.

Vaccari, J. A. (1998). Making it easy for patients to clean colostomy pouches . . . This practice may actually harm patients. *RN, 61*(12), 9–10.

Vickery, G. (1997). Basics of constipation. *Gastroenterology Nursing, 20,* 125–128.

Chapter 17

Assisting with Urinary Elimination

Techniques

OBJECTIVES

- Identify essential components of a urinary elimination history.
- Describe the steps of assisting clients with the use of a urinal.
- Identify reasons for using various types of urinary catheters or drainage systems.
- Describe insertion and removal of straight and indwelling catheters.
- Identify interventions required for clients with retention catheters.
- Discuss selected nursing interventions appropriate for caring for clients with urinary diversion ostomies.

The Urinary System

Urine is formed in the kidneys, then carried into the kidney pelvis and the ureter. The ureters extend from the kidneys to the urinary bladder. The urinary bladder lies behind the symphysis pubis. In the male, it lies in front of the rectum and above the prostate gland (Figure 17-1 ◆); in the female, it lies in front of the uterus and vagina (Figure 17-2 ◆). The urethra of the adult female is approximately 4 cm (1.5 in) in length. In the adult male, it is about 20 cm (8 in) long. The urethra extends from the bladder to the external surface of the body. This external opening is called the urinary **meatus.** In the female, it is located between the labia minora, in front of the vagina and below the clitoris (Figure 17-3 ◆); in the male, it is located at the distal end of the penis (Figure 17-1).

The urethra, in both males and females, has a continuous mucous membrane lining with the bladder and the ureters. Thus, an infection of the urethra can readily extend through the urinary tract to the kidneys.

Micturition, voiding, and **urination** all refer to the process of emptying the urinary bladder. Urine collects in the bladder until pressure stimulates special sensory nerve endings in the bladder wall called *stretch receptors.* This occurs when the adult bladder contains between 250 and 450 mL of urine. Messages sent from these nerves to the brain result in: (1) contraction of the **detrusor muscle** and (2) relaxation of the internal sphincter muscle. As a result, urine can be released from the bladder, but it is still impeded by the external urinary sphincter. If the time and place are appropriate for urination, the conscious portion of the brain relaxes the external urethral sphincter muscle, and urination takes place. If the time and place are inappropriate, the micturition reflex usually subsides until the bladder becomes more filled and the reflex is stimulated again. Table 17-1 shows variations in urinary

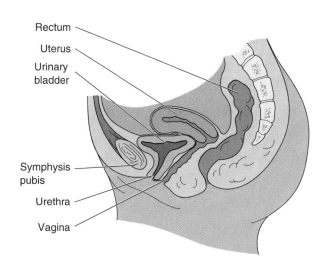

FIGURE 17-2 ◆ The female urinary system.

elimination among different age groups. In the female, the external urethral sphincter is situated at about the midpoint of the urethra; in the male, it is distal to the prostatic portion of the urethra.

Urinary Control

The nurse's role in urinary elimination may be to (1) assist the client with urinary control, (2) obtain a urine specimen (voided or catheterized), or (3) establish bladder emptiness through catheterization. Urinary control problems fall into two major categories: retention and incontinence.

Urinary retention is the accumulation of urine in the bladder and inability of the bladder to empty itself. Because urine production continues, retention results in distention of the bladder. With urinary retention, some adult bladders may distend to hold

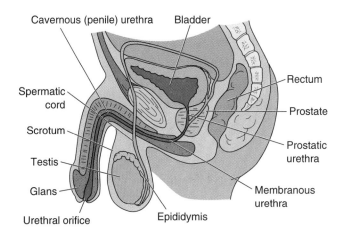

FIGURE 17-1 ◆ The male urogenital system.

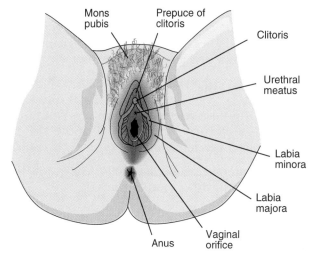

FIGURE 17-3 ◆ Location of the female urinary meatus in relation to surrounding structures.

TABLE 17-1

VARIATIONS IN URINARY ELIMINATION BY AGE

Age	Average Daily Urine Output	Other Variations
1–2 days	15–60 mL	Ability to concentrate urine is minimal; therefore, urine appears light yellow in color. Voluntary urinary control absent
3–10 days	100–300 mL	
10 days–2 months	250–450 mL	
2 months–1 year	400–500 mL	
1–3 years	500–600 mL	Urine effectively concentrated, normal amber color; voluntary control begins
3–5 years	600–700 mL	Full urinary control
5–8 years	700–1,000 mL	
8–14 years	800–1,400 mL	
Adult	1,200–1,500 mL	Kidneys continue to grow until about age 40; begin to diminish in size and function after age 50
Older adult	1,500 mL or less	Ability to concentrate urine declines

3,000 to 4,000 mL of urine. New devices can scan the bladder using ultrasound to determine bladder volume without invasive procedures (Smith, 1999).

Occasionally, a person will have urinary retention with overflow. In this situation, the bladder is holding urine, and only the overflow urine is excreted when the pressure of the urine overwhelms sphincter control. The client then voids small amounts of urine frequently or dribbles urine, while the bladder remains distended.

Urinary incontinence is a temporary or permanent inability of the external sphincter muscles to control the flow of urine from the bladder. It is the opposite of retention.

Urinals

Several designs of urinals are available: one is used for males (Figure 17-4 ◆) and one for females (Figure 17-5 ◆). Female clients most often use a bedpan for both urine and feces, while male clients generally use a urinal for urine and a bedpan for feces.

Guidelines for the Care of Urinals

The care of urinals relates largely to preventing the transmission of microorganisms and to the feelings people attach to elimination.

• To maintain medical asepsis, each client in a hospital is provided with a separate urinal.

• Urinals are stored in an appropriate place out of sight. Bedside units are often designed to provide a specific place for urinals that is not visible to others and is separate from the client's personal possessions. It is usually also separated from other equipment used for hygienic care. Medical aseptic prac-

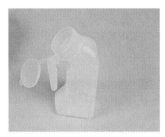

FIGURE 17-4 ◆ Male urinal.

tice prohibits the placing of a urinal on the floor under the bed or on overbed tables.

• Elimination equipment is thoroughly rinsed after use. Upon discharge, plastic urinals are generally given to the client to keep or are discarded. Metal urinals periodically need to be recycled through a central supply area for comprehensive cleaning and resterilization.

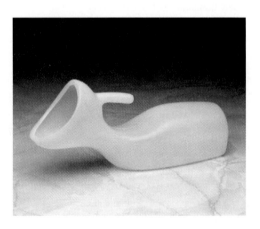

FIGURE 17-5 ◆ Female urinal.

Nursing Process: Assessment of Urinary Elimination

ASSESSMENT

The following assessment items relate to various aspects of urinary elimination. The nurse selects items appropriate to the particular technique being performed. Determine the client's usual patterns and frequency of urination. Ask the client the approximate number of times that voiding occurs each day. Determine any recent alterations in voiding in regard to:

- Passage of large amounts of urine
- Passage of small amounts of urine
- Voiding at more frequent intervals
- Trouble getting to the bathroom in time or feeling of **urgency** to void
- Painful voiding
- Difficulty starting urine stream
- Frequent dribbling of urine or feeling of bladder fullness associated with voiding small amounts of urine
- Reduced force of stream
- Accidental leakage of urine and when this occurs (e.g., when coughing, laughing, or sneezing; at night; during the day).

Obtain the medical history of elimination problems, urinary tract disease or surgery, and other diseases that may affect urinary elimination problems, including:

- Infections of the kidney, bladder, or urethra
- Urinary calculi
- Kidney surgery, bladder surgery, prostate removal, or other surgical procedures that alter urinary routes (e.g., ureterostomy)
- Cardiovascular disease, such as hypertension or heart disease
- Chronic diseases that alter urinary characteristics or impair urinary function, such as diabetes mellitus, neurologic disease (e.g., multiple sclerosis), and cancer

Assess the volume and characteristics of the client's urine:

- When the client last voided and the amount (Unanticipated volumes of less than 30 mL or more than 500 mL per hour must be reported immediately.)
- Dark, cloudy, or discolored urine
- Presence of mucous plugs
- Offensive odor

Determine any factors influencing urinary elimination:

- *Medications:* Any medications that could increase urinary output (e.g., diuretic), cause retention of urine (e.g., anticholinergic–antispasmodic, antidepressant–antipsychotic, anti-parkinsonism drugs, antihistamines, antihypertensives), or discolor urine (e.g., multivitamins, chemotherapy)
- *Fluid intake:* Amount and kind of fluid taken each day (e.g., six glasses of water, five cups of coffee, three cola drinks with or without caffeine)
- *Environmental factors:* Any problems with toileting (mobility, dexterity with clothing, toilet seat too low, facility without grab bar)
- *Disease:* Any illnesses other than urinary tract disease that may affect urinary function, such as hypertension, heart disease, neurologic disease (e.g., multiple sclerosis), cancer, prostatic enlargement, diabetes mellitus, or diabetes insipidus
- *Diagnostic procedures:* Recent procedures such as a cystoscopy or spinal anesthetic.

Determine the presence of pain:

- *Bladder pain:* Pain over the suprapubic region
- *Kidney or flank pain:* Pain between ribs and ileum that may spread to the abdomen and be associated with nausea and vomiting
  or
- *Pain at costovertebral angle,* which may radiate to the umbilicus
- *Ureteral pain:* Pain in back, which may radiate to abdomen, upper thigh, testes, or labia.

Review of data from diagnostic tests and examinations:

- **Urine pH** under 4.5 or over 8
- Specific gravity under 1.010 or over 1.025
- Presence of glucose or acetone in the urine
- Presence of occult or visible blood in the urine
- Presence of protein, urobilinogen, or nitrite in the urine
- Presence of microorganisms in the urine
- Blood serum: blood urea nitrogen (BUN), creatinine, sodium, potassium

PLANNING

Review the client record for presence of urinary tract obstructions. Determine if there are any restrictions in positioning the client. Inquire whether the client has used a urinal previously. If so, determine if the client has any unique needs related to the use of the urinal. Locate the client's urinal.

Delegation

Assisting the client with a urinal is often delegated to unlicensed assistive personnel (UAP). The nurse must determine if the specific client has unique needs that would require special training of the UAP in the use of the urinal. Ensure that UAP are aware of any specimens that need to be collected. Abnormal findings must be validated and interpreted by the nurse.

IMPLEMENTATION:
TECHNIQUE 17-1 ASSISTING WITH A URINAL

Equipment

- Clean urinal
- Toilet tissue
- Equipment for a specimen if required (see Techniques 4-4 through 4-7)

Preparation

Assist the client to an appropriate position.

1. Both males and females confined to bed may prefer a semi-Fowler's position, or the male may prefer a standing position at the side of the bed if health permits.

Performance

1. Explain to the client what you are going to do, why it is necessary, and how he or she can cooperate. Discuss how the results will be used in planning further care or treatments.

2. Wash hands and observe appropriate infection control procedures.

3. Provide for client privacy.

4. Assist the client with using the urinal.
   - Offer the urinal so that the client can position it independently.

   or

   - Place the urinal between the client's legs with the handle uppermost so that urine will flow into it.

- Leave the signal cord within reach of the person. *The client can then call for assistance if required.*
- Leave for 2 to 3 minutes or until the client signals.

  or

- Remain if the client needs support to stand at the bedside or other assistance.

5. Assist the client with removing the urinal as needed.
   - If wet, wipe the area around the urethral orifice with a tissue.
   - Make sure the perineum is dry.
   - Offer a dampened washcloth or water, soap, and a towel to wash and dry hands.
   - Change the drawsheet if it is wet.

6. Attend to the urine as required.
   - Measure the urine if the client is on monitored intake and output, and provide a specimen if required.
   - Empty and rinse out the urinal, and return it to the bedside unit. For males, the urinal may be hung on the side rail by its handle for easy access. Wash your hands.

7. **Document** findings in the client record using forms or checklists supplemented by narrative notes when appropriate. Record the amount of urine, if it was measured, and all assessment data (e.g., cloudy urine, reddened perineum).

AGE-RELATED CONSIDERATIONS

The Urinary System

Infant

- Babies have no conscious control, and the urine is released after a small amount accumulates in the bladder.

Child

- In children, 50 to 200 mL stimulates stretch receptors in the bladder.
- Urinary control normally takes place between 2 and 4½ years of age. Boys are usually slower than girls in developing this control.

Elders

- Bladder capacity decreases, as does ability to completely empty the bladder.
- Decreased muscle tone may lead to nocturia, frequency, and increased residual.
- Altered mobility or cognition may lead to incontinence.

- Perform a detailed follow-up based on findings that deviated from expected or normal for the client. Relate findings to previous assessment data if available.
- Report significant deviations from normal to the physician.

Applying an External Urinary Device

The application of a **condom catheter**, also referred to as a **urinary sheath** or **external catheter**, attached to a urinary drainage system is commonly prescribed for incontinent males. Use of a condom appliance is preferable to insertion of a retention catheter because it avoids entrance into the urethra and bladder and minimizes the risk of urethral or bladder infection. Some clients may require a condom appliance at night only, others continuously.

Nursing Process: Applying an External Urinary Device

ASSESSMENT

Review the client record to determine a pattern to voiding and other pertinent data. Apply clean gloves and examine the client's penis for swelling or excoriation that would contraindicate use of the condom catheter.

PLANNING

Delegation

Applying a condom catheter may be delegated to UAP. However, the nurse must determine if the specific client has unique needs that would require special training of the UAP in the use of the condom catheter. Abnormal findings must be validated and interpreted by the nurse. ◆

IMPLEMENTATION:
TECHNIQUE 17-2 APPLYING AN EXTERNAL CATHETER

Equipment

- Leg drainage bag with tubing or urinary drainage bag with tubing
- Condom sheath
- Bath blanket
- Disposable gloves
- Basin of warm water and soap
- Washcloth and towel
- Elastic tape or Velcro strap

Preparation

- Assemble the leg drainage bag or urinary drainage bag for attachment to the condom sheath.
- Roll the condom outward onto itself to facilitate easier application (Figure 17-6 ◆). On some models, an inner flap will be exposed. This flap is applied around the urinary meatus to prevent the reflux of urine.
- Position the client in either a supine or a sitting position.

Performance

1. Explain to the client what you are going to do, why it is necessary, and how he or she can cooperate.

2. Discuss how the results will be used in planning further care or treatments.

3. Wash hands, apply clean gloves, and observe appropriate infection control procedures.

4. Provide for client privacy.
   - Drape the client appropriately with the bath blanket, exposing only the penis.

5. Inspect and clean the penis.
   - Clean the genital area, and dry it thoroughly. *This minimizes skin irritation and excoriation after the condom is applied.*

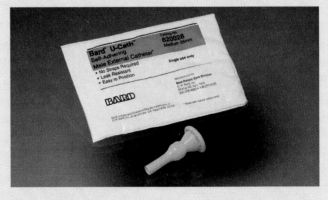

FIGURE 17-6 ◆ Before application, roll the condom outward onto itself.

6. Apply and secure the condom.
   - Roll the condom smoothly over the penis, leaving 2.5 cm (1 in) between the end of the penis and the rubber or plastic connecting tube (Figure 17-7 ◆). *This space prevents irritation of the tip of the penis and provides for full drainage of urine.*
   - Secure the condom firmly, but not too tightly, to the penis. Some condoms have an adhesive inside the proximal end that adheres to the skin of the base of the penis. Many condoms are packaged with special tape. If neither is present, use a strip of elastic tape or Velcro around the base of the penis over the condom. Ordinary tape is contraindicated because it is not flexible and can stop blood flow.

7. Securely attach the urinary drainage system.
   - Make sure that the tip of the penis is not touching the condom and that the condom is not twisted. *A twisted condom could obstruct the flow of urine.*
   - Attach the urinary drainage system to the condom.
   - Remove the gloves and wash your hands.
   - If the client is to remain in bed, attach the urinary drainage bag to the bed frame.
   - If the client is ambulatory, attach the bag to the client's leg (Figure 17-8 ◆). *Attaching the drainage*

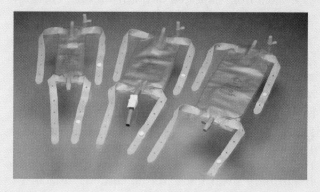

FIGURE 17-8 ◆ Urinary drainage leg bags.

bag to the leg helps control the movement of the tubing and prevents twisting of the thin material of the condom appliance at the tip of the penis.

8. Teach the client about the drainage system.
   - Instruct the client to keep the drainage bag below the level of the condom and to avoid loops or kinks in the tubing.

9. Inspect the penis 30 minutes following the condom application, and check urine flow.
   - Assess the penis for swelling and discoloration, *which indicates that the condom is too tight.*
   - Assess urine flow if the client has voided. Normally, some urine is present in the tube if the flow is not obstructed.

10. Change the condom daily, and provide skin care.
    - Remove the elastic or Velcro strip, apply clean gloves, and roll off the condom.
    - Wash the penis with soapy water, rinse, and dry it thoroughly.
    - Assess the foreskin for signs of irritation, swelling, and discoloration.
    - Reapply a new condom.

11. **Document** findings in the client record using forms or checklists supplemented by narrative notes when appropriate. Record the application of the condom, the time, and pertinent observations, such as irritated areas on the penis.

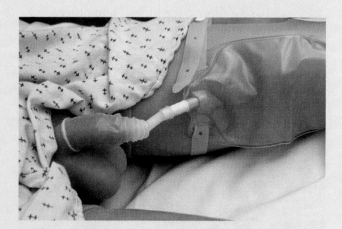

FIGURE 17-7 ◆ The condom rolled over the penis.

EVALUATION

- Perform a detailed follow-up based on findings that deviated from expected or normal for the client. Relate findings to previous assessment data if available.

- Report significant deviations from normal to the physician.

Urinary Catheterization

Urinary catheterization is the introduction of a **catheter** through the urethra into the urinary bladder. This is usually performed only when absolutely necessary, because the danger exists of introducing microorganisms into the bladder. Thus, strict sterile technique is used for catheterization.

Another hazard is trauma, particularly in the male client, whose urethra is longer and more tortuous. It is important to insert a catheter along the normal contour of the urethra. Damage to the urethra can occur if the catheter is forced through **strictures** or at an incorrect angle. In females, the urethra lies posteriorly, then takes a slightly anterior direction toward the bladder (see Figure 17-2). In males, the urethra is normally curved (see Figure 17-1), but it can be straightened by elevating the penis to a position perpendicular to the body.

Catheters are sized by the diameter of the lumen and are graded on a French scale of numbers; the larger the number, the larger the lumen. Sizes 14, 16, and 18 are commonly used for adults. Men frequently require a larger size than women. Only even numbers are available.

Two categories of urethral catheters are straight catheters and retention catheters. The straight catheter, or **Robinson catheter,** is a single-lumen tube with a small eye or opening about 1¼ cm (½ in) from the insertion tip (Figure 17-9 ◆). The retention catheter, or **Foley catheter,** contains a second, smaller tube throughout its length on the inside. This tube is connected to a balloon near the insertion tip. After catheter insertion, the balloon is inflated to hold the catheter in place within the bladder. The outside end

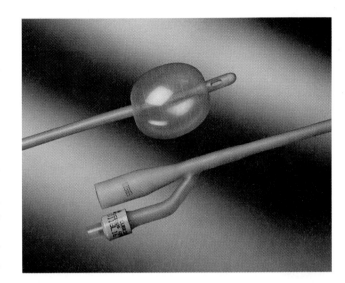

FIGURE 17-10 ◆ A retention (Foley) catheter with the balloon inflated.

of the retention catheter is bifurcated, that is, it has two openings, one to drain the urine, the other to inflate the balloon (Figure 17-10 ◆).

Another type of catheter is the coudé (elbowed) catheter, which has a curved tip (Figure 17-11 ◆). This is sometimes used for elderly men who have a hypertrophied prostate, because its passage is often less traumatic to the gland than the passage of a straight catheter. It is somewhat stiff and is more readily controlled.

For a client requiring continual or periodic bladder irrigations, the three-way Foley catheter is used (Figure 17-12 ◆). It is similar to the two-way Foley catheter described earlier, except that it has a third channel through which sterile fluid can flow into the urinary bladder. From the bladder, the fluid then flows through a second channel into a receptacle.

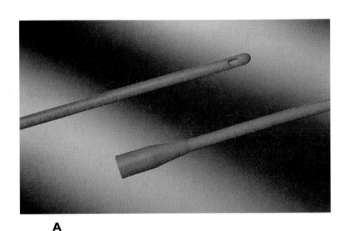

A

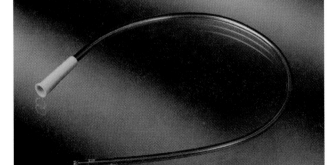

B

FIGURE 17-9 ◆ Straight (Robinson) catheters.

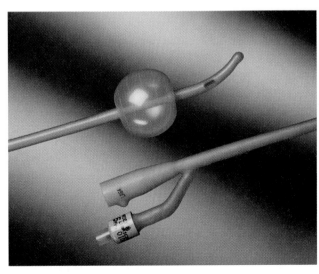

FIGURE 17-11 ◆ Coudé catheter tip.

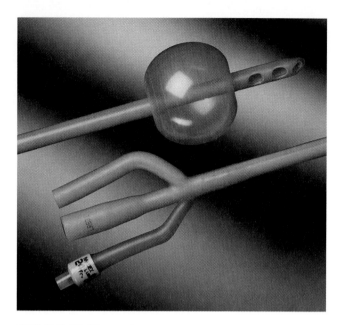

FIGURE 17-12 ◆ Three-way Foley catheter.

The balloons of retention catheters are sized by the volume of fluid or air used to inflate them. The two commonly used sizes are 5-mL and 30-mL balloons. The size of the balloon is indicated on the catheter along with the diameter (e.g., #18 Fr—5 mL). See Box 17-1 for guidelines in selecting an appropriate catheter.

Retention catheters are usually connected to a closed gravity drainage system. This system consists of the catheter, draining/collecting tubing, and the drainage/collecting bag. A closed system reduces the risk of microorganisms entering the urinary tract since it should not be opened at any point.

Nursing Process: Urinary Catheterization

ASSESSMENT

- Determine the most appropriate method of catheterization based on the purpose and any criteria specified in the order such as total amount of urine to be removed or size of catheter to be used.

- Use a straight catheter if only a spot urine specimen is needed, if amount of residual urine is being measured, or if temporary decompression/emptying of the bladder is required.

- Use an indwelling/retention catheter if the bladder must remain empty or continuous urine measurement/collection is needed.

- Assess the client's overall condition. Determine if the client is able to cooperate and hold still during the procedure, and if the client can be positioned supine with head relatively flat.

- Determine when the client last voided or was last catheterized.

- Percuss the bladder to check for fullness or distension.

PLANNING

Allow adequate time to perform the catheterization. Although the entire procedure can require as little as 15 minutes, several sources of difficulty could result in a much longer time. If possible, it should not be performed just prior to or after the client eats.

Delegation

Due to the need for sterile technique and detailed knowledge of anatomy, insertion of a urinary catheter is not delegated to UAP.

Box 17-1 *Selecting an Appropriate Catheter*

- Select the type of material in accordance with the estimated length of the catheterization period.

  a. Use *plastic* catheters for short periods only (e.g., 1 week or less), because they are inflexible.

  b. Use a *latex* or *rubber* catheter for periods of 2 or 3 weeks.

  c. Use *silicone* catheters for long-term use (e.g., 2 to 3 months) because they create less encrustation at the urethral meatus. However, they are expensive.

  d. Use *PVC* catheters for 4- to 6-week periods. They soften at body temperature and conform to the urethra.

- Determine appropriate catheter length by the client's gender. For adult females, use a 22-cm catheter; for adult males, a 40-cm catheter.

- Determine appropriate catheter size by the size of the urethral canal. Use sizes such as 8 or 10 for children, 14 or 16 for adults. Men frequently require a larger size than women, for example, 18.

- Select the appropriate balloon size. For adults, use a 5-mL balloon to facilitate optimal urine drainage. The smaller balloons allow more complete bladder emptying because the catheter tip is closer to the urethral opening in the bladder. However, a 30-mL balloon or larger is commonly used to achieve hemostasis of the prostatic area following a prostatectomy. Use 3-mL balloons for children.

From *Fundamentals of nursing: Concepts, process, and practice*, 6th ed., by B. Kozier, G. Erb, A. Berman, & K. Burke, 2000, Upper Saddle River, NJ: Prentice Hall Health.

Equipment

- Sterile catheter of appropriate size. An extra catheter should also be at hand.
- Catheterization kit (Figure 17-13 ◆) or individual sterile items:
  - 1 to 2 pairs of sterile gloves
  - Waterproof drape(s)
  - Antiseptic solution
  - Cleansing balls
  - Forceps
  - Water-soluble lubricant
  - Urine receptacle
  - Specimen container
- For an indwelling catheter:
  - Syringe prefilled with sterile water in amount specified by catheter manufacturer
  - Collection bag and tubing
- 2 percent Xylocaine gel (if agency permits)

- Disposable clean gloves
- Supplies for performing perineal cleansing
- Bath blanket or sheet for draping the client
- Ensure that there is adequate lighting—obtain a flashlight or lamp if necessary

Preparation

If using a catheterization kit, read the label carefully to be sure all necessary items are included. Apply clean gloves and perform routine perineal care to cleanse the meatus from gross contamination. For women, use this time to locate the urinary meatus relative to surrounding structures (see Figure 17-14 ◆).

Performance

1. Explain to the client what you are going to do, why it is necessary, and how he or she can cooperate. Explain that catheter insertion causes the sensation of voiding and, possibly, a burning feeling. Discuss how the results of the catheterization will be used in planning further care or treatments.

2. Wash hands and observe appropriate infection control procedures.

3. Provide for client privacy.

4. Place the client in the appropriate position and drape all areas except the perineum.
   a. Female: supine with knees flexed and externally rotated
   b. Male: supine, legs slightly abducted

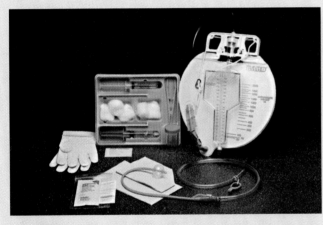

A

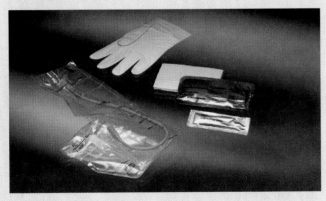

B

FIGURE 17-13 ◆ Catheter insertion kits: (A) indwelling; (B) straight.

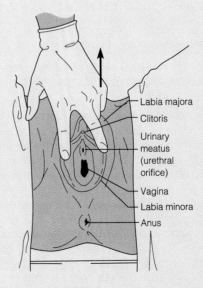

Labia majora
Clitoris
Urinary meatus (urethral orifice)
Vagina
Labia minora
Anus

FIGURE 17-14 ◆ To expose the urinary meatus, separate the labia minora and retract the tissue upward.

5. Establish adequate lighting. Stand on the client's right if you are right-handed, on the client's left if you are left-handed.

6. If using a collecting bag and it is not contained within the catheterization kit, open the drainage package and place the end of the tubing within reach. *Since one hand is needed to hold the catheter once it is in place, open the package while two hands are still available.*

7. If agency policy permits, apply clean gloves and inject 10 to 15 mL Xylocaine gel into the urethra. In the male, wipe the underside of the shaft to distribute the gel up the urethra. Wait at least 5 minutes for the gel to take effect before inserting the catheter.

8. Open the catheterization kit. Place a waterproof drape under the buttocks (female) or penis (male) without contaminating the center of the drape with your hands.

9. Apply sterile gloves.

10. Organize the remaining supplies:
    - Saturate the cleansing balls with the antiseptic solution.
    - Open the lubricant package.
    - Remove the specimen container and place it nearby with the lid loosely on top.

11. Attach the prefilled syringe to the indwelling catheter inflation hub and test the balloon. *If the balloon malfunctions, it is important to replace it prior to use.*

12. Lubricate the catheter (1 to 2 inches for females, 6 to 7 inches for males) and place it with the drainage end inside the collection container.

13. If desired, place the fenestrated drape over the perineum, exposing the urinary meatus.

14. Cleanse the meatus. *Note:* The nondominant hand is considered contaminated once it touches the client's skin.

    a. Female: Use your nondominant hand to spread the labia. Establish a firm but gentle position. The antiseptic may make the tissues slippery but the labia must not be allowed to return over the cleaned meatus. Pick up a cleansing ball with the forceps in your dominant hand and wipe one side of the labia majora in an anteroposterior direction (Figure 17-15 ◆). Use great care that wiping the client does not contaminate this sterile hand. Use a new ball for the opposite side. Repeat for the labia minora. Use the last ball to cleanse directly over the meatus.

    b. Male: Use your nondominant hand to grasp the penis just below the glans. If necessary,

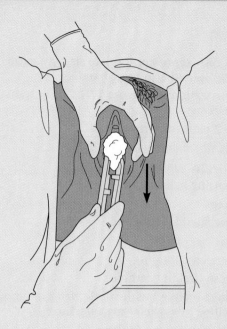

FIGURE 17-15 ◆ When cleaning the labia minora, move the swab downward.

retract the foreskin. Hold the penis firmly upright, with slight tension. *Lifting the penis in this manner helps straighten the urethra.* Pick up a cleansing ball with the forceps in your dominant hand and wipe from the center of the meatus in a circular motion around the glans. Use great care that wiping the client does not contaminate this sterile hand. Use a new ball and repeat three more times. The antiseptic may make the tissues slippery but the foreskin must not be allowed to return over the cleaned meatus nor the penis be dropped.

15. Insert the catheter.
    - Grasp the catheter firmly 2 to 3 inches from the tip. Ask the client to take a slow deep breath and insert the catheter as the client exhales. Slight resistance is expected as the catheter passes through the sphincters. If necessary, twist the catheter or hold pressure on the catheter until the sphincter relaxes.
    - Advance the catheter 2 inches further after the urine begins to flow through it to be sure it is fully in the bladder.
    - If the catheter accidentally contacts the labia or slips into the vagina, it is considered contaminated and a new, sterile catheter must be used. The contaminated catheter may be left in the vagina until the new catheter is inserted to help avoid mistaking the vaginal opening for the urethral meatus.

16. Hold the catheter with the nondominant hand. In males, lay the penis down onto the drape, being careful that the catheter does not pull out.

17. For an indwelling catheter, inflate the retention balloon with the designated volume.

   • Without releasing the catheter, hold the inflation valve between two fingers of your nondominant hand while you attach the syringe and inflate with your dominant hand. If the client complains of discomfort, immediately withdraw the instilled fluid, advance the catheter further, and attempt to inflate the balloon again.

   • Pull gently on the catheter until resistance is felt to ensure that the balloon has inflated and to place it in the **trigone** of the bladder (Figure 17-16 ◆ A and B).

18. Collect a urine specimen if needed. Allow 20 to 30 mL to flow into the bottle without touching the catheter to the bottle.

19. Allow the straight catheter to continue draining. If necessary, attach the drainage end of an indwelling catheter to the collecting tubing and bag.

20. Examine and measure the urine. In some cases, only 750 to 1,000 mL of urine are to be drained from the bladder at one time. Check agency policy for further instructions if this should occur.

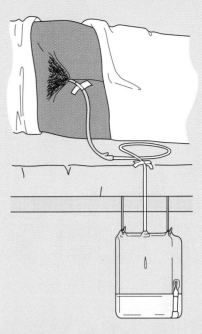

FIGURE 17-17 ◆ Tape the catheter to the inside of a female's thigh.

21. Remove the straight catheter when urine flow stops.

   For an indwelling catheter, secure the catheter tubing to the inner thigh for females (Figure 17-17 ◆) or the upper thigh/abdomen for males (Figure 17-18 ◆) with enough slack to allow usual movement. Also secure the collecting tubing to the bed linens and hang the bag below the level of the bladder. No tubing should fall below the top of the bag (Figure 17-19 ◆).

22. Wipe the perineal area of any remaining antiseptic or lubricant. Return the client to a comfortable position.

23. Discard all used supplies in appropriate receptacles and wash your hands.

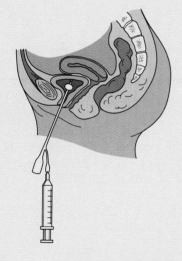

A

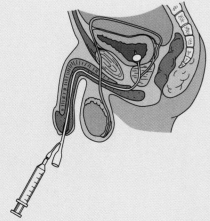

B

FIGURE 17-16 ◆ Placement of catheter and inflated balloon. (A) female client; (B) male client.

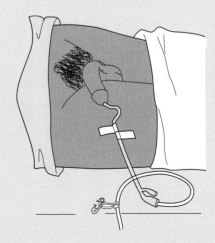

FIGURE 17-18 ◆ Tape the catheter to the thigh or abdomen of a male client.

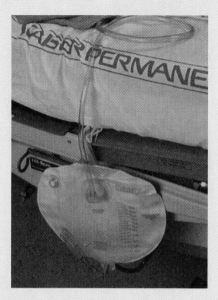

FIGURE 17-19 ◆ Correct position for urine drainage bag and tubing.

24. **Document** the catheterization procedure including catheter size and results in the client record using forms or checklists supplemented by narrative notes when appropriate.

EVALUATION

• Conduct appropriate follow-up such as notifying the physician of the catheterization results.

• Perform a detailed follow-up based on findings that deviated from expected or normal for the client. Relate findings to previous assessment data if available.

• Teach the client how to care for the indwelling catheter, to drink more fluids, and other appropriate instructions.

Catheter Care and Removal

Nursing care for a client with an indwelling catheter consists primarily of steps to reduce the chance of developing a urinary tract infection. It includes performing steps and client and family teaching about maintaining adequate fluid intake (3 L/day if possible), emptying and recording urine output, and maintaining the patency and cleanliness of the drainage system.

Perineal care practices for clients with indwelling catheters vary significantly according to agency policy. In general, routine perineal care involving washing with soap and water and removing discharge or crusts that may form around the catheter is considered sufficient.

Some clients may have a **suprapubic catheter,** an indwelling catheter that has been surgically placed in the bladder through the abdominal wall (Figure 17-20 ◆), either with or without a urethrally placed

catheter. Client teaching and care of the suprapubic system is substantially the same as for a catheter inserted through the urethra. However, the abdominal insertion site dressing must be treated as a sterile wound (see Chapter 30), and only the physician or specially trained nurse removes the catheter.

An indwelling catheter may be removed when the reason for its insertion is no longer present or a new or different type of catheter is indicated.

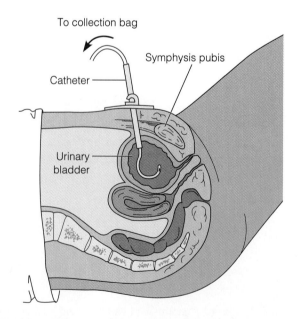

FIGURE 17-20 ◆ Suprapubic catheter in place.

Nursing Process: Catheter Care and Removal

ASSESSMENT

- Review the client record to determine the length of time the catheter has been in place and any difficulties reported with the system. Routine changing of the catheter and tubing is not recommended. If there are significant sediment, blood, or mucous threads in the tubing or the system is not draining adequately, the catheter may need to be replaced.

- Assess the client for any complaints of discomfort from the catheter. The initial sensation of the need to void is common after insertion and should diminish.

- Examine the perineal area for redness, discharge, or lesions.

PLANNING

If the catheter requires changing, an entire new system with collecting bag must be used.

Delegation

Routine care of the client with an indwelling catheter may be delegated to UAP. Abnormal findings must be validated and interpreted by the nurse. Removal of an indwelling catheter may be performed by UAP according to agency policy, provided they have been thoroughly trained in the procedure and are aware of conditions that could arise that require the assistance of a nurse.

IMPLEMENTATION:
TECHNIQUE 17-4 PERFORMING CATHETER CARE AND REMOVAL

Equipment

- Clean gloves
- Washcloth, soap, and towels

For catheter removal:
- Paper towel or waste receptacle
- Luer-Lok syringe at least as large as the size of the retention balloon (printed on the inflation port)

Preparation

Determine an appropriate time for catheter care or removal.

Performance

1. Explain to the client what you are going to do, why it is necessary, and how he or she can cooperate. Discuss how the results will be used in planning further care or treatments.

2. Wash hands and observe appropriate infection control procedures.

3. Provide for client privacy.

4. Prepare the client.
   - Ask the client to assume a back-lying position.
   - Obtain a sterile urine specimen if ordered or recommended by agency protocol.
   - If removing the catheter, remove the tape attaching the catheter to the client.

5. Perform catheter care.
   - Don gloves.
   - Wash the urinary meatus and the proximal catheter with soap and water. Dry gently.

6. Empty the collection bag at least every 8 hours.
   - Apply clean gloves.
   - Obtain the graduated container used for measuring urine for that client.
   - Remove the end of the drainage tube from its protective housing without touching the end.
   - Point the tube into the container and release the clamp.
   - After the bag is completely emptied, cleanse the end of the tube according to agency policy (e.g., with an alcohol swab) and replace it into the protective housing.
   - Note the volume and characteristics of the urine. Empty the container into the toilet if the urine does not need to be saved.
   - Rinse the container and return it to its storage location.
   - Remove gloves and wash your hands.

7. Remove the catheter.
   - Place a paper towel or receptacle between the client's legs.
   - Insert the hub of the syringe into the inflation tube of the catheter.
   - Withdraw all the fluid from the balloon. *This will permit the balloon to deflate.* If not all the fluid can be removed report this fact to the nurse in charge before proceeding. *Do not* pull the catheter while the balloon is inflated. *The urethra may be injured.*
   - Gently withdraw the catheter, observe for intactness, and place in the paper towel or waste receptacle. *If the catheter is not intact, parts may remain in the bladder. Report this immediately to the nurse in charge or physician.*
   - Wash and dry the perineal area.

8. Measure the urine in the drainage bag (see step 6 above).

9. Discard all used supplies in appropriate receptacles, remove gloves, and wash your hands.

10. Document the procedure and assessment data.
    - Record the time the catheter was removed; the intactness of the catheter; and the amount, color, and clarity of the urine.

11. Determine time of first voiding and the amount voided over the first 8 hours. Compare this with the fluid intake. *When the fluid output is considerably less than the fluid intake the bladder may be retaining urine.* If urine retention is suspected, palpate the bladder for fullness. Notify the physician if the client has not voided in 8 hours (or another interval specified by policy).

 12. **Document** findings in the client record using forms or checklists supplemented by narrative notes when appropriate.

AMBULATORY AND COMMUNITY SETTINGS

Urinary Catheterization

- Clients with spinal cord injuries who are unable to stimulate voiding may use intermittent straight catheterization every few hours. The client or another caregiver can perform this procedure once taught by a nurse. Often, the client will use clean rather than sterile technique and reuse equipment since the microorganisms to which the client is exposed are his or her own.

- For ambulatory clients, those in the home, or those in wheelchairs who have indwelling catheters, modifications are needed in securing the catheter and maintaining the collection bag below bladder level (Figure 17-21 ◆). A leg bag may substitute for a hanging bag for those who are upright.

- Clients who have indwelling catheters for lengthy periods of time need to have the catheter and bag changed at regular intervals. Changing equipment once a month is often the standard although agency policy may differ.

- Discuss with the client and family ways to minimize urinary tract infections in those requiring frequent catheterization. Increased fluid intake and urine acidification through drinking cranberry juice are two examples. Also discuss modifications in hygiene and sexual intercourse that may be indicated for persons with indwelling catheters.

- Teach the client and family when and how to empty the collection bag and to assess the urine for signs of infection, bleeding, or other complications.

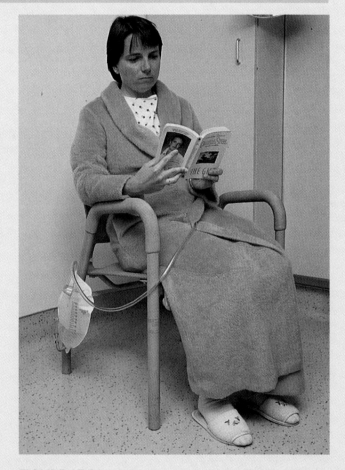

FIGURE 17-21 ◆ Positioning the collecting bag and tubing when sitting in a chair.

EVALUATION

- Perform detailed follow-up based on findings that deviated from expected or normal for the client.

Relate findings to previous assessment data if available.

- Report significant deviations from normal to the physician.

Urinary Irrigations

Irrigation is a flushing or washing out with a specified solution. Bladder irrigation is carried out on a physician's order, usually to wash out the bladder and/or apply an antiseptic solution to the bladder lining to treat a bladder infection. Sterile technique is used. Catheter irrigations are usually carried out to maintain or restore the patency of a catheter, for example, to remove blood clots that have formed in the bladder and are blocking the catheter. A physician's order may or may not be required, depending on agency protocol.

There are three ways of irrigating a catheter or bladder for a client with an indwelling catheter: (1) closed intermittent irrigation maintains the closed system by injecting the solution through an aspiration port, (2) closed intermittent or continuous irrigation irrigates through a three-way catheter (see Figure 17-12), and (3) an open intermittent system irrigates through a catheter after separating the catheter and tubing. Closed sterile drainage systems are recommended. To irrigate an adult bladder, 1,000 mL is commonly used; for catheter irrigation, 200 mL is normally required.

Nursing Process: Urinary Irrigations

ASSESSMENT

Determine the client's current urinary drainage system. Review the client record for recent intake and output and any difficulties the client has been experiencing with the system. Review the results of previous irrigations.

Assess the client for any discomfort, bladder spasms, or distended bladder.

PLANNING

Before irrigating a catheter or bladder, check (1) the reason for the irrigation; (2) the order authorizing the continuous or intermittent irrigation (in most agencies, a physician's order is required); (3) the type of sterile solution, the amount, and strength to be used, and the rate (if continuous); and (4) the type of catheter in place. If these are not specified on the client's chart, check agency protocol.

Delegation

Due to the need for sterile technique, urinary irrigation is generally not delegated to UAP. If the client has continuous irrigation, the UAP may care for the client and note abnormal findings. These must be validated and interpreted by the nurse.

IMPLEMENTATION:
TECHNIQUE 17-5 PERFORMING BLADDER IRRIGATION

Equipment

- Clean gloves
- Retention catheter in place
- Drainage tubing and bag (if not in place)
- Drainage tubing clamp
- Antiseptic swabs
- Sterile receptacle
- Sterile irrigating solution warmed or at room temperature

Label the irrigant clearly with the words *Bladder Irrigation,* including the information about any medications that have been added to the original solution.

- Infusion tubing
- IV pole

Performance

1. Explain to the client what you are going to do, why it is necessary, and how he or she can cooperate. The irrigation should not be painful or uncomfortable. Discuss how the results will be used in planning further care or treatments.

2. Wash hands and observe appropriate infection control procedures.

3. Provide for client privacy.

4. Apply clean gloves.

5. Empty, measure, and record the amount and appearance of urine present in the drainage bag. Discard urine and gloves. *Emptying the drainage bag allows more accurate measurement of urinary output after the irrigation is in place or completed. Assessing the character of the urine provides baseline data for later comparison.*

6. Prepare the equipment.
   - Wash hands.
   - Connect the irrigation infusion tubing to the irrigating solution and flush the tubing with solution, keeping the tip sterile. *Flushing the tubing removes air and prevents it from being instilled into the bladder.*
   - Apply clean gloves and cleanse the port with antiseptic swabs.
   - Connect the irrigation tubing to the input port of the three-way catheter.

- Connect the drainage bag and tubing to the urinary drainage port if not already in place.

- Remove the gloves and wash your hands.

7. Irrigate the bladder.

 a. For continuous irrigation, open the flow clamp on the urinary drainage tubing (if present). *This allows the irrigating solution to flow out of the bladder continuously.*

  - Open the regulating clamp on the irrigating tubing and adjust the flow rate as prescribed by the physician or to 40 to 60 drops per minute if not specified.

  - Assess the drainage for amount, color, and clarity. The amount of drainage should equal the amount of irrigant entering the bladder plus expected urine output.

 b. For intermittent irrigation, determine whether the solution is to remain in the bladder for a specified time.

  - If the solution is to remain in the bladder (a bladder irrigation or instillation), apply the flow clamp to the urinary drainage tubing. *Closing the flow clamp allows the solution to be retained in the bladder and in contact with bladder walls.*

  - If the solution is being instilled to irrigate the catheter, open the flow clamp on the urinary drainage tubing. *Irrigating solution will flow through the urinary drainage port and tubing, removing mucous shreds or clots.*

  - Open the flow clamp on the irrigating tubing, allowing the specified amount of solution to infuse. Clamp the tubing.

  - After the specified period the solution is to be retained, open the drainage tubing flow clamp and allow the bladder to empty.

  - Assess the drainage for amount, color, and clarity. The amount of drainage should equal the amount of irrigant entering the bladder plus expected urine output.

8. Assess the client and the urinary output.

 - Assess the client's comfort.

 - Empty the drainage bag and measure the contents (see step 6 of Technique 17-4). Subtract the amount of irrigant instilled from the total volume of drainage to obtain the volume of urine output.

 9. **Document** findings in the client record using forms or checklists supplemented by narrative notes when appropriate.

 - Note any abnormal constituents such as blood clots, pus, or mucous shreds.

Variation: Closed Irrigation Using a Two-Way Indwelling Catheter

1. Assemble the equipment. Use an irrigation tray (Figure 17-22 ◆) or assemble individual items, including:

 - Clean gloves
 - Disposable water-resistant towel
 - Sterile irrigating solution
 - Sterile basin
 - Sterile 30- to 50-mL syringe with a 18- or 19-gauge needle
 - Antiseptic swabs

2. Prepare the client (see steps 1 through 5 of main procedure for catheter irrigation).

3. Prepare the equipment.

 - Wash hands and don gloves.

 - Place the disposable water-resistant towel under the catheter.

 - Clamp the drainage tubing distal to the injection port on the tubing or catheter. *Clamping prevents the urine and solution from draining into the drainage bag.*

 - Using aseptic technique, open supplies and pour the irrigating solution into the sterile basin or receptacle. *Aseptic technique is vital to reduce the risk of instilling microorganisms into the urinary tract during the irrigation.*

 - Remove the cap from the needle and draw the prescribed amount of irrigating solution into the syringe, maintaining the sterility of the syringe and solution.

 - Using the antiseptic swab, clean the port on the catheter or drainage tubing through which the solution will be instilled.

4. Irrigate the bladder.

 - Insert the needle into the port.

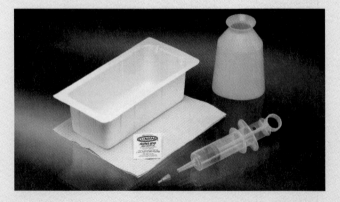

FIGURE 17-22 ◆ Irrigation tray.

- Gently inject the solution into the catheter. In adults, about 30 to 40 mL generally is instilled for catheter irrigations; 100 to 200 mL may be instilled for bladder irrigation or instillation. *Gentle instillation reduces the risks of injury to bladder mucosa and of bladder spasms.*
- For catheter irrigation, open the drainage tubing clamp *to allow the irrigant to flow back through the catheter.*
- When the total amount to be instilled has been injected (or for catheter irrigation, when urine is flowing freely), remove the needle from the port and discard the syringe and needle in an appropriate receptacle (sharps container). *Safe disposal of the syringe and needle is important to minimize the risk of needle-stick injury.*
- Remove gloves and wash your hands.
- After the prescribed dwelling time for bladder irrigation, remove the clamp from the drainage tubing and allow the urine and irrigating solution to drain into the drainage bag.
- Assess the drainage for amount, color, and clarity. The amount of drainage should equal the amount of irrigant entering the bladder plus expected urine output.

5. Assess the client and the urinary output and document the procedure as in steps 8 and 9 above.

EVALUATION

- Perform detailed follow-up based on findings that deviated from expected or normal for the client. Relate findings to previous assessment data if available.
- Report significant deviations from normal to the physician.

Urinary Diversion

A urinary diversion is the surgical rerouting of the urine produced in the kidneys to a site other than the bladder. Permanent urinary diversions are indicated for any condition that requires a total cystectomy (e.g., cancer of the bladder). Temporary urinary diversion stomas are indicated for any condition requiring partial cystectomy, trauma to the lower urinary tract, or severe chronic urinary tract infections.

With the most common type of urinary diversion, the **ileal conduit** or **ileal loop** (Figure 17-23 ◆), the client must wear an external pouch over the stoma to collect the continuous flow of urine. The person with an ileal bladder conduit or Kock pouch has had a reservoir for urine created from a piece of bowel (Figure 17-24 ◆). This diversion also has valves that close as the reservoir fills, preventing urine leakage. In this case, the client inserts a catheter into the valve several times each day to empty the urine. Between catheterizations, the client wears a small dressing over the stoma to protect the clothing from mucous drainage.

Application of a urinary diversion ostomy appliance is similar to application of a bowel diversion ostomy (see Technique 16-4). Essential interventions include peristomal care, application of a clean appliance when required, and teaching the client and support persons self-care.

Temporary disposable urinary diversion appliances are often attached to a urinary drainage system, especially during the night, to prevent accumulation and stagnation of urine in the appliance. To avoid separation of the appliance from the skin, pouches that are not attached to a drainage system must be emptied several times a day when they are one-third to one-half full.

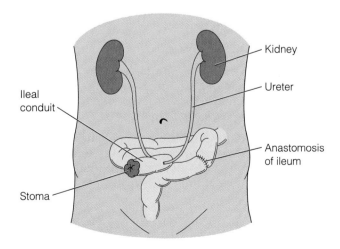

FIGURE 17-23 ◆ An ileal conduit urinary diversion.

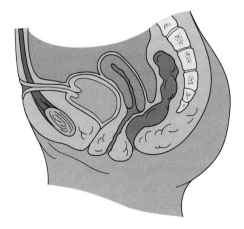

FIGURE 17-24 ◆ An ileal bladder conduit (continent urostomy/Kock pouch).

Peristomal skin barriers such as Skin Prep liquid or wipes or a similar product, or ready-made wafer-type or disc-type barriers are used according to the manufacturer's directions. The Karaya ring seal, although effective in protecting the skin, is less effective with urinary ostomies than with bowel ostomies because urine tends to melt the product.

The client will also need to learn ways to reduce the odor of urine. Use of deodorant tablets in the appliance, soaking a reusable pouch in dilute vinegar solution, a diet that makes the urine more acid, and drinking plenty of fluids all help control odor. Information about ostomy clubs and other community services available should also be included.

Nursing Process: Urinary Diversion

ASSESSMENT

Assess the amount and character of urine drainage; stoma size, shape, and color; status of the peristomal skin; allergies to tape; and the learning needs of the client and support persons.

PLANNING

Review the client's record to determine the type of urinary diversion. Determine when the device was last changed and any pertinent findings at that time. Generally, a urinary diversion appliance adheres to the client's skin for 3 to 5 days.

Delegation

Due to the complexity of the procedure, the need for assessment skills, and use of aseptic technique, changing a urostomy device is not delegated to UAP. However, aspects of ostomy function are observed during usual care and may be recorded by persons other than the nurse. Abnormal findings must be validated and interpreted by the nurse.

IMPLEMENTATION:
TECHNIQUE 17-6 PERFORMING URINARY OSTOMY CARE

Equipment (See Figure 17-25 ◆ A and B)

- One- or two-piece urinary pouch
- Tail closure clamp
- Clean gloves
- Cleaning materials, including tissues, warm water, mild soap (optional), washcloth or gauze pads, towel
- Skin barrier (gel, liquid, or film)
- Stoma measuring guide
- Pen or pencil and scissors
- Deodorant (liquid or tablet)
- Bedpan or graduated cylinder

Preparation

1. Determine the need for an appliance change.
   - Assess the used appliance for leakage of urine. *Urine irritates the peristomal skin.*
   - Ask the client about any discomfort at or around the stoma. *A burning sensation may indicate breakdown beneath the faceplate of the pouch.*
   - Assess the fullness of the pouch. *The weight of an overly full bag may loosen the faceplate and separate it from the skin, causing the urine to leak and irritate the peristomal skin.*
2. If there is pouch leakage or discomfort at or around the stoma, change the appliance.
3. Select an appropriate time to change the appliance.

- Avoid times close to meal or visiting hours. *Ostomy odor may reduce appetite or embarrass the client.*

Performance

1. Explain to the client what you are going to do, why it is necessary, and how he or she can cooperate. Discuss how the results will be used in planning further care or treatments. Changing an ostomy appliance should not cause discomfort, but it may be distasteful to the client. Communicate acceptance and support to the client. It is important to change the appliance competently and quickly. Include support persons as appropriate.

2. Wash hands and observe appropriate infection control procedures.

3. Provide for client privacy.

4. Assist the client to a comfortable sitting or lying position in bed or a sitting or standing position in the bathroom. *Lying or standing positions may facilitate smoother pouch application.*

5. Empty and remove the ostomy appliance. *Note:* Since urine flows continuously, if the stoma can be measured for the new appliance without removing the appliance, perform step 8 first.
   - Don gloves.
   - Empty the pouch through the bottom opening into a bedpan or graduated cylinder. *Emptying before removing the pouch prevents spillage of urine onto the client's skin.*

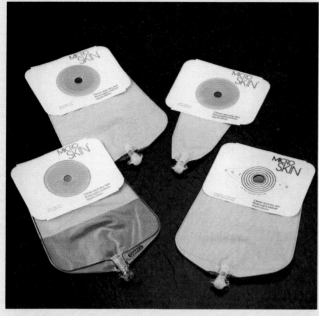

A

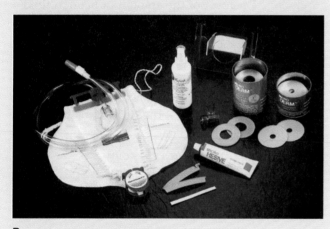

B

FIGURE 17-25 ◆ (A) one-piece urostomy system; (B) urostomy supplies.

• Peel the bag off slowly while holding the client's skin taut. *Holding the skin taut minimizes client discomfort and prevents abrasion of the skin.*

• Place tissues or gauze pads over the stoma, and change as needed. *This absorbs urine seepage from the stoma.*

6. Clean and dry the peristomal skin and stoma.

• Use warm water, mild soap (optional), and cotton balls or a washcloth and towel to clean the skin and stoma. Check agency practice on the use of soap. *Soap is sometimes not advised because it can be irritating to the skin.*

• Dry the area thoroughly by patting with a towel or cotton balls. *Excess rubbing can abrade the skin.*

7. Assess the stoma and peristomal skin.

• Inspect the stoma for color, size, shape, and bleeding.

• Inspect the peristomal skin for any redness, ulceration, or irritation. Transient redness after the removal of adhesive is normal.

8. Prepare and apply the new pouch.

• Measure the stoma size and cut the adhesive ring no more than ⅛ inch larger than the stoma. *This minimizes the risk of urine contacting peristomal skin or the ring cutting into the stoma.*

• Remove the backing to expose the sticky adhesive side of the barrier.

• Apply the peristomal skin barrier to the faceplate of the ostomy appliance or around the stoma.

• Center the faceplate over the stoma, and gently press it onto the client's skin, smoothing out any wrinkles or bubbles.

• Remove the air from the pouch. *Removing the air helps the pouch lie flat against the abdomen.*

• Place a deodorant on the pouch (optional).

• Close the pouch by turning up the bottom a few times, fanfolding its end lengthwise, and securing it with a tail closure clamp or replacing the drainage outlet cap (see Figure 17-25A).

• Discard all used supplies in appropriate receptacles, remove gloves, and wash your hands.

 9. **Document** findings in the client record using forms or checklists supplemented by narrative notes when appropriate.

EVALUATION

• Perform detailed follow-up based on findings that deviated from expected or normal for the client. Relate findings to previous assessment data if available.

• Report significant deviations from normal to the physician.

Chapter Summary

TERMINOLOGY

catheter
condom catheter
detrusor muscle
external catheter
Foley catheter
ileal conduit
ileal loop

irrigation
meatus
micturition
Robinson catheter
stricture
suprapubic catheter
trigone

urgency
urinary incontinence
urinary retention
urinary sheath
urine pH
urination
voiding

FORMING CLINICAL JUDGMENTS

Consider This:

1. An elderly male client requests that the urinal be left in place between his legs at all times. How would you respond?

2. Needing to use the urinal every 30 to 60 minutes around the clock has exhausted an 85-year-old man. However, he voids only 15 to 30 mL each time. Is a condom catheter an appropriate solution?

3. The order reads: "Catheterize for residual urine. If return is greater than 100 mL, leave catheter in place." What method will you use?

4. While removing an indwelling catheter, only about 75 percent of the amount of balloon fluid indicated on the catheter is retrieved. How would you proceed?

5. Following a transurethral resection of the prostate gland (TURP), significant bleeding may occur. The physician may order "irrigate catheter PRN." How would you determine if the catheter requires irrigating?

6. The hospitalized client's urostomy bag was last emptied 4 hours ago at 4 A.M. It now contains 100 mL. Is this acceptable? If not, what steps would you take.

RELATED RESEARCH

Adams, F., & Cooke, M. (1998). Evidence-based practice: Implementing evidence-based practice for urinary catheterization. *British Journal of Nursing, 7*(22), 1393–1394, 1396, 1398–1399.

REFERENCES

Colley, W. (1998). Practical procedures for nurses. Catheter care—1, no. 13.6. *Nursing Times, 94*(24), insert 2p.

Colley, W. (1998). Practical procedures for nurses. Catheter care—2, no. 13.7. *Nursing Times, 94*(25), insert 2p.

Evans, E. (1999). Indwelling catheter care: Dispelling the misconceptions. *Geriatric Nursing: American Journal of Care for the Aging, 20*(2), 85–89, inside back cover.

Laurent, C. (1998). Preventing infection from indwelling catheters. *Nursing Times, 94*(25), 60, 62, 64.

McMahon-Parkes, K. (1998). Management of suprapubic catheters. *Nursing Times, 94*(25), 49–51.

Newman, D. K. (1998). Managing indwelling urethral catheters. *Ostomy Wound Management, 44*(12), 26–28, 30, 32.

Pomfret, I. (2000). Catheter care in the community. *Nursing Standard, 14*(27), 46–53.

Sedor, J., & Mulholland, S. G. (1999). Hospital-acquired urinary tract infections associated with the indwelling catheter. *Urologic Clinics of North America, 26*(4), 821–828.

Sienty, M. K., & Dawson, N. (1999). Preventing urosepsis from indwelling urinary catheters. *American Journal of Nursing, 99*(1 part 1); 24C, 24F, 24H.

Smith, D. (1999). Gauging bladder volume. *Nursing, 29*(12), 52–53.

Wells, M. (1998). Coping with common catheter care problems. *Community Nurse, 4*(3), 22–24.

Winder, A. (1999). Female urinary catheterization. *Community Nurse, 5*(10), 33–34, 36.

Chapter **18**

Caring for the Client with Peritoneal Dialysis

Techniques

OBJECTIVES

- Describe essential aspects of peritoneal dialysis.
- Identify key elements of assisting the physician with insertion of a peritoneal dialysis catheter.
- Discuss care of the client undergoing intermittent or continuous peritoneal dialysis.

Peritoneal Dialysis

A nuria (lack of urine production), **oliguria** (inadequate urine production), and both acute and chronic **renal failure** can occur as a result of kidney disease, severe heart failure, burns, and shock. These conditions can be fatal if some other means is not used to remove the body wastes.

Peritoneal dialysis, also referred to as **peritoneal exchange**, is used as a temporary or permanent measure when kidney function is impaired. Peritoneal dialysis is the instillation and drainage of a solution (a **dialysate**) using the peritoneal cavity. Its purpose is to remove impurities, excess fluid, and electrolytes from the blood that would normally be excreted through the kidneys. The peritoneum is used as the dialyzing surface.

The dialysate solution contains water, glucose, and normal serum. When the solution is instilled into the peritoneal cavity, the body's waste products, excess electrolytes, and excess fluids pass by diffusion and osmosis across the semipermeable peritoneal membrane to the dialysate. The dialysate containing these waste products is then removed from the peritoneal cavity and replaced with fresh dialysate. This process replaces kidney function and permits the kidneys to rest.

For peritoneal dialysis, the physician inserts a catheter (commonly the **Tenckhoff catheter**) into the peritoneal cavity. This may be done at the bedside or in the operating room. Nurses assist with the insertion of the catheter, change the dressing at the catheter site, perform fluid exchanges, and assist with removal of the catheter. The basic peritoneal dialysis system and its components are shown in Figure 18-1 ◆.

There are currently three major types of peritoneal dialysis: intermittent peritoneal dialysis (IPD), continuous ambulatory peritoneal dialysis (CAPD), and continuous cycling peritoneal dialysis (CCPD). Intermittent peritoneal dialysis is performed within the acute care setting. IPD involves the infusion of one bag of dialysate solution at a time. The CAPD technique is performed by clients and allows the clients to go home with a peritoneal catheter in place and perform the exchange on themselves. The client is ambulatory and free to resume normal activities between exchanges. With CAPD, the focus of nursing care is on teaching the client and family to perform the **dialysis** treatments at home. CCPD is performed both in the acute care setting and at home by some clients who are capable of operating the cyclers. CCPD (also called automated peritoneal dialysis, or APD) involves the cycling of dialysate

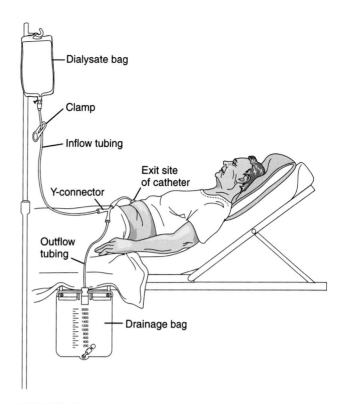

FIGURE 18-1 ◆ Peritoneal dialysis equipment.

infused through a mechanical fluid regulator and warmer.

Nursing Process: Beginning Peritoneal Dialysis

ASSESSMENT

- Vital signs and weight for baseline data and subsequent comparisons
- Abdominal girth, as an indication of fluid retention
- Respiratory status (rate, character, and breath sounds) as an indication of fluid retention
- Presence of edema
- Status of electrolytes, blood glucose level, and hematology profile studies

PLANNING

Confirm the physician's order for peritoneal dialysis and determine the type of catheter and insertion equipment preferred by this physician for the client.

Delegation

Assisting with peritoneal catheter insertion is a sterile procedure and not delegated to unlicensed assistive personnel (UAP).

Equipment

- Sterile gloves, masks, caps, goggles, and gowns for physician, nurse, and anyone assisting; mask for client and family
- Sterile peritoneal dialysis set containing
  - Peritoneal catheter: single-use (for less than 30 days use) or long-term catheter (for longer than 30 days use)
  - Local anesthetic (e.g., lidocaine), 25-gauge ⅝-inch needle, and 3-mL syringe
  - Alcohol sponges
  - Scalpel with a blade
  - Precut gauze to place around the catheter
  - Drape
  - Tubing and clamp
  - Dialysate filter (if specified by agency policy)
  - Sutures, needles, and needle driver
  - Trocar
  - Connector
  - 4" × 4" gauze square
  - Specimen container
  - Antiseptic ointment (e.g., povidone–iodine)
  - Protective catheter cap
  - 10-mL syringe and 1½-inch needle
  - Scissors
- Skin preparation set containing
  - Chlorhexidine, hydrogen peroxide, povidone–iodine, saline, or other disinfecting solution
  - Razor and blade
  - Gauze sponges
  - Nonallergenic tape

Preparation

Although the physician will have already done initial client and family teaching, the nurse reinforces key elements. Review the technique of peritoneal dialysis and its purpose with the client and family.

- Explain that since the kidneys are not functioning properly, this procedure will rid the blood and body of excess waste and fluid that are normally excreted by the kidneys.
- Explain that inserting the trocar (which is the physician's responsibility) may be uncomfortable. If the client tenses the abdominal muscles as if for a bowel movement, the discomfort can be reduced.
- Explain that the purpose of the masks, gowns, gloves, and caps is to reduce the possibility of infection. Then explain that the client and any family in the room will also need to wear masks.

Performance

1. Explain to the client what your role will be, why it is necessary, and how he or she can cooperate.

2. Wash hands and observe appropriate infection control procedures throughout the various phases of the procedure. Provide masks for the client and family.

3. Provide for client privacy.

4. Prepare the client.
   - Ask the client to urinate before the procedure. *Emptying the bladder lessens the danger that it will be punctured by the trocar.*
   - Assist the client to a supine position, and arrange the bedding to expose the area around the umbilicus. *The insertion site is usually in the midline just below the umbilicus.*

5. Prepare the solution and the tubing (see Technique 18-2).

6. Implement surgical aseptic practices and body fluid precautions according to agency protocol.
   - Don masks. *Applying masks prior to breaking the seals on the packages reduces the chance of contamination.*
   - Don a cap, a gown, and goggles.
   - Open the dialysis set and any sterile supplies not part of the set (see the techniques in Chapter 12).
   - Don sterile gloves.

7. Assist the physician as needed during and after the catheter insertion.
   - Connect the end of the tubing from the solution to the catheter.
   - Connect the drainage receptacle to the outflow tubing. Close the outflow tubing clamp.
   - Cover the catheter site with the precut sterile gauze, and tape the dressing in place.

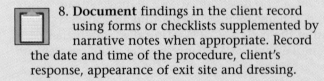 8. **Document** findings in the client record using forms or checklists supplemented by narrative notes when appropriate. Record the date and time of the procedure, client's response, appearance of exit site and dressing.

EVALUATION

Perform detailed follow-up based on findings that deviated from expected or normal for the client.

Nursing Process: Performing Peritoneal Dialysis

ASSESSMENT

Each time dialysis is begun, and periodically during continuous dialysis:

- Assess vital signs and weight for baseline data and subsequent comparisons
- Abdominal girth, as an indication of fluid retention
- Respiratory status (rate, character, and breath sounds) as an indication of fluid retention
- Presence of edema
- Status of electrolytes, blood glucose level, and hematology profile studies

PLANNING (IPD)

Review the client record for information about previous dialysis procedures. Note any complications and how these were managed and may be prevented. Before initiating dialysis, determine the physician's order specifying the amount and type of solution for each peritoneal exchange, the number of exchanges, the length of time the fluid is to remain in the peritoneal cavity, and the amount of fluid to be withdrawn from the peritoneal cavity.

Delegation

Conducting peritoneal dialysis procedures is not delegated to UAP. However, the client's status is observed during usual care and may be recorded by persons other than the nurse. Abnormal findings must be validated and interpreted by the nurse.

IMPLEMENTATION:
TECHNIQUE 18-2 CONDUCTING PERITONEAL DIALYSIS PROCEDURES

Equipment

For Infusing the Dialysate

- 1,000- or 2,000-mL container of peritoneal solution at body temperature, of the amount and kind ordered by the physician
- IV pole
- Drainage bag
- Sterile peritoneal dialysis administration set (separate or combined pieces)
  - Y connector
  - IV-type tubing for dialysate
  - Drainage bag with tubing
- Dialysis log or flow sheet
- Clean gloves, mask, goggles, gown
- Povidone–iodine swabs (or other antiseptic per agency protocol)

For Changing the Catheter Site Dressing

- Sterile gloves and masks (gowns and goggles as needed)
- Sterile cotton-tipped applicators
- Hydrogen peroxide, povidone–iodine solution, or soap and water as specified by agency protocol
- Povidone–iodine ointment
- Precut sterile 2″ × 2″ gauze or slit transparent occlusive dressing
- Nonallergenic tape

Preparation

Determine when the last dressing change was performed. The dressing should be changed when wet, soiled, loose, every 24 to 48 hours, or at intervals specified by agency policy.

Performance

1. Explain to the client what you are going to do, why it is necessary, and how he or she can cooperate. Discuss how the results will be used in planning further care or treatments.

2. Wash hands and observe appropriate infection control procedures.

3. Provide for client privacy.

4. Prepare the solution and the tubing.
   - Examine the label on the solution container and the solution itself. The solution should be clear and the seals unbroken. Check the expiration date.
   - Warm the dialysate using an approved warmer (not a microwave oven) to at least body temperature. *Warmed solution enhances exchange and is more comfortable for the client.*
   - Add any prescribed medication to the dialysate solution. Heparin is sometimes added *to prevent the accumulation of fibrin in the catheter;* povidone–iodine solution or antibiotics may be added *to prevent the growth of microorganisms;* potassium is often added *to prevent excessive loss of potassium.*
   - Spike the solution container, close the clamp, and hang the container on the IV pole.
   - Prime the tubing: remove the protective cap and hold the tubing over a cup or basin. Maintain the sterility of the end of the tubing and the cap. Open the clamp and let the fluid run

through the tubing, removing all bubbles. Close the tubing clamp. *This rids the tubing of air that could enter the peritoneal cavity, causing discomfort and preventing free drainage outflow.*

5. Connect the solution to the catheter.

   • Apply sterile gloves and free the catheter end from the dressing if necessary. Otherwise, clean gloves may be used.

   • Cleanse the catheter end with povidone–iodine or other specified disinfectant for the time listed in the agency protocol (usually 5 to 10 minutes). Attach the Y connector and end of the tubing from the solution to the catheter.

   • Connect the drainage receptacle to the outflow tubing. Close the outflow tubing clamp.

   • If necessary, cover the catheter site with the pre-cut sterile gauze, and tape the dressing in place.

   • Remove the gloves and wash your hands.

6. Infuse the peritoneal dialysate.

   • Open the clamp on the inflow tubing so that the dialysate can flow into the peritoneal cavity for the time period specified by the order. If no rate is specified, the client can usually tolerate a steady open flow.

   • After the fluid has infused, clamp the inflow tubing. *With the tubing clamped, air will not enter the peritoneal cavity.*

   • Leave the fluid in the cavity for the designated time period. This **dwell** time may range from 10 minutes to 4 hours.

7. Ensure client comfort and safety.

   • Assist the client into a comfortable position.

   • Place the call light within the client's reach, lift all bed rails, and lower the bed to its lowest position.

   • Monitor the client's vital signs every 15 minutes for the first exchange and hourly on subsequent exchanges.

   • Periodically assess the client's respiratory status and the status of comfort or discomfort during the dwell time.

8. Remove the fluid.

   • Unclamp the outflow tubing, and permit the fluid to drain into the drainage bag by gravity for about 30 minutes.

   • If the fluid does not drain freely, assist the client to change position, or raise the head of the bed. Drain only the amount specified by the order.

9. Assess the outflow fluid.

   • Assess the appearance of the outflow fluid. *A cloudy, pink-tinged, or blood-tinged return may indicate peritonitis.* During the first two to four exchanges, the return may be blood-tinged but should quickly progress to a straw-color return.

   • Apply clean gloves.

   • Measure the amount of outflow fluid, and discard the fluid and used supplies in an appropriate area.

10. Calculate the fluid balance for each exchange.

    • Compare the amount of outflow fluid with the amount of solution infused for each exchange.

    • If more fluid was infused than removed, the client's fluid balance is positive (+); if more fluid was removed than infused, the fluid balance is negative (–).

    Example:

    + 2,000 mL 2.5% dialysate solution infused

    – 1,500 mL dialysate fluid returned in drainage bag

    + 500 mL balance for this exchange

    • Repeat steps for each exchange.

11. Calculate the cumulative fluid balance. The cumulative fluid balance should be negative.

    • Add the balance from each exchange (from step 10) to the total exchange balance:

    Example:

Previous cumulative exchange balance	– 100 mL
Present exchange balance	+ 500 mL
Cumulative exchange balance	+ 400 mL

12. Check the dressing at the catheter site.

    • Wear a mask and sterile gloves when assessing the dryness or wetness of the dressing. *The dressing should remain dry during dialysis.*

    • To change the catheter site dressing, use the supplies listed above and follow Technique 30-3, pages 629–630. Do not forcibly remove crusts or scabs since *this may irritate skin and increase the risk of exit site infection.* Dressings may not be necessary for well-healed insertion sites.

13. Disconnect the catheter from the tubing, and cover the end of the catheter with a new sterile cap. *This allows the catheter to remain in place between each of the exchanges without contamination of the catheter.*

14. **Document** findings in the client record using forms or checklists supplemented by narrative notes when appropriate. Include the time during which the fluid infused; exchange number; dialysate and additives used; details of the exchange balance; color of outflow dialysate return from client; client's response; appearance of exit site and dressing; and client's weight before and after the set of exchanges.

Continuous Ambulatory Peritoneal Dialysis (CAPD)

The majority of the principles and infection control precautions that apply to IPD apply to CAPD. However, in CAPD, the empty dialysate solution bag is kept attached to the catheter during dwelling and is then used as the drainage bag. The client wears a special belt that stabilizes the catheter and holds the administration set between uses (Figure 18-2 ◆). Clients and family members require several teaching sessions to ensure they are capable of performing the techniques at home.

• In the home, warm the dialysate using a heating pad for about 1 hour.

• Hang dialysate bag at approximately shoulder height for infusion.

• After the fluid is infused, roll the empty bag and secure it using the waist pouch (Figure 18-2).

• Dwell the dialysate about 4 hours and overnight.

• After dwell is completed, unfold the dialysate bag and lower it to below the client's abdomen level. The dialysate returns by gravity flow.

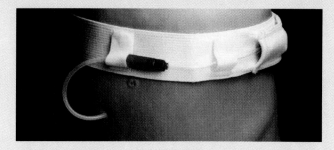

FIGURE 18-2 ◆ Peritoneal dialysis belt with tubing and pouch stored in place.

• Using clean technique, disconnect the bag from the tubing, drain into the toilet, and discard in an appropriate biohazard container.

• Hang and infuse new dialysate bag.

• Change tubing at least every 24 hours.

EVALUATION

• Perform detailed follow-up based on findings that deviated from expected or normal for the client.

Relate findings to previous assessment data if available.

• Report significant deviations from normal to the physician.

Chapter Summary

TERMINOLOGY

anuria	dwell	peritoneal exchange
dialysate	oliguria	renal failure
dialysis	peritoneal dialysis	Tenckhoff catheter

FORMING CLINICAL JUDGMENTS

Consider This:

1. As you prepare to assist with the procedure of insertion of the peritoneal dialysis catheter, the client expresses relief that the catheter will be in place for only 24 hours. How would you respond?

2. The client on continuous ambulatory peritoneal dialysis is to have daily weights taken. When would be an appropriate time to record the weight?

RELATED RESEARCH

Lindqvist, R., & Sjoden, P. (1998). Coping strategies and quality of life among patients on continuous ambulatory peritoneal dialysis (CAPD). *Journal of Advanced Nursing, 27,* 312–319.

Price, C. A., & Akin, B. (1999). A clinical project to evaluate reuse of a CAPD disconnect system minicap as a safe, effective practice. *ANNA Journal, 26,* 573–576.

REFERENCES

Bernardini, J. (1998). Establish protocols of patient care based on published research. *Peritoneal Dialysis International, 19,* 98.

Gokal, R., Alexander, S., Ash, S., Chen, T. W., Danielson, A., Holmes, C., Joffe, P., Moncrief, J., Nichols, K., Piraino, B., Prowant, B., Slingeneyer, A., Stegmayr, B., Twardowski, Z., & Vas, S. (1998). Peritoneal catheters and exit-site practices toward optimum peritoneal access: 1998 update: Official Report from the International Society for Peritoneal Dialysis. *Peritoneal Dialysis International, 18,* 11–33.

Gokal, R., & Mallick, N, P. (1999). Peritoneal dialysis. *Lancet, 353*(9155), 823–828.

Williams, J. (1998). "A change for the better": A nursing innovation for change in the CAPD catheter exit site care. *EDT-NAERCA Journal, 24,* 23–25.

Chapter 19

Promoting Circulation

Techniques

OBJECTIVES

- Describe two measures to help prevent venous stasis.
- Apply antiemboli stockings effectively.
- Apply a sequential compression device to the leg effectively.

Preventing Venous Stasis

When clients have limited mobility or are confined to bed, venous return to the heart is impaired and the risk of venous stasis increases. Immobility is a problem not only for ill or debilitated clients but also for some travelers who sit with legs dependent for long periods in a motor vehicle or an airplane. Venous stasis can lead to thrombus formation and edema of the extremities. Preventing venous stasis is an important nursing intervention to reduce the risk of complications following surgery, trauma, or major medical problems. Antiemboli stockings and sequential compression devices are measures to help prevent venous stasis and the potential complications of **deep vein thrombosis (DVT)** and **pulmonary embolism (PE)**.

Antiemboli Stockings

Antiemboli (elastic) stockings are firm elastic hosiery that exert external pressure to compress the veins of the legs, decrease venous blood from pooling in the extremities, and thereby facilitate the return of venous blood to the heart. They also improve arterial circulation to the feet and prevent edema of the legs and feet. They frequently are used for clients with limited mobility, either because of restricted activities or because of prolonged standing (e.g., supermarket checkers, surgeons, and surgery technicians). These stockings are frequently used postoperatively to avoid complications such as DVT and PE.

There are several types of stockings. One type extends from the foot to the knee and another from the foot to midthigh. These stockings usually have a partial foot that exposes the toes so that extremity circulation can be assessed. Elastic stockings usually come in small, medium, and large sizes. Some clients may require custom-made stockings. When obtaining antiemboli stockings for a client, follow the manufacturer's recommendations for measuring and fitting the stockings. See Technique 19-1 on applying antiemboli stockings.

Nursing Process: Preventing Venous Stasis

ASSESSMENT

Assess both lower extremities for:

- Rates, volumes, and rhythms of posterior tibial and dorsalis pedis pulses
- Skin color (note pallor, cyanosis, or other pigmentation)
- Skin temperature
- Presence of distended veins or edema
- Skin condition (e.g., thickened, shiny, taut)
- **Homans' sign** (pain in calf with passive dorsiflexion of the foot)

PLANNING

Before applying antiemboli stockings, determine any potential or present circulatory problems and the surgeon's orders involving the lower extremities.

Delegation

Unlicensed assistive personnel (UAP) frequently remove and apply antiemboli stockings as part of morning and evening hygiene care. The nurse should stress the importance of removing and reapplying the stockings and reporting any changes in the client's skin to the nurse.

IMPLEMENTATION:
TECHNIQUE 19-1 APPLYING ANTIEMBOLI STOCKINGS

Equipment

- Tape measure
- Clean antiemboli stockings of appropriate size and of the type ordered
- Talcum powder or cornstarch (check if the client has an allergy to the powder)

Preparation

Take measurements as needed to obtain the appropriate size stockings.

- Measure the length of both legs from the heel to the gluteal fold (for thigh-length stockings) or from the heel to the popliteal space (for knee-length stockings).
- Measure the circumference of each calf and each thigh at the widest point.
- Compare the measurements to the size chart to obtain stockings of correct size. Obtain two sizes if there is a significant difference. *Stockings that are too large for the client do not place adequate pressure on the legs to facilitate venous return, and may bunch, increasing the risk of pressure and skin irritation. Stockings that are too small may impede blood flow to the feet and cause discomfort.*

Performance

1. Explain to the client what you are going to do, why it is necessary, and how he or she can cooperate.
2. Wash hands and observe other appropriate infection control procedures.

3. Provide for client privacy.

4. Select an appropriate time to apply the stockings.

- Apply stockings in the morning, if possible, before the client arises. *In sitting and standing positions, the veins can become distended so that edema occurs; the stockings should be applied before this happens.*

- Assist the client who has been ambulating to lie down and elevate the legs for 15 to 30 minutes before applying the stockings. *This facilitates venous return and reduces swelling.*

5. Prepare the client.

- Assist the client to a lying position in bed.
- Wash and dry their legs as needed.
- Dust the ankles with talcum powder or cornstarch. *This eases application.*

6. Apply the stockings.

- Reach inside the stocking from the top, and grasping the heel, turn the upper portion of the stocking inside out so the foot portion is inside the stocking leg. *Firm elastic stockings are easier to fit over the foot and calf when inverted in this manner rather than bunching up the stocking.*

- Ask the client to point their toes, then position the stocking on the client's foot. With the heel of the stocking down and stretching each side of the stocking, ease the stocking over the toes taking care to place the toe and heel portions of the stocking appropriately (Figure 19-1 ◆). *Pointing the toes makes application easier.*

- Grasp the loose portion of the stocking at the ankle and gently pull the stocking over the leg, turning it right side out in the process (Figure 19-2 ◆).

- Inspect the client's leg and stocking, smoothing any folds or creases. Ensure that the stocking is not rolled down or bunched at the top or ankle. *Folds and creases can cause skin irritation under the stocking; bunching of the stocking can further impair venous return.*

- Remove the stockings for 30 minutes every 8 hours, inspecting the legs and skin while the stockings are off.

- Soiled stockings may be laundered by hand with warm water and mild soap. Hang to dry.

 7. **Document** the procedure. Record the procedure, your assessment data, and when the stockings are removed and reapplied.

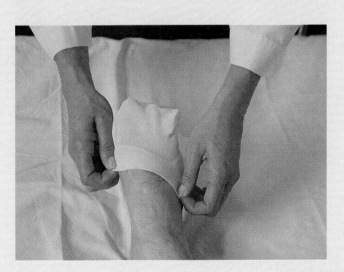

FIGURE 19-1 ◆ Applying the inverted stocking over the toes.

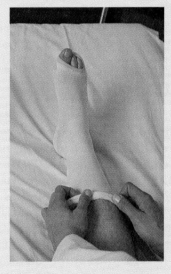

FIGURE 19-2 ◆ Pulling the stocking snugly over the leg.

AMBULATORY AND COMMUNITY SETTINGS

Antiemboli Stockings

- Teach the client or caregiver how to apply the antiemboli stockings.

- Stress the importance of no wrinkles or rolling down of the stockings and the rationale.

- Instruct the client or caregiver to remove the stockings regularly and inspect the skin on the legs.

- Provide instructions about:
  - Laundering the stockings
  - The need for two pairs of stockings to allow for one pair to be worn while the other is being laundered
  - Replacing the stockings when they lose their elasticity

AGE-RELATED CONSIDERATIONS

Antiemboli Stockings

Children

- Antiemboli stockings are infrequently used on children.

Elders

- Because the elastic is quite strong in antiemboli stockings, the older adult may need assistance with putting on the stockings. Clients with arthritis may need to have another person put the stockings on for them.

- Many elderly clients have circulation problems and wear antiemboli stockings. It is important to check for wrinkles in the stockings and/or to see if the stocking has rolled down or twisted. If so, correct immediately because the stockings must be evenly distributed over the limb to promote rather than hinder circulation.

EVALUATION

- Conduct appropriate follow-up at least every 4 hours.

- Note the appearance of the legs and skin integrity, any edema, peripheral pulses, skin color and temperature, and compare to previous assessment data, if available.

- If complications occur, remove the stockings and report significant deviations from normal to the physician.

Sequential Compression Devices

Clients who are undergoing surgery or who are immobilized because of illness or injury may benefit from a **sequential compression device (SCD)**, also known as **pneumatic compression device (PCD)**, to promote venous return from the legs. SCDs inflate and deflate plastic sleeves wrapped around the legs to promote venous flow. The plastic sleeves are attached by tubing to an air pump that alternately inflates and deflates portions of the sleeve to a specified pressure. The ankle area inflates first, followed by the calf region and then the thigh area. This sequential inflation and deflation counteracts blood stasis in the lower extremities and increases venous blood flow toward the heart (Figure 19-3 ◆).

Sequential compression therapy often complements other preventive measures. The client's risk level for DVT or PE often determines the preventive measures used. For example, clients at low risk may require only antiemboli stockings. Clients at moderate risk may have both antiemboli stockings and sequential therapy as part of their treatment. The physician may order antiemboli stockings, sequential therapy, and anticoagulation therapy for the high-risk client.

The SCD is available in knee-length or thigh-length sleeves. One research review (Vanek, 1998) found that SCD was effective in decreasing the incidence of DVT;

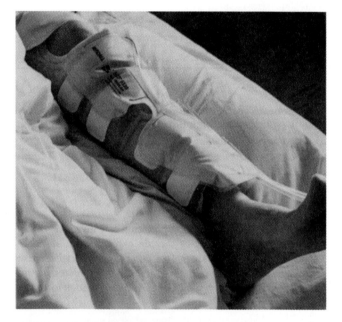

FIGURE 19-3 ◆ The sequential venous compression device enhances venous return. They are available in knee-high or above the knee length.

however, the data comparing knee-high versus thigh-high sleeves was sparse and conflicting. On the other hand, Elliott and colleagues (1999) found that thigh-high SCD was more effective than calf-high SCD after major trauma without lower-extremity injuries.

Antiembolism stockings are worn under the SCD to provide added support and protect the skin from irritation by the plastic. The SCD is removed for ambulation and is usually discontinued when the client resumes walking activities. SCDs are useful in *preventing* thrombi and edema from venous stasis, but they are not used for clients who have arterial insufficiency, cellulitis, infection of the extremity, or preexisting venous thrombosis. Technique 19-2 outlines how to apply a sequential compression device.

Nursing Process: Sequential Compression Devices

ASSESSMENT

Assess for baseline data:

- Cardiovascular status, including heart rate and rhythm, peripheral pulses, and capillary refill
- Color and temperature of extremities
- Movement and sensation of feet and lower extremities and Homan's sign

PLANNING

Delegation

UAP often remove and reapply the SCD when performing hygiene care. The nurse should check that the UAP knows the correct application process for the SCD. Remind the UAP that the client should not have the SCD removed for long periods of time as the purpose of the SCD is to promote circulation.

IMPLEMENTATION:
TECHNIQUE 19-2 APPLYING A SEQUENTIAL COMPRESSION DEVICE

Equipment

- Measuring tape
- Antiemboli stockings
- SCD, including disposable sleeves, air pump, and tubing

Preparation

Check the physician's order for type of SCD sleeve. *Both knee- and thigh-length sleeves are available.*

Performance

1. Explain to the client what you are going to do, why it is necessary, and the procedure for applying the sequential compression device. *The client's cooperation and comfort will be increased by understanding the rationale for applying the SCD.*

2. Observe appropriate infection control procedures.

3. Provide for client privacy and drape the client appropriately.

4. Prepare the client.
   - Place the client in a dorsal recumbent or semi-Fowler's position.
   - Measure the client's legs as recommended by the manufacturer if a thigh-length sleeve is required. *Knee-length sleeves come in just one size; the thigh circumference determines the size needed for a thigh-length sleeve.*
   - Apply antiemboli stockings (see Technique 19-1). Make sure there are no wrinkles or folds in the stockings. *Antiemboli stockings provide added support and reduce skin irritation from the compression sleeve.*

5. Apply the sequential compression sleeves.
   - Place a sleeve under each leg with the opening at the knee.
   - Wrap the sleeve securely around the leg, securing the Velcro tabs (Figure 19-4 ◆). Allow two fingers

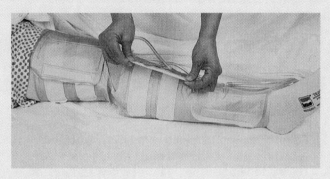

FIGURE 19-4 ◆ Applying a sequential compression device to the leg.

to fit between the leg and the sleeve. *This amount of space ensures that the sleeve does not impair circulation when inflated.*

6. Connect the sleeves to the control unit and adjust the pressure as needed.
   - Connect the tubing to the sleeves and control unit, ensuring that arrows on the plug and the connector are in alignment and that the tubing is not kinked or twisted. *Improper alignment or obstruction of the tubing by kinks or twists will interfere with operation of the SCD.*
   - Turn on the control unit and adjust the alarms and pressures as needed. The sleeve cooling control and alarm should be "on"; ankle pressure is usually set at 35 to 55 mm Hg. *It is important to have the sleeve cooling control on for comfort and to reduce the risk of skin irritation from moisture under the sleeve. Alarms warn of possible control unit malfunctions.*

7. **Document** the procedure.
   - Record baseline assessment data and application of the SCD. Note control unit settings.
   - Assess and document skin integrity and neurovascular status at least every 8 hours while the

SCD is in place. Remove the unit and notify the physician if the client complains of numbness and tingling or leg pain. These may be symptoms of nerve compression.

AMBULATORY AND COMMUNITY SETTINGS

Sequential Compression Device

• A sequential compression device may be used in the home. Inform the client or caregiver how to apply the device correctly and how to operate the system, including how to respond to the alarm.

AGE-RELATED CONSIDERATIONS

Sequential Compression Device

Children

• The SCD is rarely used on children.

Elders

• The SCD sleeves may become loose as clients move around in bed. Check that the sleeves are secure and properly positioned.

EVALUATION

• Perform appropriate follow-up assessments, such as cardiovascular status including pedal pulses, skin color and temperature, skin integrity, and neurovascular status, including movement and sensation.

• Compare to the baseline data, if available.
• Report significant deviations from normal to the physician.

Chapter Summary

TERMINOLOGY

antiemboli (elastic) stockings
deep vein thrombosis (DVT)
Homans' sign

pneumatic compression device
(PCD)
pulmonary embolism (PE)

sequential compression device
(SCD)

FORMING CLINICAL JUDGMENTS

Consider This:

1. The client brought her own antiemboli stockings from home. The UAP tells you that the client's stockings are loose and do not stay up. What will you do?

2. The client is on a sequential compression device and you are monitoring neurovascular checks every 2 hours. During this last check, the client states that his leg is starting to feel numb. What action, if any, do you take?

Related Research

Elliott, C. G., Dudney, T. M., Egger, M., Orme, J. F., Clemmer, T. P., Horn, S. D., Weaver, L., Handrahan, D., Thomas, F., Merrell, S., Kitterman, N., & Yeates, S. (1999). Calf-thigh sequential pneumatic compression compared with plantar venous pneumatic compression to prevent deep-vein thrombosis after non-lower extremity trauma. *Journal of Trauma, 47*(1), 25–32.

Siddiqui, A. U., Buchman, T. G., & Hotchkiss, R. S. (2000). Pulmonary embolism as a consequence of applying sequential compression device on legs in a patient asymptomatic of deep vein thrombosis. *Anesthesiology, 92*(3), 880–882.

Vanek, V. W. (1998). Meta-analysis of effectiveness of intermittent pneumatic compression devices with a comparison of thigh-high to knee-high sleeves. *American Surgeon, 64*(11), 1050–1058.

Weiss, R. A., & Duffy, D. (1999). Clinical benefits of lightweight compression: reduction of venous-related symptoms by ready-to-wear lightweight gradient compression hosiery. *Dermatology Surgery, 25*(9), 701–704.

Winemiller, M. H., Stolp-Smith, K. A., & Silverstein, M. D. (1999). Prevention of venous thromboembolism in patients with spinal cord injury: Effects of sequential pneumatic compression and heparin. *Journal of Spinal Cord Medicine, 22*(3), 182–191.

References

Springhouse (1996). Getting a leg up on sequential compression therapy. *Nursing, 26*(10), 56–58.

Chapter 20

Breathing Exercises

Techniques

OBJECTIVES

- Identify the purposes of breathing exercises.
- State assessment data relevant to oxygenation.
- Demonstrate abdominal (diaphragmatic) and pursed-lip breathing exercises.
- Assist clients to use incentive spirometer devices.

20-1 Teaching Abdominal (Diaphragmatic) Breathing

20-2 Using an Incentive Spirometer

Promoting Oxygenation

Most people in good health give little thought to their respiratory function. Changing position frequently, ambulating, and exercising usually maintain adequate ventilation and gas exchange. When people become ill, however, their respiratory function may be inhibited for such reasons as pain and immobility. Shallow respirations inhibit both diaphragmatic excursion and lung distensibility. The result of inadequate chest expansion is stasis and pooling of respiratory secretions, which ultimately harbor microorganisms and promote infection. This situation is often compounded by giving narcotics for pain because narcotics further depress the rate and depth of respiration.

Interventions by the nurse to maintain the normal respirations of clients include:

- Positioning the client to allow for maximum chest expansion
- Encouraging or providing frequent changes in position
- Encouraging ambulation
- Implementing measures that promote comfort such as giving pain medication

The semi-Fowler's or high-Fowler's position allows maximum chest expansion in bed-confined clients, particularly dyspneic clients. The nurse also encourages clients to turn from side to side frequently so that alternate sides of the chest are permitted maximum expansion. People in respiratory distress often sit upright and lean on their arms or elbows. This position is called the **tripod position** (Figure 20-1 ◆). Dyspneic clients often sit in bed and lean over their overbed tables (which are raised to a suitable height), usually with a pillow for support. This **orthopneic position** is an adaptation of the high-Fowler's position. It has a further advantage in that, unlike in high-Fowler's, the abdominal organs are not pressing on the diaphragm. Also, a client in the orthopneic position can press the lower part of the chest against the table to help in exhaling (Figure 20-2 ◆).

Deep Breathing and Coughing

The nurse can facilitate respiratory functioning by encouraging deep breathing exercises and coughing to remove secretions. Breathing exercises are frequently indicated for clients with restricted chest expansion, such as people with **chronic obstructive pulmonary disease (COPD)** or clients recovering from thoracic or abdominal surgery. Instructing and encouraging the client to take sustained deep breaths is among the

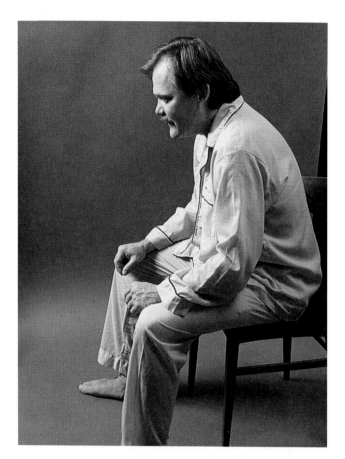

FIGURE 20-1 ◆ Tripod position to assist breathing.

safest, most effective, and least expensive strategies for keeping the lungs expanded (Fink & Hunt, 1999, p. 356).

A commonly employed breathing exercise is abdominal (diaphragmatic) and pursed-lip breathing. **Abdominal (diaphragmatic) breathing** permits deep, full breaths with little effort. **Pursed-lip breathing** helps the client develop control over breathing. The pursed lips create a resistance to the air flowing out of the lungs, thereby prolonging exhalation and preventing airway collapse by maintaining positive airway pressure. A deep breath is an important factor for a normal, effective cough. Forceful coughing often is less effective than using **controlled** or **huff coughing** techniques. Technique 20-1 explains how to teach clients to perform abdominal (diaphragmatic) breathing exercises and instructions for coughing techniques.

Nursing Process: Deep Breathing and Coughing

ASSESSMENT

The following items relate to various aspects of the history and assessment of clients relative to respiratory techniques. The nurse selects items appropriate to the particular technique being performed. Also see Technique 3-11 Assessing the Thorax and Lungs.

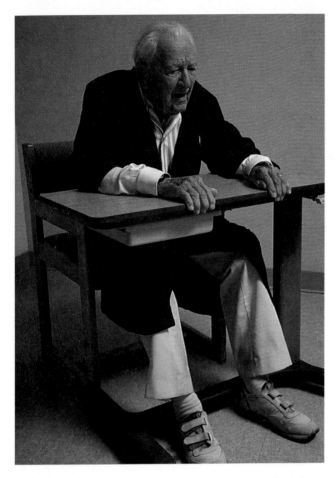

FIGURE 20-2 ◆ Clients in respiratory distress find that resting their arms on an overbed table helps them to breathe more effectively.

Determine:

- *Current respiratory problems:* What recent changes has the client experienced in breathing pattern (e.g., shortness of breath, difficulty breathing, need to be in an upright position to breathe, or rapid and shallow breathing)? Which activities might cause the above symptom(s) to occur? What pollutants has the client been exposed to?
- *History of respiratory disease:* Has the client had colds, allergies, asthma, tuberculosis, bronchitis, pneumonia, or emphysema? How frequently have these occurred? How long did they last? And, how were they treated?
- *Presence of a cough:* Is it productive or nonproductive? If a cough is productive, when is sputum produced? What are the amount, color, thickness, and odor (e.g., thick, frothy, pink, rusty, or blood-tinged)?
- *Lifestyle:* Does the client smoke? If so, how much? Does any member of the client's family smoke? Are there any occupational hazards (e.g., inhaling fumes)?
- *Pain:* Does the client experience any pain associated with breathing or activity? Where is the pain located? What words does the client use to describe the pain? How long does it last, and how does it affect breathing? What activities precede the pain?

- *Medication history:* Has the client taken or does the client take any over-the-counter or prescription medications for breathing? Which ones? What are the dosages, times taken, and effects on the client, including side effects?

Observe (see Box 20-1 for definitions and description of terms):

- Breathing pattern (rate, rhythm, depth, and quality). Note any signs of hyperventilation, hypoventilation, tachypnea, bradypnea.
- Ease or effort of breathing and posture assumed for breathing (e.g., orthopneic)
- Breath sounds audible without amplification (e.g., stridor, wheezes)
- Chest movements (e.g., retractions, flail chest, or paradoxical breathing). Note the specific location of retractions: intercostals, substernal, suprasternal, supraclavicular, or tracheal tug
- Clinical signs of hypoxia or anoxia (e.g., increased pulse rate, rapid or deep respirations, cyanosis of the skin and nailbeds, restlessness, anxiety, dizziness [vertigo], or faintness [syncope]).
- The location of any surgical incision in relation to the muscles needed for breathing. An incision can impede appropriate lung expansion.

Palpate for:

- Respiratory excursion (see Chapter 3)
- Lungs for vocal (tactile) fremitus (see Chapter 3)

Percuss the chest for:

- Diaphragmatic excursion (see Chapter 3).
- Chest sounds (flatness, dullness, resonance, hyperresonance, tympany).

Auscultate the lungs for:

- Breath sounds (normal, adventitious, or absent) (see Tables 3-6 and 3-7 in Chapter 3)

Determine the results of:

- Sputum analysis
- Venous blood samples (e.g., complete blood count).
- Arterial blood samples (blood gases)
- Pulmonary function tests
- Pulse oximetry

PLANNING

Delegation

Unlicensed assistive personnel (UAP) can reinforce and assist clients in performing breathing exercises. However, it is the responsibility of the nurse to teach

Box 20-1 *Abnormal Breathing Patterns and Sounds*

Breathing Patterns

Rate

- *Tachypnea*—rapid respiration marked by quick, shallow breaths
- *Bradypnea*—abnormally slow breathing
- *Apnea*—cessation of breathing

Volume/Depth

- *Hyperventilation*—an increase in the amount of air in the lungs; characterized by prolonged and deep breaths
- *Hypoventilation*—reduction in the amount of air in the lungs; characterized by shallow respirations

Rhythm

- *Cheyne–Stokes breathing*—rhythmic waxing and waning of respirations, from very deep to very shallow breathing and temporary apnea

Ease or Effort

- *Dyspnea*—difficult and labored breathing during which the individual has a persistent, unsatisfied need for air and feels distressed
- *Orthopnea*—ability to breathe only in upright sitting or standing positions

Breath Sounds

Audible Without Amplification

- *Stridor*—a shrill, harsh sound heard during inspiration with laryngeal obstruction
- *Stertor*—snoring or sonorous respiration, usually due to a partial obstruction of the upper airway
- *Wheeze*—continuous, high-pitched musical squeak or whistling sound occurring on expiration and sometimes on inspiration when air moves through a narrowed or partially obstructed airway
- *Bubbling*—gurgling sounds heard as air passes through moist secretions in the respiratory tract

Audible by Stethoscope

- *Crackles (rales)*—dry or wet crackling sounds simulated by rolling a lock of hair near the ear; generally heard on inspiration as air moves through accumulated moist secretions. *Fine to medium crackles* occur when air passes through moisture in small air passages and alveoli; *medium to coarse crackles* occur when air passes through moisture in the bronchioles, bronchi, and trachea
- *Gurgles (rhonchi)*—continuous, coarse, low-pitched, harsh, moaning or snoring sound more audible during expiration as the air moves through tenacious mucus or narrowed bronchi
- *Pleural friction rub*—coarse, leathery, or grating sound produced by the rubbing together of inflamed pleura

Chest Movements

- *Intercostal retraction*—indrawing between the ribs
- *Substernal retraction*—indrawing beneath the breastbone
- *Suprasternal retraction*—indrawing above the breastbone
- *Supraclavicular retraction*—indrawing above the clavicles
- *Tracheal tug*—indrawing and downward pull of the trachea during inspiration
- *Flail chest*—the ballooning out of the chest wall through injured rib spaces; results in *paradoxical breathing*, during which the chest wall balloons on expiration but is depressed or sucked inward on inspiration

Secretions and Coughing

- *Hemoptysis*—the presence of blood in the sputum
- *Productive cough*—a cough accompanied by expectorated secretions
- *Nonproductive cough*—a dry, harsh cough without secretions

the client the breathing exercises, to evaluate the effectiveness of the teaching, and to assess the outcomes of the breathing exercises (e.g., ease of breathing, effectiveness of cough, breath sounds).

IMPLEMENTATION:
TECHNIQUE 20-1 TEACHING ABDOMINAL (DIAPHRAGMATIC) BREATHING

Equipment

- None
- Pillow optional (for splinting abdominal or thoracic incision)

Preparation

Before starting to teach breathing exercises, determine the location of a surgical incision that could impede lung expansion and need for analgesia as incisional pain and splinting may make deep breathing painful after surgery.

Performance

1. Explain to the client what you are going to do, why it is necessary, and how he or she can cooperate. Discuss how deep breathing and coughing will help keep the lungs expanded and clear of secretions.

2. Wash hands and observe other appropriate infection control procedures.

3. Provide for client privacy.

4. Prepare the client.
   - Assist the client to assume a comfortable sitting position or a semi-Fowler's position if a sitting position is not possible or a lying position in bed with one pillow.
   - Have the client flex the knees *to relax the muscles of the abdomen.*
   - Have the client place one or both hands on the abdomen just below the ribs.

5. Perform abdominal breathing.
   - Instruct the client to breathe in deeply through the nose with the mouth closed, to stay relaxed, not to arch the back, and to concentrate on feeling the abdomen rise as far as possible. *When a person breathes in, the diaphragm contracts (drops), the lungs fill with air, and the abdomen rises or protrudes.*
   - If the client has difficulty raising the abdomen, instruct the person to take a quick, forceful inhalation through the nose. *With a quick sniff, the client will feel the abdomen rise.*
   - Ask the client to perform relaxed diaphragmatic breathing for a few minutes.

6. Perform controlled and huff coughing as the next step, if needed.
   - For clients who have had thoracic or abdominal surgery, instruct them to place their hands or a pillow over the incisional site and to apply gentle pressure while deep breathing or coughing.
   - Instruct the client to take three to four slow deep breaths, inhaling through the nose and exhaling through pursed lips as if gently blowing out a candle. *Increasing lung volume increases air flow through the small airways, expands the lungs, and helps mobilize secretions on expiration.* Limit the active deep breaths *to avoid fatigue and hyperventilation.*

- Ask the client to inhale deeply and hold his or her breath for a few seconds.
- Instruct the client to cough twice while exhaling. *The first cough loosens the mucus; the second expels the secretions.*
- For huff coughing, the client leans forward and exhales sharply with a "huff" sound. *This helps keep the airways open while moving secretions up and out of the lungs.*
- Have the client inhale by taking rapid short breaths in succession ("sniffing") *to prevent mucus from moving back into smaller airways.*
- Allow the client to rest. Try to avoid prolonged episodes of coughing *as these may cause fatigue and hypoxia.*
- Instruct the client to perform several relaxed diaphragmatic breaths before the next cough effort.

 7. **Document** the teaching and assessments for the exercises performed and the client's response.

Variation: Pursed-Lip Breathing

- Teach the client to inhale through the nose and pursing lips, as if about to whistle, and breathe out slowly and gently, making a slow "whooshing" sound without puffing out their cheeks. *This pursed-lip breathing creates a resistance to air flowing out of the lungs, increases pressure within the bronchi (main air passages), and minimizes collapse of smaller airways, a common problem for people with COPD.*
- Instruct the client to inhale deeply through their nose and count to 3.
- Have the client concentrate on tightening their abdominal muscles while breathing out slowly and evenly through their pursed lips while counting to 7 or until they can't exhale any more. *Tightening the abdominal muscles and leaning forward helps compress the lungs and enhances effective exhalation.*
- Teach the client how to perform pursed-lip breathing while walking: Inhale while taking two steps, then exhale through pursed lips while taking the next four steps (McConnell, 1999, p. 18).
- Instruct the client to use this exercise whenever feeling short of breath and to increase gradually to 5 to 10 minutes four times a day. *Regular practice will help the client do this type of breathing without conscious effort.*

- Determine the client's ability to perform the breathing exercises and compliance to the instructions.
- Relate current assessment data (e.g., ease of breathing, cough, secretions) to prior assessment data from before teaching the breathing exercises.
- Report significant deviations from normal to the physician.

Incentive Spirometry

Incentive spirometers, also referred to as **sustained maximal inspiration devices (SMIs),** are used to:

- Improve pulmonary ventilation
- Counteract the effects of anesthesia or hypoventilation
- Loosen respiratory secretions
- Facilitate respiratory gaseous exchange
- Expand collapsed alveoli

Incentive spirometry is designed to mimic natural sighing or yawning by encouraging the client to take long, slow, deep breaths. Incentive spirometers measure the flow of air inhaled through the mouthpiece and, therefore, offer an incentive to improve inhalation. Two general types are the flow-oriented spirometer and the volume-oriented spirometer.

The **flow-oriented SMI** consists of one or more clear plastic chambers containing freely moveable colored balls or discs. The balls or discs are elevated as the client inhales. The client is asked to keep them elevated as long as possible with a maximal sustained inhalation (Figure 20-3 ◆). The longer the inspiratory flow is maintained, the larger is the volume, so the client is encouraged to take slow deep breaths. Unfortunately, a client can generate a high flow (with low volume) by taking a quick, forceful inhalation. When doing this, the client does not meet the therapeutic volume or deep-breathing objectives. Therefore, effective client education is necessary. Flow-oriented SMIs are low-cost devices, are often disposable, and can be used independently by clients. They do not, however, measure the specific volume of air inhaled.

Volume-oriented SMIs, in contrast, measure the inhalation volume maintained by the client. A plastic disposable device is shown in Figure 20-4 ◆. When the client inhales, a pistonlike plate or accordion-pleated cylinder rises as the client inspires, and markings on the side indicate the volume of inspiration achieved by the client.

More expensive, nondisposable volume-oriented SMIs can precisely measure the inhalation volume maintained by the client. These devices contain pis-

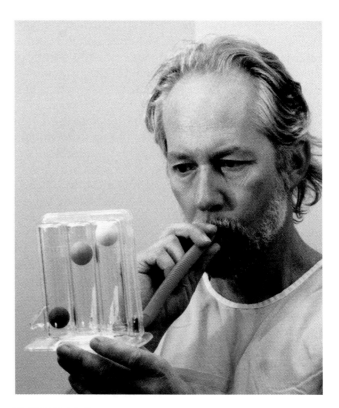

FIGURE 20-3 ◆ Flow-oriented SMI or incentive spirometer.

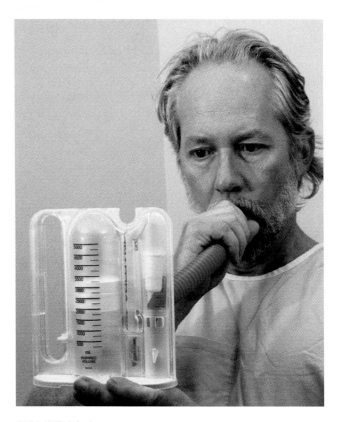

FIGURE 20-4 ◆ Plastic disposable volume-oriented SMI.

tons or bellows that are raised by the client's inhalation to a predetermined volume. Some volume-oriented devices feature an achievement counter or light. The light will not turn on until the inspiration is held at the minimum predetermined volume for a specified time period.

When using an incentive spirometer, the client should be assisted into a position, preferably an upright sitting position in bed or a chair. This position facilitates maximum ventilation. Technique 20-2 describes how to assist a client with an incentive spirometer or SMI.

Incentive spirometry is widely used in the United States. In comparison, the United Kingdom has a reported lower usage citing reasons of cost and questionable effectiveness (Brooks-Brunn, 1995). A number of recent studies (Gosselink et al., 2000; Crowe & Bradley, 1997; Weiner et al., 1997; Tan, 1995; Thomas & McIntosh, 1994) compared clients who received deep breathing exercises alone versus clients who received deep breathing exercises and incentive spirometry. The results were mixed with some studies stating that the addition of incentive spirometry did improve lung function, reduce pulmonary complications, and shorten hospital stay. Other studies, however, stated there was no significant difference in outcomes between deep breathing exercises and incentive spirometry. Given the changing health care environment and increasing economic constraints in health care, it is possible that incentive spirometers may not be prescribed on a routine basis but primarily for clients who are at high risk for pulmonary complications.

Nursing Process: Incentive Spirometry

ASSESSMENT

- Auscultate the client's lungs before use of the incentive spirometer.
- Note the location of a surgical incision that could impede lung expansion. If so, assess pain level and determine if an analgesic may facilitate use of the SMI device.
- Determine the client's knowledge level pertaining to correct use of the device.

PLANNING

Before assisting a client to use an SMI device, determine the prescribed inspiratory volume level.

Delegation

It is the responsibility of the nurse to teach the client how to use the incentive spirometer, assess the client's performance, and evaluate the outcomes of the therapy. UAP, however, can reinforce and assist clients in using the incentive spirometer. The nurse should inform the UAP of the key points to using the incentive spirometer correctly.

IMPLEMENTATION:
TECHNIQUE 20-2 USING AN INCENTIVE SPIROMETER

Equipment

- Flow-oriented or volume-oriented SMI
- Mouthpiece or breathing tube
- Label for mouthpiece
- Progress chart
- Nose clip (optional)

Preparation

- Determine if the client has a disposable SMI at the bedside.
- This technique should not be performed immediately after a meal or other physically stressful activity.

Performance

1. Explain to the client what you are going to do, why it is necessary, and how he or she can cooperate. Discuss how the results will be used in planning further care or treatments.

2. Wash hands and observe other appropriate infection control procedures.

3. Provide for client privacy.

4. Prepare the client
   - Assist the client to an upright position in bed or in a chair. If the person is unable to assume a sitting position for a flow spirometer, have the person assume any position. *A sitting position facilitates maximum ventilation of the lungs.*

For a Flow-Oriented SMI

5. Set the spirometer
   - If the spirometer has an inspiratory volume–level pointer, set the pointer at the prescribed level. The physician's or respiratory therapist's order should indicate the level.

6. Instruct the client to use the spirometer as follows:
   - Hold the spirometer in the upright position. *A tilted spirometer requires less effort to raise the balls or discs.*

- Exhale normally.
- Seal the lips tightly around the mouthpiece, take in a slow deep breath to elevate the balls and then hold the breath for two seconds initially, increasing to six seconds (optimum) to keep the balls elevated if possible. Instruct the client to avoid brisk low-volume breaths that snap the balls to the top of the chamber. The client may use a nose clip if the person has difficulty breathing only through the mouth. *A slow, deep breath ensures maximal ventilation. Greater lung expansion is achieved with a very slow inspiration than with a brisk shallow breath. Sustained elevation of the balls ensures adequate ventilation of the alveoli (lung air sacs).*
- Remove the mouthpiece and exhale normally.
- Cough productively, if possible and not contraindicated, after using the spirometer. *Deep ventilation may loosen secretions and coughing can facilitate their removal.*
- Relax and take several normal breaths before using the spirometer again.
- Repeat the procedure to a total of 10 breaths encouraging the client to take progressively deeper breaths up to the maximal goal (Fink & Hunt, 1999, p. 361).
- Repeat series of breaths once each hour while awake. *Practice increases inspiratory volume, maintains alveolar ventilation, and prevents* **atelectasis** *(collapse of the air sacs).*

For a Volume-Oriented SMI

7. Set the spirometer.
- Set the spirometer to the predetermined volume. Check the physician's or respiratory therapist's order.
- Since some SMIs are battery operated, ensure that the spirometer is functioning. Place the device on the client's bedside table.

8. Instruct the client to use the spirometer as follows:
- Exhale normally.
- Seal the lips tightly around the mouthpiece and take in a slow, deep breath until the piston is elevated to the predetermined level. The piston level may be visible to the client or there may be lights or the word *Hold* illuminated to identify the volume obtained.

- Hold the breath for 6 seconds to ensure maximal alveolar ventilation.
- Remove the mouthpiece and exhale normally.
- Cough productively, if possible and not contraindicated, after using the spirometer. *Deep ventilation may loosen secretions and coughing can facilitate their removal.*
- Relax and take several normal breaths before using the spirometer again.
- Repeat the procedure to a total of 10 breaths, encouraging the client to take progressively deeper breaths up to the maximal goal (Fink & Hunt, 1999, p. 361).
- Repeat series of breaths once each hour while awake. *Practice increases inspiratory volume, maintains alveolar ventilation, and prevents atelectasis.*
- Encourage the client to record the top volume achieved at each hour he or she performed the technique. *This facilitates cooperation of the client and assists in evaluating outcomes of the technique.*

For All Devices

9. Clean the equipment.
- Clean the mouthpiece with water and shake it dry. Label the mouthpiece and a disposable SMI with the client's name. A disposable SMI may be left at the bedside for the client to use as prescribed. *Only the mouthpiece of a nondisposable volume SMI is stored with the client because volume SMIs are used by many clients.* Change the disposable mouthpieces every 24 hours.

10. **Document** all relevant information.
- Record the technique including type of spirometer, number of breaths taken, volume or flow levels achieved, client response, and results of auscultation. Also include, when appropriate, client education and the ability of the client to perform the procedure without prompting.
- For a flow SMI, calculate the volume achieved by multiplying the setting by the length of time the client kept the balls elevated. For example, if the setting was 500 mL and the balls were suspended for 2 seconds, the volume is 500×2 or 1,000 mL.
- For a volume SMI, take the volume directly from the spirometer (e.g., 1,500 mL).

AMBULATORY AND COMMUNITY SETTINGS

SMI Device
- Show the client how to use and clean the SMI device.
- Make certain the client understands how often to use the SMI and how to document the volume achieved.

- Evaluate the client's ability and willingness to follow instructions and comply with treatment.

AGE-RELATED CONSIDERATIONS

Breathing Exercises

Child

- Consider the developmental level of the child when choosing a method to promote breathing exercises. Examples include an incentive spirometer, pinwheels, or other blow toys.

- The SMI device can be a game for young clients. Demonstrate the procedure beforehand and show the child how to take slow, deep breaths.

- Nasal clips may be needed if the younger client doesn't understand how to prevent breathing through the nose.

- A child may want to hold a favorite stuffed animal instead of a pillow to help support the incision when deep breathing after abdominal or thoracic surgery.

Elders

- Older adults may have trouble sealing their lips around the mouthpiece of a spirometer because of dentures or a dry mouth.

EVALUATION

- Conduct appropriate follow-up, such as:
  - Auscultating lung sounds and comparing to sounds heard before the procedure
  - Client's color, heart rate, respiratory rate
  - Degree of dyspnea before, during, and after the use of the incentive spirometer. Watch for fatigue or dizziness in the client.

- Relate current findings to previous inspiratory volume levels and note the trend of the data.
- Report significant deviations from normal to the physician.

Chapter Summary

TERMINOLOGY

abdominal (diaphragmatic)
   breathing
atelectasis
chronic obstructive pulmonary disease (COPD)
controlled coughing

flow-oriented SMI
huff coughing
incentive spirometer
orthopneic position
pursed-lip breathing

sustained maximal inspiration
   devices (SMIs)
tripod position
volume-oriented SMI

FORMING CLINICAL JUDGMENTS

Consider This:

1. Your assigned client, a 45-year-old male, had emergency abdominal surgery last night. He smoked one pack of cigarettes a day prior to surgery. Because of the emergency nature of the surgery, he received no preoperative teaching about deep breathing, coughing, or the incentive spirometer that is sitting at his bedside. He refuses to perform any breathing exercises or to use the incentive spirometer. What will you do?

2. At your next visit after instructing and observing the client in the proper use of a flow-oriented SMI, you ask the client how it is working. The client reports that since coughing after its use was nonproductive, the client stopped using it. What would you say to the client?

RELATED RESEARCH

Crowe, J. M., & Bradley, C.A. (1997). The effectiveness of incentive spirometry with physical therapy for high-risk patients after coronary artery bypass surgery. *Physical Therapy, 77*(3), 260–268.

Gosselink, R., Schrever, K., Cops, P., Witvrouwen, H., DeLeyn, P., Troosters, T., Lerut, A., Deneffe, G., & Decramer, M. (2000). Incentive spirometry does not enhance recovery after thoracic surgery. *Critical Care Medicine, 28*(3), 679–683.

Tan, A. K. (1995). Incentive spirometry for tracheostomy and laryngectomy patients. *Journal of Otolaryngology, 24*(5), 292–294.

Thomas, J. A., & McIntosh, J. M. (1994). Are incentive spirometry, intermittent positive pressure breathing, and deep breathing exercises effective in the prevention of postoperative pulmonary complications after upper abdominal surgery? A systematic overview and meta-analysis. *Physical Therapy, 74*(1), 3–10.

Weiner, P., Man, A., Weiner, M., Rabner, M., Waizman, J., Magadle, R., Zamir, D., & Greiff, Y. (1997). The effect of incentive spirometry and inspiratory muscle training on pulmonary function after lung resection. *Journal of Thoracic Cardiovascular Surgery, 113*(3), 552–557.

REFERENCES

Brenner, Z. R. (1999). Preventing postoperative complications: What's old, what's new, what's tried-and-true. *Nursing, 29* (10), 34–39.

Brooks-Brunn, J. (1995). Postoperative atelectasis and pneumonia. *Heart & Lung, 24*(2), 94–111.

Fink, J. B., & Hunt, G. E. (1999). *Clinical Practice in Respiratory Care.* Philadelphia: Lippincott Williams & Wilkins.

Jackson, B. (1994). How to use a volume incentive spirometer. *Nursing, 24*(11), 32T.

Lezon, K. (1999). Teaching incentive spirometry. *Nursing, 29*(1), 60–61.

McConnell, E. A. (1999). Do's & don'ts: Teaching pursed-lip breathing. *Nursing, 29*(9), 18.

Chapter 21

Oxygen Therapy

Techniques

OBJECTIVES

- Identify essential assessment data required during oxygen therapy.
- Describe various methods used to administer oxygen.
- Outline safety precautions necessary during oxygen therapy.
- Administer oxygen by cannula, mask, and face tent safely and effectively.
- Describe the technique of measuring peak expiratory air flow.

21-1 Administering Oxygen by Cannula, Face Mask, or Face Tent

21-2 Measuring Peak Expiratory Flow

Oxygen Therapy

Supplemental oxygen is indicated for numerous clients who have **hypoxemia** (low partial pressure of oxygen or low saturation of oxyhemoglobin in the arterial blood), for example, people who have reduced lung diffusion of oxygen through the respiratory membrane, heart failure leading to inadequate transport of oxygen, or substantial loss of lung tissue due to tumors or surgery. Oxygen therapy is prescribed by the physician, who specifies the specific concentration, method, and liter flow per minute (L/min). The order may also call for the nurse to titrate the oxygen to achieve a desired saturation level as measured by pulse oximetry (see Technique 2-7). When the administration of oxygen is an emergency measure, the nurse may initiate the therapy.

Oxygen is supplied in two ways in health care facilities: by portable systems—cylinders or tanks—and from wall outlets. Generally, oxygen cylinders are encased in metal carriers equipped with wheels for transport and a broad flat base on which the cylinder stands at the bedside to prevent it from falling. When not in use, a cap on the top protects the valves and outlets. Accidentally opened outlets can turn a tank into a dangerous projectile. They should be placed away from traffic areas and heaters.

A **regulator** that releases oxygen at a safe level and at a desirable rate must be attached before the oxygen supply is used. On a cylinder, the regulator has two gauges: the contents gauge indicates the pressure or amount of oxygen remaining in the tank; the flow meter gauge or flow indicator gauge indicates the gas flow in L/min (Figure 21-1 ◆). A flow meter is also required for wall outlet systems.

Oxygen administered from a cylinder or wall-outlet system is dry. Dry gases dehydrate the respiratory mucous membranes. Humidifying devices that add water vapor to inspired air are thus an essential adjunct of oxygen therapy, particularly for liter flows over 2 L/min. These devices provide 20 to 40 percent humidity. A **humidifier** bottle is attached below the flow meter gauge so that the oxygen passes through water and then through the specific oxygen tubing and equipment prescribed for the client (e.g., nasal cannula or mask) (Figure 21-2 ◆).

Safety Precautions for Oxygen Therapy

Safety precautions are essential during oxygen therapy (see Box 21-1). Although oxygen by itself will not burn or explode, it does facilitate combustion. For example, a bedsheet ordinarily burns slowly when ignited in the atmosphere; however, if saturated with free-flowing oxygen and ignited by a spark, it will burn rapidly and explosively. The greater the concentration of the oxygen, the more rapidly fires start and burn, and such fires are difficult to extinguish. Because oxygen is colorless, odorless, and tasteless, people are often unaware of its presence.

Like any medication, oxygen is not completely harmless to the client. Oxygen concentrations greater than 50 percent can lead to **oxygen toxicity**, noted by

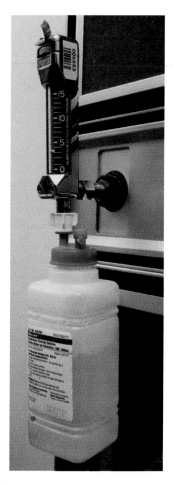

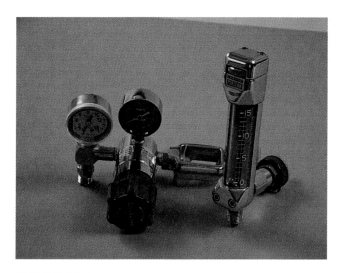

FIGURE 21-1 ◆ An oxygen tank regulator and wall flow meter.

FIGURE 21-2 ◆ An oxygen humidifier attached to a wall outlet oxygen flow meter.

Box 21-1 *Oxygen Therapy Safety Precautions*

- Place cautionary signs reading "No Smoking: Oxygen in Use" on the client's door, at the foot or head of the bed, and on the oxygen equipment.
- Instruct the client and visitors about the hazard of smoking with oxygen in use.
- Make sure that electrical equipment (e.g., razors, hearing aids, radios, televisions, and heating pads) is in good working order to prevent the occurrence of short-circuit sparks.
- Avoid materials that generate static electricity, such as woolen blankets and synthetic fabrics. Cotton blankets are used, and nurses are advised to wear cotton fabrics.
- Avoid the use of volatile, flammable materials, such as oils, greases, alcohol, and ether, near clients receiving oxygen. Avoid alcohol back rubs, and take nail polish removers and the like away from the immediate vicinity.
- Ground electric monitoring equipment, suction machines, and portable diagnostic machines.
- Make known the location of fire extinguishers, and make sure personnel are trained in their use.

substernal pain, cough, sore throat, dyspnea, and pulmonary edema. The lowest concentration needed to achieve the desired arterial blood oxygen saturation should be used.

Oxygen Delivery Equipment

In low-flow systems, oxygen is delivered via small-bore tubing. Low-flow administration devices include the nasal cannula, face masks, oxygen tents, and transtracheal catheters. Because room air is also inhaled along with oxygen, the fraction of inspired oxygen (FiO_2) will vary depending on the respiratory rate, tidal volume, and liter flow. Low-flow systems are generally used for clients who have a respiratory rate below 25 per minute and a regular and consistent respiratory pattern. They are contraindicated for clients who require carefully monitored concentrations of oxygen.

High-flow systems supply all of the gas required during ventilation in precise amounts, regardless of the client's respiratory status. The ratio of room air to oxygen is regulated and does not vary with the client's respirations. Thus, it is a precise and consistent method for controlling the client's FiO_2. In high-flow systems, gas is delivered via a Venturi device and large-bore tubing.

Cannula

The **nasal cannula (prongs)** is the most common inexpensive low-flow device used to administer oxygen. It consists of a tube that extends around the face, with 0.6- to 1.3-cm (¼- to ½-in) curved prongs that fit into the nostrils. One side of the tube connects to the oxygen tubing and oxygen supply. The cannula is often held in place by an elastic band that fits around the client's head or under the chin (Figure 21-3 ◆). As long as the nasal airway is patent, the cannula will deliver adequate oxygen, even to clients who breathe primarily through the mouth.

It delivers a relatively low concentration of oxygen (24 to 44 percent) at flow rates of 2 to 6 L/min. However, above 6 L/min, there is a tendency for the client to swallow air and for the nasal and pharyngeal mucosa to become irritated. In addition, the FiO_2 is *not* increased.

Face Mask

Face masks that cover the client's nose and mouth may be used for oxygen inhalation. Most masks are made of clear, pliable plastic that can be molded to fit the face. They are held to the client's head with elastic

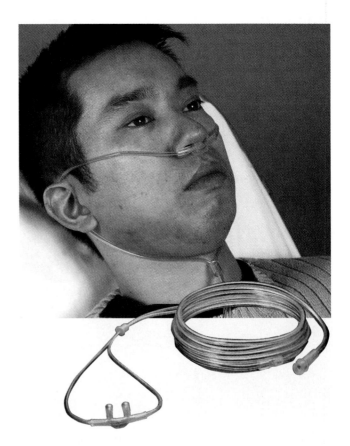

FIGURE 21-3 ◆ A nasal cannula.

bands. Some have a metal clip that can be bent over the bridge of the nose for a snug fit. There are several holes in the sides of the mask (exhalation ports) to allow the escape of exhaled carbon dioxide. To avoid the client's rebreathing carbon dioxide while wearing a mask, a minimum of 5 L/min oxygen flow rate is required.

Some masks have reservoir bags, which provide higher oxygen concentrations to the client. A portion of the client's expired air is directed into the bag. Because this air comes from the upper respiratory passages (e.g., the trachea and bronchi), where it does not take part in gaseous exchange, its oxygen concentration remains the same as that of inspired air.

A variety of oxygen masks are marketed:

- The *simple face mask* delivers oxygen concentrations from 40 to 60 percent at liter flows of 5 to 8 L/min, respectively (Figure 21-4 ◆).

- The **partial rebreather mask** delivers oxygen concentrations of 40 to 60 percent at liter flows of 6 to 10 L/min. The oxygen reservoir bag that is attached allows the client to rebreathe about the first third of the exhaled air in conjunction with oxygen (Figure 21-5 ◆). The partial rebreather bag must not totally deflate during inspiration to avoid carbon dioxide buildup. If this problem occurs, the liter flow of oxygen needs to be increased.

- The **nonrebreather mask** delivers the highest oxygen concentration possible by means other than intubation or mechanical ventilation (i.e., 95 to 100 percent, at liter flows of 10 to 15 L/min). Using a nonrebreather mask, the client breathes only the source gas from the bag. One-way valves on the mask and between the reservoir bag and the mask prevent the room air and the client's exhaled air from entering the bag (Figure 21-6 ◆). To prevent carbon dioxide buildup, the nonrebreather bag

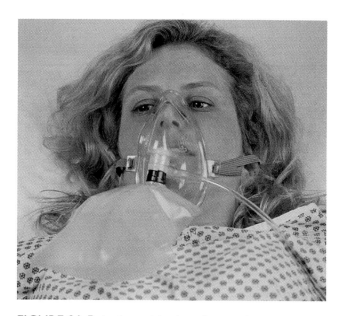

FIGURE 21-5 ◆ A partial rebreather mask.

must not totally deflate during inspiration. If it does, the nurse can correct this problem by increasing the liter flow of oxygen.

- The **Venturi mask** delivers precise oxygen concentrations (Figure 21-7 ◆). Oxygen concentrations vary from 24 to 50 percent delivered through wide-

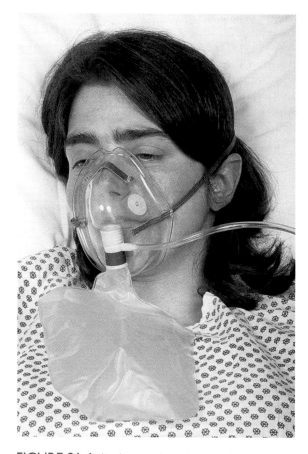

FIGURE 21-6 ◆ A nonrebreather mask.

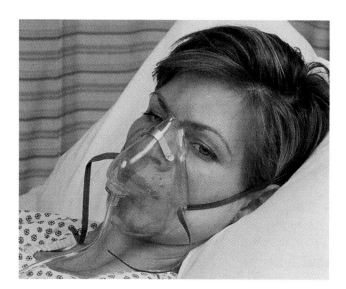

FIGURE 21-4 ◆ A simple face mask.

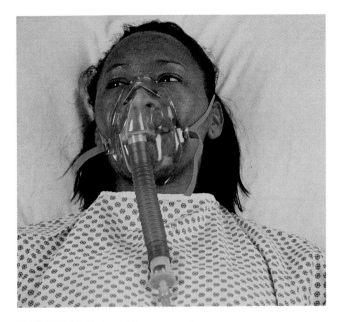

FIGURE 21-7 ◆ A Venturi mask.

bore tubing and jet adapters. The oxygen concentration is specified on the mask. Turning the flow rate higher than specified will not increase the concentration delivered to the client.

Face Tent

Face tents (Figure 21-8 ◆) can replace oxygen masks when clients poorly tolerate masks. When a face tent alone is used to supply oxygen, the concentration of oxygen varies; therefore, it is often used in conjunction with a Venturi system. Face tents provide varying concentrations of oxygen (e.g., 30 to 50 percent concentration of oxygen at 4 to 8 L/min).

Transtracheal Catheter

A **transtracheal catheter** is placed through a surgically created tract in the lower neck directly into the

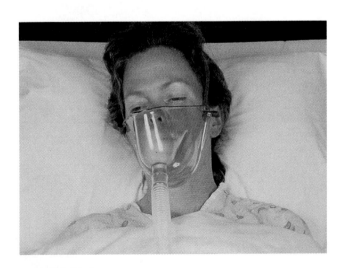

FIGURE 21-8 ◆ An oxygen face tent.

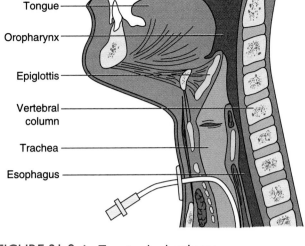

FIGURE 21-9 ◆ Transtracheal catheter.

trachea (Figure 21-9 ◆). Once the tract has matured, the client removes and cleans the catheter two to four times per day. Oxygen applied to the catheter at less than 1 L/min need not be humidified, and rates over 5 L/min can be administered.

Nursing Process: Oxygen Delivery Equipment

ASSESSMENT

See also Technique 3-11 Assessing the Thorax and Lungs.

Observe:

- *Skin and mucous membrane color:* Note whether cyanosis is present.
- *Breathing patterns:* Note depth of respirations and presence of tachypnea, bradypnea, orthopnea.
- *Chest movements:* Note whether there are any intercostal, substernal, suprasternal, supraclavicular, or tracheal retractions during inspiration or expiration.
- *Chest wall configuration* (e.g., kyphosis).
- *Lung sounds* audible by auscultating the chest and by ear.
- *Presence of clinical signs of hypoxemia:* tachycardia, tachypnea, restlessness, dyspnea, cyanosis, and confusion. Tachycardia and tachypnea are often early signs. Confusion is a later sign of severe oxygen deprivation.
- *Presence of clinical signs of* **hypercarbia (hypercapnia):** restlessness, hypertension, headache, lethargy, tremor.
- *Presence of clinical signs of oxygen toxicity:* tracheal irritation and cough, dyspnea, and decreased pulmonary ventilation.

Determine:

- Vital signs, especially pulse rate and quality, and respiratory rate, rhythm, and depth

- Whether the client has chronic obstructive pulmonary disease (COPD). A high carbon dioxide level in the blood is the normal stimulus to breathe. However, people with COPD may have a chronically high carbon dioxide level, and their stimulus to breathe is hypoxemia. Low flows of oxygen (2 L/min) stimulate breathing for such persons by maintaining slight hypoxemia. During continuous oxygen administration, arterial blood gas levels of oxygen (PO_2) and carbon dioxide (PCO_2) are measured periodically to monitor hypoxemia.
- Results of diagnostic studies
- Hemoglobin, hematocrit, complete blood count
- Arterial blood gases
- Pulmonary function tests

PLANNING

Consult with a respiratory therapist as needed in the beginning and ongoing care of clients receiving oxygen therapy. In many agencies, the therapist establishes the initial equipment and client teaching.

Delegation

Initiating the administration of oxygen is considered similar to administering a medication and is not delegated to unlicensed assistive personnel (UAP). However, reapplying the oxygen delivery device may be performed by the UAP and many aspects of the client's response to oxygen therapy are observed during usual care and may be recorded by persons other than the nurse. Abnormal findings must be validated and interpreted by the nurse. The nurse is also responsible to ensure that the correct delivery method is being used.

IMPLEMENTATION:

TECHNIQUE 21-1 ADMINISTERING OXYGEN BY CANNULA, FACE MASK, OR FACE TENT

Equipment

Cannula
- Oxygen supply with a flow meter and adapter
- Humidifier with distilled water or tap water according to agency protocol
- Nasal cannula and tubing
- Tape
- Padding for the elastic band

Face Mask
- Oxygen supply with a flow meter and adapter
- Humidifier with distilled water or tap water according to agency protocol
- Prescribed face mask of the appropriate size
- Padding for the elastic band

Face Tent
- Oxygen supply with a flow meter and adapter
- Humidifier with distilled water or tap water according to agency protocol
- Face tent of the appropriate size

Preparation

1. Determine the need for oxygen therapy, and verify the order for the therapy.
   - Perform a respiratory assessment to develop baseline data if not already available.
2. Prepare the client and support people.
   - Assist the client to a semi-Fowler's position if possible. *This position permits easier chest expansion and hence easier breathing.*

- Explain that oxygen is not dangerous when safety precautions are observed. Inform the client and support people about the safety precautions connected with oxygen use.

Performance

1. Explain to the client what you are going to do, why it is necessary, and how he or she can cooperate. Discuss how the effects of the oxygen therapy will be used in planning further care or treatments.
2. Wash hands and observe appropriate infection control procedures.
3. Provide for client privacy, if appropriate.
4. Set up the oxygen equipment and the humidifier.
   - Attach the flow meter to the wall outlet or tank. The flow meter should be in the OFF position.
   - If needed, fill the humidifier bottle. (This can be done before coming to the bedside.)
   - Attach the humidifier bottle to the base of the flow meter.
   - Attach the prescribed oxygen tubing and delivery device to the humidifier.
5. Turn on the oxygen at the prescribed rate, and ensure proper functioning.
   - Check that the oxygen is flowing freely through the tubing. There should be no kinks in the tubing, and the connections should be airtight. There should be bubbles in the humidifier as the oxygen flows through. You should feel the oxygen at the outlets of the cannula, mask, or tent.
   - Set the oxygen at the flow rate ordered, for example.
6. Apply the appropriate oxygen delivery device.

Cannula

- Put the cannula over the client's face, with the outlet prongs fitting into the nares and the elastic band around the head (see Figure 21-3). Some models have a strap to adjust under the chin.

- If the cannula will not stay in place, tape it at the sides of the face.

- Pad the tubing and band over the ears and cheekbones as needed.

Face Mask

- Guide the mask toward the client's face, and apply it from the nose downward.

- Fit the mask to the contours of the client's face (see Figure 21-4). *The mask should mold to the face, so that very little oxygen escapes into the eyes or around the cheeks and chin.*

- Secure the elastic band around the client's head so that the mask is comfortable but snug.

- Pad the band behind the ears and over bony prominences. *Padding will prevent irritation from the mask.*

Face Tent

- Place the tent over the client's face, and secure the ties around the head (Figure 21-8).

7. Assess the client regularly.

- Assess the client's vital signs, level of anxiety, color, and ease of respirations, and provide support while the client adjusts to the device.

- Assess the client in 15 to 30 minutes, depending on the client's condition, and regularly thereafter.

- Assess the client regularly for clinical signs of hypoxia, tachycardia, confusion, dyspnea, restlessness, and cyanosis. Review arterial blood gas results if they are available.

Nasal Cannula

- Assess the client's nares for encrustations and irritation. Apply a water-soluble lubricant as required to soothe the mucous membranes.

Face Mask or Tent

- Inspect the facial skin frequently for dampness or chafing, and dry and treat it as needed.

8. Inspect the equipment on a regular basis.

- Check the liter flow and the level of water in the humidifier in 30 minutes and whenever providing care to the client.

- Make sure that safety precautions are being followed.

9. **Document** findings in the client record using forms or checklists supplemented by narrative notes when appropriate.

AMBULATORY AND COMMUNITY SETTINGS

Home Care Equipment

Three major oxygen systems for home care use are available in most communities: cylinders or tanks of compressed gas, liquid (cryogenic) oxygen, and oxygen concentrators.

1. *Cylinders ("green tanks"):* These are the system of choice for clients who need oxygen episodically (e.g., on a PRN basis). Advantages are that cylinders deliver all liter flows (1 to 15 L/min), and oxygen evaporation does not occur during storage. Disadvantages are that the cylinders are heavy and awkward to move, the supply company must be notified when a refill is needed, and they are costly for the high-use client. A size "D" tank weighs about 8 pounds and stores 425 L of oxygen, an "E" tank hold 680 L and is transported on wheels (Figure 21-10 ◆). The large "H" tank weighs 150 pounds. The gauge on a full tank reads a pressure of at least 2,000 pounds per square inch (PSI), and a tank is considered empty when it reads less than 500 PSI.

2. *Liquid oxygen:* Liquid systems have two parts—a large stationary container and a portable unit with a small lightweight tank, refilled from the stationary unit. Liquid reservoirs store oxygen at −212°C (−350°F) in a smaller amount of space than compressed gas. Advantages are that these reservoirs are lighter in weight and cleaner in appearance than cylinders and they are not as difficult to operate. Disadvantages of liquid oxygen are that many home care medical supply and service companies are not able to handle it, oxygen evaporation occurs when the unit is not used, only low flows (1 to 4 L/min) can be used or freezing occurs, and the portable unit designed to be carried over the shoulder weighs 8 to 10 pounds, a possible burden to the typical COPD client (Figure 21-11 ◆). A wheeled cart can be used to carry the unit but may be awkward.

3. *Oxygen concentrators.* Concentrators are electrically powered systems that manufacture oxygen from room air. At 1 L/min, such a system can

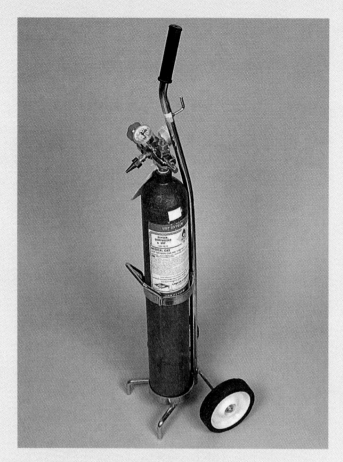

FIGURE 21-10 ◆ "E" cylinder oxygen on a stand.

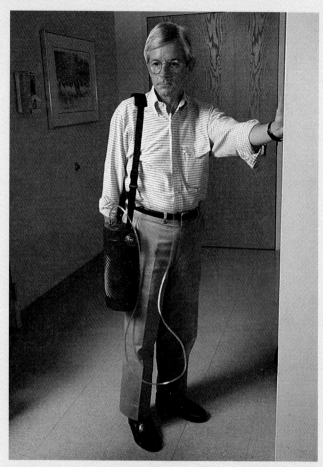

FIGURE 21-11 ◆ A portable liquid oxygen supply.

deliver a concentration of about 95 percent oxygen, but the concentration drops when the flow rate increases (e.g., 75 percent concentration at 4 L/min). Advantages are that they are more attractive in appearance, resembling furniture rather than medical equipment; they eliminate the need for regular delivery of oxygen or refilling of cylinders; because the supply of oxygen is constant, they alleviate the client's anxiety about running out of oxygen; and they are the most economical system when continuous use is required. Major disadvantages of a concentrator are that it is expensive; lacks real portability (small units weigh 28 pounds); tends to be noisy; is powered by electricity; an emergency backup unit (e.g., an oxygen tank) must be provided for clients for whom a power failure could be life threatening; and heat produced by the concentrator motor is a problem for those who live in trailers, small houses, or warm climates, where air conditioners are required. The oxygen concentrator must also be checked periodically with an O_2 analyzer to ensure that it is providing an adequate delivery of oxygen.

Another type of oxygen concentrator is the *oxygen enricher*. It uses a plastic membrane that allows water vapor to pass through with the oxygen, thus eliminating the need for a humidifying device. It is also thought to filter out bacteria present in the air. The enricher provides an O_2 concentration of 40

percent at all flow rates, it tends to be quieter than the concentrator, there is less chance of combustion (since the gas is only 40 percent oxygen), it has only two moving parts (thus decreasing the risk of something going wrong), and a nebulizer can be operated off the enricher because of the high flow rate.

The nurse needs to ensure that the client has appropriate help in choosing a reputable home oxygen vendor. Services furnished should include:

• A 24-hour emergency service
• Trained personnel to make the initial delivery and instruct the client in safe, appropriate use of the oxygen and maintenance of the equipment
• At least monthly follow-up visits to check the equipment and reinstruct the client as necessary
• A regular cost review to ensure that the system is the most cost effective one for that client, with routine notification of the physician or home care professional if it seems that another system is more appropriate

The nurse needs to also ensure that the client knows about the financial reimbursements available from Medicare and Medicaid or other insurance agencies. In Canada's system of socialized health care, the cost of home oxygen therapy is fully covered.

AGE-RELATED CONSIDERATIONS

Oxygen Delivery Equipment

Infant

Oxygen Hood

- An oxygen hood is a rigid plastic dome that encloses an infant's head. It provides precise oxygen levels and high humidity.
- The gas should not be allowed to blow directly into the infant's face, and the hood should not rub against the infant's neck, chin, or shoulder.

Child

Oxygen Tent (Figure 21-12 ◆)

- The tent consists of a rectangular, clear, plastic canopy with outlets that connect to an oxygen or compressed air source and to a humidifier that moisturizes the air or oxygen.
- Because the enclosed tent becomes very warm, some type of cooling mechanism such as an ice chamber or a refrigeration unit is provided to maintain the temperature at 20 to 21°C (68 to 70°F).
- Cover the child with a gown or a cotton blanket. Some agencies provide gowns with hoods, or a small towel may be wrapped around the head. *The child needs protection from chilling and from the dampness and condensation in the tent.*

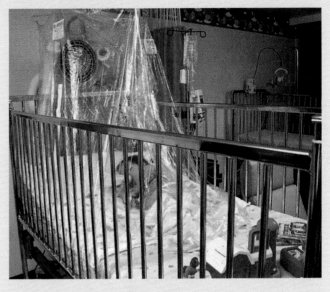

FIGURE 21-12 ◆ Pediatric oxygen tent.

- Flood the tent with oxygen by setting the flow meter at 15 L/min for about 5 minutes. Then, adjust the flow meter according to orders (e.g., 10 to 15 L/min). *Flooding the tent quickly increases the oxygen to the desired level.*
- The tent can deliver approximately 30 percent oxygen.

EVALUATION

- Perform follow-up based on findings that deviated from expected or normal for the client. Relate findings to previous data if available.
- Report significant deviations from normal to the physician.

Peak Expiratory Flow

Some clients have acute or chronic respiratory disorders, such as asthma or COPD, that affect the amount of air that is able to be expired from the lungs. In these situations, the measurement of the maximum amount the client can expire may be helpful in directing therapy. This measurement is the **peak expiratory flow rate (PEFR)**. Measuring PEFR before and after a breathing treatment, for example, can assist the health care team in determining whether additional respiratory therapy is needed.

Nursing Process: Peak Expiratory Flow

ASSESSMENT

Perform a thorough respiratory and chest assessment (see Technique 3-11 Assessing the Thorax and Lungs). Examine blood gas results and other relevant laboratory values (e.g., hemoglobin).

PLANNING

Review the client record for previous assessments, results of PEFR measurements, and resultant changes in therapy.

Delegation

PEFR measurement may be delegated to trained UAP. The nurse must interpret the findings. Modifications in the treatment regimen may not be initiated by the UAP.

Equipment

- Peak flow meter

Performance

1. Explain to the client what you are going to do, why it is necessary, and how he or she can cooperate. Discuss how the results will be used in planning further care or treatments.

2. Wash hands and observe appropriate infection control procedures.

3. Provide for client privacy.

4. Position the client.
   - If possible, the client should be sitting with the chest free from contact with the bed or chair. If not possible, place the client in semi-Fowler's or high-Fowler's position.

5. Reset the marker on the flow meter to the zero position (Figure 21-13 ◆).

6. Assist the client to use the flow meter.
   - Ask the client to take a deep breath in (Figure 21-14 ◆).
   - Client places the mouthpiece in the mouth with the teeth around the opening and lips forming a tight seal.
   - Have the client exhale as quickly and forcefully as possible. If you suspect the client is exhaling a significant amount of air through the nose, apply a nose clip.

7. Perform step 6 twice more. Record the highest level achieved.

 8. **Document** findings in the client record using forms or checklists supplemented by narrative notes when appropriate.

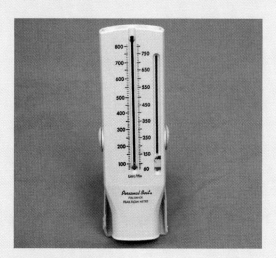

FIGURE 21-13 ◆ Peak flow meter with marker in the zero position.

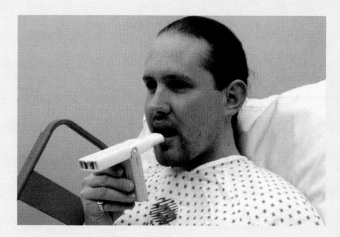

FIGURE 21-14 ◆ PEFR measurement.

EVALUATION

- Perform follow-up based on findings that deviated from expected or normal for the client. Relate findings to previous assessment data if available.

- Report significant deviations from normal to the physician.

Chapter Summary

TERMINOLOGY

face mask

face tent

hypercapnia

hypercarbia

hypoxemia

humidifier

nasal cannula (prongs)

nonrebreather mask

oxygen concentrator

oxygen toxicity

partial rebreather mask

peak expiratory flow rate (PEFR)

regulator

transtracheal catheter

Venturi mask

FORMING CLINICAL JUDGMENTS

Consider This:

1. The client has a physician's order for "oxygen by mask at 6 L/min." However, the client complains of feeling as though not enough air is being delivered and frequently removes the mask. What alternatives might the nurse suggest?

2. The hospitalized client's PEFR is markedly lower in the morning than it was the previous evening. What might explain this finding, and how would the nurse respond?

RELATED RESEARCH

Ring, L., & Danielson, E. (1997). Patients' experiences of long-term oxygen therapy. *Journal of Advanced Nursing, 26,* 337–344.

REFERENCES

Conway, M. E., Pontius, T., & Abalos, D. (1997). Home care: An update for case managers—home respiratory therapy. *Case-Manager, 8*(5), 65–67.

Dunn, L., & Chisholm, H. (1998). RCN continuing education: Oxygen therapy. *Nursing Standard, 13*(7), 57–60, 63–64.

Harman, R. (1999). Management of COPD with oxygen therapy at home. *Community Nurse, 5*(7), 25–26.

Information from your doctor: Using oxygen at home. (2000). *Patient Care, 34*(10), 74.

Mathews, P. J. (1997). Using a peak flowmeter: Monitoring the air waves. *Nursing, 27*(6), 57–59.

McConnell, E. A. (1997). Administering oxygen by mask. *Nursing, 27*(9), 26.

Smith, T, & Matti, A. M. (1999). Respiratory care: Air apparent . . . long-term oxygen therapy. *Nursing Times, 95*(41), 59, 62.

Chapter 22

Suctioning

Techniques

OBJECTIVES

- Describe four types of artificial airways.
- Describe the purposes of suctioning.
- Differentiate oropharyngeal, nasopharyngeal, endotracheal, and tracheostomy suctioning.
- Identify indications for suctioning.
- Compare and contrast open and closed airway/tracheal suction systems.
- Discuss complications associated with suctioning.
- Identify essential assessment data required before and after suctioning.
- Perform oropharyngeal, nasopharyngeal, endotracheal, and tracheostomy suctioning safely and effectively.

22-1 Suctioning the Upper Airway

22-2 Suctioning a Tracheostomy or Endotracheal Tube

Artificial Airways

Artificial airways are inserted to maintain a patent air passage for clients whose airways have become or may become obstructed. A patent airways is necessary so that air can flow to and from the lungs. Four of the more common types of airways are oropharyngeal, nasopharyngeal, endotracheal, and tracheostomy.

Oropharyngeal and Nasopharyngeal Airways

Oropharyngeal and nasopharyngeal airways are used to keep the upper air passages open when they may become obstructed by secretions or the tongue. These airways are easy to insert and have a low risk of complications. Sizes vary and should be appropriate to the size and age of the client. The airway should be well lubricated with water-soluble gel prior to insertion.

Oropharyngeal airways (Figure 22-1 ◆) stimulate the gag reflex and are only used for clients with altered levels of consciousness (e.g., because of general anesthesia, overdose, or head injury). To insert the airway:

- Place the client in a supine or semi-Fowler's position.
- Put on clean gloves.
- Hold the lubricated airway by the outer flange with the distal end pointing up.
- Open the client's mouth and insert the airway along the top of the tongue.
- When the distal end of the airway reaches the soft palate at the back of the mouth, rotate the airway 180 degrees downward and slip it past the uvula into the oral pharynx.
- If not contraindicated, place the client in a side-lying position or with the head turned to the side to allow secretions to drain out of the mouth.
- The oropharynx may be suctioned as needed by inserting the suction catheter alongside the airway.
- Do not tape the airway in place; remove it when the client begins to cough or gag.

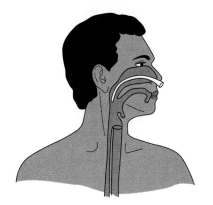

FIGURE 22-2 ◆ A nasopharyngeal airway in place.

- Provide mouth care at least every 2 to 4 hours, keeping suction available at the bedside.

Nasopharyngeal airways are tolerated better by alert clients. They are inserted through the **nares**, terminating in the oropharynx (Figure 22-2 ◆). When caring for a client with a nasopharyngeal airway, provide frequent oral and nares care, repositioning the airway in the other **naris** (nostril) every 8 hours or as ordered to prevent necrosis of the mucosa.

Endotracheal Tubes

Endotracheal tubes are most commonly inserted for clients who have had general anesthetics or for those in emergency situations in which mechanical ventilation is required. The physician or nurse with specialized education inserts an endotracheal tube through either the mouth or the nose and into the trachea with the guide of a laryngoscope (Figure 22-3 ◆). The tube terminates just superior to the bifurcation of the trachea into the bronchi. The tube may have an air-filled cuff to prevent air leakage around it. Because an endotracheal tube passes through the epiglottis and glottis, the client is unable to speak while it is in place. Nursing interventions for clients with endotracheal tubes are shown in Box 22-1.

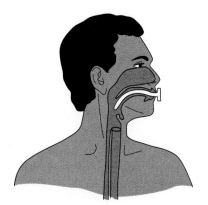

FIGURE 22-1 ◆ An oropharyngeal airway in place.

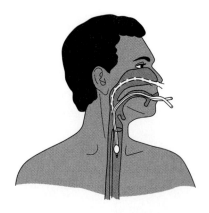

FIGURE 22-3 ◆ An endotracheal tube in place.

Box 22-1 *Nursing Interventions for Clients with Endotracheal Tubes*

- Assess the client's respiratory status at least every 4 hours, or more frequently if indicated. Include respiratory rate, rhythm, depth, equality of chest excursion, and lung sounds; level of consciousness; and skin color in your assessment.

- Frequently assess nasal and oral mucosa for redness and irritation. Report any abnormal findings to the physician.

- Secure the endotracheal tube with tape to prevent accidental movement of the tube further into or out of the trachea. Assess the position of the tube frequently. Notify the physician immediately if the tube is dislodged out of the airway. If the tube advances into a main bronchus, it may need to be slightly withdrawn to ensure ventilation of both lungs.

- Unless contraindicated, place the client in a side-lying or semiprone position as tolerated to prevent aspiration of oral secretions.

- Using sterile technique, suction the endotracheal tube as needed to remove excessive secretions.

- Closely monitor cuff pressure, maintaining a pressure of 20 to 25 mm Hg (or as recommended by the tube manufacturer) to minimize the risk of tracheal tissue necrosis. If recommended, deflate the cuff periodically.

- Provide oral and nasal care every 2 to 4 hours. Use an oropharyngeal airway to prevent the client from biting down on an oral endotracheal tube. Move oral endotracheal tubes to the opposite side of the mouth every 8 hours or per agency protocol, taking care to maintain the position of the tube in the trachea.

- Provide humidified air or oxygen because the upper airways which normally moisten the air are by-passed by the endotracheal tube.

- If the client is on mechanical ventilation, ensure that all alarms are enabled at all times as the client cannot call for help should an emergency occur.

- Communicate frequently with the client, providing a note pad or picture board for the client to use in communicating.

From *Fundamentals of nursing: Concepts, process, and practice,* 6th ed., by B. Kozier, G. Erb, A. Berman, & K. Burke, 2000, Upper Saddle River, NJ: Prentice Hall Health.

Tracheostomy

Clients who need long-term airway support may have a **tracheostomy**, a surgical incision in the trachea just below the larynx. A curved tracheostomy tube is inserted to extend through the stoma into the trachea (Figure 22-4 ◆). Tracheostomy tubes may be either plastic or metal and are available in different sizes.

Upper Airway Suctioning

When clients have difficulty handling their secretions or an airway is in place, suctioning may be necessary to clear air passages. **Suctioning** is aspirating secretions through a catheter connected to a suction machine or wall suction outlet. Even though the upper airways (the oropharynx and nasopharynx) are not sterile, sterile technique is recommended for all suctioning to avoid introducing pathogens into the airways in the event the catheter slips into the lower airway. It is best to check the agency's policy as some facilities may use clean rather than sterile technique for **nasopharyngeal** and **oropharyngeal suctioning** with the rationale that the catheter does not extend down to the lower airway.

Suction catheters are flexible, plastic, and may be either open-tipped or whistle-tipped (Figure 22-5 ◆). The **whistle-tipped catheter** is less irritating to respiratory tissues, although the **open-tipped catheter** may be more effective for removing thick mucus plugs. A rigid, plastic tube, called a Yankauer, is sometimes used for secretions in the oral cavity (Figure 22-6 ◆). Alert clients can be taught how to use this method of oral suction-

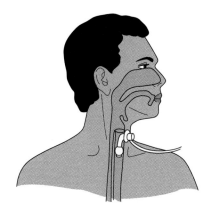

FIGURE 22-4 ◆ A tracheostomy tube in place.

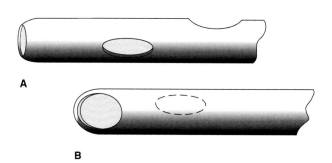

FIGURE 22-5 ◆ Types of suction catheters. A, open-tipped; B, whistle-tipped.

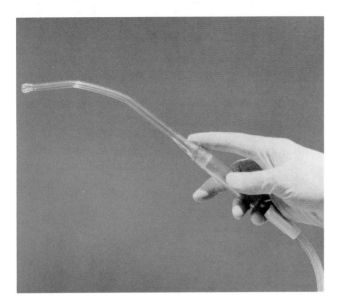

FIGURE 22-6 ◆ Yankauer suction tube.

ing. Most suction catheters have a thumb port on the side to control the suction. The catheter is connected to suction tubing that is connected to a collection chamber and suction control gauge (Figure 22-7 ◆).

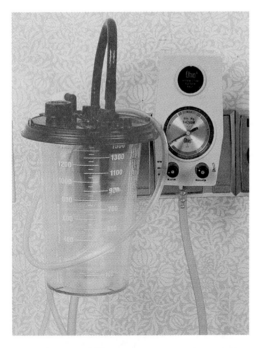

FIGURE 22-7 ◆ A wall suction unit.

Oropharyngeal or nasopharyngeal suctioning removes secretions from the upper respiratory tract. In contrast, tracheal suctioning is used to remove secretions from the trachea and bronchi or the lower respiratory tract. The nurse decides when suctioning is needed by assessing the client for signs of respiratory distress or evidence that the client is unable to cough up and expectorate secretions. Dyspnea, bubbling or rattling breath sounds, poor skin color (cyanosis), or decreased SaO_2 levels (also called O_2 sats) may indicate the need for suctioning. Good nursing judgment is necessary as suctioning irritates mucous membranes and can increase secretions if performed too frequently. In addition to removing secretions that obstruct the airway and facilitating ventilation, suctioning can be performed to obtain secretions for diagnostic purposes and to prevent infection that may result from accumulated secretions. Technique 22-1 outlines oropharyngeal and nasopharyngeal suctioning using sterile technique.

Nursing Process: Upper Airway Suctioning

ASSESSMENT

Assess for clinical signs indicating the need for suctioning:

- Restlessness
- Gurgling sounds during respiration
- **Adventitious** (abnormal) breath sounds when the chest is auscultated
- Change in mental status
- Skin color
- Rate and pattern of respirations
- Pulse rate and rhythm

PLANNING

Delegation

Oral or oropharyngeal suctioning using a **Yankauer suction tube** can be delegated to unlicensed assistive personnel (UAP) and to the client or family, if appropriate. The nurse needs to review the technique and important points such as not applying suction during insertion of the tube to avoid trauma to the mucous membrane. In contrast, nasopharyngeal suction or oropharyngeal suction that uses sterile technique requires application of knowledge and problem solving and should be performed by the nurse.

IMPLEMENTATION:
TECHNIQUE 22-1 SUCTIONING THE UPPER AIRWAY

Equipment

- Towel or moisture-resistant pad

- Portable or wall suction machine with tubing and collection receptacle
- Sterile disposable container for fluids

- Sterile normal saline or water
- Sterile gloves
- Goggles or face shield, if appropriate
- Sterile suction catheter kit (#12 to #18 Fr for adults; #8 to #10 Fr for children, and #5 to #8 Fr for infants); if both the oropharynx and the nasopharynx are to be suctioned, one sterile catheter is required for each
- Water-soluble lubricant (for nasopharyngeal suctioning)
- Y-connector
- Sterile gauzes
- Moisture-resistant disposal bag
- Sputum trap, if specimen is to be collected

Performance

1. Explain to the client what you are going to do, why it is necessary, and how he or she can cooperate. Inform the client that suctioning will relieve breathing difficulty and that the procedure is painless but may be uncomfortable and stimulate the cough, gag, or sneeze reflex. *Knowing that the procedure will relieve breathing problems is often reassuring and enlists the client's cooperation.*

2. Wash hands and observe other appropriate infection control procedures.

3. Provide for client privacy.

4. Prepare the client.
   - Position a conscious person who has a functional gag reflex in the semi-Fowler's position with the head turned to one side for oral suctioning or with the neck hyperextended for nasal suctioning. *These positions facilitate the insertion of the catheter and help prevent aspiration of secretions.*
   - Position an unconscious client in the lateral position, facing you. *This position allows the tongue to fall forward, so that it will not obstruct the catheter on insertion. The lateral position also facilitates drainage of secretions from the pharynx and prevents the possibility of aspiration.*
   - Place the towel or moisture-resistant pad over the pillow or under the chin.

5. Prepare the equipment.
   - Set the pressure on the suction gauge, and turn on the suction. Many suction devices are calibrated to three pressure ranges:

   Wall Unit
   Adult: 100 to 120 mm Hg
   Child: 95 to 110 mm Hg
   Infant: 50 to 95 mm Hg

   Portable Unit
   Adult: 10 to 15 mm Hg

Child: 5 to 10 mm Hg
Infant: 2 to 5 mm Hg

   - Open the lubricant if performing nasopharyngeal suctioning
   - Open the sterile suction package.

   a. Set up the cup or container, touching only the outside.

   b. Pour sterile water or saline into the container.

   c. Put on the sterile gloves, or put on a nonsterile glove on the nondominant hand and then a sterile glove on the dominant hand. *The sterile gloved hand maintains the sterility of the suction catheter, and the unsterile glove prevents the transmission of the microorganisms to the nurse.*

   - With your sterile gloved hand, pick up the catheter, and attach it to the suction unit (Figure 22-8 ◆).

6. Make an approximate measure of the depth for the insertion of the catheter and test the equipment.
   - Measure the distance between the tip of the client's nose and the earlobe, or about 13 cm (5 in) for an adult.
   - Mark the position on the tube with the fingers of the sterile gloved hand.
   - Test the pressure of the suction and the patency of the catheter by applying your sterile gloved finger or thumb to the port or open branch of the Y-connector (the suction control) to create suction.

7. Lubricate and introduce the catheter.
   - For nasopharyngeal suction, lubricate the catheter tip with sterile water, saline, or water-soluble lubricant; for oropharyngeal suction, moisten the tip with sterile water or saline. *This reduces friction and eases insertion.*

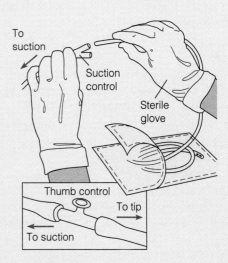

FIGURE 22-8 ◆ Attaching the catheter to the suction unit.

For an Oropharyngeal Suction

- Pull the tongue forward, if necessary, using gauze.
- Do not apply suction (that is, leave your finger off the port) during insertion. *Applying suction during insertion causes trauma to the mucous membrane.*
- Advance the catheter about 10 to 15 cm (4 to 6 in) along one side of the mouth into the oropharynx. *Directing the catheter along the side prevents gagging.*

For a Nasopharyngeal Suction

- Without applying suction, insert the catheter the premeasured or recommended distance into either naris and advance it along the floor of the nasal cavity. *This avoids the nasal turbinates.*
- Never force the catheter against an obstruction. If one nostril is obstructed, try the other.

8. Perform suctioning.
   - Apply your finger to the suction control port to start suction, and gently rotate the catheter. *Gentle rotation of the catheter ensures that all surfaces are reached and prevents trauma to any one area of the respiratory mucosa due to prolonged suction.*
   - Apply suction for 5 to 10 seconds while slowly withdrawing the catheter, then remove your finger from the control, and remove the catheter.
   - A suction attempt should last only 10 to 15 seconds. During this time, the catheter is inserted, the suction applied and discontinued, and the catheter removed.
   - It may be necessary during oropharyngeal suctioning to apply suction to secretions that collect in the vestibule of the mouth and beneath the tongue.

9. Clean the catheter, and repeat suctioning as above.
   - Wipe off the catheter with sterile gauze if it is thickly coated with secretions. Dispose of the used gauze in a moisture-resistant bag.
   - Flush the catheter with sterile water or saline.
   - Relubricate the catheter, and repeat suctioning until the air passage is clear.
   - Allow 20- to 30-second intervals between each suction and limit suctioning to 5 minutes in total. *Applying suction for too long may cause secretion to increase or decrease the client's oxygen supply.*
   - Alternate nares for repeat suctioning.
   - Encourage the client to breathe deeply and to cough between suctions. *Coughing and deep breathing help carry secretions from the trachea and bronchi into the pharynx, where they can be reached with the suction catheter.*

10. Obtain a specimen if required. Use a sputum trap (Figure 22-9 ◆) as follows:
    - Attach the suction catheter to the rubber tubing of the sputum trap.
    - Attach the suction tubing to the sputum trap air vent.
    - Suction the client's nasopharynx or oropharynx. The sputum trap will collect the mucus during suctioning.
    - Remove the catheter from the client. Disconnect the sputum trap rubber tubing from the suction catheter. Remove the suction tubing from the trap air vent.
    - Connect the rubber tubing of the sputum trap to the air vent. *This retains any microorganisms in the sputum trap.*
    - Connect the suction catheter to the tubing.
    - Flush the catheter to remove secretions from the tubing.

11. Promote client comfort.
    - Offer to assist the client with oral or nasal hygiene.
    - Assist the client to a position that facilitates breathing.

12. Dispose of equipment and ensure availability for the next suction.
    - Dispose of the catheter, gloves, water, and waste container. Wrap the catheter around your sterile gloved hand and hold the catheter as the glove is removed over it for disposal.
    - Rinse the suction tubing as needed by inserting the end of the tubing into the used water con-

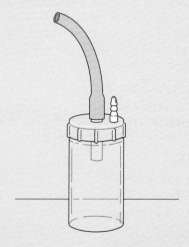

FIGURE 22-9 ◆ A sputum collection trap.

tainer. Empty and rinse the suction collection container as needed or indicated by protocol. Change the suction tubing and container daily.

- Ensure that supplies are available for the next suctioning (suction kit, gloves, water or normal saline).

13. Assess the effectiveness of suctioning.

- Auscultate the client's breath sounds to ensure they are clear of secretions. Observe skin color, dyspnea, and level of anxiety.

14. **Document** relevant data.

- Record the procedure: the amount, consistency, color, and odor of sputum (e.g., foamy, white mucus; thick, green-tinged mucus; or blood-flecked mucus) and the client's breathing status before and after the procedure.
- If the technique is carried out frequently (e.g., every hour), it may be appropriate to record only once, at the end of the shift; however, the frequency of the suctioning must be recorded.

AMBULATORY AND COMMUNITY SETTINGS

Upper Airway Suctioning

- Teach clients and families that the most important aspect of infection control is frequent handwashing.
- Airway suctioning in the home is considered a clean procedure (Humphrey, 1998).
- The catheter or Yankauer should be flushed by suctioning recently boiled or distilled water to rinse away mucus, followed by the suctioning of air through the device to dry the internal surface and,

thus, discourage bacterial growth. The outer surface of the device may be wiped with alcohol or hydrogen peroxide. The suction catheter or Yankauer should be allowed to dry and then be stored in a clean, dry area (American Association for Respiratory Care, 1999, p. 100).

- Suction catheters treated in the manner described above may be reused. It is recommended that catheters be discarded after 24 hours. Yankauer suction tubes may be cleaned, boiled, and reused indefinitely (AARC, 1999, p. 100).

AGE-RELATED CONSIDERATIONS

Suctioning the Upper Airway

Infant

- A bulb syringe is used to remove secretions from an infant's nose or mouth. Care needs to be taken to avoid stimulating the gag reflex.

Child

- A catheter is used to remove secretions from an older child's mouth or nose.

EVALUATION

- Conduct appropriate follow-up, such as: appearance of secretions suctioned; breath sounds; respiratory rate, rhythm, and depth; pulse rate and rhythm; and skin color.
- Compare findings to previous assessment data if available.
- Report significant deviations from normal to the physician.

Tracheostomy or Endotracheal Tube Suctioning

Following endotracheal intubation or a tracheostomy, the trachea and surrounding respiratory tissues are irritated and react by producing excessive secretions. Suctioning is necessary to remove these secretions, maintain a patent airway, and prevent pneumonia that may result from accumulated secretions. The fre-

quency of suctioning depends on the client's health and how recently the intubation was done. Technique 22-2 describes how to suction a tracheostomy or endotracheal tube.

Open Airway Suction System

The traditional method of suctioning an endotracheal tube or tracheostomy is sometimes referred to as an "open" method. If a client is connected to a ventilator, the nurse disconnects the client from the ventilator, suctions the airway, reconnects the client to the ventilator, and discards the suction catheter.

Suctioning, by itself, causes hypoxemia or low oxygen in the blood. The repeated disconnecting of the client from the ventilator can also contribute to hypoxemia. Other drawbacks to the **open airway suction system** include the nurse needing to wear personal protective equipment (e.g., goggles or face shield, gown) to avoid exposure to the client's sputum and the potential cost of one-time catheter use, especially if the client requires frequent suctioning (Carroll, 1998).

Closed Airway/Tracheal Suction System or "In-Line" Suctioning

With the **closed airway/tracheal suction system ("in-line" suctioning)** (Figure 22-10 ◆), the suction catheter attaches to the ventilator tubing and the client does not need to be disconnected from the ventilator. The nurse is not exposed to any secretions because the suction catheter is enclosed in a plastic sheath. The catheter can be reused as many times as necessary until the system is changed. Manufacturers recommend changing closed suction catheter systems on a daily basis. Some studies, however, challenge this recommendation with showing no difference in specified factors such as ventilator-associated pneumonia and length of hospital stay for clients who had the closed system changed daily versus once a week (Hess, 1999) or the system changed on an as-needed basis (Little, 1998). The closed catheter system costs many times more than a conventional suction catheter. However, an increase in closed suctioning is becoming more common in health care settings given the benefit of using the catheter multiple times along with other recent studies indicating a cost-saving with weekly or as-needed changing of the system. The nurse needs to inquire about the agency's policy for changing the closed suction system.

Complications of Suctioning

Suctioning is associated with several complications: **hypoxemia,** trauma to the airway, nosocomial infection, and cardiac dysrhythmia, which is related to the hypoxemia. Techniques to minimize or decrease these complications include:

- *Suction only as needed.* Because suctioning the client with an endotracheal tube or tracheostomy is uncomfortable for the client and potentially hazardous, it should be performed only when indicated and not at a fixed frequency (Hess, 1999).

- *Sterile technique.* Infection of the lower respiratory tract can occur during tracheal suctioning. The nurse using sterile technique during the suctioning process can prevent this complication.

- *Hyperinflation.* This involves giving the client breaths that are 1 to 1.5 times the tidal volume set on the ventilator through the ventilator circuit or via a manual resuscitation bag. Three to five breaths are delivered before and after each pass of the suction catheter.

- *Hyperoxygenation.* Hyperoxygenation is the best technique to avoid suction-related hypoxemia and should be used with all suction procedures (Hess, 1999, p. 764). This can be done with a manual resuscitation bag or through the ventilator and is performed by increasing the oxygen flow (usually to 100 percent) before suctioning and between suction attempts.

- *Safe catheter size.* For tracheostomy and **endotracheal suctioning,** the diameter of the suction catheter should be about half the inside diameter of the tracheostomy or endotracheal tube to allow air to enter around the catheter during suctioning so that hypoxia can be prevented. A rule of thumb to determine suction catheter size is to double the millimeter size of the artificial airway. For example, an artificial airway (e.g., tracheostomy) diameter of 8 mm × 2 = 16. A size 16 French suction catheter would be the largest size catheter that would be safe to use.

- *No saline instillation.* Instilling normal saline into the airway was a common practice and a routine

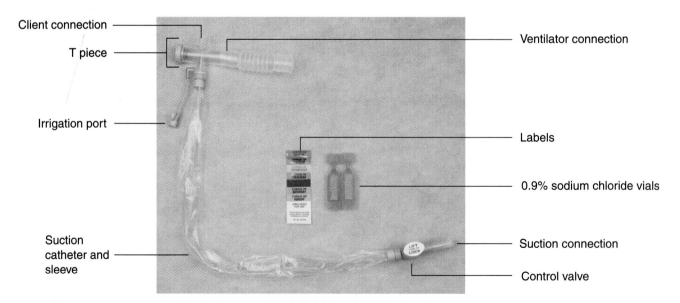

Client connection —
T piece —
Irrigation port —
Suction catheter and sleeve —

Ventilator connection
Labels
0.9% sodium chloride vials
Suction connection
Control valve

FIGURE 22-10 ◆ Closed airway/tracheal system ("in-line" suction).

part of the suctioning procedure. It was thought that the saline would facilitate removal of secretions and improve the client's oxygenation status. Recent studies (Kinloch, 1999; Ackerman & Mick, 1998; Hess, 1999) report just the opposite—that is, instillation of saline promotes adverse effects for the client. Results indicated that oxygen saturation decreased and took longer to return to baseline value when saline was used. The saline can dislodge bacteria from the inside of the artificial airway, thus predisposing the client to lower respiratory infection. Saline instillation should *not* be a routine component of suctioning.

Nursing Process: Tracheostomy or Endotracheal Tube Suctioning

ASSESSMENT

Assess the client for the presence of congestion on auscultation of the thorax. Note the client's ability or inability to remove the secretions through coughing.

PLANNING

Delegation

Suctioning a tracheostomy or endotracheal tube is a sterile, invasive technique requiring application of scientific knowledge and problem solving. This skill is performed by a nurse or respiratory therapist and is not delegated to UAP.

IMPLEMENTATION:
TECHNIQUE 22-2 SUCTIONING A TRACHEOSTOMY OR ENDOTRACHEAL TUBE

Equipment

- Resuscitation bag (Ambu bag) connected to 100 percent oxygen
- Sterile towel (optional)
- Equipment for suctioning the oropharyngeal cavity (see Technique 21-1)
- Goggles and mask if necessary
- Gown (if necessary)
- Sterile gloves
- Moisture-resistant bag

Performance

1. Explain to the client what you are going to do, why it is necessary, and how he or she can cooperate. Inform the client that suctioning usually causes some intermittent coughing and that this assists in removing the secretions.

2. Wash hands and observe other appropriate infection control procedures (e.g., gloves, goggles).

3. Provide for client privacy.

4. Prepare the client.
   - If not contraindicated because of health, place the client in the semi-Fowler's position to promote deep breathing, maximum lung expansion, and productive coughing. *Deep breathing oxygenates the lungs, counteracts the hypoxic effects of suctioning, and may induce coughing. Coughing helps to loosen and move secretions.*
   - If necessary, provide analgesia prior to suctioning. Endotracheal suctioning stimulates the cough reflex, which can cause pain for clients who have had thoracic or abdominal surgery or who have experienced traumatic injury.

Premedication can increase the client's comfort during the suctioning procedure.

5. Prepare the equipment.
   - Attach the resuscitation apparatus to the oxygen source (Figure 22-11 ◆). Adjust the oxygen flow to "100 percent flush."
   - Open the sterile supplies in readiness for use.
   - Place the sterile towel, if used, across the client's chest below the tracheostomy.
   - Turn on the suction, and set the pressure in accordance with agency policy. For a wall unit, a pressure setting of about 100 to 120 mm Hg is normally used for adults, 50 to 95 mm Hg for infants and children.
   - Put on goggles, mask, and gown if necessary.
   - Put on sterile gloves. Some agencies recommend putting a sterile glove on the dominant hand and an unsterile glove on the nondominant hand to protect the nurse.

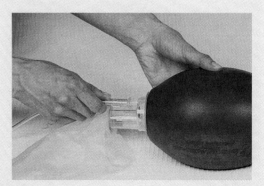

FIGURE 22-11 ◆ Attaching the resuscitation apparatus to the oxygen source.

- Holding the catheter in the dominant hand and the connector in the nondominant hand, attach the suction catheter to the suction tubing (see Figure 22-8).

6. Flush and lubricate the catheter.

   - Using the dominant hand, place the catheter tip in the sterile saline solution.
   - Using the thumb of the nondominant hand, occlude the thumb control and suction a small amount of the sterile solution through the catheter. *This determines that the suction equipment is working properly and lubricates the outside and the lumen of the catheter. Lubrication eases insertion and reduces tissue trauma during insertion. Lubricating the lumen also helps prevent secretions from sticking to the inside of the catheter.*

7. If the client does not have copious secretions, hyperventilate the lungs with a resuscitation bag before suctioning.

   - Summon an assistant, if one is available, for this step.
   - Using your nondominant hand, turn on the oxygen to 12 to 15 L/min.
   - If the client is receiving oxygen, disconnect the oxygen source from the tracheostomy tube using your nondominant hand.
   - Attach the resuscitator to the tracheostomy or endotracheal tube (Figure 22-12 ◆).
   - Compress the Ambu bag three to five times as the client inhales. This is best done by a second person who can use both hands to compress the bag, thus, providing a greater inflation volume.
   - Observe the rise and fall of the client's chest to assess the adequacy of each ventilation.
   - Remove the resuscitation device and place it on the bed or the client's chest with the connector facing up.

Variation

If the client is on a ventilator, use the ventilator for hyperventilation and hyperoxygenation. Newer models have a mode that provides 100 percent oxygen for 2 minutes and then switches back to the previous oxygen setting as well as a "manual breath" or "sigh" button. *The use of ventilator settings provides more consistent delivery of oxygenation and hyperinflation than a resuscitation device.*

8. If the client has copious secretions, do not hyperventilate with a resuscitator.

   Instead:

   - Keep the regular oxygen delivery device on and increase the liter flow or adjust the FiO_2 to 100 percent for several breaths before suctioning. *Hyperventilating a client who has copious secretions can force the secretions deeper into the respiratory tract.*

9. Quickly but gently insert the catheter *without applying any suction*.

   - With your nondominant thumb off the suction port, quickly but gently insert the catheter into the trachea through the tracheostomy tube (Figure 22-13 ◆). *To prevent tissue trauma and oxygen loss, suction is not applied during insertion of the catheter.*
   - Insert the catheter about 12.5 cm (5 in) for adults, less for children, or until the client coughs or you feel resistance. *Resistance usually means that the catheter tip has reached the bifurcation of the trachea.* To prevent damaging the mucous membranes at the bifurcation, withdraw the catheter about 1 to 2 cm (0.4 to 0.8 in) before applying suction.

10. Perform suctioning.

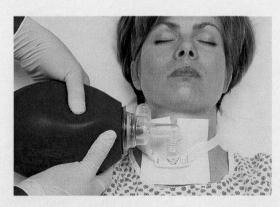

FIGURE 22-12 ◆ Attaching the resuscitator to the tracheostomy.

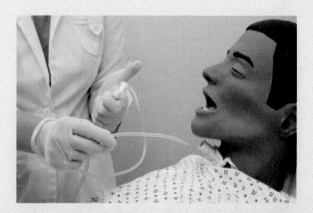

FIGURE 22-13 ◆ Inserting the catheter into the trachea through the tracheostomy tube. *Note:* Suction is *not* being applied when inserting the catheter.

- Apply intermittent suction for 5 to 10 seconds by placing the nondominant thumb over the thumb port. *Suction time is restricted to 10 seconds or less to minimize oxygen loss.*
- Rotate the catheter by rolling it between your thumb and forefinger while slowly withdrawing it. *This prevents tissue trauma by minimizing the suction time against any part of the trachea.*
- Withdraw the catheter completely, and release the suction.
- Hyperventilate the client.
- Then suction again.

11. Reassess the client's oxygenation status and repeat suctioning.
    - Observe the client's respirations and skin color. Check the client's pulse if necessary, using your nondominant hand.
    - Encourage the client to breathe deeply and to cough between suctions.
    - Allow 2 to 3 minutes between suctions when possible. *This provides an opportunity for reoxygenation of the lungs.*
    - Flush the catheter, and repeat suctioning until the air passage is clear and the breathing is relatively effortless and quiet.
    - After each suction, pick up the resuscitation bag with your nondominant hand and ventilate the client with no more than three breaths.

12. Dispose of equipment and ensure availability for the next suction.
    - Flush the catheter and suction tubing.
    - Turn off the suction, and disconnect the catheter from the suction tubing.
    - Wrap the catheter around your sterile hand, and peel the glove off so that it turns inside out over the catheter.
    - Discard the glove and the catheter in the moisture-resistant bag.
    - Replenish the sterile fluid and supplies so that the suction is ready for use again. *Clients who require suctioning often require it quickly, so it is essential to leave the equipment at the bedside ready for use.*

13. Provide for client comfort and safety.
    - Assist the client to a comfortable, safe position that aids breathing. If the person is conscious, a semi-Fowler's position is frequently indicated. If the person is unconscious, the Sims' position aids in the drainage of secretions from the mouth.

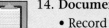 14. **Document** relevant data.
    - Record the suctioning, including the amount and description of suction returns and any other relevant assessments.

Variation: Closed Airway/Tracheal Suction System ("In-Line" Catheter)

- If a catheter is not attached, put on clean gloves, aseptically open a new closed catheter set, and attach the ventilator connection on the T piece to the ventilator tubing. Attach the client connection to the endotracheal tube or tracheostomy.
- Attach one end of the suction connecting tubing to the suction connection port of the closed system and the other end of the connecting tubing to the suction device.
- Turn suction on, occlude or kink tubing, and depress suction control valve (on closed catheter system) to set suction to the appropriate level. Release the suction control valve.
- Use the ventilator to hyperoxygenate and hyperinflate the client's lungs.
- Unlock suction control mechanism if required by the manufacturer.
- Advance the suction catheter enclosed in plastic sheath with dominant hand. Steady the T piece with the nondominant hand.
- Depress the suction control valve and apply suction for no more than 10 seconds and gently withdraw the catheter.
- Repeat as needed remembering to provide hyperoxygenation and hyperinflation as needed.
- When completed suctioning, withdraw the catheter into its sleeve and close the access valve, if appropriate. *If the system does not have an access valve on the client connector, the nurse needs to observe for the potential of the catheter migrating into the airway and partially obstructing the artificial airway.*
- **Lavage** or flush the catheter by instilling normal saline into the irrigation port and applying suction. Repeat until the catheter is clear.
- Close the irrigation port and close the suction valve.

AMBULATORY AND COMMUNITY SETTINGS

Suctioning a Tracheostomy or Endotracheal Tube

- Whenever possible, the client should be encouraged to clear their airway by coughing.
- Clients may need to learn to suction their secretions if they cannot cough effectively.
- Clean gloves should be used when endotracheal suctioning is performed in the home environment (AARC, 1999).
- The nurse needs to instruct the caregiver on how to determine the need for suctioning and the correct process of suctioning to avoid potential complications of suctioning.
- Stress the importance of adequate hydration as it thins secretions, which can aid in the removal of secretions by coughing or suctioning.

AGE-RELATED CONSIDERATIONS

Suctioning a Tracheostomy or Endotracheal Tube

Infant and Child

- Have an assistant gently restrain the child to keep the child's hands out of the way. The assistant will need to keep the child's head in the midline position. The intubated child is frequently sedated (Bindler & Ball, 1999, p. 97).

Elders

- Older adults often have cardiac and/or pulmonary disease, thus increasing their susceptibility to hypoxemia related to suctioning. Watch closely for signs of hypoxemia. If noted, stop suctioning and hyperoxygenate.

EVALUATION

- Perform a follow-up examination of the client to determine the effectiveness of the suctioning (e.g., respiratory rate, depth, and character; breath sounds; color of skin and nailbeds; character and amount of secretions suctioned; changes in vital signs).
- Relate findings to previous assessment data if available.
- Report significant deviations from normal to the physician.

Chapter Summary

TERMINOLOGY

adventitious
artificial airway
closed airway suction system
closed tracheal suction system
endotracheal suctioning
endotracheal tube
hyperinflation
hyperoxygenation

hypoxemia
"in-line" suctioning
lavage
nares
naris
nasopharyngeal airway
nasopharyngeal suctioning
open airway suction system

open-tipped catheter
oropharyngeal airway
oropharyngeal suctioning
suctioning
tracheostomy
whistle-tipped catheter
Yankauer suction tube

FORMING CLINICAL JUDGMENTS

Consider This:

1. A client who has a history of coronary artery disease (CAD) and chronic pulmonary disease recently had major abdominal surgery and is currently on a ventilator. He has copious amounts of secretions and requires frequent suctioning. The nurses are using the open suction system. Upon suctioning the client becomes restless and anxious, his heart rate decreases, and the cardiac monitor shows an occasional missed and extra beat. What actions would you take when caring for this client?

2. You have just suctioned and cleared a client's endotracheal tube of secretions. You assessed the client's need for upper airway suctioning and removed a small amount of oral secretions. As you start to remove your gloves and discard the catheter, the client begins coughing and loosens

up a moderate amount of secretions from his lower airway. How do you proceed?

3. A client requires nasopharyngeal suctioning. You notice that the client's right naris is reddened and sore, and minimal bleeding occurs after suctioning. What actions would you take to promote both comfort and oxygenation needs for this client?

Related Research

Ackerman, M. H., & Mick, D. J. (1998). Instillation of normal saline before suctioning in patients with pulmonary infections: A prospective randomized controlled trial. *American Journal of Critical Care, 7*(4), 261–266.

Kinloch, D. (1999). Instillation of normal saline during endotracheal suctioning: Effects on mixed venous oxygen saturation. *American Journal of Critical Care, 8*(4), 231–242.

Little, K. (1998). As needed in line suction catheter changes were as safe as and less expensive than daily scheduled catheter changes during mechanical ventilation. *Evidence Based Nursing, 1*(3), 82.

Paul-Allen, J., & Ostrow, C. L. (2000). Survey of nursing practices with closed-system suctioning. *American Journal of Critical Care, 9*(1), 9–17.

References

AARC. (1999). AARC Clinical practice guideline: Suctioning of the patient in the home. *Respiratory Care, 44*(1), 99–104.

Bindler, R., & Ball, J. (1999). *Quick Reference to Pediatric Clinical Skills.* Stamford, CT: Appleton & Lange.

Carroll, P. (1998). Closing in on safer suctioning. *RN, 61*(5), 22–26.

Fink, J. B., & Hunt, G. E. (1999). *Clinical Practice in Respiratory Care.* Philadelphia: Lippincott Williams & Wilkins.

Galvin, W. F. (1998). Making a clean sweep: Using a closed tracheal suction system. *Nursing, 28*(6), 50–51.

Glass, C. A., & Grap, M. J. (1995). Ten tips for safer suctioning. *American Journal of Nursing, 95*(5), 51–53.

Griggs, A. (1999). Tracheostomy: Suctioning and humidification. *Emergency Nurse, 6*(9), 33–40.

Hess, D. R. (1999). Managing the artificial airway. *Respiratory Care, 44*(7), 759–776.

Humphrey, C. J. (1998). *Home Care Nursing Handbook* (3rd ed.). Gaithersburg, MD: Aspen.

McConnell, E. A. (2000). Do's & don'ts: Suctioning a tracheostomy tube. *Nursing, 30*(1), 80.

Chapter 23

Caring for the Client with a Tracheostomy

Techniques

OBJECTIVES

- List three types of tracheostomy tubes.
- Identify parts of a tracheostomy tube and their purposes.
- Describe methods for facilitating communication for a client with a tracheostomy.
- Describe the reason for and process of plugging a tracheostomy tube.
- Provide safe and effective tracheostomy care.

Tracheostomy

Clients who need long-term airway support may have a **tracheostomy**, a surgical incision in the trachea just below the larynx. Advantages of a tracheostomy include improved client comfort and reduced laryngeal, pharyngeal, oral, and nasal damage that can be caused by long-term endotracheal tube placement (Fink & Hunt, 1999). Other advantages include: the use of nasogastric or nasoenteric tubes for nutrition may not be necessary because a client can swallow effectively with a tracheostomy tube in place; management of oral secretions is improved with a tracheostomy tube; and clients, with the use of adaptive devices, are able to speak with tracheostomy tubes.

Tracheostomy tubes (Figure 23-1 ◆) have an **outer cannula** that is inserted into the trachea, with a **flange** that rests against the neck that allows the tube to be secured in place with tape or ties. All tubes also have an **obturator** that is used to insert the outer cannula and is then removed. The obturator is kept at the client's bedside in case the tube becomes dislodged and needs to be reinserted. Some tracheostomy tubes have an inner cannula that may be removed for periodic cleaning.

Three types of tracheostomy tubes are available: uncuffed, cuffed, and fenestrated. An uncuffed tube may be plastic or metal, which allows for air to flow around the tube. A person with a permanent tracheostomy may use an **uncuffed tracheostomy tube.** **Cuffed tracheostomy tubes** (Figure 23-2 ◆) are surrounded by an inflatable cuff that produces an airtight seal between the tube and the trachea. This seal prevents aspiration of oropharyngeal secretions and air leakage between the tube and the trachea. Cuffed tubes are often used immediately after a tracheostomy and are essential when ventilating a tracheostomy client with a mechanical ventilator. Children do not

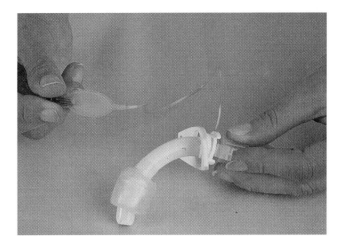

FIGURE 23-2 ◆ A tracheostomy tube with a low-pressure cuff.

require cuffed tubes because their tracheas are resilient enough to seal the air space around the tube.

Low-pressure cuffs are commonly used to distribute a low, even pressure against the trachea, thus decreasing the risk of tracheal tissue necrosis. They do not need to be deflated periodically to reduce pressure on the tracheal wall. The foam cuff does not require injected air; instead when the port is opened, ambient air enters the balloon, which then conforms to the client's trachea (Figure 23-3 ◆). Air is removed from the cuff prior to insertion or removal of the tube.

The **fenestrated tracheostomy tube** has holes in the outer cannula (Figure 23-4 ◆). The **inner cannula** is in place when the client is on mechanical ventilation. When the client is being **weaned** (gradual discontinuation of mechanical support), the inner cannula is removed, the cuff deflated, and the external opening of the tracheostomy tube plugged. The client can now breathe around the tube and through the fenestration

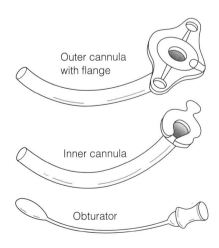

FIGURE 23-1 ◆ Components of an uncuffed tracheostomy tube.

Outer cannula with flange

Inner cannula

Obturator

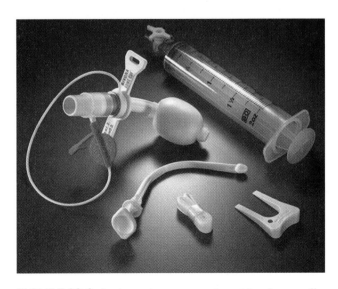

FIGURE 23-3 ◆ A tracheostomy tube with a foam cuff.

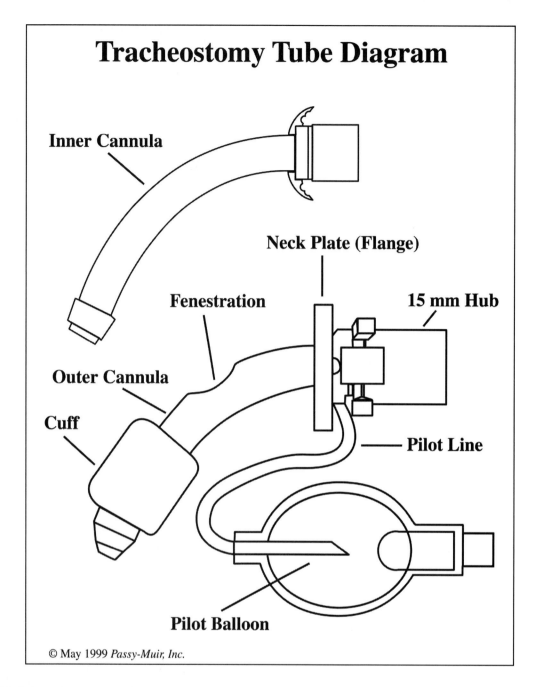

Tracheostomy Tube Diagram

Inner Cannula

Neck Plate (Flange)

Fenestration

15 mm Hub

Outer Cannula

Cuff

Pilot Line

Pilot Balloon

© May 1999 *Passy-Muir, Inc.*

FIGURE 23-4 ◆ A fenestrated tracheostomy tube.

and also talk because the tracheostomy tube is plugged. If the client tires and needs to return to using the ventilator, the nurse can easily do this by inserting the inner cannula (which occludes the fenestration), inflate the cuff, unplug the tracheostomy tube, and attach the ventilator.

The nurse provides tracheostomy care for the client with a new or recent tracheostomy to maintain patency of the tube and reduce the risk of infection. Initially, a tracheostomy may need to be suctioned (see Chapter 22) and cleaned as often as every 1 to 2 hours. After the initial inflammatory response subsides, tracheostomy care may need to be done only once or

twice a day, depending on the client. For clients with a new tracheostomy, aseptic technique should be used when providing tracheostomy care in order to prevent infection. After the stoma has healed, clean gloves can be used while changing the dressing and tie tapes. Technique 23-1 describes tracheostomy care.

Tracheostomy Dressing and Tie Tapes

As part of tracheostomy care, the tracheostomy dressing and the tie tapes need to be changed whenever they become soiled. Soiled dressings harbor microorganisms and can be a potential source of skin excoriation, breakdown, and infection around the tracheostomy incision. Usually, the dressing is changed after the cannula is cleaned, but a more frequent dressing change may be necessary. The dressing technique is described in Technique 23-1.

Before applying a new dressing, the nurse needs to check any special orders or agency protocol regarding application of solutions around the tracheostomy site. Noncotton-filled 4″ × 4″ gauze dressings are used. Do not cut the gauze square because gauze fibers can be aspirated.

If the tracheostomy ties need to be changed, have an assistant put on gloves and hold the tracheostomy tube in place. This prevents the tracheostomy tube from becoming accidentally dislodged if the client moves or starts coughing when the ties are not secure. If an assistant is not available, leave the old ties in place while securing the clean ties to prevent inadvertent dislodging of the tracheostomy tube.

Nursing Process: Tracheostomy

ASSESSMENT

Assess:

- Respiratory status including ease of breathing, rate, rhythm, depth, and lung sounds
- Pulse rate
- Character and amount of secretions from tracheostomy site
- Presence of drainage on tracheostomy dressing or ties
- Appearance of incision (note any redness, swelling, purulent discharge, or odor)

PLANNING

Delegation

Tracheostomy care involves application of scientific knowledge, sterile technique, and problem solving, and therefore needs to be performed by a nurse.

IMPLEMENTATION:
TECHNIQUE 23-1 PROVIDING TRACHEOSTOMY CARE

Equipment

- Sterile disposable tracheostomy cleaning kit or supplies including sterile containers, sterile nylon brush and/or pipe cleaners, sterile applicators, gauze squares
- Towel or drape to protect bed linens
- Sterile suction catheter kit (suction catheter and sterile container for solution)
- Hydrogen peroxide and sterile normal saline
- Sterile gloves (2 pairs)
- Clean gloves
- Moistureproof bag
- Commercially prepared sterile tracheostomy dressing or sterile 4″ × 4″ gauze dressing
- Cotton twill ties
- Clean scissors

Performance

1. Explain to the client what you are going to do, why it is necessary, and how he or she can cooperate. Provide for a means of communication, such as eye blinking or raising a finger, to indicate pain or distress.

2. Wash hands and observe other appropriate infection control procedures.

3. Provide for client privacy.

4. Prepare the client and the equipment.
   - Assist the client to a semi-Fowler's or Fowler's position *to promote lung expansion.*
   - Open the tracheostomy kit or sterile basins. Pour hydrogen peroxide and sterile normal saline into separate containers.
   - Establish a sterile field.
   - Open other sterile supplies as needed including sterile applicators, suction kit, and tracheostomy dressing.

5. Suction the tracheostomy tube.
   - Put a clean glove on your nondominant hand and a sterile glove on your dominant hand (or put on a pair of sterile gloves).
   - Suction the full length of the tracheostomy tube to remove secretions and ensure a patent airway (see Technique 22-2).
   - Rinse the suction catheter and wrap the catheter around your hand, and peel the glove off so that it turns inside out over the catheter.
   - Using the gloved hand, unlock the inner cannula (if present) and remove it by gently pulling it out toward you in line with its curvature. Place the inner cannula in the hydrogen peroxide solution. *This moistens and loosens dried secretions.*
   - Remove the soiled tracheostomy dressing. Place the soiled dressing in your gloved hand and peel the glove off so that it turns inside out over the dressing. Discard the glove and the dressing.

- Put on sterile gloves. Keep your dominant hand sterile during the technique.

6. Clean the inner cannula.

- Remove the inner cannula from the soaking solution.

- Clean the lumen and entire inner cannula thoroughly using the brush or pipe cleaners moistened with sterile normal saline (Figure 23-5 ◆). Inspect the cannula for cleanliness by holding it at eye level and looking through it into the light.

- Rinse the inner cannula thoroughly in the sterile normal saline. *Thorough rinsing is important to remove the hydrogen peroxide from the inner cannula.*

- After rinsing, gently tap the cannula against the inside edge of the sterile saline container. Use a pipe cleaner folded in half to dry only the inside of the cannula; do not dry the outside. *This removes excess liquid from the cannula and prevents possible aspiration by the client, while leaving a film of moisture on the outer surface to lubricate the cannula for reinsertion.*

- Using sterile technique, suction the outer cannula. *Suctioning removes secretions from the outer cannula.*

7. Replace the inner cannula, securing it in place.

- Insert the inner cannula by grasping the outer flange and inserting the cannula in the direction of its curvature.

- Lock the cannula in place by turning the lock (if present) into position to secure the flange of the inner cannula to the outer cannula.

8. Clean the incision site and tube flange.

- Using sterile applicators or gauze dressings moistened with normal saline, clean the incision site (Figure 23-6 ◆). Handle the sterile supplies with your dominant hand. Use each applicator or gauze dressing only once and then discard. *This*

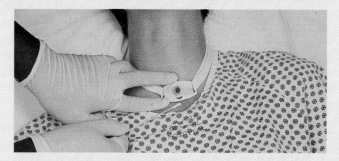

FIGURE 23-6 ◆ Using an applicator stick to clean the tracheostomy site.

avoids contaminating a clean area with a soiled gauze dressing or applicator.

- Hydrogen peroxide may be used (usually in a half-strength solution mixed with sterile normal saline—use a separate sterile container if this is necessary) to remove crusty secretions. Thoroughly rinse the cleaned area using gauze squares moistened with sterile normal saline. *Hydrogen peroxide can be irritating to the skin and inhibit healing if not thoroughly removed.*

- Clean the flange of the tube in the same manner.

- Thoroughly dry the client's skin and tube flanges with dry gauze squares.

9. Apply a sterile dressing

- Use a commercially prepared tracheostomy dressing of nonraveling material or open and refold a 4″ × 4″ gauze dressing into a V shape as shown in Figure 23-7 ◆ A through D. Avoid using cotton-filled gauze squares or cutting the 4″ × 4″ gauze. *Cotton lint or gauze fibers can be aspirated by the client, potentially creating a tracheal abscess.*

- Place the dressing under the flange of the tracheostomy tube as shown in Figure 23-7E.

- While applying the dressing, ensure that the tracheostomy tube is securely supported. *Excessive movement of the tracheostomy tube irritates the trachea.*

10. Change the tracheostomy ties.

Two-Strip Method

- Cut two unequal strips of twill tape, one approximately 25 cm (10 in) long and the other about 50 cm (20 in) long. *Cutting one tape longer than the other allows them to be fastened at the side of the neck for easy access and to avoid the pressure of a knot on the skin at the back of the neck.*

- Cut a 1-cm (0.5-in) lengthwise slit approximately 2.5 cm (1 in) from one end of each strip. To do this, fold the end of the tape back onto itself about 2.5 cm (1 in), then cut a slit in the middle of the tape from its folded edge.

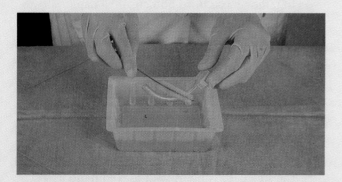

FIGURE 23-5 ◆ Cleaning the inner cannula with a brush.

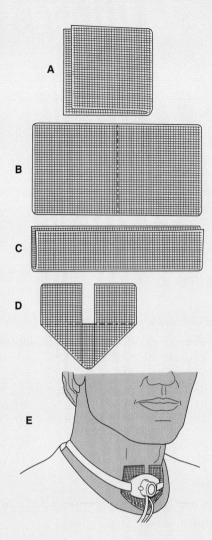

FIGURE 23-7 ◆ Folding a 4" × 4" gauze to make a tracheostomy dressing.

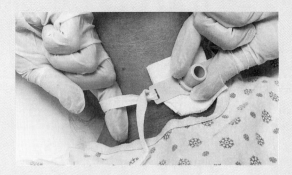

FIGURE 23-8 ◆ Placing a finger underneath the tie tape before tying it.

interfere with coughing or place pressure on the jugular veins.

- Tie the ends of the tapes using square knots. Cut off any long ends, leaving approximately 1 to 2 cm (0.5 in). *Square knots prevent slippage and loosening. Adequate ends beyond the knot prevent the knot from inadvertently untying.*

- Once the clean ties are secured, remove the soiled ties and discard.

One-Strip Method

- Cut a length of twill tape 2.5 times the length needed to go around the client's neck from one tube flange to the other.

- Thread one end of the tape into the slot on one side of the flange.

- Bring both ends of the tape together, take them around the client's neck, keeping them flat and untwisted.

- Thread the end of the tape next to the client's neck through the slot from the back to the front.

- Have the client flex the neck. Tie the loose ends with a square knot at the side of the client's neck, allowing for slack by placing two fingers under the ties as with the two-strip method. Cut off long ends.

11. Tape and pad the tie knot.

- Place a folded 4" × 4" gauze square under the tie knot, and apply tape over the knot. *This reduces skin irritation from the knot and prevents confusing the knot with the client's gown ties.*

12. Check the tightness of the ties.

- Frequently check the tightness of the tracheostomy ties and position of the tracheostomy tube. *Swelling of the neck may cause the ties to become too tight, interfering with coughing and circulation. Ties can loosen in restless clients, allowing the tracheostomy tube to extrude from the stoma.*

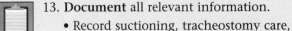 13. **Document** all relevant information.

- Record suctioning, tracheostomy care, and the dressing change, noting your assessments.

- Leaving the old ties in place, thread the slit end of one clean tape through the eye of the tracheostomy flange from the bottom side; then thread the long end of the tape through the slit, pulling it tight until it is securely fastened to the flange. *Leaving the old ties in place while securing the clean ties prevents inadvertent dislodging of the tracheostomy tube. Securing tapes in this manner avoids the use of knots, which can come untied or cause pressure and irritation.*

- If old ties are very soiled or it is difficult to thread new ties onto the tracheostomy flange with old ties in place, have an assistant put on a sterile glove and hold the tracheostomy in place while you replace the ties.

- Repeat the process for the second tie.

- Ask the client to flex the neck. Slip the longer tape under the client's neck, place two fingers between the tape and the client's neck (Figure 23-8 ◆), and tie the tapes together at the side of the neck. *Flexing the neck increases its circumference the way coughing does. Placing two fingers under the ties prevents making the ties too tight, which could*

Variation: Using a Disposable Inner Cannula

- Check policy for frequency of changing inner cannula *as standards vary among institutions.*
- Open new cannula package.
- Using a gloved hand, unlock the current inner cannula (if present) and remove it by gently pulling it out toward you in line with its curvature.

- Check the cannula for amount and type of secretions and discard properly.
- Pick up the new inner cannula touching only the outer locking portion.
- Insert the new inner cannula into the tracheostomy.
- Lock the cannula in place by turning the lock (if present).

AMBULATORY AND COMMUNITY SETTINGS

Tracheostomy Care

- For tracheostomies older than one month, clean technique is used for tracheostomy care (Humphrey, 1998).
- Stress the importance of good handwashing technique to the caregiver.
- Tap water may be used for rinsing the inner cannula.

- Teach the caregiver the tracheostomy care technique and observe a return demonstration.
- Inform the caregiver of the signs and symptoms that may indicate an infection of the stoma site or lower airway.
- Names and telephone numbers of health care personnel who can be reached for emergencies or advice must be available to the client and/or caregiver.

AGE-RELATED CONSIDERATIONS

Tracheostomy Care

Infant & Child

- An assistant should *always* be present while tracheostomy care is performed.
- Always keep a sterile, packaged tracheostomy tube taped to the child's bed so that if the tube dislodges, a new one is available for immediate reintubation (Bindler & Ball, 1999, p. 84).

Elder

- Older adult skin is more fragile and prone to breakdown. Care of the skin at the tracheostomy stoma is very important.

EVALUATION

- Perform appropriate follow-up such as: character and amount of secretions; drainage from the tracheostomy; appearance of the tracheostomy incision; pulse rate and respiratory status compared to baseline data; complaints of pain or discomfort at the tracheostomy site.
- Relate findings to previous assessment data if available.
- Report significant deviations from normal to the physician.

Humidification

When the client breathes through a tracheostomy, air is no longer filtered and humidified as it is when passing through the upper airways; therefore, special precautions are necessary. Humidity may be provided with a tracheostomy mist collar (Figure 23-9 ◆). Clients with long-term tracheostomies may wear a light scarf or a 4″ × 4″ gauze held in place with a cotton tie over the stoma to filter air as it enters the tracheostomy.

Plugging a Tracheostomy Tube

A client may have the tracheostomy tube plugged during the weaning process of discontinuing mechanical ventilation. The purpose of plugging the tracheostomy tube is to establish ventilation through the natural airway. It is important for the nurse to monitor the client closely because if the client's respiratory status deteriorates, mechanical support will need to be restarted. Technique 23-2 describes the process for plugging a tracheostomy tube. Once clients can suc-

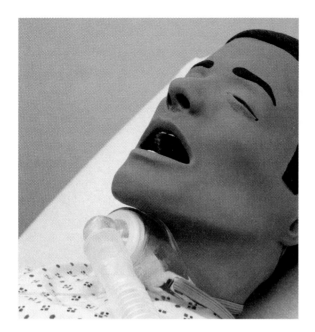

FIGURE 23-9 ◆ Tracheostomy mist collar.

cessfully breathe spontaneously on their own without respiratory compromise, they are taken off of mechanical support. This does not mean, however, that the tracheostomy tube is automatically removed. The health care team (physician, nurse, respiratory therapist) must determine whether or not there is a need to maintain an artificial airway.

Nursing Process: Plugging a Tracheostomy Tube

ASSESSMENT

Assess vital signs and respiratory effort before plugging the tube. Note the presence of excessive secretions in the respiratory tract as this may contraindicate plugging of the tube.

PLANNING

Delegation

Plugging a tracheostomy involves the application of scientific knowledge, assessment skills, and problem solving, and therefore needs to be performed by a nurse or a respiratory therapist.

IMPLEMENTATION:
TECHNIQUE 23-2 PLUGGING A TRACHEOSTOMY TUBE

Equipment

- Suction apparatus
- Sterile suction catheters
- Sterile 10-mL syringe
- Sterile gloves
- Sterile tracheostomy plug

Performance

1. Explain to the client what you are going to do, why it is necessary, and how he or she can cooperate.

2. Wash hands and observe other appropriate infection control procedures.

3. Provide for client privacy.

4. Position the client
   - Assist the client to a semi-Fowler's position if not contraindicated. *This position enhances lung expansion and may decrease fears about not being able to breathe.*

5. Suction the airways.
   - Suction the client's nasopharynx and oropharynx if there are any secretions present.
   - Change suction catheters and use a new sterile catheter to suction the tracheostomy. If there are excessive secretions, report this finding to the nurse in charge or physician to determine whether to proceed with the procedure.

6. Deflate the tracheal cuff if ordered.
   - Suction the tracheostomy tube again if secretions are present.

7. Insert the tracheostomy plug.
   - Using sterile gloves, fit the tracheostomy plug into either the inner or the outer cannula, depending on whether the tracheostomy tube has a double or single cannula.
   - Monitor the client closely for ten minutes for signs of respiratory distress, such as noisy and/or rapid respirations and use of accessory muscles for breathing. At the first signs of distress, remove the tracheostomy plug and suction the tracheostomy if necessary.
   - Clean the inner cannula, if it was removed, so that it is ready to be reinserted.
   - Observe the client frequently while the tube is plugged.

8. Remove the plug at the designated time.
   - After removing the plug, suction the tracheostomy if indicated, and replace the inner cannula if removed.
   - Reinflate the cuff if ordered.

9. **Document** all relevant information.
   - Document the amount, color, and consistency of the secretions; the times the plug was inserted and removed; and your assessments.

AMBULATORY AND COMMUNITY SETTINGS

Plugging a Tracheostomy Tube

- Suction equipment should be available in the home when performing this technique.
- Use a clean, private area of the home for the procedure and place the equipment on a clean towel or drape.

- Stay with the client while the tracheostomy is plugged and observe for signs of respiratory distress.
- Don't perform the procedure at home if the client is short of breath or extremely anxious. Have a plan of action in case problems occur, and notify the physician immediately.

AGE-RELATED CONSIDERATIONS

Plugging a Tracheostomy Tube

Elders

- Observe the older client carefully for signs of respiratory distress and stress the importance of slow, deep breathing. *Decreased lung compliance is part of the aging process.*

- Teach the older client how to cough and breathe deeply to keep the airway clear. *Decreased ability to cough occurs with aging.*

EVALUATION

- Conduct appropriate follow-up such as assessing respiratory status while the tube is plugged (e.g., breath sounds, respiratory rate, and the use of accessory muscles for breathing).
- Compare to previous assessment data if available.
- Keep the physician informed of the client's progress in the weaning process.

Facilitating Communication

A client with a tracheostomy tube cannot speak because the vocal cords are above the level of the tracheostomy tube (Craven & Hirnle, 2000). Alternate methods for communication are necessary to avoid client frustration. Writing materials can be used if the client has the strength and coordination. Some clients may prefer a communication board that contains pictures or phrases on it to allow the client to communicate by pointing to the appropriate picture or phrase.

Some clients use their finger to occlude the tracheostomy tube to allow them to speak. This method, however, can lead to an infection of the airway. A more reliable method is to use a commercially available tracheostomy speaking valve. These devices are one-way valves that are connected to the tracheostomy tube opening. The device opens during inspiration but closes during expiration, forcing exha-

lation to occur around the tube and past the vocal cords (Fink & Hunt, 1999, p. 400). One example is the Passy–Muir valve (Figure 23-10 ◆). The nurse should suction the tracheostomy tube and mouth, if needed, before using the valve. If the client has a cuffed tracheostomy tube, it is mandatory that the cuff is deflated while the client uses the valve. The client will be unable to breathe if the cuff is not completely deflated. Airway patency is a key factor when using a one-way speaking valve.

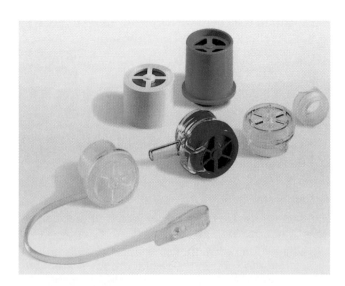

FIGURE 23-10 ◆ A Passy–Muir valve. Examples of a tracheostomy speaking valve.

Chapter Summary

TERMINOLOGY

cuffed tracheostomy tube

fenestrated tracheostomy tube

flange

inner cannula

obturator

outer cannula

tracheostomy

uncuffed tracheostomy tube

wean

FORMING CLINICAL JUDGMENTS

Consider This:

1. The nurse informs you that the client frequently starts coughing when the inner cannula is removed. You are now performing tracheostomy care for this client. As you are cleaning the inner cannula, the client begins to cough and bring up secretions. What will you do?

2. You are assigned to provide nursing care for a client who had an emergency tracheostomy performed the previous day. What equipment will you ensure is available in the client's room?

RELATED RESEARCH

Burns, S. M., Spilman, M., Wilmoth, D., Carpenter, R., Turrentine, B., Wiley, B., Marshall, M., Martens, S., Burns, J. E., & Truwit, J. D. (1998). Are frequent inner cannula changes necessary?: A pilot study. *Heart & Lung, 27*(1), 58–62.

REFERENCES

Bindler, R., & Ball, J. (1999). *Quick Reference to Pediatric Clinical Skills*. Stamford, CT: Appleton & Lange.

Craven, R. F., & Hirnle, C. J. (2000). *Fundamentals of Nursing—Human Health and Function* (3rd ed.). Philadelphia: Lippincott.

Fink, J. B., & Hunt, G. E. (1999). *Clinical Practice in Respiratory Care*. Philadelphia: Lippincott Williams & Wilkins.

Griggs, A. (1999). Tracheostomy: Suctioning and humidification. *Emergency Nurse, 6*(9), 33–40.

Humphrey, C. J. (1998). *Home Care Nursing Handbook* (3rd ed.). Gaithersburg, MD: Aspen.

Theaker, C. (1999). How to guide: Pitfalls in tracheostomy care. *Care of the Critically Ill, 15*(5).

Chapter 24

Caring for the Client with Chest Tube Drainage

Techniques

OBJECTIVES

- Identify assessment data essential for clients with chest drainage.
- Describe how various types of chest drainage systems operate.
- Monitor clients with chest drainage effectively.
- Identify the steps of assisting with chest tube insertion and removal.

Chest Tubes

Chest tubes are usually inserted through an intercostal space into the pleural cavity. They are used following chest surgery or trauma and for pneumothorax or hemothorax. A **pneumothorax** is a collection of air or other gas in the pleural space that causes the lung to collapse. A **hemothorax** is the accumulation of blood and fluid in the pleural cavity, usually as a result of trauma or surgery. Chest tubes used to remove air are usually inserted in the upper anterior chest (i.e., through the second intercostal space) because air rises in the pleural cavity. Tubes used to drain fluids are inserted more inferiorly, often in the eighth or ninth intercostal space, and more posteriorly (see Figure 24-1 ◆).

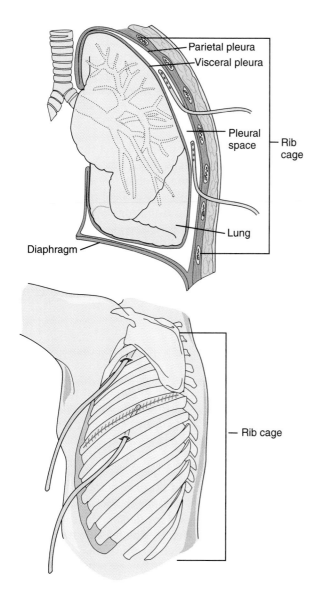

Placement of chest tubes.

FIGURE 24-1 ◆ **Chest tubes in the pleural spaces.**

Drainage Systems

Because the pleural cavity normally has negative pressure that allows lung expansion, any tube connected to it must be sealed so that air or liquid cannot enter. The tube may be connected to a one-way valve or to water-sealed (underwater) drainage. In water-sealed drainage, fluid in the bottom of the container prevents air from entering the chest tube and pleural cavity when the client inhales.

Drainage systems use three mechanisms to drain fluid and air from the pleural cavity; positive expiratory pressure, gravity, and suction. When the pleural cavity contains air or fluid, a positive pressure develops during expiration. This positive pressure is abnormal, but it helps expel the air and some fluid from the space. Placing the tubing so that it descends from the insertion site to the drainage receptacle allows gravity to act as an evacuation force. Suction is used in conjunction with the other two forces in some drainage systems.

There are several kinds of water-sealed drainage systems: one- and two-bottle gravity systems, two- and three-bottle suction systems, and sterile disposable unit systems (most common).

Bottle Systems

In a *one-bottle system,* the air or fluid enters through the collection inlet, which terminates under sterile water (the seal). Air exits through the water and then the air vent; the fluid remains in the bottle (Figure 24-2A ◆). The one-bottle system depends on gravity and positive expiratory pressure for drainage.

A *two-bottle system* uses bottle 1 to receive the fluid or air from the client and bottle 2 to create the water seal (Figure 24-2B). The air or fluid from the pleural cavity is received into bottle 1. The air from bottle 1 is passed into bottle 2, exits through the water and then the air vent. The fluid from the pleural cavity remains in bottle 1. This system uses gravity and positive expiratory pressure for drainage.

The *three-bottle system* has a collection bottle (1), a water-seal bottle (2), and a suction-control bottle (3) (Figure 24-2C). Bottles 1 and 2 function the same as they do in a two-bottle system except that bottle 2 is connected to bottle 3. Bottle 3 has a manometer control tube submerged in sterile water. The depth to which this tube is submerged determines the amount of suction exerted on the pleural cavity. The suction-control bottle has another inlet, for suction. This system uses positive expiratory pressure, gravity, and suction for drainage.

Disposable Unit Systems

Disposable unit systems consist of three chambers (Figure 24-3 ◆): the collection chamber with sub-

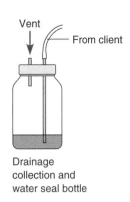

Drainage
collection and
water seal bottle

A

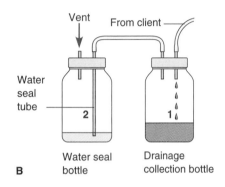

B

Water seal
bottle

Drainage
collection bottle

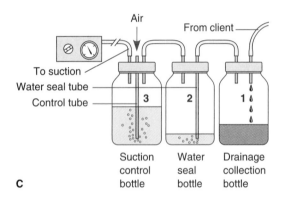

C

Suction
control
bottle

Water
seal
bottle

Drainage
collection
bottle

FIGURE 24-2 ◆ Drainage systems for chest tubes: (A) one-bottle system; (B) two-bottle system; (C) three-bottle system.

chambers; the **water-seal** chamber; and the suction chamber. The height of the fluid in the suction chamber determines the amount of suction pressure exerted upon the client. The exact configuration of these chambers varies by manufacturer. In some, when the collection chamber is filled with drainage, it can be changed or replaced without interrupting the entire system.

Assisting with Chest Tubes

Chest tubes are inserted and removed by the physician with the nurse assisting. Both procedures require sterile technique and must be done without introducing

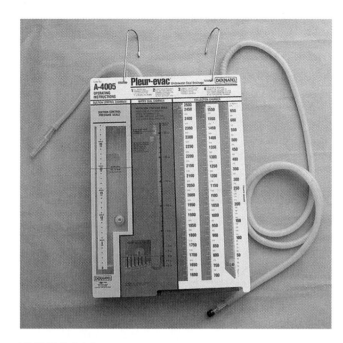

FIGURE 24-3 ◆ A disposable chest drainage system. Fluid and blood collect in the white calibrated chambers. The red chamber provides the water seal and the blue chamber is the suction control.

air or microorganisms into the pleural cavity. After the insertion, an x-ray film is taken to confirm the position of the tube. The major objective of nursing care of clients with chest tubes is to facilitate drainage of fluid and air, thus promoting lung reexpansion.

Nursing Process: Assisting with Chest Tubes

ASSESSMENT

See also Technique 3-11 Assessing the Thorax and Lungs.

Obtain:

- Vital signs for baseline data and then every 4 hours.
- Breath sounds. Auscultate bilaterally for baseline data. *Diminished or absent breath sounds after chest drainage is established indicate inadequate lung expansion.*

Examine for:

- Clinical signs of pneumothorax before and after chest tube insertion. *Leakage or blockage of a chest tube can seriously impair ventilation.* Signs include sharp pain on the affected side; weak, rapid pulse; pallor; vertigo; faintness; dyspnea; diaphoresis; excessive coughing; and blood-tinged sputum.
- Chest expansion (respiratory excursion). See Chapter 3, page 93 and Figures 3-52 and 3-56.
- Chest movements, such as retractions, flail chest, or paradoxical breathing.

Set Up the Drainage System (Disposable Water-Seal)

Nurses must follow strict surgical aseptic technique when setting up chest drainage to prevent microorganisms from entering the system and subsequently entering the client's pleural cavity. To set up the system:

- Open the packaged unit.
- Remove the cap on the water-seal chamber (Figure 24-4 ◆).
- Using a 50-mL irrigating syringe with the plunger removed, fill the water-seal chamber with sterile water up to the 2-cm mark or as specified (Figure 24-5 ◆). Then reattach the plastic connector.

or

- Inject the required amount of water into the self-sealing port of the water-seal chamber using a syringe and needle.
- If the physician has ordered suction, remove the diaphragm (cap) on the suction-control chamber and use the 50-mL syringe to fill the suction-control chamber with sterile water to the ordered level or 20 to 25 cm, and replace the cap.

or

- Set the suction control dial to the ordered amount.
- Place the system in the rack supplied, or attach it to the bed frame.

Delegation

Assisting the physician with insertion of a chest tube is not delegated to unlicensed assistive personnel (UAP).

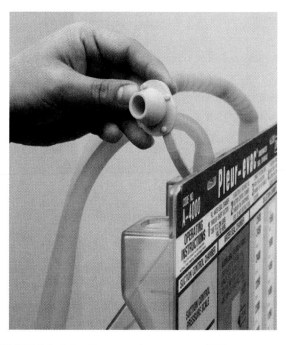

FIGURE 24-4 ◆ Opening the water-seal filling port.

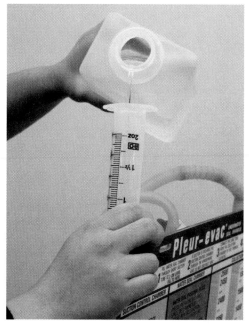

FIGURE 24-5 ◆ Filling the water-seal chamber with sterile water.

IMPLEMENTATION:
TECHNIQUE 24-1 ASSISTING WITH CHEST TUBE INSERTION

Equipment

- Sterile chest tube tray that includes:
  - Drapes
  - 10-mL syringe
  - Gauze sponges
  - 22-gauge needle
  - 25-gauge needle

- #11 blade scalpel
- Forceps
- 2 rubber-tipped tube clamps
- Extra 4" × 4" gauze sponges
- Split drain sponges
- Chest tube and trocar
- Suture materials
- Drainage system

- Sterile gloves (for physician and nurse)
- Local anesthetic vial
- Skin cleansing solution (e.g., povidone–iodine)
- Adhesive tape
- Petrolatum gauze (optional)

Preparation

1. Although the physician will have already done initial client and family teaching, the nurse reinforces key elements. Review the technique of chest tube insertion and its purpose with the client and family.

2. Confirm with the physician the desired types and numbers of equipment needed. Physicians have personal preferences for styles and sizes of chest tubes, and needs vary with the purpose of the tube.

Performance

1. Explain to the client what your role will be, why it is necessary, and how he or she can cooperate. Discuss how the results will be used in planning further care or treatments.

2. Observe appropriate infection control procedures.

3. Provide for client privacy.

4. Position the client as directed by the physician
   - The area receiving the tube should be facing upward.
   - The client may be placed supine or semi-Fowler's. *The supine position is preferred for insertion into the second or third intercostal space, a semi-Fowler's position is preferred for insertion into the sixth to eighth intercostal space.*

5. Prepare for the insertion.
   - Open the chest tube tray and sterile gloves on the overbed table.
   - Assist the physician to clean the insertion site.
   - Assist the physician to draw up the local anesthetic.

6. Provide emotional support and monitor the client during insertion.

7. Dress the site.
   - Don sterile gloves and wrap the petrolatum gauze (if desired) around the tube at the insertion site.
   - Place drain gauze around the tube, one from the top and one from the bottom.
   - Place several additional gauze squares over the drain gauze. *These gauze pieces form an airtight seal at the insertion site.*

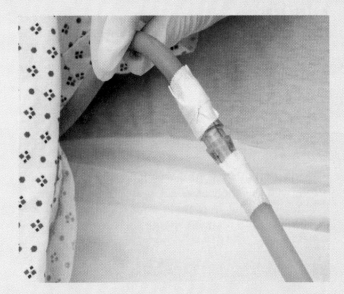

FIGURE 24-6 ◆ Taped tubing connection with the connector exposed for observation of drainage.

8. Secure the tube.
   - Assist with clamping or connecting the tube to the valve or drainage system.
   - Attach the longer tube from the collection chamber to the client's chest tube.
   - Tape the tube to the client's skin.
   - Tape all connections using spiral turns, but do not completely cover the tubing with tape (Figure 24-6 ◆). *Taping prevents inadvertent separation. Not covering all the tubing allows drainage to be seen.*
   - Coil the drainage tubing and secure it to the linen, ensuring slack for the client to turn and move (Figure 24-7 ◆). *This prevents kinking of the tubing and impairment of drainage.*

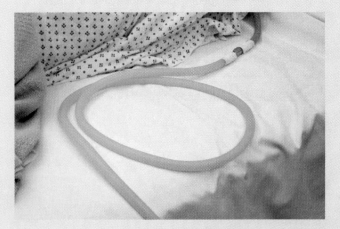

FIGURE 24-7 ◆ Coiled drainage tubing on the bed linen.

- If suction is ordered, attach the remaining shorter tube to the suction source, and turn it on. Inspect the suction chamber for bubbling. Gentle bubbling indicates an appropriate suction level.
- If suction has not been ordered, keep the shorter rubber tube unclamped. This maintains negative or equal pressure in the system.

9. When all drainage connections are complete, ask the client to take a deep breath and hold it for a few seconds, then slowly exhale. These actions facilitate drainage from the pleural space and lung reexpansion.

10. Prepare the client for a chest x-ray *to check for placement of the tube and lung expansion.*

11. Ensure client safety.
- Keep rubber-tipped chest tube clamps at the bedside. *These are used to clamp the chest tube and prevent pneumothorax if the tube becomes discon-nected from the drainage system or the system breaks or cracks.*
- Assess the client for signs of pneumothorax and subcutaneous emphysema. Palpate around the dressing site, and listen for a crackling sound indicative of subcutaneous emphysema. *Subcutaneous emphysema can result from a poor seal at the chest tube insertion site.* This is not an emergency but should be reported, documented, and monitored.
- Assess drainage and vital signs every 15 minutes for the first hour and then as ordered. Report bleeding or drainage greater than 100 mL/hr.

12. **Document** the insertion in the client record using forms or checklists supplemented by narrative notes when appropriate. Include the name of the physician, site of placement, type of tube, type of drainage system, characteristics of the immediate drainage, and other assessment findings.

EVALUATION

- Perform a detailed follow-up based on findings that deviated from expected or normal for the client. Relate findings to previous assessment data if available.
- Report significant deviations from normal to the physician.

Managing a Client with Chest Drainage

Once a client has had a chest tube inserted, the nurse is responsible for maintaining patency of the chest drainage system, facilitating lung reexpansion, and preventing complications associated with chest drainage (e.g., infection).

ASSESSMENT

See Technique 3-11 Assessing the Thorax and Lungs and the assessments listed with Technique 24-1 on page 472.

PLANNING

Review the client record for previous data regarding the condition, output, and client tolerance of the chest tube.

Delegation

Care of chest tubes is not delegated to UAP. However, aspects of the client's condition are observed during usual care and may be recorded by persons other than the nurse. Abnormal findings must be validated and interpreted by the nurse.

IMPLEMENTATION:
TECHNIQUE 24-2 MAINTAINING CHEST TUBE DRAINAGE

Equipment

- Sterile gloves
- 2 rubber-tipped tube clamps
- Petrolatum gauze (optional)
- 4″ × 4″ gauze sponges
- Split drain sponges
- Drainage system
- Skin cleansing solution (e.g., povidone–iodine)
- Adhesive tape

Preparation

Determine when the last dressing change was performed.

Performance

1. Explain to the client what you are going to do, why it is necessary, and how he or she can cooperate. Discuss how the results will be used in planning further care or treatments.

2. Observe appropriate infection control procedures.

3. Provide for client privacy.

4. Assess the client.

- Determine ease of respirations, breath sounds, respiratory rate and depth, and chest movements.

- Observe the dressing site. Inspect the dressing for excessive and abnormal drainage, such as bleeding or foul-smelling discharge. Palpate around the dressing site, and listen for a crackling sound indicative of subcutaneous emphysema. *Subcutaneous emphysema can result from a poor seal at the chest tube insertion site.*

- Determine level of discomfort with and without activity. *Analgesics may need to be administered before the client moves or does deep-breathing and coughing exercises.*

5. Implement all necessary safety precautions.

- Keep two 15- to 18-cm (6- to 7-in) rubber-tipped clamps within reach at the bedside, to clamp the chest tube in an emergency.

- Keep one sterile petrolatum gauze within reach at the bedside to use with an air-occlusive material if the chest tube becomes dislodged.

- Keep an extra drainage system unit available in the client's room. To change the drainage system:

  a. Clamp the chest tube close to the insertion site with two rubber-tipped clamps placed in opposite directions (Figure 24-8 ◆).

  b. Reestablish a water-sealed drainage system and remove the clamps.

- Keep the drainage system below chest level and upright at all times, unless the chest tubes are clamped. *Keeping the unit below chest level prevents backflow of fluid from the drainage chamber into the pleural space. Keeping the unit upright maintains the glass tube below the water level, forming the water seal.*

6. Maintain the patency of the drainage system.

- Check that all connections are secured with tape *to ensure that the system is airtight.*

- Inspect the drainage tubing for kinks or loops dangling below the entry level of the drainage system.

- Coil the drainage tubing and secure it to the bed linen, ensuring enough slack for the client to turn and move (Figure 24-7). *This prevents kinking of the tubing and impairment of the drainage system.*

- Inspect the air vent in the system periodically to make sure it is not occluded. A vent must be present to allow air to escape. *Obstruction of the air vent causes an increased pressure in the system that could result in pneumothorax.*

- **Milk (strip) the chest tubing** as ordered and only in accordance with agency protocol. *Too vigorous milking can create excessive negative pressure that can harm the pleural membranes and/or surrounding tissues.* Always verify the physician's orders before milking the tube; milking of only short segments of the tube may be specified (e.g., 10 to 20 cm, or 4 to 8 in). To milk a chest tube, follow these steps:

  a. Lubricate about 10 to 20 cm (4 to 8 in) of the drainage tubing with lubricating gel, soap, or hand lotion, or hold an alcohol sponge between your fingers and the tube. *Lubrication reduces friction and facilitates the milking process.*

  b. With one hand, securely stabilize and pinch the tube at the insertion site.

  c. Compress the tube with the thumb and forefinger of your other hand and milk it by sliding them down the tube, moving away from the insertion site. *Milking the tubing dislodges obstructions, such as blood clots. Milking from the insertion site downward prevents movement of the obstructive material into the pleural space.* Gently release the hand pinching the tube.

  d. If the entire tube is to be milked, reposition your hands farther along the tubing, and repeat steps a through c in progressive overlapping steps, until you reach the end of the tubing.

7. Assess any fluid level fluctuations and bubbling in the drainage system.

- In gravity drainage systems, check for fluctuation (**tidaling**) of the fluid level in the water-seal chamber as the client breathes. Normally, fluctuations of 5 to 10 cm (2 to 4 in) occur until the lung has reexpanded. In suction drainage systems, the fluid line remains constant. *Fluctuations reflect the pressure changes in the pleu-*

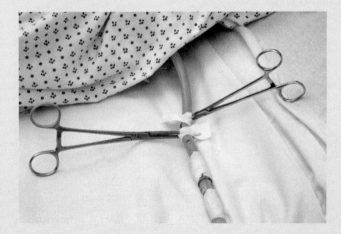

FIGURE 24-8 ◆ Clamping a chest tube.

ral space during inhalation and exhalation. The fluid level rises when the client inhales and falls when the client exhales. The absence of fluctuations may indicate tubing obstruction from a kink, dependent loop, blood clot, or outside pressure (e.g., because the client is lying on the tubing), or may indicate that full lung reexpansion has occurred.

- To check for fluctuation in suction systems, temporarily turn off the suction. Then observe the fluctuation.
- Check for intermittent bubbling in the water of the water-seal chamber. *Intermittent bubbling normally occurs when the system removes air from the pleural space, especially when the client takes a deep breath or coughs. Absence of bubbling indicates that the pleural space has healed and is sealed. Continuous bubbling or a sudden change from an established pattern can indicate a break in the system (i.e., an air leak) and should be reported immediately.*
- Check for gentle bubbling in the suction-control bottle or chamber. *Gentle bubbling indicates proper suction pressure.*

8. Assess the drainage.
- Inspect the drainage in the collection container at least every 30 minutes during the first 2 hours after chest tube insertion and every 2 hours thereafter.
- Every 8 hours, mark the time, date, and drainage level on a piece of adhesive tape affixed to the container, or mark it directly on a disposable container (Figure 24-9 ◆).
- Note any sudden change in the amount or color of the drainage.

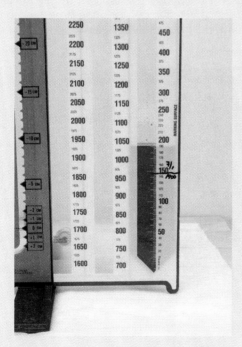

FIGURE 24-9 ◆ Marking the date, time, and drainage level.

- If drainage exceeds 100 mL/hr or if a color change indicates hemorrhage, notify the physician immediately.

9. Watch for dislodgement of the tubes, and remedy the problem promptly.
- If the chest tube becomes disconnected from the drainage system,
  a. Have the client exhale fully.
  b. Clamp the chest tube close to the insertion site with two rubber-tipped clamps placed in opposite directions. *Clamping the tube prevents external air from entering the pleural space. Two clamps ensure complete closure of the tube.*
  c. Quickly clean the ends of the tubing with an antiseptic, reconnect them, and tape them securely.
  d. Unclamp the tube as soon as possible. *Having the client exhale and clamping the tube for no longer than necessary prevents an air or fluid buildup in the pleural space, which can cause further lung collapse.*
  e. Assess the client closely for respiratory distress (dyspnea, pallor, diaphoresis, blood-tinged sputum, or chest pain).
  f. Check vital signs every 10 minutes.
- If the chest tube becomes dislodged from the insertion site:
  a. Remove the dressing, and immediately apply pressure with the petrolatum gauze, your hand, or a towel.
  b. Cover the site with sterile 4″ × 4″ gauze squares.
  c. Tape the dressings with air-occlusive tape.
  d. Notify the physician immediately.
  e. Assess the client for respiratory distress every 10 to 15 minutes or as client condition indicates.
- If the drainage system is accidentally tipped over:
  a. Immediately return it to the upright position.
  b. Ask the client to take several deep breaths. *Deep breaths help force air out of the pleural cavity that might have entered when the water seal was not intact.*
  c. Notify the physician.
  d. Assess the client for respiratory distress.

10. If continuous bubbling persists in the water-seal collection chamber, indicating an air leak, determine its source. Continuous bubbling in the water-seal collection chamber normally occurs for only a few minutes after a chest tube is attached to drainage, because fluid and air initially rush out from the intrapleural space under high pressure.
- To detect an air leak, follow the next steps sequentially:

a. Check the tubing connection sites. Tighten and retape any connection that seems loose. *The tubing connection sites are the most likely places for leaks to occur.*

b. If bubbling continues, clamp the chest tube near the insertion site, and see whether the bubbling stops while the client takes several deep breaths. *Clamping the chest will determine whether the leak is proximal or distal to the clamp. Chest tube clamping must be done only for a few seconds at a time. Clamping for long periods can aggravate an existing pneumothorax or lead to a recurrent pneumothorax.*

c. If bubbling stops, proceed with the next step. The source of the air leak is above the clamp (i.e., between the clamp and the client). It may be either at the insertion site or inside the client.

d. If bubbling continues, the source of the air leak is below the clamp (i.e., in the drainage system below the clamp). See next step below.

• To determine whether the air leak is at the insertion site or inside the client:

a. Unclamp the tube and palpate gently around the insertion site. If the bubbling stops, the leak is at the insertion site. To remedy this situation, apply a petrolatum gauze and a 4" × 4" gauze around the insertion site, and secure these dressings with adhesive tape.

b. If the leak is not at the insertion site, it is inside the client and may indicate a dislodged tube or a new pneumothorax. In this instance, leave the tube unclamped, notify the physician, and monitor the client for signs of respiratory distress.

• To locate an air leak below the chest tube clamp:

a. Move the clamp a few inches farther down and keep moving it downward a few inches at a time. Each time the clamp is moved, check the water-seal collection chamber for bubbling. *The bubbling will stop as soon as the clamp is placed between the air leak and the water-seal drainage.*

b. Seal the leak when you locate it by applying tape to that portion of the drainage tube.

c. If bubbling continues after the entire length of the tube is clamped, the air leak is in the drainage device. To remedy this situation, replace the drainage system according to agency protocol.

11. Take a specimen of the chest drainage as required.

• Specimens of chest drainage may be taken from a disposable chest drainage system because these systems are equipped with self-sealing ports. If a specimen is required:

a. Use a povidone–iodine swab to wipe the self-sealing diaphragm on the back of the drainage collection chamber. Allow it to dry.

b. Attach a sterile 18- or 20-gauge needle to a syringe, and insert the needle into the diaphragm (Figure 24-10 ◆).

c. Aspirate the specimen, discard the needle in the appropriate container, label the syringe, and send it to the laboratory with the appropriate requisition form.

12. Ensure essential client care.

• Encourage deep-breathing and coughing exercises every 2 hours, if indicated (this may be contraindicated in clients with a lobectomy). Have the client sit upright to perform the exercises, and splint the tube insertion site with a pillow or with a hand to minimize discomfort. *Deep breathing and coughing help remove accumulations from the pleural space, facilitate drainage, and help the lung to reexpand.*

• While the client takes deep breaths, palpate the chest for thoracic excursion.

• Reposition the client every 2 hours. When the client is lying on the affected side, place rolled towels beside the tubing. *Frequent position changes promote drainage, prevent complications, and provide comfort. Rolled towels prevent occlusion of the chest tube by the client's weight.*

• Assist the client with range-of-motion exercises of the affected shoulder three times per day to maintain joint mobility.

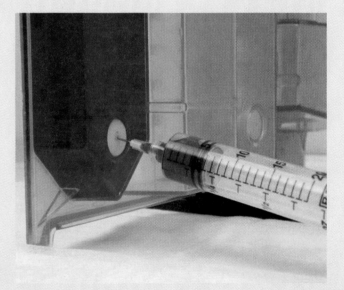

FIGURE 24-10 ◆ Obtaining a specimen through a self-sealing port.

- When transporting and ambulating the client:
  a. Attach rubber-tipped forceps to the client's gown for emergency use.
  b. Keep the water-seal unit below chest level and upright.
  c. Disconnect the drainage system from the suction apparatus before moving the client, and make sure the air vent is open.

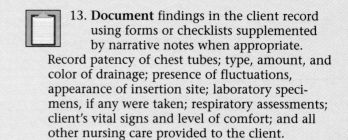 13. **Document** findings in the client record using forms or checklists supplemented by narrative notes when appropriate. Record patency of chest tubes; type, amount, and color of drainage; presence of fluctuations, appearance of insertion site; laboratory specimens, if any were taken; respiratory assessments; client's vital signs and level of comfort; and all other nursing care provided to the client.

AGE-RELATED CONSIDERATIONS

Maintaining Chest Tube Drainage

Older Adult

- Coughing and deep breathing exercises are particularly important since shallow breathing and decreased ability to cough may occur with aging.
- Encourage the client to take pain medication when needed. Older adults may be reluctant to take pain medication.

- Use special care of the client's skin due to the possibility of skin tears from tape and increased risk of skin breakdown over bony prominences as skin becomes thinner and less elastic.
- The older client is at increased risk for respiratory distress due to decreased lung compliance.

EVALUATION

- Perform detailed follow-up based on findings that deviated from expected or normal for the client. Relate findings to previous assessment data if available.
- Report significant deviations from normal to the physician.

Chest Tube Removal

Nursing Process: Chest Tube Removal

ASSESSMENT

See also Technique 3-11 Assessing the Thorax and Lungs.

Chest tube removal can be a very painful procedure. Determine when the client was last medicated for pain.

PLANNING

The physician will determine when the chest tube is to be removed. Arrange the client's other activities around this.

Delegation

Assisting with the removal of a chest tube is not delegated to UAP. However, many effects of the removal may be observed during usual care and may be recorded by persons other than the nurse. Abnormal findings must be validated and interpreted by the nurse.

IMPLEMENTATION:
TECHNIQUE 24-3 ASSISTING WITH CHEST TUBE REMOVAL

Equipment

- Nonsterile gloves
- Sterile gloves
- Suture removal set with forceps and scissors
- Sterile petrolatum gauze
- 4" × 4" gauze sponges
- Adhesive tape

- Moistureproof bag
- Linen-saver pad

Preparation

Ensure that the client has been informed that the chest tube will be removed and when. Clamp the tube, if ordered. Administer an analgesic, if ordered, 30 minutes prior to removal of the chest tube.

Performance

1. Explain to the client what you are going to do, why it is necessary, and how he or she can cooperate. Discuss how the results will be used in planning further care or treatments.

2. Observe appropriate infection control procedures.

3. Provide for client privacy.

4. Prepare the client:

   - Assist the client to a side-lying or semi-Fowler's position with the chest tube site exposed.
   - Place the linen-saver pad under the client, beneath the chest tube *to protect the bed linens and provide a place for the chest tube after removal.*
   - Instruct the client how to hold the breath during removal. Some experts recommend holding a full inhalation while others recommend holding a full exhalation.

5. Prepare the sterile field and supplies. Have the petrolatum gauze opened and ready for quick application.

6. Remove the dressing around the chest tube.

   - Apply clean gloves and dispose of the dressing in the moistureproof bag.

7. Assist with removal of the tube.

   - Assist the client with the breathing technique and provide emotional support during the physician's removal of the sutures and tube.
   - Immediately apply the petrolatum gauze, and cover it with dry gauze and adhesive tape *to form an airtight bandage.*

8. Assess and monitor the client's response to tube removal.

   - Obtain vital signs every 15 minutes for the first hour and, if stable, then as indicated.
   - Auscultate lung sounds every hour for the first 4 hours *to determine that the lung is remaining inflated.*
   - Observe for signs of pneumothorax.

9. **Document** the date and time of removal, any drainage noted, and the client's response to the procedure in the client record using forms or checklists supplemented by narrative notes when appropriate.

10. Prepare the client for a chest x-ray 1 to 2 hours after chest tube removal.

EVALUATION

- Perform detailed follow-up based on findings that deviated from expected or normal for the client. Relate findings to previous assessment data if available.

- Report significant deviations from normal to the physician.

Chapter Summary

TERMINOLOGY

hemothorax

pneumothorax

water-seal

milk (strip) tubing

tidaling

FORMING CLINICAL JUDGMENTS

Consider This:

1. A client with a pneumothorax has had a chest tube inserted into the second intercostal space. After 1 hour, there is no drainage in the system. How do you explain this finding?

2. A client who had open heart surgery 48 hours ago has a chest tube in place that exits from the seventh intercostal space. Why is the chest tube in place? What might be the reasons that the chest tube stops draining?

3. The nurse on the off-going shift reports that there may be an air leak in the client's chest tube system but has not had time to completely assess the problem. How would you proceed?

RELATED RESEARCH

Fox, V., Gould, D., Davies, N., & Owen, S. (1999). Patients' experiences of having an underwater seal chest drain: A replication study. *Journal of Clinical Nursing, 8,* 684–692.

Houston, S., & Jesurum, J. (1999). The quick relaxation technique: Effect on pain associated with chest tube removal. *Applied Nursing Research, 12,* 196–205.

Schmelz, J. O., Johnson, D., Norton, J. M., Andrews, M., & Gordon, P. A. (1999). Effects of position of chest drainage tube on volume drained and pressure. *American Journal of Critical Care, 8,* 319–323.

REFERENCES

Faries, J. Controlling pain: Managing pain during chest tube insertion. *Nursing, 27*(11), 28

Kirkwood, P. (2000). Ask the experts: Gentle versus vigorous chest tube bubbling. *Critical Care Nurse, 30*(3), 98.

Pettinicchi, T. A. Trouble shooting chest tubes. *Nursing, 28*(3), 58–59.

Shuster, P. M. (1998). News, notes, and tips. Chest tubes: To clamp or not to clamp. *Nurse Educator, 23*(3), 9, 13.

Chapter 25

Administering Basic Life Support to the Hospitalized Client

Techniques

OBJECTIVES

- Describe the role of the nurse in initiating and participating in a cardiopulmonary arrest situation in a hospital.
- List the steps to take in clearing an obstructed airway.
- Identify the process of establishing a patent airway and performing rescue breathing.
- Explain the steps of administering external cardiac compression.
- Discuss the use of an automated external defibrillator.

M edical emergencies of different types occur regularly in hospital, long-term care, outpatient, and community settings. The most serious of these is cardiac or cardiopulmonary arrest. All health care workers are trained in **cardiopulmonary resuscitation (CPR)**, which can be used in any setting. However, the events surrounding an arrest in the hospital are somewhat different due to the presence of numbers of highly skilled health care workers and the availability of diagnostic and therapeutic services. Whether the nurse is a member of a specially trained arrest team or the nurse who happens to discover a client who has arrested, it is a time of high anxiety and requires the nurse to be able to recall the appropriate steps to take from memory.

Each health care facility has policies and procedures for announcing an arrest and initiating interventions. In many locations, a cardiac or respiratory arrest is called a **Code Blue**, and announcing the arrest may be referred to as "Calling a Code." The nurse is required to know how this is handled in each facility and each area within the facility. For example, there may be a special Code button in the client's room, a special red or orange telephone at the nurse's station used only for such emergencies, or a specific phone number to call from any phone that the operator knows to answer immediately so that the Code can be announced over the public address system to summon the arrest team. Outside the hospital, the nurse's only resource may be the public emergency medical system (EMS) phone number, such as 911.

In most hospitals and some extended care facilities, specific personnel are designated as members of the Code Blue Team. Persons are needed to perform breathing, deliver chest compressions, administer medications, and record the Code activities. If possible, additional persons should handle the emergency cart and equipment, support the family and clients who may be in the room, and care for other clients of nurses participating in the Code. One person must be designated as the Code Leader—the person who directs the activities of the other team members. An ideal Code team would include a physician familiar with code procedures (e.g., emergency room MD or intensivist), respiratory therapist, critical care nurses, electrocardiography technician, laboratory technician (to draw blood specimens), chaplain, and the client's nurse.

Some clients have chosen to request that, should they arrest, they not be resuscitated. After discussion with the physician, and following agency policies, the client record can be marked with the designation **No Code Blue**, "no CPR," or **Do Not Resuscitate (DNR)**. Under most circumstances, if there is no DNR order in the record, all clients who arrest will have resuscitation efforts begun. Both legally and ethically, there is no such thing as a "partial code," "slow code," or "mini code."

Obstructed Airway

There are several possible causes of airway obstruction and, as a result, several different ways of clearing an **obstructed airway.** Causes include:

- Aspirated food, mucous plug, or foreign bodies, such as partial dentures. Food is the most common cause of choking, particularly meat that has been ineffectively chewed.
- Unconsciousness or seizures, which cause the tongue to fall back and block the airway.
- Severe trauma to the nose, mouth, or neck that produces blood clots that obstruct the airway, especially in unconscious victims.
- Acute edema of the trachea, from smoke inhalation, facial and neck burns, or anaphylaxis. In these instances, a tracheostomy is often indicated.

Nursing Process: Obstructed Airway

ASSESSMENT

Foreign bodies may cause either partial or complete airway obstruction. When an airway is partially obstructed, the victim may have either good air exchange or poor air exchange. If sufficient air is obtained, even though there is frequent wheezing between coughs, do not interfere with the victim's attempts to expel the foreign object. Partial obstructions with inadequate air exchange are dealt with in the same manner as complete obstructions. The victim with complete airway obstruction is unable to speak, breathe, or cough and may clutch at the neck.

PLANNING

The nurse should be prepared for a client to develop an obstructed airway at any time. In the hospital, all nurses and other available health care workers automatically come to the nurse's assistance and work as a team to provide care to the client and to the other clients while the nurse is unavailable.

Delegation

Although unlicensed assistive personnel (UAP) cannot perform all aspects of a hospital code situation, they are trained in CPR and can perform obstructed airway techniques. If they are the first responders, UAP should initiate the intervention and not wait for a nurse.

Equipment

- Standard Precautions supplies including gloves, masks, gowns, and protective eyewear should always be easily accessible.

Performance

Abdominal Thrusts to a Conscious Standing or Sitting Victim

1. Explain to the client that you are trained to help, what you are going to do, and how he or she can cooperate. Speak slowly, clearly, and with confidence.

2. Observe appropriate infection control procedures as much as possible.

3. Provide for client privacy. If another person is present and can cooperate, have that person get help. If family members are present, the nurse may request they leave for the moment.

4. Give abdominal thrusts.

- Stand behind the victim, and wrap your arms around the victim's waist.

- Make a fist with one hand, tuck the thumb inside the fist, and place the flexed thumb just above the victim's navel and below the xiphoid process. *A protruding thumb could inflict injury.*

- With the other hand, grasp the fist (see Figure 25-1 ◆) and press it into the victim's abdomen with a firm, quick upward thrust (see Figure 25-2 ◆). Avoid tightening the arms around the rib cage.

- Deliver successive thrusts as separate and complete movements until the victim's airway clears or the victim becomes unconscious.

- If the victim becomes unconscious, lower the person carefully to the floor, supporting the head and neck to prevent injury.

Abdominal Thrusts to an Unconscious Victim

5. Open the airway.

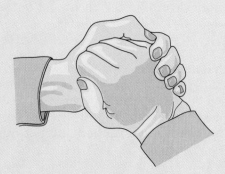

FIGURE 25-1 ◆ The hand and fist position used for abdominal thrusts in a conscious victim.

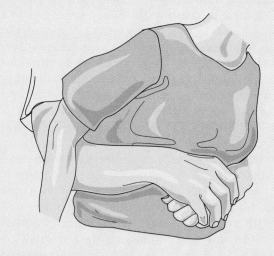

FIGURE 25-2 ◆ The position to provide abdominal thrusts to a conscious victim.

- Tilt the victim's head back, lift the chin, and pinch the nose shut. Put on mouth shield, if available.

- Give two slow breaths.

- If unable to ventilate, retilt the head and repeat breaths.

6. Give abdominal thrusts.

- Straddle the victim's legs.

- Place the heel of one hand slightly above the victim's navel and well below the xiphoid process.

- Place the other hand directly on top of the first. Your shoulders should be over the victim's abdomen and your elbows should be straight.

- Point the fingers of both hands toward the victim's head and give five quick inward and upward abdominal thrusts. See Figure 25-3 ◆. Perform the thrusts to the middle of the abdomen, not to the left or right.

7. Check for foreign objects.

- If foreign material is visible in the mouth, it must be expediently removed. The finger sweep maneuver should be used only on unconscious persons and with extreme caution since the foreign material can be pushed back into the airway, causing increased obstruction.

- Open the person's mouth by grasping the tongue and lower jaw between the thumb and fingers and lifting the jaw upward (see Figure 25-4 ◆). *This pulls the tongue away from the back of the throat.*

- To remove solid material, insert the index finger of your free hand along the inside of the person's cheek and deep into the throat. With your finger hooked, use a sweeping motion to try to dislodge and lift out the foreign object.

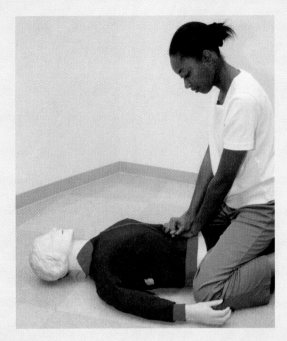

FIGURE 25-3 ◆ The position to provide abdominal thrusts to an unconscious victim.

- After removing the foreign object, clear out liquid material, such as mucus, blood, or emesis, with a scooping motion, using two fingers wrapped with a gauze pad, tissue, or piece of cloth.

8. Repeat ventilation attempts, abdominal thrusts, and foreign object checks until the airway clears or the victim breathes.

Chest Thrusts to a Conscious Standing or Sitting Victim

Chest thrusts are to be administered only to women in advanced stages of pregnancy and markedly obese persons who cannot receive abdominal thrusts.

See steps 1–3 on page 482.

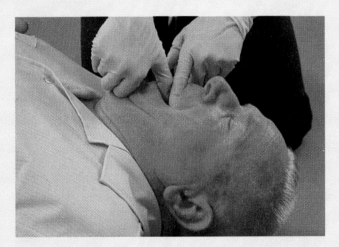

FIGURE 25-4 ◆ The finger sweep maneuver.

4. To administer chest thrusts:
   - Place the thumb side of the fist on the middle of the breastbone, not on the xiphoid process.
   - Grab the fist with the other hand and deliver a quick backward thrust.
   - Repeat thrusts until the obstruction is relieved or the victim becomes unconscious.

Chest Thrusts to an Unconscious Victim Lying Flat

Chest thrusts to unconscious victims lying on the ground are administered only to women in advanced stages of pregnancy or markedly obese persons. After attempting to ventilate:

5. Deliver thrusts.
   - Position the victim supine and kneel close to the side of the victim's trunk.
   - Position the hands as for cardiac compression with the heel of the hand on the lower half of the sternum (see Procedure 25-3, step 4).
   - Deliver five thrusts.

6. Check for foreign objects.
   - If foreign material is visible in the mouth, it must be expediently removed. The finger sweep maneuver should be used only on unconscious persons and with extreme caution since the foreign material can be pushed back into the airway, causing increased obstruction.
   - Open the person's mouth by grasping the tongue and lower jaw between the thumb and fingers, and lifting the jaw upward (see Figure 25-4). *This pulls the tongue away from the back of the throat.*
   - To remove solid material, insert the index finger of your free hand along the inside of the person's cheek and deep into the throat. With your finger hooked, use a sweeping motion to try to dislodge and lift out the foreign object. If these measures fail, try more abdominal thrusts in adults.
   - After removing the foreign object, clear out liquid material, such as mucus, blood, or emesis, with a scooping motion, using two fingers wrapped with a gauze pad, tissue, or piece of cloth.

7. Repeat airway maneuvers, chest thrusts, and foreign object checks until the airway clears or the person breathes.

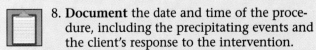 8. **Document** the date and time of the procedure, including the precipitating events and the client's response to the intervention.
   - Describe the type of the procedure, the duration of breathlessness, and the type and size of any foreign object.
   - Note vital signs, any complications, and type of follow-up care.

AMBULATORY AND COMMUNITY SETTINGS

Obstructed Airway

- Stay with the individual and call the emergency medical service (EMS).
- Any individual who receives intervention to treat an obstructed airway should seek immediate follow-up medical evaluation, even if the person remains conscious and the airway is cleared with abdominal thrusts.
- After removal of an airway obstruction at home, the client should receive a medical evaluation. The client may have aspirated foreign material, which can cause airway edema and infection.

- If the person becomes unconscious, activate the EMS.

Family Role

- If a client has difficulty swallowing, teach the caregiver how to clear an obstructed airway.
- Young children are most likely to choke on objects such as small toys. Children don't understand the danger of placing objects in the mouth. Teach parents how to clear an obstructed airway and emphasize the importance of keeping small objects away from a young child.

AGE-RELATED CONSIDERATIONS

Obstructed Airway

Infant

Back Blows and Chest Thrusts

To administer a combination of back blows and chest thrusts to infants:

1. Deliver back blows.
   - Straddle the infant over your forearm with his or her head lower than the trunk.
   - Support the infant's head by firmly holding the jaw in the hand.
   - Rest your forearm on your thigh.
   - With the heel of the free hand, deliver five sharp blows to the back over the spine between the shoulder blades (see Figure 25-5 ◆).

2. Deliver chest thrusts.
   - Turn the infant as a unit to the supine position:
   a. Place the free hand on the infant's back.

   b. While continuing to support the jaw, neck, and chest with the other hand, turn and place the infant on the thigh with the baby's head lower than the trunk.

- Using two fingers, administer five chest thrusts over the sternum in the same location as external chest compression for cardiac massage, one finger-width below the nipple line (see Figure 25-6 ◆).
- For a conscious infant, continue chest thrusts and back blows until the airway is cleared or the infant becomes unconscious.
- If the infant is unconscious, assess the airway and give two breaths. If unable to ventilate, retilt the infant's head and try to give two breaths. If the air does not go in, then give back blows and chest thrusts (see above). Following the chest thrusts, lift the jaw and tongue and check for foreign object. If an object is noted, sweep it out with finger. Repeat this sequence of breaths, for-

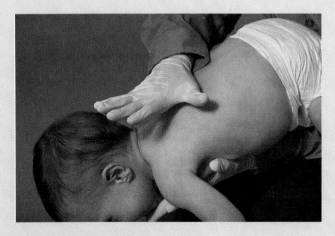

FIGURE 25-5 ◆ Infant back blows.

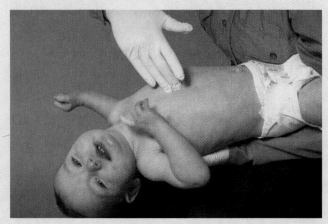

FIGURE 25-6 ◆ Infant chest thrusts.

eign object checks, back blows, and chest thrusts until the airway clears or the infant begins to breathe.

Child

- For conscious children ages 1 to 8 who are choking, perform the **Heimlich maneuver** as for adults (Technique 25-1) (see Figure 25-7 ◆).

- If unable to clear the airway and the child becomes unconscious, perform abdominal thrusts in the supine position (Figure 25-8 ◆).

Elders

- Older clients have a decreased gag reflex.
- Older clients can be injured by incorrect placement of the rescuer's hands. The sternum becomes more brittle with aging.

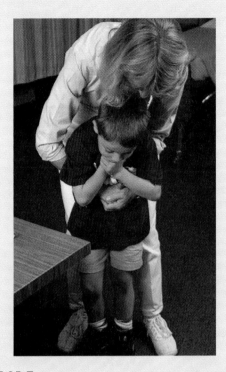

FIGURE 25-7 ◆ Conscious child abdominal thrusts.

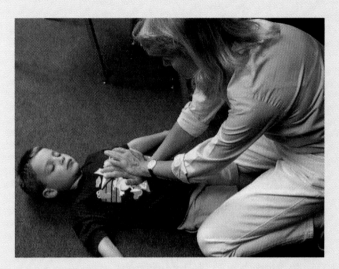

FIGURE 25-8 ◆ Unconscious child abdominal thrusts.

EVALUATION

- Report to the physician the relevant events.
- Conduct appropriate follow-up such as teaching or other interventions that could prevent an airway obstruction in the future.

Respiratory Arrest

A **respiratory arrest** is defined as the absence of breathing. It can be caused by an obstructed airway, suppression of the respiratory center of the brain due to medication overdose, poisoning, **asphyxiation** (suffocation), acid–base or electrolyte imbalance, seizure, drowning, or electric shock. The heart can continue to beat for only a few minutes after breathing stops.

PLANNING

The nurse should be prepared to deliver rescue breathing at any time. In the hospital, all nurses and other available health care workers automatically come to the nurse's assistance and work as a team to provide care to the client and to the other clients while the nurse is unavailable.

Delegation

Although UAP cannot perform all aspects of a hospital code situation, they are trained in CPR and can perform rescue breathing techniques. If they are the first responders, UAP should initiate the intervention and not wait for a nurse.

Equipment

- Standard Precautions supplies including gloves, masks, gowns, and protective eyewear should always be easily accessible.

- Emergency equipment such as an Ambu bag and defibrillation and intubation equipment should be centrally located.

- Pocket face mask with one-way valve or mouth shields, or hand-compressible Ambu bag with mask with one-way valve (see Figure 25-9 ◆).

Performance

1. Determine that the client is unresponsive.

2. If victim does not respond, call a "code" or follow agency protocol to call for assistance. If another person is present and can cooperate, have that person go get help. Tell the person to return and let you know that help has been called.

3. Observe appropriate infection control procedures as much as possible.

4. Provide for client privacy. If family members are present, the nurse may request that they leave for the moment.

5. Position the client appropriately.
   - If the victim is lying on one side or face down, turn the client onto the back as a unit, while supporting the head and neck. Kneel beside the head.

6. Open the airway.
   - Use the head tilt–chin lift maneuver, or the jaw-thrust maneuver. A modified jaw thrust is used for victims with suspected neck injury. In unconscious victims, the tongue lacks sufficient muscle tone, falls to the back of the throat, and obstructs the pharynx. *Because the tongue is attached to the lower jaw, moving the lower jaw forward and tilting the head backward lifts the tongue away from the pharynx and opens the airway* (see Figure 25-10 ◆).

Head Tilt–Chin Lift Maneuver

- Place one hand palm downward on the forehead.
- Place the fingers of the other hand under the bony part of the lower jaw near the chin. The teeth should then be almost closed. The mouth should not be closed completely.
- Simultaneously press down on the forehead with one hand, and lift the victim's chin upward with the other (see Figure 25-11 ◆). Avoid pressing the fingers deeply into the soft tissues under the

chin, since too much pressure can obstruct the airway.

- Open the victim's mouth by pressing the jaw downward with the thumb after tilting the head.

- Remove dentures if they cannot be maintained in place. However, dentures that can be maintained in place make a mouth-to-mouth seal easier should rescue breathing be required.

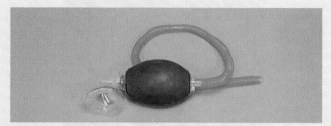

A

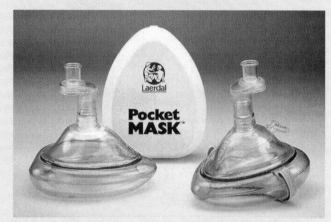

B

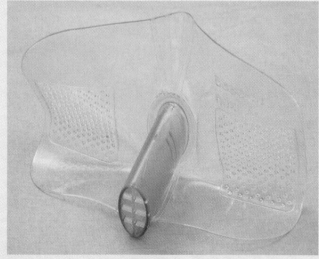

C

FIGURE 25-9 ◆ Facemasks: (A) Ambu bag; (B) pocket mask with one-way valve; (C) face shield.

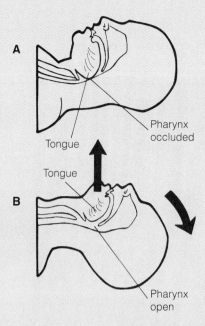

FIGURE 25-10 ◆ The position of an unconscious person's tongue: (A) airway occluded; (B) airway open.

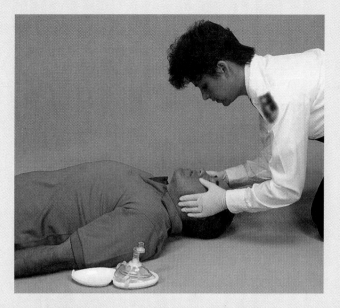

FIGURE 25-12 ◆ Jaw-thrust maneuver.

Jaw-Thrust Maneuver

- Kneel at the top of the victim's head.
- Grasp the angle of the mandible directly below the earlobe between your thumb and forefinger on each side of the victim's head.
- While tilting the head backward, lift the lower jaw until it juts forward and is higher than the upper jaw (see Figure 25-12 ◆).
- Rest your elbows on the surface on which the victim is lying.
- Retract the lower lip with the thumbs prior to giving artificial respiration.
- If the victim is suspected of having a spinal neck injury, do not hyperextend the neck.

7. Determine if the victim is breathing. This takes 3 to 5 seconds.
   - Place your ear and cheek close to the victim's mouth and nose.
   - Look at the chest and abdomen for rising and falling movement.

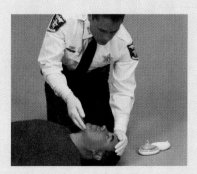

FIGURE 25-11 ◆ Head tilt–chin lift maneuver.

- Listen for air escaping during exhalation.
- Feel for air escaping against your cheek.

8. If no breathing is evident, provide rescue breathing.

Mouth-to-Mouth Method

- If available, put on a mouth shield (Figure 25-9).
- Maintain the open airway by using the head tilt–chin lift maneuver.
- Pinch the victim's nostrils with the index finger and thumb of the hand on the victim's forehead. *Pinching closes the nostrils and prevents resuscitation air from escaping through them.*
- Take a deep breath, and place the mouth, opened widely, around the victim's mouth. Ensure an airtight seal (see Figure 25-13 ◆).
- Give two full breaths (1½ seconds per breath). Pause and take a breath after the first ventilation. *The 1½-second time span closely matches the victim's inspiratory time, allows adequate time to provide good chest expansion, and decreases the possibility of gastric distention. Excessive air volumes and rapid inspiratory flow rates can cause pharyngeal pressures that are great enough to open the esophagus, thus allowing air to enter the stomach.*
- Ensure adequate ventilation by observing the victim's chest rise and fall and by assessing the person's breathing as outlined in step 7.
- If the initial ventilation attempt is unsuccessful, reposition the victim's head and repeat the rescue breathing as above.
- If the victim still cannot be ventilated, proceed to clear the airway of any foreign bodies using the finger sweep, abdominal thrusts, or chest thrusts described earlier (Technique 25-1).

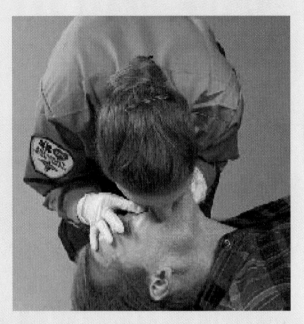

FIGURE 25-13 ◆ Mouth-to-mouth rescue breathing.

Mouth-to-Nose Method

This method can be used when there is an injury to the mouth or jaw or when the client is edentulous (toothless), making it difficult to achieve a tight seal over the mouth.

- Maintain the head tilt–chin lift position.
- Close the victim's mouth by pressing the palm of your hand against the victim's chin. The thumb of the same hand may be used to hold the bottom lip closed.
- Take a deep breath, and seal your lips around the victim's nose. Ensure a tight seal by making contact with the cheeks around the nose.
- Deliver two full breaths of 1½ seconds each, and pause to inhale before delivering the second breath.
- Remove your mouth from the nose, and allow the victim to exhale passively. It may be necessary to separate the victim's lips or to open the mouth for exhaling, since the nasal passages may be obstructed during exhalation.

Mouth-to-Mask Method

- Remove the mask from its case and push out the dome.
- Connect the one-way valve to the mask port.
- Position yourself at the top of the victim's head, and open the airway using the jaw-thrust maneuver.
- Place the bottom rim of the mask between the victim's lower lip and chin. Place the rest of the mask over the face using your thumbs on each

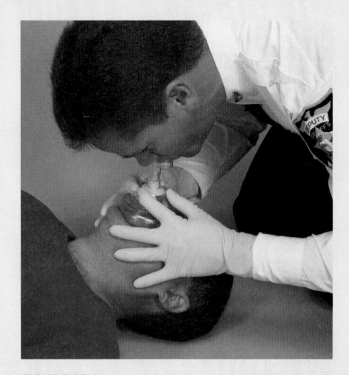

FIGURE 25-14 ◆ Mouth-to-mask rescue breathing.

side of the mask to hold it in place. This keeps the mouth open under the mask (Figure 25-14 ◆).

Hand-Compressible Breathing Bag (Ambu) Method

- Use one hand to secure the mask at the top and bottom and to hold the victim's jaw forward. Use the other hand to squeeze and release the bag (see Figure 25-2 ◆).

9. After delivering two successful breaths, determine the presence of a carotid pulse.

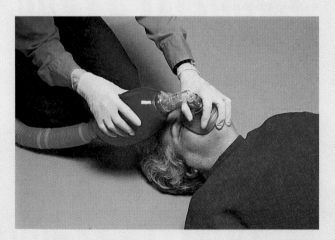

FIGURE 25-15 ◆ Ambu bag-to-mask breathing.

- Take about 5 to 10 seconds for this pulse check. Adequate time is needed since the victim's pulse may be very weak and rapid, irregular, or slow.
- To palpate the carotid artery, first locate the larynx, then slide your fingers alongside it into the groove between the larynx and the neck muscles on the same side you are (see Figure 25-16 ◆). Use gentle pressure. *This avoids compressing the artery. The carotid pulse site is used because it is easy to reach and can often be palpated when more peripheral pulses, such as the radial, are imperceptible.*

10. If the carotid pulse is palpable, but breathing is not restored, repeat rescue breathing.
- Inflate at the rate of 12 breaths per minute (1 breath every 5 seconds).
- Blow slowly but forcibly enough to make the victim's chest rise.
- If chest expansion fails to occur, ensure that the head is hyperextended and the jaw lifted upward, or check again for the presence of obstructive material, fluid, or vomitus.
- After each inflation, move your mouth away from the victim's mouth by turning your head toward the victim's chest. *This movement allows the air to escape when the victim exhales. It also gives the nurse time to inhale and to watch for chest expansion.*

11. Reassess the carotid pulse after 12 inflations (1 minute) and every few minutes thereafter.

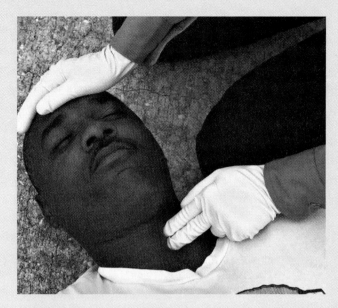

FIGURE 25-16 ◆ Checking the carotid pulse.

- If you cannot locate the pulse, the victim's heart has stopped. Provide cardiac compression (see Procedure 25-3).
- **Document** the date and time of the arrest, including the precipitating events, the duration of breathlessness, and the client's response to the breathing.
- Notify the physician of the relevant events.

AMBULATORY AND COMMUNITY SETTINGS

Respiratory Arrest

- If a client has cardiac or breathing problems, encourage the caregiver to learn cardiopulmonary resuscitation.
- Carry a pocket mask in the home care nursing bag at all times.
- Activate the emergency medical system and contact the physician. In most cases of respiratory arrest the client will need oxygen, respiratory support, and ambulance transport to the emergency room.
- Assist the ambulance crew as needed and provide information about the client's history.

- Once the client is en route to the hospital, call the emergency room and give the report to the nurse in charge, including:
  - A brief health history
  - Medications the client takes at home
  - Findings prior to the respiratory arrest
  - Duration of respiratory arrest and the client's response to resuscitation
  - Vital signs
- Provide emotional support to family members. If the client lives alone, contact family members, as needed.

AGE-RELATED CONSIDERATIONS

Respiratory Arrest

Infant

- Airway obstruction by a foreign body is the most common cause of respiratory arrest in children.

- Acute epiglottitis can lead to upper airway obstruction in children. Symptoms usually occur suddenly and include drooling, difficulty swallowing, and a croaking sound with inspiration.

Respiratory Arrest (continued)

Rescue Breathing

- Place one hand on the infant's forehead and tilt the head back gently. Do not hyperextend the neck as this can cause the soft trachea to collapse (Figure 25-17 ◆).
- The jaw-thrust maneuver can also be used if a neck injury is suspected (Figure 25-18 ◆).
- Assess breathing (Figure 25-19 ◆).
- When performing mouth-to-mouth breathing, cover both the mouth and nose of the infant (Figure 25-20 ◆).
- If an appropriate size mask and bag are available, they may be used (Figure 25-21 ◆). The mask should reach from the bridge of the nose to the chin but not cover the eyes.

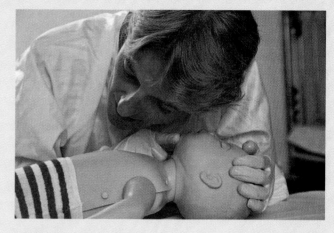

FIGURE 25-19 ◆ Infant assessment of breathing.

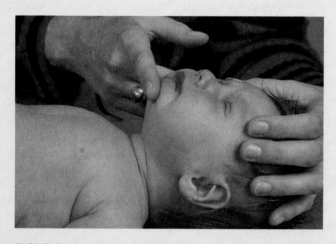

FIGURE 25-17 ◆ Infant head tilt–chin lift maneuver.

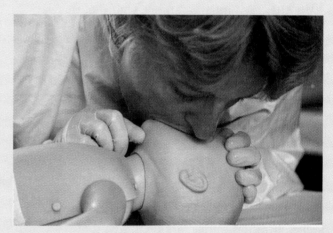

FIGURE 25-20 ◆ Infant mouth-to-mouth rescue breathing.

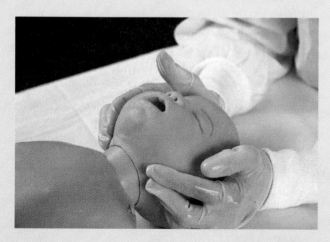

FIGURE 25-18 ◆ Infant jaw-thrust maneuver.

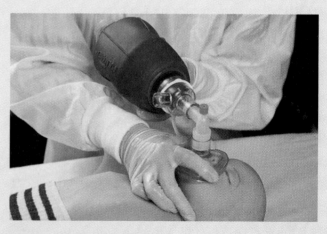

FIGURE 25-21 ◆ Infant Ambu bag-to-mask breathing.

Respiratory Arrest (continued)

- Following two successful breaths, check the brachial pulse (Figure 25-22 ◆).
- If breathing is absent but pulse is present, deliver one breath every 3 seconds.

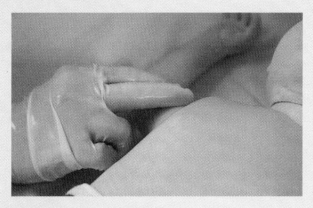

FIGURE 25-22 ◆ Checking the brachial pulse on an infant.

EVALUATION

In a health care setting, a review of the emergency event and the staff's response are commonly performed to see if there are indications for improvement in procedures. Mock arrests may be planned to assist the staff in practicing their skills.

Pulselessness and Cardiac Arrest

Several conditions can cause the heart to develop a lethal arrhythmia or to stop beating. When blood supply to the heart muscle is interrupted, such as occurs during a myocardial infarct (heart attack), the heart may develop ventricular tachycardia or ventricular fibrillation, both rhythms that cannot support life. Other causes of inadequate cardiac contraction that result in insufficient flow of blood throughout the body (pulselessness) include respiratory arrest, electric shock, electrolyte imbalances, and other cardiac diseases.

Nursing Process: Pulselessness and Cardiac Arrest

ASSESSMENT

Pulselessness is generally detected as a result of assessment of an unconscious client. An unresponsive client is first examined for patency of airway (Technique 25-1) and then for breathing (Technique 25-2). If rescue breathing is indicated, the next step is to assess for a pulse.

PLANNING

The nurse should be prepared to provide external cardiac compressions at any time.

Delegation

Although UAP cannot perform all aspects of a hospital code situation, they are trained in CPR and can perform external cardiac compression techniques. If they are the first responders, UAP should initiate the intervention and not wait for a nurse.

IMPLEMENTATION:
TECHNIQUE 25-3 ADMINISTERING EXTERNAL CARDIAC COMPRESSIONS

Equipment

- Standard Precautions supplies including gloves, masks, gowns, and protective eyewear should always be easily accessible.
- Emergency equipment such as an Ambu bag and defibrillation and intubation equipment should be centrally located.
- Pocket face mask with one-way valve or mouth shields, or hand-compressible Ambu bag with mask with one-way valve (see Figure 25-9).
- A hard surface, such as a cardiac board or the floor, on which to place the victim

Performance

1. Determine that the client is unresponsive.
2. If victim does not respond, call a "Code" or follow agency protocol to call for assistance. If another person is present and can cooperate, have that person go get help. Tell the person to return and let you know that help has been called.
3. Observe appropriate infection control procedures as much as possible.
4. Provide for client privacy. If family members are present, the nurse may request they leave for the moment.

5. Position the victim appropriately if not already done.

   • Place the victim supine on a firm surface. *Blood flow to the brain will be inadequate during CPR if the victim's head is positioned higher than the thorax. A hard surface facilitates compression of the heart between the sternum and the hard surface.*

   • If the victim is in bed, place a cardiac board—preferably the full width of the bed—under the back. If necessary, place the victim on the floor.

   • If the victim must be turned, turn the body as a unit while firmly supporting the head and neck so that the head does not roll, twist, or tilt backward or forward. *Turning the person as a unit prevents further injury (if present) to the neck or spine.*

6. Assess airway, breathing, and circulation (see Techniques 25-1 and 25-2).

7. Position the hands on the sternum. Proper hand placement is essential for effective cardiac compression. Position the hands as follows:

   • With the hand nearest the victim's legs, use your middle and index fingers to locate the lower margin of the rib cage.

   • Move the fingers up the rib cage to the notch where the lower ribs meet the sternum. See Figure 25-23 ◆.

   • Place the heel of the other hand (nearest the person's head) along the lower half of the victim's sternum, close to the index finger that is next to the middle finger in the costal–sternal notch. *Proper positioning of the hands during cardiac compression prevents injury to underlying organs and the ribs* (see Figure 25-24 ◆). *Compression directly over the xiphoid process can lacerate the victim's liver.*

   • Then place the first hand on top of the second hand so that both hands are parallel. The fin-

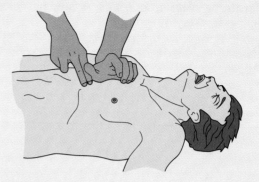

FIGURE 25-24 ◆ Proper positioning of the hands during external cardiac compression.

gers may be extended or interlaced. Compression occurs only on the sternum and through the heels of the hands.

8. Administer cardiac compression.

   • Lock your elbows into position, straighten your arms, and position your shoulders directly over your hands. See Figure 25-25 ◆.

   • For each compression, thrust straight down on the sternum. For an adult of normal size, depress the sternum 3.8 to 5.1 cm (1.5 to 2 in). *The muscle force of both arms is needed for adequate cardiac compression of an adult. The weight of your shoulders and trunk supplies power for compression. Extension of the elbows ensures an adequate and even force throughout compression.*

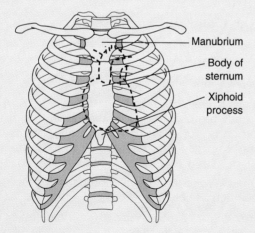

FIGURE 25-23 ◆ The sternum and ribs.

Manubrium

Body of sternum

Xiphoid process

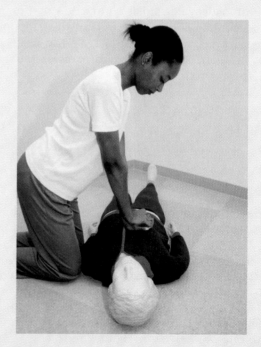

FIGURE 25-25 ◆ Arm and hand position for external cardiac compression.

- Between compressions, completely release the compression pressure. However, do not lift your hands from the chest or change their position. *Releasing the pressure allows the sternum to return to its normal position and allows the heart chambers to fill with blood. Leaving the hands on the chest prevents taking a malposition between compressions and possibly injuring the person.*

- Provide external cardiac compressions at the rate of 80 to 100 per minute. Maintain the rhythm by counting "one and, two and," and so on. *The specified compression rate and rhythm simulate normal heart contractions.*

- Administer 5 or 15 external compressions, depending on the number of rescuers, and coordinate them with rescue breathing. See CPR performed by one rescuer or by two rescuers, next.

Variation: CPR Performed by One Rescuer

- Perform chest compression: 15 external chest compressions at the rate of 80 to 100 per minute. Count "One and, two and, three and . . ." up to 15.

- Open the airway and give two rescue breaths.

- Repeat four complete cycles of 15 compressions and two ventilations.

- Assess the victim's carotid pulse. If there is no pulse, continue with CPR and check for the return of the pulse every few minutes.

Variation: CPR Performed by Two Rescuers

- When help arrives, one rescuer can provide external cardiac compression, and the other can provide pulmonary resuscitation, inflating the lungs once after every five compressions, a 5:1 ratio.

- The first rescuer completes a cycle of 15 compressions and two breaths, and the second rescuer gets into position to give compression.

- The first rescuer assesses the carotid pulse for 5 to 10 seconds and if there is no pulse, gives one breath and then states, "No pulse, continue CPR."

- The second rescuer then:
  a. Provides compression.
  b. Sets the pace, counting aloud, "One and, two and, three and, four and, five and." Pause for the breath to be delivered.

- The first rescuer:
  a. Provides one ventilation after every five chest compressions.
  b. Observes each breath for effectiveness.

c. Assesses the carotid pulse frequently between breaths to assess the effectiveness of cardiac compression.

d. Observes for abdominal (gastric) distention, which can result from overinflation of the lungs. If distention occurs, the rescuer reduces the force of the ventilations, but ensures sufficient ventilation to elevate the ribs.

- When the person compressing the chest becomes fatigued, positions should be changed. To initiate a change in position, the person compressing states, "Change and, two and, three and, four and, five and"; moves to the person's head; and counts the pulse for 5 seconds.

- The person ventilating gives the breath and moves into position to provide compression.

- If there is no pulse, the original person compressing states, "No pulse—start compression," and CPR is continued.

9. When relieved from CPR

- Stand by to assist. Often a person is needed to take notes, document the actions taken, and record the drugs given by the cardiac arrest team.

- Provide emotional support to the victim's family members and any others who may have witnessed the cardiac arrest. This is often a frightening experience for others because it is so sudden and so serious.

10. Terminating CPR

A Rescuer Terminates CPR Only When One of the Following Events Occurs:

- Another trained individual takes over.

- The victim's heartbeat and breathing are reestablished.

- Adjunctive life-support measures are initiated.

- A physician states that the victim is dead and that CPR is to be discontinued.

- The rescuer becomes exhausted, and there is no one to take over.

11. **Document** the date and time of the arrest, including the precipitating events, the duration of respiratory and cardiac arrest and resuscitation efforts, and the client's response.

- Record any advanced cardiac life support interventions such as defibrillation or initiation of intravenous therapy.

- Document vital signs, rhythm strips, any complications, and type of follow-up care. Notify the physician of the relevant events.

AMBULATORY AND COMMUNITY SETTINGS

Administering External Cardiac Compressions

- Always carry a pocket mask in the home care nursing bag.
- Survey the scene for safety hazards, presence of bystanders, and other victims.
- Call for help or have another person call for EMS or 911.
- The person who calls the local EMS must be able to impart all of the following information:
  - Location of the emergency
  - Telephone number from which the call is being made
  - What happened
  - Number of people needing assistance
  - Condition of the victim(s)
  - What aid is being given
  - Any other information that is requested
- If the rescuer is alone, summon help and then perform CPR.
- Have a bystander elevate the lower extremities (optional). This may promote venous return and augment circulation during external cardiac compressions.

- If a second person identifies himself or herself as a trained rescuer, have that person verify that EMS has been notified. If EMS has been notified, the second rescuer offers to help with CPR.
- After activating the emergency response system, continue resuscitation until the ambulance arrives. Be prepared to give report to the ambulance crew and assist them as needed.
- While the client is en route to the hospital, contact the emergency room and report the following to the nurse in charge:
  - A brief health history
  - Medications the client takes at home
  - Findings prior to the cardiopulmonary arrest
  - Duration of the cardiopulmonary arrest and the client's response to resuscitation
- Provide emotional support to family members. If the client is alone, contact family members or neighbors, as needed.
- Advise elderly clients to talk with the physician about preparing an advanced directive for life support measures.
- Encourage caregivers or family members to learn cardiopulmonary resuscitation.

AGE-RELATED CONSIDERATIONS

Administering External Cardiac Compressions

Infant

- Check carefully for airway obstruction in children with **cardiac arrest.** Cardiac arrest in children most often occurs after an initial respiratory arrest.
- To find the position for compressions, place your index finger on the sternum at the nipple line. Place your middle and ring fingers on the sternum next to your index finger, then lift your index finger.
- Compress the chest 1.25 to 2.5 cm (½ to 1 in) straight down using the pads of two fingers. Keep your fingers in the compression position while the other hand remains on the forehead, maintaining the open airway.
- Give compressions at a rate of up to 120 compressions/minute with cycles of five compressions and one breath. See Figure 25-26 ◆.

Child

- Check carefully for airway obstruction in children

with cardiac arrest. Cardiac arrest in children most often occurs after an initial respiratory arrest.

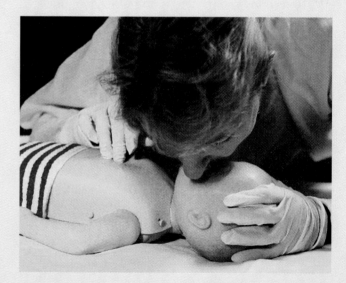

FIGURE 25-26 ◆ CPR on an infant.

- In children, to find the hand position for compressions, run your index and middle fingers up the ribs until you locate the sternal notch. With those two fingers on the lower end of the sternum look at the loction of the index finger and lift fingers off sternum and put the heel of the same hand on the sternum just above the location of the index finger (Figure 25-27 ◆). The other hand should remain on the child's forehead so as to maintain an open airway.
- Use the heel of one hand for compressions, keeping the fingers off the chest. Compression depth is 2.5 to 3.8 cm (1 to 1½ in). Never lift the hand off the chest.
- CPR for a child is given at the following rate: 100 compressions/min with cycles of five compressions and one breath.

Elders

- Older clients are most likely to be injured by incorrect placement of the rescuer's hands. The sternum becomes more brittle with aging.

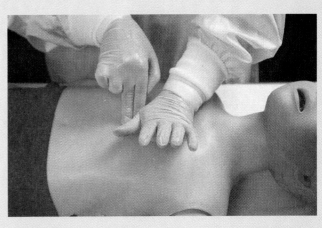

FIGURE 25-27 ◆ Locating the site for chest compressions on a child.

- The older client may have an advanced directive, or living will, expressing his wishes for life support.

EVALUATION

In a health care setting, a review of the emergency event and the staff's response are commonly performed to see if there are indications for improvement in procedures. Mock arrests may be planned to assist the staff in practicing their skills.

Automated External Defibrillation

The most common arrhythmia in sudden cardiac arrest is **ventricular fibrillation (VF)**, a quivering, nonfunctional beat, which, if untreated, coverts to **asystole** (no heartbeat). The best treatment for VF is electric shock defibrillation. Since the early 1990s it has become clear that, in both the hospital and community settings, early defibrillation provides the greatest chance for survival and can be implemented easily. The **automated external defibrillator (AED)** is a relatively small, battery-operated device that senses the cardiac rhythm through two adhesive pads (Figure 25-28 ◆ and 25-29 ◆). If the AED detects a rhythm that should be treated with electric shock, it can either deliver that shock automatically or indicate to the operator that a shock is advised. The latter is preferred because it allows the operator to determine that delivery of the shock is safe at that moment.

Nursing Process: Automated External Defibrillation

ASSESSMENT

Determine that the client is in cardiac arrest.

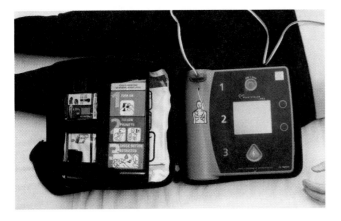

FIGURE 25-28 ◆ An automated external defibrillator (AED).

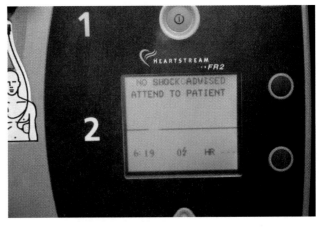

FIGURE 25-29 ◆ An AED readout.

PLANNING

An AED should be available on those nursing units where the full "crash cart" with defibrillator is not available.

Delegation

Any person who has been trained in its use can apply and activate the AED.

IMPLEMENTATION:

TECHNIQUE 25-4 ADMINISTERING AUTOMATED EXTERNAL DEFIBRILLATION

Equipment

- AED with all components including the automatic override key, event documentation module or tape, electrodes and cables, and charged battery pack. Brands and models differ in their features.

Performance

1. Follow steps 1 through 9 of Technique 25-3. Traditional CPR must be performed until the AED can be attached.

2. Attached the AED.
   - Turn on the power of the AED.
   - Apply the electrode pads to dry skin: one in the upper right chest near the clavicle and the other in the lower left chest, below the nipple (Figure 25-30 ◆).

3. Initiate rhythm analysis. In most models, this also charges the AED.

4. Defibrillate as indicated.
   - Before delivering the shock, state loudly "Clear" and ensure that no one is touching the client.
   - Press the shock button and observe for the brief contraction of the client's muscles that indicates the shock has been delivered.
   - Immediately press the analyze button again.
   - Repeat the shock and analyze sequence for a total of three shocks if the AED indicates the rhythm is treatable.

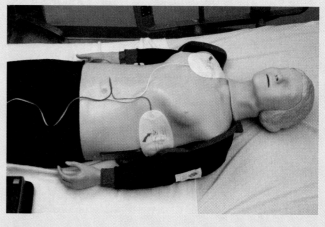

FIGURE 25-30 ◆ Placement of AED electrode pads.

5. Check the carotid pulse. If the pulse is present and breathing is absent, perform rescue breathing. If there is no pulse, perform CPR for one minute then recheck the carotid pulse.

6. If there is no pulse after one minute of CPR, repeat steps 3, 4, and 5.

7. Continue the sequence of CPR, pulse checks, and defibrillation until the AED specifies that no shock is indicated, the client converts to a functional rhythm (pulse is felt), or the code team takes over.

8. Document the events as in Technique 25-3 above including data provided by the AED. Attach electrocardiogram strips or other records made by the AED.

AMBULATORY AND COMMUNITY SETTINGS

Automated External Defibrillation

- Training in the use of AEDs should be conducted in all health care facilities including clinics, long-term care facilities, and urgent care centers.
- AEDs can be used by trained lay rescuers.
- Use of the AED takes priority over CPR. The sequence of events is:

- Determine unresponsiveness, absence of breathing, and pulse.
- Activate the emergency medical services (EMS) notification system (e.g., call 911).
- Start CPR until the AED can be attached.
- Defibrillate if indicated.

Automated External Defibrillation

Infant

• AED is not recommended. VF is rare in infants and children, and the AED is usually not equipped to deliver the lower shock setting that would be needed.

Child

• Follow the steps of adult AED use in children over age 8 or weighing at least 25 kg (55 lb).

EVALUATION

In a health care setting, a review of the emergency event and the staff's response is commonly performed to see if there are indications for improvement in procedures. Review of the use of the AED may be indicated. Mock arrests may be planned to assist the staff in practicing their skills.

Chapter Summary

TERMINOLOGY

asphyxiation
asystole
automated external defibrillator
  (AED)
cardiac arrest

cardiopulmonary resuscitation
  (CPR)
Code Blue
Do Not Resuscitate (DNR)
Heimlich maneuver

No Code Blue
obstructed airway
respiratory arrest
ventricular fibrillation (VF)

FORMING CLINICAL JUDGMENTS

Consider This:

1. You answer a patient's call light and find the adult client coughing forcefully with the lunch tray thrown to the floor. On inspiration, there is an audible wheeze, the client's face is ruddy, and the eyes are wide. You ask: "Can you speak?" The client shakes the head "no" and continues to cough. When you approach the client and start to put your arms around the chest to attempt a Heimlich maneuver, the client waves the arms broadly, pushing you away. What should you do next?

2. You are administering medication to a client who suddenly has a grand mal seizure. At the end of the seizure, the client does not regain consciousness. Would you *first* (a) call a Code, (b) begin mouth-to-mouth resuscitation, (c) begin CPR, or (d) do something different?

3. You find a client slumped in the hospital bedside chair. The client is unresponsive to verbal stimuli and touch and is not breathing. After calling a Code, establishing an open airway, and giving two breaths, you are unable to feel a carotid pulse. Describe your next steps.

4. After applying an AED and delivering three shocks, a pulse check indicates that the heart has not resumed a normal rhythm. What are the steps you should take next?

Related Research

Marik, P. E., & Craft, M. (1997). An outcomes analysis of in-hospital cardiopulmonary resuscitation: The futility rationale for do not resuscitate orders. *Journal of Critical Care, 12,* 142–146.

References

Chandra, N. C., & Hazinski, M. F. (eds.). (1997). *Basic life support for healthcare providers.* Dallas, TX: American Heart Association.

Lezon, K. (1998). Code blue: Defibrillate. *Nursing, 28*(4), 58–60.

Little, C. (2000). Manual ventilation: Find out how to perform rescue breathing with a manual resuscitator. *Nursing, 30*(3), 50–51.

Meyers, T. A., Eichhorn, D. J., Guzzetta, C. E., Clark, A. P., Klein, J. D., Taliaferro, E., & Calvin, A. (2000). Family presence during invasive procedures and resuscitation: The experience of family members, nurses, and physicians. *American Journal of Nursing, 100*(2), 32–43.

Oliver, J. E., & Fruth, R. (2000). Family presence during resuscitation. *American Journal of Nursing, 100*(5 Suppl.), 15–18, 47–50.

Turjanica, M. A. (1999). Anatomy of a code: How do you feel at the start of a code blue? *Nursing Management, 30*(11), 44–50.

Walker, W. M. (1999). Do relatives have a right to witness resuscitation? *Journal of Clinical Nursing, 8*(6), 625–630.

Chapter 26

Administering Oral/Enteral Medications

Techniques

OBJECTIVES

- Identify various types of drug preparations.
- Describe legal aspects of administering medications.
- Compare and contrast the advantages and disadvantages of the oral and enteral routes of medication administration.
- Identify the essential parts of a medication order.
- Give examples of various types of medication orders.
- List six essential steps to follow when administering medication.
- State the five "rights" of medication administration.
- Administer oral medications safely.
- Outline steps required for nasogastric and gastrostomy tube medication administration.

A medication is a substance administered for the diagnosis, cure, treatment, mitigation (relief), or prevention of disease. In the health care context, the words *medication* and *drug* are generally used interchangeably. The term **drug** also has the connotation of an illicitly obtained substance such as heroin, cocaine, or amphetamines. Medications have been known and used since antiquity. Crude drugs, such as opium, castor oil, and vinegar, were used in ancient times. Over the centuries, the number of drugs available has increased greatly and knowledge about these drugs has become correspondingly more accurate and detailed.

In the United States and Canada, medications are usually dispensed on the order of physicians and dentists. In some states, specially qualified nurse practitioners and physicians' assistants may prescribe drugs. The written direction for the preparation and administration of a drug is called a **prescription.** One drug can have as many as four kinds of names: its generic name, official name, chemical name, and trademark or brand name. The **generic name** is given before a drug becomes official. The **official name** is the name under which it is listed in one of the official publications (e.g., the *United States Pharmacopeia*). The **chemical name** is the name by which a chemist knows it; this name describes the constituents of the drug precisely. The **trademark** or **brand name** is the name given by the drug manufacturer. Because several companies may manufacture one drug, it can have several trade names; for example, the drug ibuprofen (official name) is known by the trade names Advil and Motrin. Medications are often available in a variety of forms (see Table 26-1).

Legal Aspects of Drug Administration

The administration of drugs in both the United States and Canada is controlled by law. See Table 26-2 for a

TABLE 26-1	TYPES OF DRUG PREPARATIONS		
Type	**Description**	**Type**	**Description**
Aerosol spray or foam	A liquid, powder, or foam deposited in a thin layer on the skin by air pressure	Paste	A preparation like an ointment, but thicker and stiff, that penetrates the skin less than an ointment
Aqueous solution	One or more drugs dissolved in water	Pill	One or more drugs mixed with a cohesive material, in oval, round, or flattened shapes
Aqueous suspension	One or more drugs finely divided in a liquid such as water	Powder	A finely ground drug or drugs; some are used internally, others externally
Caplet	A solid form, shaped like a capsule, coated and easily swallowed	Suppository	One or several drugs mixed with a firm base such as gelatin and shaped for insertion into the body (e.g., the rectum); the base dissolves gradually at body temperature, releasing the drug
Capsule	A gelatinous container to hold a drug in powder, liquid, or oil form		
Cream	A nongreasy, semisolid preparation used on the skin		
Elixir	A sweetened and aromatic solution of alcohol used as a vehicle for medicinal agents	Syrup	An aqueous solution of sugar often used to disguise unpleasant-tasting drugs
Extract	A concentrated form of a drug made from vegetables or animals	Tablet	A powdered drug compressed into a hard small disc; some are readily broken along a scored line; others are enteric coated to prevent them from dissolving in the stomach
Gel or jelly	A clear or translucent semisolid that liquefies when applied to the skin		
Liniment	A medication mixed with alcohol, oil, or soapy emollient and applied to the skin	Tincture	An alcoholic or water-and-alcohol solution prepared from drugs derived from plants
Lotion	A medication in a liquid suspension applied to the skin	Transdermal patch	A semipermeable membrane shaped in the form of a disc or patch that contains a drug to be absorbed through the skin over a long period of time
Lozenge (troche)	A flat, round, or oval preparation that dissolves and releases a drug when held in the mouth		
Ointment (salve, unction)	A semisolid preparation of one or more drugs used for application to the skin and mucous membrane		

From *Fundamentals of nursing: Concepts, process, and practice,* 6th ed., by B. Kozier, G. Erb, A. Berman, & K. Burke, 2000, Upper Saddle River, NJ: Prentice Hall Health.

TABLE 26-2	UNITED STATES DRUG LEGISLATION	
Legislation	**Content**	
Food, Drug, and Cosmetic Act (1938)	Implemented by Food and Drug Administration (FDA); requires that labels be accurate and that all drugs be tested for harmful effects.	
Durkham–Humphrey Amendment (1952)	Clearly differentiates drugs that can be sold only with a prescription, those that can be sold without a prescription, and those that should not be refilled without a new prescription.	
Kefauver–Harris Amendment (1962)	Requires proof of safety and efficacy of a drug for approval.	
Comprehensive Drug Abuse Prevention and Control Act (1970) (Controlled Substances Act)	Categorizes controlled substances and limits how often a prescription can be filled; established government-funded programs to prevent and treat drug dependence.	

From *Fundamentals of nursing: Concepts, process, and practice*, 6th ed., by B. Kozier, G. Erb, A. Berman, & K. Burke, 2000, Upper Saddle River, NJ: Prentice Hall Health.

summary of U.S. drug legislation. Table 26-3 provides a summary of Canadian drug legislation.

Nurses need to (1) know how nursing practice acts in their areas define and limit their functions and (2) recognize the limits of their own knowledge and skill. To function beyond the limits of nursing practice acts or one's ability is to endanger clients' lives and expose oneself to malpractice lawsuits. Under the law, nurses are responsible for their own actions regardless of whether there is a written order. If a physician writes an incorrect order (e.g., Demerol 500 mg instead of Demerol 50 mg), *a nurse who administers the written incorrect dosage is responsible for the error as well as the physician*. Therefore, nurses must question any order that appears unreasonable and refuse to give the medication until the order is clarified.

Another aspect of nursing practice governed by law is the use of controlled substances. In hospitals, controlled substances are kept in a locked drawer, cupboard, medication cart, or computer-controlled dispensing system. Agencies may have special inventory forms for recording the use of controlled substances. The information required usually includes the name of the client, the date and time of administration, the name of the drug, the dosage, and the signature of the person who prepared and gave the drug. The name of the physician who ordered the drug may also be part of the record. Before removing a controlled substance, the nurse verifies the number actually available to the number indicated on the narcotic or controlled substance inventory record (Figure 26-1 ◆). If the number is not the same, the nurse must investigate and correct the discrepancy before proceeding.

Included on the record are the controlled substances wasted during preparation. When a portion or all of a controlled substance dose is discarded, the nurse must ask a second nurse to witness the discarding. Both nurses must sign the control inventory form.

In most agencies, counts of controlled substances are taken at the end of each shift. The count total must tally with the total at the end of the last shift minus the number used. If the totals do not tally and the discrepancy cannot be resolved, it must be reported immediately to the nurse manager, nursing supervisor, and pharmacy according to agency policy. In facilities that use a computerized dispensing system, manual counts are not required, because the dispensing system runs a continuous count; however, discrepancies must still be accounted for.

Routes of Administration

Pharmaceutical preparations are generally designed for one or two specific routes of administration. The

TABLE 26-3	CANADIAN DRUG LEGISLATION	
Legislation	**Content**	
Proprietary or Patent Medicine Act (1908)	Protects the public against unsafe and ineffective over-the-counter drugs.	
Canada Food and Drugs Act (1953)	Prohibits advertising any food, drug, cosmetic, or device as a cure for certain specified diseases. Sets standards for manufacture, distribution, and sale of all drugs, with the exception of narcotics.	
Canadian Narcotic Control Act (1961)	Allows only authorized people to possess narcotics. Specifies records about narcotics that must be kept.	

From *Fundamentals of nursing: Concepts, process, and practice*, 6th ed., by B. Kozier, G. Erb, A. Berman, & K. Burke, 2000, Upper Saddle River, NJ: Prentice Hall Health.

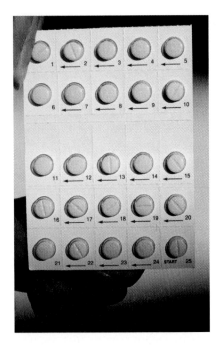

FIGURE 26-1 ◆ Some narcotics are kept in specially designed packages or plastic containers that are sectioned and numbered.

route of administration should be indicated when the drug is ordered. When administering a drug, the nurse should ensure that the pharmaceutical preparation is appropriate for the route specified. Numerous routes exist for medication administration. This chapter describes the oral route and subsequent chapters discuss other routes.

Oral

Oral administration is the most common, least expensive, and most convenient route for most clients. In oral administration, the drug is swallowed. Because the skin is not broken as it is for an injection, oral administration is also a safe method.

The major disadvantages are possible unpleasant taste of the drugs, irritation of the gastric mucosa, irregular absorption from the gastrointestinal tract, slow absorption, and in some cases, harm to the client's teeth.

Sublingual

In **sublingual** administration, a drug is placed under the tongue, where it dissolves (Figure 26-2 ◆). In a relatively short time, the drug is largely absorbed into the blood vessels on the underside of the tongue. The medications should not be swallowed. Nitroglycerin is one example of a drug commonly given in this manner.

Buccal

Buccal means "pertaining to the cheek." In buccal administration, a medication (e.g., a tablet) is held in

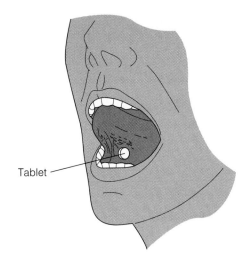

FIGURE 26-2 ◆ Sublingual administration of a tablet.

the mouth against the mucous membranes of the cheek until the drug dissolves (Figure 26-3 ◆). The drug may act locally on the mucous membranes of the mouth or systemically when it is swallowed in the saliva.

Enteral

Oral medications can also be administered into feeding or enteral tubes. See Technique 26-2.

Medication Orders

A physician usually determines the client's medication needs and orders medications, although in some settings nurse practitioners and physician's assistants now order some drugs. Each health agency will have its own policies. Typically, the order is written, although telephone and verbal orders are acceptable in a number of agencies. Nursing students must know

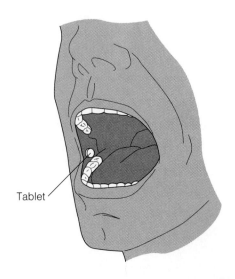

FIGURE 26-3 ◆ Buccal administration of a tablet.

the agency policies about medication orders. In some hospitals, for example, only licensed nurses are permitted to accept telephone and verbal orders.

Policies about physicians' orders vary considerably from agency to agency. For example, a client's orders are frequently automatically canceled after surgery or an examination involving an anesthetic agent. New orders must then be written. Most agencies also have lists of abbreviations officially accepted for use in the agency. Both nurses and physicians may need to refer to these lists if they have been working in a different agency. These abbreviations can be used on legal documents, such as clients' chart (Table 26-4).

Types of Medication Orders

Four common medication orders are the stat order, the single order, the standing order, and the PRN order.

TABLE 26-4		COMMON ABBREVIATIONS USED IN MEDICATION ORDERS			
Abbreviation	**Explanation**	**Example of Administration Time**	**Abbreviation**	**Explanation**	**Example of Administration Time**
ac	before meals	0700, 1100, and 1700 hours	po or PO	by mouth	
			prn	when needed	
ad lib	freely, as desired		q	every	
aq	water		qAM (om)	every morning	1000 hours
bid	twice a day	0900 and 2100 hours	qh (q1h)	every hour	
c̄	with		q2h	every 2 hours	0800, 1000, 1200 hours, and so on
cap	capsule				
dil	dissolve, dilute		q3h	every 3 hours	0900, 1200, 1500 hours, and so on
ʒ	dram				
elix	elixir		q4h	every 4 hours	1000, 1400, 1800 hours, and so on
g, gm, or Gm	gram				
gr	grain		q6h	every 6 hours	0600, 1200, 1800, 2400 hours
gtt	drop				
h	an hour		qid	four times a day	1000, 1400, 1800, 2200 hours
hs	at bedtime (hour of sleep)		qod	every other day	0900 hours on odd dates
ID	intradermal		qs	sufficient quantity	
IM	intramuscular		rept	may be repeated	
IV	intravenous		Rx	take	
kg or Kg	kilogram		s̄	without	
l or L	liter		sc, Sc, or SQ	subcutaneous	
M or m	mix		Sig or S	label	
mcg or μg	microgram		sos	if it is needed	
mg or mgm	milligram		ss or s̄s̄	one half	
no.	number		stat	at once	
non rep	do not repeat		sup or supp	suppository	
OD	right eye		susp	suspension	
OS	left eye		tab	tablet	
OU	both eyes		tid	three times a day	1000, 1400, and 1800 hours
ʒ	ounce				
pc	after meals	0900, 1300, and 1900 hours	Tr or tinct	tincture	

From *Fundamentals of nursing: Concepts, process, and practice*, 6th ed., by B. Kozier, G. Erb, A. Berman, & K. Burke, 2000, Upper Saddle River, NJ: Prentice Hall Health.

1. A **stat order** indicates that the medication is to be given immediately and only once (e.g., Demerol 100 mg IM stat).

2. The **single order** or "one-time order" is for medication to be given once at a specified time (e.g., Seconal 100 mg hs before surgery).

3. The **standing order** may or may not have a termination date. A standing order may be carried out indefinitely (e.g., multiple vitamins daily) until an order is written to cancel it or it may be carried out for a specified number of days (e.g., Demerol 100 mg IM q4h × 5 days). In some agencies, standing orders are automatically canceled after a specified number of days and must be reordered.

4. A **PRN order** or "as needed order" permits the nurse to give a medication when, in the nurse's judgment, the client requires it (e.g., Amphojel 15 mL PRN). The nurse must use good judgment about when the medication is needed and when it can be safely administered.

Essential Parts of a Drug Order

The drug order has seven essential parts as listed in Box 26-1. In addition, unless it is a standing order, it should state the number of doses or the number of days the drug is to be administered.

The *client's full name,* that is, the first and last names and middle initial or name, should always be used to avoid confusion between two clients who have the same last names. In some agencies, the client's identification number and physician's name are put on the order as further identification. Some hospitals imprint the client's name, identification number, and room number on all forms, while some agencies use stickers with similar client information.

In addition to *the day, the month, and the year* the order was written, some agencies also require that the *time of day* be written. Writing the time of day on the order can eliminate errors when nursing shifts change and makes

---

Box 26-1 *Essential Parts of a Drug Order*

- Full name of the client
- Date and time the order is written
- Name of the drug to be administered
- Dosage of the drug
- Route of administration
- Frequency of administration
- Signature of the person writing the order

From *Fundamentals of nursing: Concepts, process, and practice,* 6th ed., by B. Kozier, G. Erb, A. Berman, & K. Burke, 2000, Upper Saddle River, NJ: Prentice Hall Health.

---

clear when certain orders automatically terminate. For example, in some settings, narcotics can be ordered only for 48 hours after surgery. Therefore, a drug that is ordered at 1600 hours February 1, 2002, is automatically canceled at 1600 hours February 3, 2002. Many health agencies use the 24-hour clock, which eliminates confusion between morning and afternoon times. Time with the 24-hour clock starts at midnight, which is 0000 hours.

The *name of the drug to be administered* must be clearly written. In some settings, only generic names are permitted; however, trade names are widely used in hospitals and health agencies.

The *dosage of the drug* includes the amount, the times or frequency of administration, and in many instances the strength; for example, tetracycline *250 mg* (the amount) *four times a day* (frequency); hydrochloric acid *10%* (strength) *5 mL* (amount) *three times a day with meals* (time and frequency). Dosages can be written in apothecaries' or metric systems.

Also included in the order is the *route of administration* of the drug. This part of the order, like other parts, is frequently abbreviated. See Table 26-4 for abbreviations of routes of administration. It is not unusual for a drug to have several possible routes of administration; therefore, it is important that the *route* be included in the order.

The *signature* of the ordering physician or nurse makes the drug order a legal request. *An unsigned order has no validity,* and the ordering physician or nurse needs to be notified if the order is unsigned.

Communicating a Medication Order

A drug order is written on the client's chart by a physician or by a nurse receiving a telephone or verbal order from a physician. Most acute care agencies have a specified time frame (e.g., 24 or 48 hours) in which the physician issuing the telephone or verbal order must cosign the order written by the nurse. A nurse or clerk copies the medication order to a Kardex or **medication administration record (MAR).** Increasingly, nurses are being provided with computer printouts of a client's medications instead of copying the physician's order. This method avoids errors of copying and saves nursing time.

Medication administration records (Figure 26-4 ◆) vary in form, but all include the client's name, room number, and bed number; drug name and dose; and times and method of administration. In some agencies, the date the order was prescribed and the date the order expires are also included.

The nurse must always question the physician about any order that is ambiguous, unusual (e.g., an abnormally high dosage of a medication), or contraindicated by the client's condition. When the nurse judges a physician-ordered medication inappropriate, the following actions are *required:*

MEDICATION ADMINISTRATION RECORD

PRN#:
MRN#:   AGE:
ADM: 08-04-01   SEX:
DOB: HT:
DR.   HT:

VERIFIED BY: _____ DATE: _____

DIAGNOSIS: *#ALOC
            *#PNEUMONIA

ALLERGIES: NO KNOWN DRUG ALLERGIES

GENERATED: 08-07-01   07:32am
FOR PERIOD: 08-07-01 08:00
THROUGH: 08-08-01 07:59

START	STOP	MEDICATION/I.V./IVPB/IRRIGATION		0800-1559	1600-2359	0000-0759
08-06 17	09-05 16	FERROUS SULFATE 300MG=5ML TWICE A DAY PO (FES04)	(973539)	09	17	
08-06 17	09-05 16	DOCUSATE SODIUM 100MG=1UDCUP TWICE A DAY PO (COLACE) 100MG/30ML UD HOLD FOR LOOSE STOOL	(973532)	09	17	
08-05 09	09-04 08	ASCORBIC ACID 500MG=1TAB TWICE A DAY PO (VITAMIN C) 500MG TAB	(972096)	09	17	
08-05 09	09-04 08	LEVOTHYROXINE 0.05MG=1TABDAILY PO (SYNTHROID) 0.05MG TAB	(972095)	09		
08-05 09	09-04 08	ASPIRIN 325MG=1 TAB DAILY PO (ASPIRIN) 325MG TAB *W/FOOD TO AVOID GI UPSET	(972094)	09		
08-04 23	08-14 22	CEFUROXIME ADDV. 1.500GM=1VIAL EVERY 8 HOUS IV (KEFUROX) 1.5GM ADDV *ATTACH TO D5W 50ML ADDV BAG *ACTIVATE BEFORE UNFUSION* * INFUSE OVER 30 MINS*	(971776)	14	22	06
		——— PRN ORDERS ———				
08-04 23	09-03 22	ACETAMINOPHEN 650MG=1SUPP EVERY 4 HOURS AS NEEDED PR (TYLENOL) 650MG SUPP	(971779)			

INITIALS	SIGNATURE	SHIFT	INITIALS	SIGNATURE	SHIFT	INITIALS	SIGNATURE	SHIFT

SITE CODES:
A. Right Upper Outer Gluteus
B. Left Upper Outer Quadrant Gluteus
C. Right Outer Aspect Arm
D. Left Outer Aspect Arm
E. Right Ventrogluteal
F. Left Ventrogluteal
G. Abdomen
H. Right Thigh
J. Left Thigh

FIGURE 26-4 ◆ Sample medication administration record (MAR).

- Contact the physician and discuss the rationale for believing the medication or dosage to be inappropriate.

- Document in notes the following: when the physician was notified, what information was conveyed to the physician, and how the physician responded.

- If the physician cannot be reached, document all attempts to contact the physician and the reason for withholding the medication.
- If someone else gives the medication, document assessments pertaining to the client's condition before and after the medication.
- If an incident report is indicated, clearly document all factual information.

Systems of Measurement

Three systems of measurement are used in North America: the metric system, the apothecaries' system, and the household system, which is similar to the apothecaries' system.

Metric System

The metric system, devised by the French in the latter part of the eighteenth century, is the system prescribed by law in most European countries and Canada. The metric system is logically organized into units of 10; it is a decimal system. Basic units can be multiplied or divided by 10 to form secondary units. Multiples are calculated by moving the decimal point to the right, and divisions by moving the decimal point to the left.

Basic units of measurement are the meter, the liter, and the gram. Prefixes derived from Latin designate subdivisions of the basic unit: *deci* (1/10 or 0.1), *centi* (1/100 or 0.01), and *milli* (1/1000 or 0.001). Multiples of the basic unit are designated by prefixes derived from Greek: *deka* (10), *hecto* (100), and *kilo* (1,000). Only the measurements of volume (the liter) and weight (the gram) are discussed in this chapter. These are the measures used in medication administration. In nursing practice, the kilogram (kg) is the only multiple of the gram used, and the milligram (mg) and microgram (mcg or μg) are subdivisions. Fractional parts of the liter are usually expressed in milliliters (mL), for example, 600 mL; multiples of the liter are usually expressed as liters or milliliters, for example, 2.5 liters or 2,500 mL. Another volume measurement frequently used in practice is the cubic centimeter (cc). It is equivalent to 1 milliliter.

Apothecaries' System

The apothecaries' system, older than the metric system, was brought to the United States from England during America's colonial period. The basic unit of weight in the apothecaries' system is the *grain (gr)*, likened to a grain of wheat, and the basic unit of volume is the **minim**, a volume of water equal in weight to a grain of wheat. The word *minim* means "the least." In ascending order, the other units of weight

are the *scruple,* the *dram,* the *ounce,* and the *pound.* Today, the scruple (scr) is seldom used. The units of volume are, in ascending order, the *fluid dram, fluid ounce, pint, quart,* and *gallon.*

Quantities in the apothecaries' system are often expressed by lowercase Roman numerals, particularly when the unit of measure is abbreviated. The Roman numeral follows rather than precedes the unit of measure. For example, a fluid ounce is abbreviated as ℥. Two fluid ounces are written as ℥ ii, and 4 fluid ounces are written as ℥ iv. Quantities less than 1 are expressed as a fraction, for example, gr ⅙.

Household System

Household measures may be used when more accurate systems of measure are not required. Included in household measures are drops, teaspoons, tablespoons, cups, and glasses. Although pints and quarts are often found in the home, they are defined as apothecaries' measures.

Converting Units of Weight and Measure

When preparing client medications, a nurse may need to convert weights or volumes from one system to another. As an example, the pharmacy may dispense milligrams or grams of chloral hydrate, yet the nurse must administer an order that reads "chloral hydrate gr viiss." To prepare the correct dose, the nurse must convert from the apothecaries' to the metric system. To give clients a useful, realistic measure for home use, the nurse may have to convert from the apothecaries' or metric system to the household system. All conversions are approximate, that is, not totally precise (see Tables 26-5 and 26-6).

TABLE 26-5	APPROXIMATE VOLUME EQUIVALENTS: METRIC, APOTHECARIES', AND HOUSEHOLD SYSTEMS		

Metric		Apothecaries'	Household
1 mL	=	15 minims (min or m)	= 15 drops (gtt)
15 mL	=	4 fluid drams (℥)	= 1 tablespoon (Tbsp)
30 mL	=	1 fluid ounce (℥)	= same
500 mL	=	1 pint (pt)	= same
1,000 mL	=	1 quart (qt)	= same
4,000 mL	=	1 gallon (gal)	= same

From *Fundamentals of nursing: Concepts, process, and practice,* 6th ed., by B. Kozier, G. Erb, A. Berman, & K. Burke, 2000, Upper Saddle River, NJ: Prentice Hall Health.

TABLE 26-6	APPROXIMATE WEIGHT EQUIVALENTS: METRIC AND APOTHECARIES' SYSTEMS	
Metric		**Apothecaries'**
1 mg	=	1/60 grain
60 mg	=	1 grain
1 g	=	15 grains
4 g	=	1 dram
30 g	=	1 ounce
500 g	=	1.1 pound (lb)
1,000 g (1 kg)	=	2.2 lb

Administering Medications Safely

The nurse should always assess a client's health status and obtain a medication history prior to giving *any* medication. The extent of the assessment depends on the client's illness or current condition, the intended drug, and the route of administration. For example, the nurse assesses a dyspneic client's respirations carefully before administering any medication that might affect breathing. It is important to determine whether the route of administration is suitable. For example, a client who is nauseated may not be able to keep down a drug taken orally. In general, the nurse assesses the client *prior* to administering any medication to obtain baseline data by which to evaluate the effectiveness of the medication.

The **medication history** includes information about the drugs the client is taking currently or has taken recently. This includes prescription drugs; over-the-counter drugs such as antacids, alcohol, and tobacco; and illegal drugs such as marijuana and cocaine. Sometimes, an incompatibility with one or more of these drugs affects the choice of a new medication.

An important part of the history is clients' knowledge of their drug allergies. Some clients can tell a nurse, "I am allergic to penicillin, adhesive tape, and curry." Other clients may not be sure about allergic reactions. An illness occurring after a drug was taken may not be identified as an allergy, but the client may associate the drug with an illness or unusual reaction. The client's physician can often give information about allergies. During the history, the nurse tries to elicit information about drug dependencies. How often drugs are taken and the client's perceived need for them are measures of dependence.

Also included in the history are the client's normal eating habits. Sometimes, the medication schedule needs to be coordinated with mealtimes or the ingestion of foods. Where a medication must be taken with food on a specified schedule, clients can often adjust their mealtime or have a snack (e.g., with a bedtime medication). In addition, certain foods are incompatible with certain medications; for example, milk is incompatible with tetracycline.

Any problems the client may have in self-administering a medication must also be identified. A client with poor eyesight, for example, may require special labels for the medication container; elderly clients with unsteady hands may not be able to hold a syringe to inject themselves or another person.

Clinical guidelines for administering medications are given in Box 26-2.

Medication Dispensing Systems

Medical facilities vary in their medication dispensing systems. The systems can include:

- *Medication cart.* The medication cart is on wheels allowing the nurse to move the cart to outside the client's room. The cart contains small numbered drawers that correlate to the room numbers on the nursing unit. The small drawer is labeled with the name of the client currently in that room and holds the client's medications for the shift or 24 hours (Figure 26-5 ◆). The medication is usually in unit-dose packaging in which the drug is packaged individually and labeled with the drug name, dose, and expiration date (Figure 26-6 ◆). Controlled substances are not kept in the client's individual drawer but in a larger locked drawer in the cart. The cart may also include a supply drawer that contains client-labeled bulk containers, such as Metamucil, that are too large for the small individual drawer. The MAR is usually located in a binder on top of the medication cart. The nurse carries a key for the medication cart, as it must be kept locked when not in use (Figure 26-7 ◆).

- *Medication cabinet.* Some facilities have a locked cabinet in the client's room. This cabinet holds the client's unit-dose medications and MAR. Controlled substances are not kept in this cabinet but at another location on the nursing unit. The nurse carries a key for opening the client's medication cabinet, as it must be locked when not in use.

- *Medication room.* Depending on the facility, a medication room may be used for a variety of purposes. For example, the medication carts, when not in use, may be placed in this room. The medication room may also be the central location for stock medications, controlled medications, and/or drugs used for emergencies. The medication room is often kept locked. Check agency policy.

- *Computerized medication access system.* This system (Figure 26-8 ◆) automates the distribution, manage-

Box 26-2 *Clinical Guidelines: Administering Medications*

- Nurses who administer medications are responsible for their own actions. Question any order that is illegible or that you consider incorrect. Call the person who prescribed the medication for clarification.
- Be knowledgeable about the medications you administer. You need to know why the client is receiving the medication. Look up the necessary information if you are not familiar with the medication.
- Federal laws govern the use of narcotics and barbiturates. Keep these medications in a locked place.
- Use only medications that are in a clearly labeled container.
- Do not use liquid medications that are cloudy or have changed color.
- Calculate drug doses accurately. If you are uncertain, ask another nurse to double check your calculations.
- Administer only medications personally prepared.
- Before administering a medication, identify the client correctly using the appropriate means of identifica-

tion, such as checking the identification bracelet, asking clients to state their name, or both.
- Do not leave medications at the bedside, with certain exceptions (e.g., nitroglycerin, cough syrup). Check agency policy.
- If a client vomits after taking an oral medication, report this to the nurse in charge, or the physician, or both.
- Take special precautions when administering certain medications, for example, have another nurse check the dosages of anticoagulants, insulin, and certain IV preparations.
- Most hospital policies require new orders from the physician for the client's postsurgery care.
- When a medication is omitted for any reason, record the fact together with the reason.
- When a medication error is made, report it immediately to the nurse in charge, the physician, or both.

ment, and control of medications. Similar to automated teller machines (ATMs), the nurse uses a password to access the system and select the medication (Figure 26-9 ◆).

Process of Administering Medications

When administering any drug, regardless of the route of administration, the nurse must do the following:

1. *Identify the client.* In hospitals, most clients wear some kind of identification, such as a wristband

with name and hospital identification number. Errors can and do occur, usually because one client gets a drug intended for another. Before giving the client any drug, always check the client's identification band. As a double check, the nurse can ask the alert client to state his or her name or can ask another nurse to identify the client before

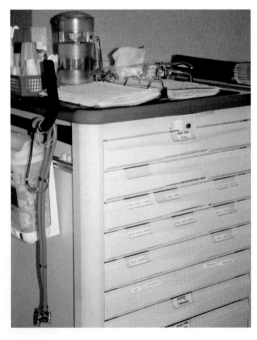

FIGURE 26-5 ◆ Medication cart.

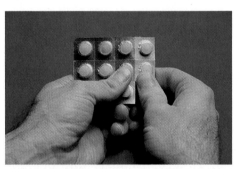

A

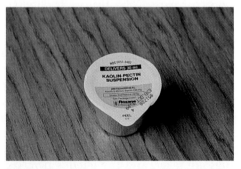

B

FIGURE 26-6 ◆ Unit-dose packages: (A) tablets; (B) liquid medications.

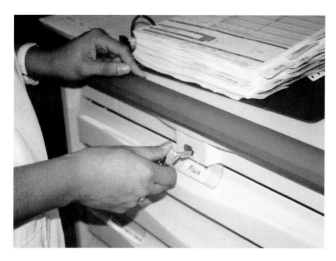

FIGURE 26-7 ◆ The medication cart is kept locked when not in use. The nurse unlocks the medication cart to access client medications.

administering any medication. Do not ask, "Are you John Jones?" because the client may answer "yes" to the wrong name.

2. *Inform the client.* If the client is unfamiliar with the medication, the nurse should explain the intended action as well as any side effects or adverse effects that might occur.

3. *Administer the drug.* Read medication orders and records carefully and check against the name on the medication envelope or on the drawer in which the client's medications are kept if a medication cart is used. Then, administer the medica-

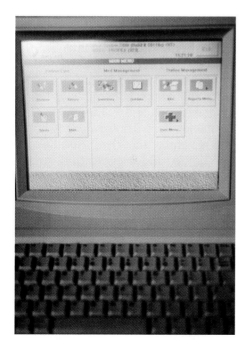

FIGURE 26-8 ◆ Computerized medication access system.

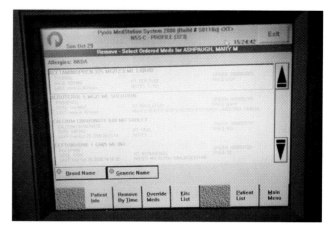

FIGURE 26-9 ◆ Client profile in a computerized medication access system.

tion in the prescribed dosage, by the route ordered, at the correct time. See Box 26-3 for the five "rights" to accurate medication administration.

4. *Provide adjunctive interventions as needed.* Clients may need help when receiving medications. They may require physical assistance, for instance, in assuming positions for intramuscular injections, or they may need guidance about measures to enhance drug effectiveness and prevent complications, such as drinking fluids. Some clients convey fear about their medications. The nurse can allay fears by listening carefully to clients' concerns and giving correct information.

5. *Record the drug administered.* The facts recorded in the chart, in ink or by computer printout, are the name of the drug, dosage, method of administration, specific relevant data such as pulse rate (taken in most settings prior to the administration of digitalis), and any other pertinent information. The record must also include the exact time of administration and the signature of the nurse providing the medication. Many medication records are designed so that the nurse signs once on the page and initials each medication administered. Often, medications that are given regularly are recorded on a special flow record. PRN (as needed) or stat (at once) medications are recorded separately.

6. *Evaluate the client's response to the drug.* The kinds of behavior that reflect the action or lack of action of a drug and its untoward effects (both minor and major) are as variable as the purposes of the drugs themselves. The anxious client may show the desired effect of a tranquilizer by behavior that reflects a lowered stress level (e.g., slower speech or fewer random movements). The effectiveness of a sedative can often be measured by how well a client slept and the effectiveness of an antispasmodic by how much pain the client feels. In all nursing activities, nurses need to be aware of the medications that a client is taking and record

Box 26-3 *Five "Rights" of Medication Administration*

- **Right medication**
  - The medication given was the medication ordered.
- **Right dose**
  - The dose ordered is appropriate for the client.
  - Give special attention if the calculation indicates multiple pills/tablets or a large quantity of a liquid medication.
  - Double check calculations that appear questionable.
  - Know the usual dosage range of the medication.
  - Question a dose outside of the usual dosage range.
- **Right time**
  - Give the medication at the right frequency and at the time ordered according to agency policy.

- Medications given within 30 minutes before or after the scheduled time are considered to meet the "right time" standard.
- **Right route**
  - Give the medication by the ordered route.
  - Make certain that the route is safe and appropriate for the client.
- **Right client**
  - Medication is given to the intended client.
  - Check the client's identification band with each administration of a medication.
  - Know the agency's "name alert" procedure when clients with the same or similar last names are on the nursing unit.

their effectiveness as assessed by the client and the nurse on the client's chart. The nurse may also report the client's response directly to the charge nurse and physician.

Oral Medications

The oral route is the most common route by which medications are given. As long as a client can swallow and retain the drug in the stomach, this is the route of choice (see Technique 26-1). Oral medications are contraindicated when a client is vomiting, has gastric or intestinal suction, or is unconscious and unable to swallow. Such clients in a hospital are usually on orders for "nothing by mouth" (Latin nil per os: **NPO**).

Nursing Process: Oral Medications

ASSESSMENT

- Assess:
  - Allergies to medication(s)
  - Client's ability to swallow the medication
  - Presence of vomiting or diarrhea that would interfere with the ability to absorb the medication

- Specific drug action, side effects, interactions, and adverse reactions
- Client's knowledge of and learning needs about the medication
- Perform appropriate assessments (e.g., vital signs, laboratory results) specific to the medication.
- Determine if the assessment data influences administration of the medication (i.e., is it appropriate to administer the medication or does the medication need to be held and/or the physician notified?).

PLANNING

Delegation

In acute care settings, the administration of oral/enteral medications is performed by the nurse and is not delegated to unlicensed assistive personnel (UAP). The nurse can inform the UAP of the intended therapeutic effects and/or specific side effects of the medication and request the UAP to report specific client observations to the nurse for follow-up. In some long-term care settings, UAP may be trained to administer certain medications to stable clients. However, it is important for the nurse to remember that the medication knowledge of the UAP is limited and *assessment and evaluation of the effectiveness of the medication remains the responsibility of the nurse.*

IMPLEMENTATION:
TECHNIQUE 26-1 ADMINISTERING ORAL MEDICATIONS

Equipment

- Medication cart
- Disposable medication cups: small paper or plastic

cups for tablets and capsules, waxed or plastic calibrated medication cups for liquids
- MAR or computer printout
- Pill crusher

- Straws to administer medications that may discolor the teeth or to facilitate the ingestion of liquid medication for certain clients
- Drinking glass and water or juice.

Preparation

1. Know the reason why the client is receiving the medication, the drug classification, contraindications, usual dosage range, side effects, and nursing considerations for administering and evaluating the intended outcomes for the medication.

2. Check the MAR
   - Check the MAR for the drug name, dosage, frequency, route of administration, and expiration date for administering the medication, if appropriate. *Certain medication (e.g., narcotics, antibiotics) have a specified time frame at which they expire and need to be reordered.*
     - If the MAR is unclear or pertinent information is missing, compare the MAR with the most recent physician's written order.
     - Report any discrepancies to the charge nurse or the physician, as agency policy dictates.

3. Verify the client's ability to take medication orally.
   - Determine whether the client can swallow, is NPO, is nauseated or vomiting, has gastric suction, or has diminished or absent bowel sounds.

4. Organize the supplies.
   - Place the medication cart outside the client's room.
   - Assemble the MAR(s) for each client together so that medications can be prepared for one client at a time. *Organization of supplies saves time and reduces the chance of error.*

Performance

1. Wash hands and observe other appropriate infection control procedures.

2. Unlock the medication cart.

3. Obtain appropriate medication.
   - Read the MAR and take the appropriate medication from the shelf, drawer, or refrigerator. The medication may be dispensed in a bottle, box, or unit-dose package.
   - Compare the label of the medication container or unit-dose package against the order on the MAR (Figure 26-10 ◆) or computer printout. *This is a safety check to ensure that the right medication is given.* If these are not identical, recheck the client's chart. If there is still a discrepancy, check with the nurse in charge or the pharmacist.
   - Check the expiration date of the medication. Return expired medications to the pharmacy. *Outdated medications are not safe to administer.*

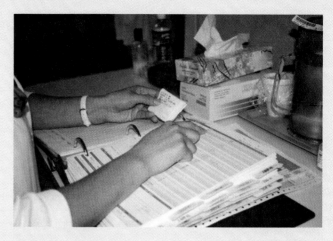

FIGURE 26-10 ◆ Compare the medication label to the MAR.

- Use only medications that have clear, legible labels *to ensure accuracy.*

4. Prepare the medication.
   - Calculate medication dosage accurately.
   - Prepare the correct amount of medication for the required dose, without contaminating the medication. *Aseptic technique maintains drug cleanliness.*
   - While preparing the medication, recheck each prepared drug and container with the MAR again. *This second safety check reduces the chance of error.*

Tablets or Capsules

- Place packaged unit-dose capsules or tablets directly into the medicine cup. Do not remove the medication from the wrapper until at the bedside. *The wrapper keeps the medication clean. Not removing the medication from the wrapper facilitates identification of the medication in the event the client refuses the drug or assessment data indicates the drug should be held. Unopened unit-dose packages can usually be returned to the medication cart.*
- If using a stock container, pour the required number into the bottle cap, and then transfer the medication to the disposable cup without touching the tablets.
- Keep narcotics and medications that require specific assessments, such as pulse measurements, respiratory rate or depth, or blood pressure, separate from the others. *This reminds the nurse to complete the needed assessment(s) in order to decide whether to give the medication or to withhold the medication if indicated.*
- Break only scored tablets if necessary to obtain the correct dosage. Use a file or cutting device if needed (Figure 26-11 ◆). Check the agency policy as to whether unused portions of a medication can be discarded and, if so, how they are to be discarded.

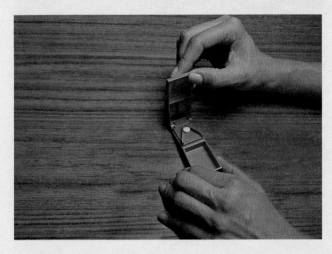

FIGURE 26-11 ◆ A cutting device can be used to divide tablets.

- If the client has difficulty swallowing, crush the tablets to a fine powder with a pill crusher or between two medication cups. Then, mix the powder with a small amount of soft food (e.g., custard, applesauce). *Note:* Check with the pharmacy before crushing tablets. Sustained-action, enteric coated, buccal, or sublingual tablets should not be crushed.

Liquid Medication

- Thoroughly mix the medication before pouring. Discard any medication that has changed color or turned cloudy.
- Remove the cap and place it upside down on the countertop *to avoid contaminating the inside of the cap.*
- Hold the bottle so the label is next to your palm and pour the medication away from the label (Figure 26-12 ◆). *This prevents the label from becoming soiled and illegible as a result of spilled liquids.*
- Hold the medication cup at eye level and fill it to the desired level, using the bottom of the **meniscus** (crescent-shaped upper surface of a column of liquid) to align with container scale (Figure 26-13 ◆). *This method ensures accuracy of measurement.*

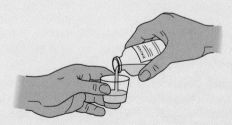

FIGURE 26-12 ◆ Pouring a liquid medication from a bottle.

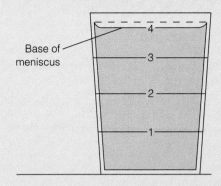

FIGURE 26-13 ◆ The bottom of the meniscus is the measuring guide.

- Before capping the bottle, wipe the lip with a paper towel. *This prevents the cap from sticking.*
- When giving small amounts of liquids (e.g., < 5 mL), prepare the medication in a sterile syringe without the needle.
- Keep unit-dose liquids in their package and open them at the bedside.

Oral Narcotics

- If an agency uses a manual recording system for controlled substances, check the narcotic record for the previous drug count and compare it with the supply available. Some medications, including narcotics, are kept in plastic containers that are sectioned and numbered.
- Remove the next available tablet and drop it in the medicine cup.
- After removing a tablet, record the necessary information on the appropriate narcotic control record and sign it.
- *Note:* Computer-controlled dispensing systems allow access only to the selected drug and automatically record its use.

All Medications

- Place the prepared medication and MAR together on the medication cart.
- Recheck the label on the container before returning the bottle, box, or envelope to its storage place. *This third check further reduces the risk of error.*
- Avoid leaving prepared medications unattended. *This precaution prevents potential mishandling errors.*
- Lock the medication cart before entering the client's room. This is a *safety measure as medication carts are not to be left open when unattended.*
- Check the room number against the MAR if agency policy does not allow the MAR to be removed from the medication cart. *This is another*

safety measure to ensure that the nurse is entering the correct client room.

5. Provide for client privacy.

6. Prepare the client.
   - Check the client's identification band. *This ensures that the right client receives the medication.*
   - Assist the client to a sitting position or, if not possible, to a side-lying position. *These positions facilitate swallowing and prevent aspiration.*
   - If not previously assessed, take the required assessment measures, such as pulse and respiratory rates or blood pressure. Take the apical pulse rate before administering digitalis preparations. Take blood pressure before giving antihypertensive drugs. Take the respiratory rate prior to administering narcotics. *Narcotics depress the respiratory center.* If any of the findings are above or below the predetermined parameters, consult the physician before administering the medication.

7. Explain the purpose of the medication and how it will help, using language that the client can understand. Include relevant information about effects; for example, tell the client receiving a diuretic to expect an increase in urine output. *Information facilitates acceptance of and compliance with the therapy.*

8. Administer the medication at the correct time.
   - Take the medication to the client within the time frame of 30 minutes before or after the scheduled time.
   - Give the client sufficient water or preferred juice to swallow the medication. Before using juice, check for any food and medication incompatibilities. *Fluids ease swallowing and facilitate absorption from the gastrointestinal tract.* Liquid medications other than antacids or cough preparations are generally diluted with 15 mL (½ oz) of water to facilitate absorption.
   - If the client is unable to hold the pill cup, use the pill cup to introduce the medication into the client's mouth, and give only one tablet or capsule at a time. *Putting the cup to the client's mouth maintains the cleanliness of the nurse's*

hands. Giving one medication at a time eases swallowing.
   - If an older child or adult has difficulty swallowing, ask the client to place the medication on the back of the tongue before taking the water. *Stimulation of the back of the tongue produces the swallowing reflex.*
   - If the medication has an objectionable taste, ask the client to suck a few ice chips beforehand, or give the medication with juice, applesauce, or bread if there are no contraindications. *The cold of the ice chips will desensitize the taste buds, and juices or bread can mask the taste of the medication.*
   - If the client says that the medication you are about to give is different from what the client has been receiving, do not give the medication without first checking the original order. *Most clients are familiar with the appearance of medications taken previously. Unfamiliar medications may signal a possible error.*
   - Stay with the client until all medications have been swallowed. *The nurse must see the client swallow the medication before the drug administration can be recorded.* A physician's order or agency policy is required for medications left at the bedside.

 9. **Document** each medication given.
   - Record the medication given, dosage, time, any complaints or assessments of the client, and your signature.
   - If medication was refused or omitted, record this fact on the appropriate record; document the reason, when possible, and the nurse's actions according to agency policy.

10. Dispose of all supplies appropriately.
   - Replenish stock (e.g., medication cups) and return the cart to the appropriate place.
   - Discard used disposable supplies.

11. Evaluate the effects of the medication.
   - Return to the client when the medication is expected to take effect (usually 30 minutes) to evaluate the effects of the medication on the client.

AMBULATORY AND COMMUNITY SETTINGS

Administering Oral/Enteral Medications
Home Care Considerations
Instruct the client to:
- Learn the names of the medications as well as their actions and possible adverse effects.
- Keep all medications out of reach of children and pets.
- If using a syringe to administer the medication to an infant or child, remove and dispose of the plas-

tic cap that fits on the end of the syringe. Infants and small children have been known to choke on these caps.
- Take the medications only as prescribed. Immediately consult the nurse, pharmacist, or physician about any problems with the medication.
- Always check the medication label to make sure the correct medication is being taken.

Administering Oral/Enteral Medications (*continued*)

- Request labels printed with larger type on medication containers if there is difficulty reading the label.
- Check the expiration date and discard outdated medications.
- Ask the pharmacist to substitute childproof caps with ones that are more easily opened, as necessary.
- If a dose or more is missed, do not take two or more doses; ask the pharmacist or physician for directions.

- Do not crush or cut a tablet or capsule without first checking with the physician or pharmacist. Doing so may affect the medication's absorption.
- Never stop taking the medication without the physician's permission.
- Always check with the pharmacist before taking any nonprescription medications. Some over-the-counter medications can interact with the prescribed medication.
- Set up a medication schedule. Weekly pill containers (available at the pharmacy) or a written plan may be helpful.

AGE-RELATED CONSIDERATIONS

Administering Oral/Enteral Medications

Infants

- A syringe or dropper provides the best control for administering medications.
- Place small amounts of liquid along the side of the infant's mouth. To prevent aspiration or spitting out, wait for the infant to swallow before giving more (Bindler & Ball, 1999, p. 49).
- Another method for giving liquid medications to infants is to have the infant suck the liquid through a nipple. Other methods should be used, however, for unpleasant tasting medicine so that the infant will not associate the unpleasant taste with the nipple. Medication should never be added to the infant's formula for the same reason.

Children

- Knowledge of growth and development is essential for the nurse administering medications to children.
- Whenever possible, give children a choice between the use of a spoon, dropper, or syringe.
- Oral medications for children are usually prepared in sweetened liquid form to make them more palatable. Crush medications that are not supplied in liquid form and mix them with substances available on most pediatric units, such as honey, flavored syrup, jam, or a fruit puree.
- Necessary foods such as milk or orange juice should not be used to mask the taste of medications because the child may develop unpleasant associations and refuse that food in the future.

- Disguise disagreeable-tasting medications with sweet-tasting substances mentioned previously. However, present any altered medication to the child honestly and not as a food or treat.
- Place the young child or toddler on your lap or the parent's lap in a sitting position.
- Administer the medication slowly with a measuring spoon, plastic syringe, or medicine cup.
- To prevent nausea, pour a carbonated beverage over finely crushed ice and give it before or immediately after the medication is administered.
- For children who take sweetened medications on a long-term basis, follow the medication administration with oral hygiene. These children are at high risk for dental caries.
- If giving several medications by an enteral tube, administer medications separately and flush with 5 to 10 mL of warm water between each medication.

Elders

- The physiologic changes associated with aging influence medication administration and effectiveness. Examples include altered memory, less acute vision, decrease in renal function, less complete and slower absorption from the gastrointestinal tract, decreased liver function. Many of these changes enhance the possibility of cumulative effects and toxicity.
- Older adults usually require smaller dosages of drugs, especially sedatives and other central nervous system depressants.
- Older adults are mature adults capable of reasoning. The nurse, therefore, needs to explain the reasons for and the effects of the client's medications.

EVALUATION

- Conduct appropriate follow up.
  - Desired effect (e.g., relief of pain or decrease in body temperature)
  - Any adverse effects or side effects (e.g., nausea, vomiting, skin rash, change in vital signs)
- Relate to previous findings, if available.
- Report significant deviations from normal to the physician.

Nasogastric and Gastrostomy Medications

For clients who cannot take anything by mouth (NPO) and have nasogastric tubes or a gastrostomy tube in place, an alternative route for administering medications is through the nasogastric or gastrostomy tube. A **nasogastric (NG) tube** is inserted by way of the nasopharynx and is placed into the client's stomach for the purpose of feeding the client or to remove gastric secretions. A **gastrostomy tube** is surgically placed directly into the client's stomach and provides another route for administering nutrition and medications. See Chapter 15 for further discussion of nasogastric and gastrostomy tubes.

When administering medications by nasogastric or gastrostomy tube, use the following guidelines:

- Administer liquid forms of medication whenever possible to avoid clogging of the enteral tube. Always check with the pharmacist to see if the client's medications are available in a liquid form.
- If medications are not available in liquid form, check with the pharmacist to see if they may be crushed. Enteric coated, sustained release, buccal, and sublingual tablets should not be crushed.
- Crush a tablet into a fine powder and dissolve in at least 30 mL of warm water. Use only water for mixing and flushing.
- Read medication labels carefully before opening a capsule. Open capsule and mix with water only with the pharmacist's advice.
- Do not administer whole or undissolved medications, as they will clog the tube.

- If the tube is connected to suction, disconnect the suction and keep the tube clamped for 20 to 30 minutes after giving the medication to enhance absorption of the medication.
- Always check and confirm tube placement before administering medications.
- Flush the tube before and after medication administration.
- If giving several medications, administer medications separately and flush with 15 to 30 mL of warm water between each medication.

Technique 26-2 provides guidelines for administering medications by enteral tube.

Nursing Process: Nasogastric and Gastrostomy Medications

ASSESSMENT

- Assess:
  - Allergies to medication(s)
  - Specific drug action, side effects, interactions, and adverse reactions
  - Client's knowledge of and learning needs about the medication
  - Whether fluid restriction or fluid overload is a concern for the client
- Perform appropriate assessments (e.g., vital signs, laboratory results) specific to the medication.
- Determine if the assessment data influences administration of the medication (i.e., is it appropriate to administer the medication or does the medication need to be held and/or the physician notified?).

PLANNING

Delegation

The administration of medications through an enteral tube is performed by the nurse and is not delegated to UAP. The nurse can inform the UAP of the intended therapeutic effects and/or specific side effects of the medication and request the UAP to report specific client observations to the nurse for follow-up.

IMPLEMENTATION:
TECHNIQUE 26-2 ADMINISTERING MEDICATIONS BY ENTERAL TUBE

Equipment

- Medication to be administered
- Disposable medication cups: small paper or plastic calibrated medication cups for liquids

- 50- to 60-mL syringe with catheter tip for large-bore tube or Luer-Lok tip for small-bore tube
- Pill crusher for medications that need to be crushed
- Tongue blade or straw to stir dissolved medication

- pH test strip
- Warm water to dissolve crushed medications
- Tap water (room temperature) for flushing tube
- Emesis basin
- Disposable gloves
- MAR or computer printout

Preparation

1. Know the reason why the client is receiving the medication, the drug classification, contraindications, usual dosage range, side effects, and nursing considerations for administering and evaluating the intended outcomes for the medication.

2. Check the MAR
   - Check the MAR for the drug name, dosage, frequency, route of administration, and expiration date for administration of the medication, if appropriate.
   - If the MAR is unclear or pertinent information is missing, compare the MAR with the most recent physician's written order.
   - Report any discrepancies to the charge nurse or the physician, as agency policy dictates.

3. Organize supplies

4. Prepare the client.
   - Assist the client to a Fowler's position in bed or a sitting position in a chair. If a sitting position is contraindicated, a slightly elevated right side-lying position is acceptable. *These positions enhance gravitational flow and prevent aspiration of fluid into the lungs.*

Performance

1. Wash hands and observe other appropriate infection control procedures (e.g., disposable gloves).

2. Provide for client privacy.

3. Explain the purpose of the medication and how it will help, using language that the client can understand. Include relevant information about effects; for example, tell the client receiving a diuretic to expect an increase in urine. *Information facilitates acceptance of and compliance with the therapy.*

4. Prepare medications for appropriate administration by enteral tube (e.g., use liquids or crush and dissolve tablets). Calculate medication dosage accurately.

5. Assess tube placement (see Chapter 15 for methods to verify tube placement).

6. Aspirate all the stomach contents and measure the residual volume.
   - Check agency policy if residual volume greater than 100 mL.

7. Check the client's identification band. *This ensures the right client receives the medication.*

8. Administer the medication(s).
   - Remove the plunger from the syringe and connect the syringe to a pinched or kinked tube. *Pinching or kinking the tube prevents excess air from entering the stomach and causing distention.*
   - Put 15 to 30 mL of water into the syringe barrel to flush the tube before administering the first medication. Raise or lower the barrel of the syringe to adjust the flow as needed. Pinch or clamp the tubing before all the water is instilled *to avoid excess air entering the stomach.*
   - Pour liquid or dissolved medication into syringe barrel and allow to flow by gravity into enteral tube.
   - If administering more than one medication, flush with 15 to 30 mL of tap water between each medication.
   - After administering the last medication, flush the tube with 15 to 30 mL of tap water *to clear the tube.*

9. **Document** each medication given.
   - Record the medication given, dosage, time, any complaints or assessments of the client, and your signature.
   - If medication was refused or omitted, record this fact on the appropriate record; document the reason, when possible, and the nurse's actions according to agency policy.
   - Record fluid intake accurately if client is on intake and output.

10. Dispose of all supplies appropriately.
    - Replenish stock (e.g., medication cups) and return cart to the appropriate place.
    - Discard used disposable supplies.

11. Evaluate the effects of the medication.
    - Return to the client when the medication is expected to take effect (usually 30 minutes) to evaluate the effects of the medication on the client.

- Conduct appropriate follow-up.
  - Desired effect (e.g., relief of pain or decrease in body temperature)
  - Any adverse effects or side effects (e.g., nausea, vomiting, skin rash, change in vital signs)

- Compare tube patency before and after medication administration
- Relate to previous findings, if available.
- Report significant deviations from normal to the physician.

Chapter Summary

TERMINOLOGY

brand name
buccal
chemical name
drug
gastrostomy tube
generic name
medication administration record
  (MAR)

medication
medication history
meniscus
minim
nasogastric (NG) tube
NPO
official name
oral

prescription
PRN order
single order
standing order
stat order
sublingual
trademark

FORMING CLINICAL JUDGMENTS

Consider This:

1. The client asks you, "Why are you checking my name band again? I haven't changed since the last time you checked!" How will you respond?

2. You are administering medication and the client asks you why he is getting a certain pill. You tell him the reason. The client says, "My pill at home is a different color." How do you respond?

3. Presume that the full name of the client is on the physician's order sheet, the date and time that the order was written and the physician's signature is all present on the order sheet. The following medications are listed on the MAR. Which, if any, would you question?

   - Lasix 40 mg STAT
   - Ampicillin 500 mg IVPB
   - Dulcolax suppository i PRN if no BM for 3 days
   - Humulin L (Lente) insulin 36 U, SC, q am, ac

   - Codeine q4–6h, PO, PRN for pain
   - KCl 40 mg IV STAT

4. You are preparing to administer a narcotic, Tylenol #3. You notice that there are 16 tablets remaining in the plastic container holding the narcotic. The narcotic inventory record, however, indicates that three of the 20 tablets in the Tylenol #3 container have been signed out. What do you do?

5. You are to administer multiple medications to a client. These medications include tablets (one is sublingual), a capsule, and a powder that needs to be mixed with juice or water. In what order will you administer these medications?

6. Your assigned client has a small-bore feeding tube in place. You note that all of the client's medications are in tablet form, with one being an enteric coated tablet. What action(s) will you take?

Related Research

Ashby, D. A. (1997). Medication calculation skills of the medical–surgical nurse. *MEDSURG Nursing, 6*(2), 90–94.

Cheek, J. (1997). Nurses and the administration of medications: Broadening the focus. *Clinical Nursing Research, 6*(3), 253–274.

Wakefield, B. J., Wakefield, D. S., Uden-Holman, T., & Blegen, M. A. (1998). Nurses' perceptions of why medication administration errors occur. *MEDSURG Nursing, 7*(1), 39–44.

References

Bindler, R., & Ball, J. (1999). *Pediatric Clinical Skills* (2nd ed.) Stamford: Appleton & Lange.

Fiesta, J. (1998). Legal aspects of medication administration. *Nursing Management, 29*(1), 22–23.

Ignatavicius, D. D. (2000). Asking the right questions about medication safety. *Nursing, 30*(9), 51–54.

Kudzma, E. C. (1999). Culturally competent drug administration. *American Journal of Nursing, 99*(8), 46–51.

Leonard, T. S. (1996). Understanding automated medication-dispensing systems. *Nursing, 26*(5), 24h–24j.

Lord, L. M. (1997). Enteral access devices. *Nursing Clinics of North America, 32*(4), 685–703.

Miller, D., & Miller, H. (2000). To crush or not to crush. *Nursing, 30*(2), 50–52.

Quillen, T. (2000). Tips and timesavers: Crushing advice. *Nursing, 30*(4), 30.

Smetzer, J. L. (1998). Beyond blaming individuals. Lesson from Colorado. *Nursing, 28*(5), 48–51.

Chapter 27

Administering Topical Medications

Techniques

OBJECTIVES

- Identify assessment data needed prior to administering topical medications.
- Identify essential guidelines in preparing, administering, and documenting topical medications and in evaluating the client's response.
- Apply dermatologic medications safely.
- Perform eye, ear, nose, vaginal, and rectal instillations and irrigations safely.
- Assist clients with metered dose nebulizers.

Topical medications are those applied locally to the skin or mucous membranes in areas such as the eye, ear, nose, vagina, and respiratory tract. Topical applications include:

- *Dermatologic preparations*—applied to the skin, including lotions, creams, ointments, pastes, gels, sprays, and powders (See Chapter 33, Table 33-1). See Box 27-1 for general guidelines for applying dermatologic medications.

- *Instillations* and *irrigations*—applied into body cavities or orifices such as the urinary bladder, eyes, ears, nose, rectum, or vagina. Irrigations may or may not be medicated.

- *Inhalations*—administered into the respiratory tract by inhalers, nebulizers, or positive pressure breathing apparatuses. Air, oxygen, and vapor are generally used to carry the drug into the lungs.

Dermatologic Medications

Medications applied to the skin may be used to decrease itching (**pruritus**), lubricate and soften the skin, cause local vasoconstriction or vasodilation, increase or decrease secretions from the skin, provide a protective coating to the skin, apply an antibiotic or antiseptic to treat or prevent infection, to reduce local inflammation, or as an entry for medications that will be absorbed into the systemic circulation.

Unless contraindicated by a specific order, the nurse washes and carefully dries the area before applying a dermatologic preparation. Skin encrustations and discharges harbor microorganisms and cause local infections. They can also prevent the medication from coming in contact with the area to be treated.

Transdermal Patches

A particular type of dermatologic medication delivery system is the **transdermal patch.** This system administers sustained-action medications (e.g., nitroglycerin, estrogen, and nicotine) via multilayered films containing the drug and an adhesive layer. The rate of delivery of the drug is controlled and varies with each product (e.g., from 12 hours to 1 week). Generally, the patch is applied to a hairless, clean area of skin that is not subject to excessive movement or wrinkling (i.e., the trunk or lower abdomen). It may also be applied on the side, lower back, or buttocks. Patches should not be applied to areas with cuts, burns, or abrasions, or on distal parts of extremities (e.g., the forearms). If hair is likely to interfere with patch adhesion or removal, clipping may be necessary before application.

Reddening of the skin with or without mild local itching or burning, as well as allergic contact dermatitis, may occasionally occur. Upon removal of the

---

Box 27-1 Guidelines for Dermatologic Medication Administration

Powder

Make sure the skin surface is dry. Spread apart any skin folds, and sprinkle the site until the area is covered with a fine *thin* layer. Cover the site with a dressing if ordered.

Suspension-Based Lotion

Shake the container before use to distribute suspended particles. Put a little lotion on a small gauze dressing or pad, and apply the lotion to the skin by stroking it evenly in the direction of the hair growth.

Creams, Ointments, Pastes, and Oil-Based Lotions

Warm and soften the preparation in the gloved hands to make it easier to apply and to prevent chilling (if a large area is to be treated). Smear it evenly over the skin using long strokes that follow the direction of the hair growth. Explain that the skin may feel somewhat greasy after application. Apply a sterile dressing if ordered by the physician.

Aerosol Spray

Shake the container well to mix the contents. Hold the spray container at the recommended distance from the area (usually about 15 to 30 cm [6 to 12 in] but check the label). Cover the client's face with a towel if the upper chest or neck is to be sprayed. Spray the medication over the specified area.

Transdermal Patches

Select a clean, dry area that is free of hair and matches the manufacturer's recommendations. Remove the patch from its protective covering, holding it without touching the adhesive edges, and apply it by pressing firmly with the palm of the hand for about 10 seconds. Advise the client to avoid using a heating pad over the area to prevent an increase in circulation and the rate of absorption. Remove the patch at the appropriate time, folding it so that the medicated side is covered.

From *Fundamentals of nursing: Concepts, process, and practice,* 6th ed., by B. Kozier, G. Erb, A. Berman, & K. Burke, 2000, Upper Saddle River, NJ: Prentice Hall Health.

patch, any slight reddening of the skin usually disappears within a few hours. All applications should be changed regularly to prevent local irritation, and each successive application should be placed on a different site. All clients need to be assessed for allergies to the drug and to materials in the patch before the patch is applied.

Nursing Process: Dermatologic Medications

ASSESSMENT

In addition to the assessment performed by the nurse related to the administration of any medication (see Chapter 26), prior to applying dermatologic medications:

- Inspect skin or mucous membrane areas for lesions, rashes, erythema, and breakdown. Note size, color, distribution, and configuration of lesions (see Technique 3-2).

- Determine the presence of symptoms of skin irritation (e.g., pruritus, burning sensation, pain).
- Note the presence of excessive body hair that may require removal before the application of a topical medication.

PLANNING

Review the client record regarding the condition of the skin area used previously for topical medication administration. If the medication is intended for systemic absorption, rotate sites used.

Delegation

Due to the need for assessment and interpretation of client status, topical medication administration is generally not delegated to unlicensed assistive personnel (UAP). In some agencies, UAP may apply lotions and creams used primarily for relieving itching or dry skin. However, responsibility for periodically assessing the area remains with the nurse.

IMPLEMENTATION:
TECHNIQUE 27-1 ADMINISTERING DERMATOLOGIC MEDICATIONS

Equipment

- Gloves (clean and sterile if required)
- Solution to wash area if indicated
- 2" × 2" gauze pads for cleaning
- Medication container
- Application tube (if required)
- Tongue blades
- Gauze to cover area (if required)

Preparation

1. Check the medication administration record (MAR).
   - Check the MAR for the drug name, strength, and prescribed frequency.
   - If the MAR is unclear or pertinent information is missing, compare it with the most recent physician's written order.
   - Report any discrepancies to the charge nurse or physician, as agency policy dictates.

2. Know the reason why the client is receiving the medication, the drug classification, contraindications, usual dose range, side effects, and nursing considerations for administering and evaluating the intended outcomes of the medication.

3. Determine whether area is to be washed or the hair clipped before applying medication.

Performance

1. Compare the label on the medication tube or jar with the medication record and check the expiration date.

2. If necessary, calculate the medication dosage.

3. Explain to the client what you are going to do, why it is necessary, and how he or she can cooperate. Discuss how the results will be used in planning further care or treatments.

4. Wash hands and observe appropriate infection control procedures. Apply clean gloves if needed to protect the hands from contact with the medication.

5. Prepare the client.
   - Check the client's identification band, and ask the client's name. *This ensures that the right client receives the medication.*
   - Assist the client to a comfortable position, either sitting or lying. Expose the area to be treated but provide for client privacy.

6. Apply the medication and dressing as ordered.
   - Place a small amount of cream on the tongue blade, and spread it evenly on the skin.
   or
   - Apply sterile gloves if indicated. Pour some lotion on the gauze, and pat the skin area with it.
   or

If a liniment is used, rub it into the skin using long, smooth strokes.

- Repeat the application until the area is completely covered.
- Apply a sterile dressing as necessary.
 or
- Apply a prepackaged transdermal patch (See Box 27-1).

7. Provide for client comfort.

- Provide a clean gown or pajamas after the application if the medication will come in contact with the clothing.

8. **Document** all assessments and interventions.

- Record the type of preparation used, the site to which it was applied, the time, and the response of the client, including data about the appearance of the site, discomfort, itching, and so on.
- Return at a time by which the preparation should have acted to assess the reaction (e.g., relief of itching, burning, swelling, or discomfort).

EVALUATION

- Perform follow-up based on findings of the effectiveness of the medication or outcomes that deviated from expected or normal for the client. Relate findings to previous data if available.
- Report significant deviations from normal to the physician.

Ophthalmic Medications

Medications may be administered to the eye using irrigations or instillations, An eye irrigation is administered to wash out the conjunctival sac. Medications for the eyes are instilled in the form of liquids or ointments. Eyedrops are packaged in monodrip plastic containers that are used to administer the preparation. Ointments are usually supplied in small tubes. All containers must state that the medication is for ophthalmic use. Usually, sterile preparations are used, but sterile technique is not always indicated. Prescribed liquids are usually dilute (e.g., less than 1 percent strength).

Nursing Process: Ophthalmic Medications

ASSESSMENT

In addition to the assessment performed by the nurse related to the administration of any medication (see Chapter 26), prior to applying ophthalmic medications, assess:

- Appearance of eye and surrounding structures for lesions, exudate, erythema, or swelling
- The location and nature of any discharge, lacrimation, and swelling of the eyelids or of the lacrimal gland
- Client complaints (e.g., itching, burning, pain, blurred vision, and photophobia)
- Client behavior (e.g., squinting, blinking excessively, frowning, or rubbing the eyes)

Determine if assessment data influences administration of the medication (i.e., is it appropriate to administer the medication or does the medication need to be held or the physician notified?).

PLANNING

Delegation

Due to the need for assessment, interpretation of client status, and use of sterile technique, ophthalmic medication administration is not delegated to UAP.

Equipment

- Clean gloves

- Sterile absorbent sponges soaked in sterile normal saline
- Medication

- Sterile eye dressing (pad) as needed and paper eye tape to secure it

For irrigation, add:

- Irrigating solution (e.g., normal saline) and irrigating syringe or tubing
- Dry sterile absorbent sponges
- Moisture-resistant towel
- Basin (e.g., emesis basin)

Preparation

1. Check the MAR.
   - Check the MAR for the drug name, dose, and strength. Also confirm the prescribed frequency of the instillation and which eye is to be treated. Abbreviations are frequently used to identify the eye: OD (right eye), OS (left eye), OU (both eyes).
   - If the MAR is unclear or pertinent information is missing, compare it with the most recent physician's written order.
   - Report any discrepancies to the charge nurse or physician, as agency policy dictates.

2. Know the reason why the client is receiving the medication, the drug classification, contraindications, usual dose range, side effects, and nursing considerations for administering and evaluating the intended outcomes of the medication.

Performance

1. Compare the label on the medication tube or bottle with the medication record and check the expiration date.

2. If necessary, calculate the medication dosage.

3. Explain to the client what you are going to do, why it is necessary, and how he or she can cooperate. The administration of an ophthalmic medication is not usually painful. Ointments are often soothing to the eye, but some liquid preparations may sting initially. Discuss how the results will be used in planning further care or treatments.

4. Wash hands and observe appropriate infection control procedures.

5. Provide for client privacy.

6. Prepare the client.
   - Check the client's identification band, and ask the client's name. *This ensures that the right client receives the medication.*
   - Assist the client to a comfortable position, either sitting or lying.

7. Clean the eyelid and the eyelashes.
   - Don clean gloves.
   - Use sterile cotton balls moistened with sterile irrigating solution or sterile normal saline, and wipe from the inner canthus to the outer can-

thus. *If not removed, material on the eyelid and lashes can be washed into the eye. Cleaning toward the outer canthus prevents contamination of the other eye and the lacrimal duct.*

8. Administer the eye medication.
   - Check the ophthalmic preparation for the name, strength, and number of drops if a liquid is used. Draw the correct number of drops into the shaft of the dropper if a dropper is used. If ointment is used, discard the first bead. *Checking medication data is essential to prevent a medication error. The first bead of ointment from a tube is considered to be contaminated.*
   - Instruct the client to look up to the ceiling. Give the client a dry sterile absorbent sponge. *The person is less likely to blink if looking up. While the client looks up, the cornea is partially protected by the upper eyelid. A sponge is needed to press on the nasolacrimal duct after a liquid instillation or to wipe excess ointment from the eyelashes after an ointment is instilled.*
   - Expose the lower conjunctival sac by placing the thumb or fingers of your nondominant hand on the client's cheekbone just below the eye and gently drawing down the skin on the cheek. If the tissues are edematous, handle the tissues carefully to avoid damaging them. *Placing the fingers on the cheekbone minimizes the possibility of touching the cornea, avoids putting any pressure on the eyeball, and prevents the person from blinking or squinting.*
   - Approach the eye from the side and instill the correct number of drops onto the outer third of the lower conjunctival sac. Hold the dropper 1 to 2 cm (0.4 to 0.8 in) above the sac (Figure 27-1 ◆). *The client is less likely to blink if a side approach is used. When instilled into the conjunctival sac, drops will not harm the cornea as they might if dropped directly on it. The dropper must not touch the sac or the cornea.*

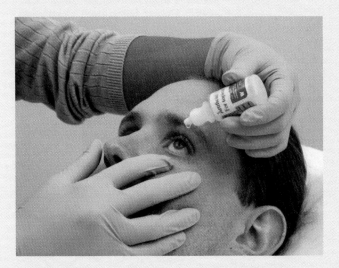

FIGURE 27-1 ◆ Instilling an eyedrop into the lower conjunctival sac.

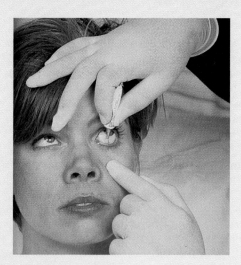

FIGURE 27-2 ◆ Instilling an eye ointment into the lower conjunctival sac.

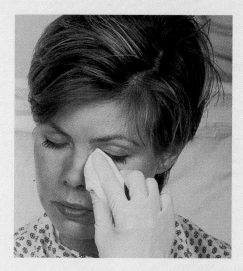

FIGURE 27-3 ◆ Pressing on the nasolabial duct.

or

- Holding the tube above the lower conjunctival sac, squeeze 2 cm (0.8 in) of ointment from the tube into the lower conjunctival sac from the inner canthus outward (Figure 27-2 ◆).

- Instruct the client to close the eyelids but not to squeeze them shut. *Closing the eye spreads the medication over the eyeball. Squeezing can injure the eye and push out the medication.*

- For liquid medications, press firmly or have the client press firmly on the nasolacrimal duct for at least 30 seconds (Figure 27-3 ◆). *Pressing on the nasolacrimal duct prevents the medication from running out of the eye and down the duct.*

Variation: Irrigation

- Place absorbent pads under the head, neck, and shoulders. Place an emesis basin next to the eye to catch drainage.

- Expose the lower conjunctival sac. Or, to irrigate in stages, first hold the lower lid down, then hold the upper lid up. Exert pressure on the bony prominences of the cheekbone and beneath the eyebrow when holding the eyelids. *Separating the lids prevents reflex blinking. Exerting pressure on the bony prominences minimizes the possibility of pressing the eyeball and causing discomfort.*

- Fill and hold the eye irrigator about 2.5 cm (1 in) above the eye. *At this height the pressure of*

the solution will not damage the eye tissue, and the irrigator will not touch the eye.

- Irrigate the eye, directing the solution onto the lower conjunctival sac and from the inner canthus to the outer canthus. *Directing the solution in this way prevents possible injury to the cornea and prevents fluid and contaminants from flowing down the nasolacrimal duct.*

- Irrigate until the solution leaving the eye is clear (no discharge is present) or until all the solution has been used.

- Instruct the client to close and move the eye periodically. *Eye closure and movement help to move secretions from the upper to the lower conjunctival sac.*

9. Clean and dry the eyelids as needed. Wipe the eyelids gently from the inner to the outer canthus to collect excess medication.

10. Apply an eye pad if needed, and secure it with paper eye tape.

11. Assess the client's response.

- Assess responses immediately after the instillation or irrigation and again after the medication should have acted.

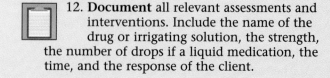

12. **Document** all relevant assessments and interventions. Include the name of the drug or irrigating solution, the strength, the number of drops if a liquid medication, the time, and the response of the client.

Administering Ophthalmic Medications

Infant/Child

- Explain the technique to the parents of an infant or child.
- For a young child or infant, enlist assistance to immobilize the arms and head. The parent may hold the infant or young child. *This prevents accidental injury during medication administration.*
- For a young child, use a doll to demonstrate the procedure. *This facilitates cooperation and decreases anxiety.*
- An intravenous (IV) bag and tubing may be used to deliver irrigating fluid to the eye (Figure 27-4 ♦).

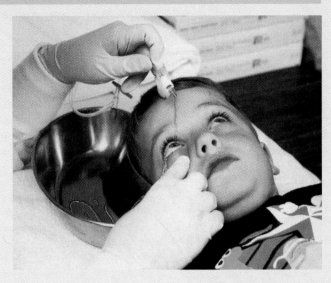

FIGURE 27-4 ♦ Eye irrigation using IV tubing.

EVALUATION

- Perform follow-up based on findings of the effectiveness of the administration or outcomes that deviated from expected or normal for the client. Relate findings to previous data if available.
- Report significant deviations from normal to the physician.

Otic Medications

Irrigations or instillations of the external auditory canal are generally carried out for cleaning purposes, although applications of heat and antiseptic solutions are sometimes prescribed. Irrigations performed in a hospital require aseptic technique so that microorganisms will not be introduced into the ear. Sterile technique is used if the eardrum is perforated. The position of the external auditory canal varies with age. In the child under 3 years of age, it is directed upward. In the adult, the external auditory canal is an S-shaped structure about 2.5 cm (1 in) long.

Nursing Process: Otic Medications

ASSESSMENT

In addition to the assessment performed by the nurse related to the administration of any medications (see Chapter 26), prior to applying otic medications, assess:

- Appearance of the pinna of the ear and meatus for signs of redness and abrasions
- Type and amount of any discharge

Determine if assessment data influences administration of the medication (i.e., is it appropriate to administer the medication or does the medication need to be held or the physician notified?).

PLANNING

Delegation

Due to the need for assessment, interpretation of client status, and use of aseptic technique, otic medication administration is not delegated to UPA.

IMPLEMENTATION:
TECHNIQUE 27-3 ADMINISTERING OTIC MEDICATIONS

Equipment

- Clean gloves
- Cotton-tipped applicator
- Correct medication bottle with a dropper
- Flexible rubber tip (optional) for the end of the

dropper, which prevents injury from sudden motion, for example, by a disoriented client
- Cotton fluff

For irrigation, add:
- Moisture-resistant towel
- Basin (e.g., emesis basin)

- Irrigating solution at the appropriate temperature, about 500 mL (16 oz) or as ordered
- Container for the irrigating solution
- Syringe (rubber bulb or Asepto syringe is frequently used)

Preparation

1. Check the MAR.

   - Check the MAR for the drug name, strength, number of drops, and prescribed frequency.

   - If the MAR is unclear or pertinent information is missing, compare it with the most recent physician's written order.

   - Report any discrepancies to the charge nurse or physician, as agency policy dictates.

2. Know the reason why the client is receiving the medication, the drug classification, contraindications, usual dose range, side effects, and nursing considerations for administering and evaluating the intended outcomes of the medication.

Performance

1. Compare the label on the medication container with the medication record and check the expiration date.

2. If necessary, calculate the medication dosage.

3. Explain to the client what you are going to do, why it is necessary, and how he or she can cooperate. The administration of an otic medication is not usually painful. Discuss how the results will be used in planning further care or treatments.

4. Wash hands and observe appropriate infection control procedures.

5. Provide for client privacy.

6. Prepare the client.

   - Check the client's identification band, and ask the client's name. *This ensures that the right client receives the medication.*

   - Assist the client to a comfortable position for eardrops, lying with the ear being treated uppermost.

7. Clean the pinna of the ear and the meatus of the ear canal.

   - Don gloves if infection is suspected.

   - Use cotton-tipped applicators and solution to wipe the pinna and auditory meatus. *This removes any discharge present before the instillation so that it won't be washed into the ear canal.*

8. Administer the ear medication.

   - Warm the medication container in your hand, or

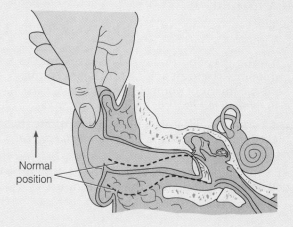

Normal position

FIGURE 27-5 ◆ Straightening the ear canal.

place it in warm water for a short time. *This promotes client comfort.*

- Partially fill the ear dropper with medication.

- Straighten the auditory canal. Pull the pinna upward and backward (Figure 27-5 ◆). *The auditory canal is straightened so that the solution can flow the entire length of the canal.*

- Instill the correct number of drops along the side of the ear canal (Figure 27-6 ◆).

- Press gently but firmly a few times on the tragus of the ear. *Pressing on the tragus assists the flow of medication into the ear canal.*

- Ask the client to remain in the side-lying position for about 5 minutes. *This prevents the drops from escaping and allows the medication to reach all sides of the canal cavity.*

- Insert a small piece of cotton fluff loosely at the meatus of the auditory canal for 15 to 20 minutes. Do not press it into the canal. *The cotton helps retain the medication when the client is up. If pressed tightly into the canal, the cotton would inter-*

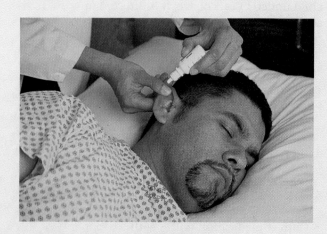

FIGURE 27-6 ◆ Instilling eardrops.

fere with the action of the drug and the outward movement of normal secretions.

Variation: Ear Irrigation

- Explain that the client may experience a feeling of fullness, warmth, and, occasionally, discomfort when the fluid comes in contact with the tympanic membrane.
- Assist the client to a sitting or lying position with head turned toward the affected ear. *The solution can then flow from the ear canal to a basin.*
- Place the moisture-resistant towel around the client's shoulder under the ear to be irrigated, and place the basin under the ear to be irrigated.
- Fill the syringe with solution.
  or
- Hang up the irrigating container, and run solution through the tubing and the nozzle. *Solution is run through to remove air from the tubing and nozzle.*
- Straighten the ear canal.
- Insert the tip of the syringe into the auditory meatus, and direct the solution gently upward against the top of the canal. *The solution will flow around the entire canal and out at the bottom. The*

solution is instilled gently because strong pressure from the fluid can cause discomfort and damage the tympanic membrane.

- Continue instilling the fluid until all the solution is used or until the canal is cleaned, depending on the purpose of the irrigation. Take care not to block the outward flow of the solution with the syringe.
- Assist the client to a side-lying position on the affected side. *Lying with the affected side down helps drain the excess fluid by gravity.*
- Place a cotton fluff in the auditory meatus to absorb the excess fluid.

9. Assess the client's response.

- Assess the character and amount of discharge, appearance of the canal, discomfort, and so on, immediately after the instillation and again when the medication is expected to act. Inspect the cotton ball for any drainage.

10. **Document** all nursing assessments and interventions relative to the procedure. Include the name of the drug or irrigating solution, the strength, the number of drops if a liquid medication, the time, and the response of the client.

AGE-RELATED CONSIDERATIONS

Administering Otic Medications

Infant/Child

- Obtain assistance to immobilize an infant or young child. This prevents accidental injury due to sudden movement during the procedure.
- In infants and children under 3 years of age, the ear canal is directed upward. For an infant, gently pull the pinna down and back (Figures 27-7 ◆ and

27-8 ◆). For a child older than 3 years of age, pull the pinna upward and backward (see Figure 27-5).

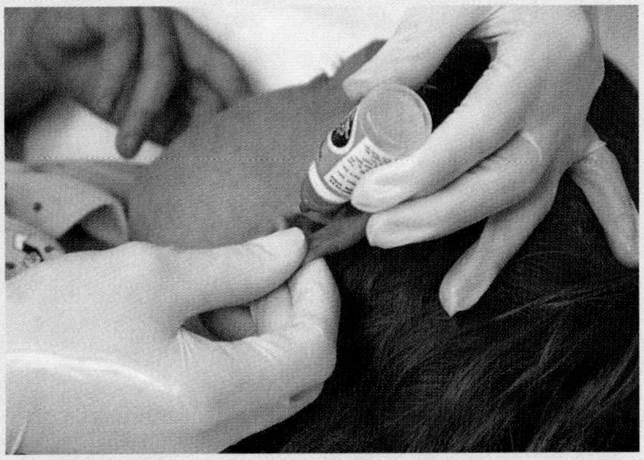

FIGURE 27-7 ◆ Straightening the ear canal of a child by pulling the pinna down and back.

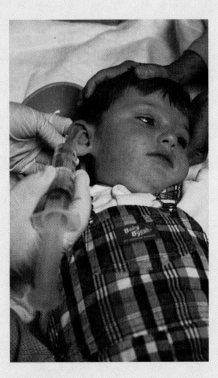

FIGURE 27-8 ◆ Ear irrigation.

EVALUATION

- Perform follow-up based on findings of the effectiveness of the administration or outcomes that deviated from expected or normal for the client. Relate findings to previous data if available.
- Report significant deviations from normal to the physician.

Nasal Medications

Nasal instillations (nose drops) usually are instilled for their astringent effect (to shrink swollen mucous membranes), to loosen secretions and facilitate drainage, or to treat infections of the nasal cavity or sinuses. Nasal instillations are sometimes intended for the nasal sinuses, which are hollow cavities in the facial bones. There are four groups of sinuses: sphenoid, ethmoid, frontal, and maxillary. The sinuses are lined with mucous membrane, which is continuous with the mucous membrane of the nasal passage.

Nursing Process: Nasal Medications

ASSESSMENT

- If nasal secretions are excessive, ask the client to blow the nose to clear the nasal passages.
- Inspect the discharge on the tissues for color, odor, and thickness.

In addition to the assessment performed by the nurse related to the administration of any medications (see Chapter 26), prior to applying nasal medications, assess:

- Appearance of nasal cavities
- Congestion of the mucous membranes and any obstruction to breathing. Ask the client to hold one nostril closed and blow out gently through the other nostril. Listen for the sound of any obstruction to the air. Repeat for the other nostril.
- Assess signs of distress when nares are occluded. Block each naris and observe for signs of greater distress when the naris is obstructed.
- Facial discomfort with or without palpation. An infected or congested sinus can cause an aching, full feeling over the area of the sinus and facial tenderness on palpation.
- Assess any crusting, redness, bleeding, or discharge of the mucous membranes of the nostrils. Use a nasal speculum. The membrane normally appears moist, pink, and shiny.

Determine if assessment data influences administration of the medication (i.e., is it appropriate to administer the medication or does the medication need to be held or the physician notified?).

PLANNING

Delegation

Due to the need for assessment and interpretation of client status, nasal medication administration is not delegated to UAP.

IMPLEMENTATION:
TECHNIQUE 27-4 ADMINISTERING NASAL MEDICATIONS

Equipment

- Tissues
- Correct medication bottle with a dropper

Preparation

1. Check the MAR.
   - Check the MAR for the drug name, strength, and number of drops. Also confirm the prescribed frequency of the instillation and which side of the nose is to be treated.
   - If the MAR is unclear or pertinent information is missing, compare it with the most recent physician's written order.
   - Report any discrepancies to the charge nurse or physician, as agency policy dictates.
2. Know the reason why the client is receiving the medication, the drug classification, contraindications, usual dose range, side effects, and nursing considerations for administering and evaluating the intended outcomes of the medication.

Performance

1. Compare the label on the medication container with the medication record and check the expiration date.
2. If necessary, calculate the medication dosage.
3. Explain to the client what you are going to do, why it is necessary, and how he or she can cooperate. The administration of nasal medication is not usually painful. Discuss how the results will be used in planning further care or treatments.
4. Wash hands and observe appropriate infection control procedures.
5. Provide for client privacy.

6. Prepare the client.
   - Check the client's identification band, and ask the client's name. *This ensures that the right client receives the medication.*
7. Assist the client to a comfortable position.
   - To treat the opening of the eustachian tube, have the client assume a back-lying position. *The drops will flow into the nasopharynx, where the eustachian tube opens.*
   - To treat the ethmoid and sphenoid sinuses, have the client take a back-lying position with the head over the edge of the bed or a pillow under the shoulders so that the head is tipped backward. This is called the *Proetz position* (Figure 27-9 ◆).
   - To treat the maxillary and frontal sinuses, have the client assume the same back-lying position, with the head turned toward the side to be treated. This is called the *Parkinson position* (Figure 27-10 ◆). If only one side is to be treated, be sure the person is positioned so that the correct side is accessible. If the client's head is over the edge of the bed, support it with your hand so that the neck muscles are not strained.

8. Administer the medication.
   - Draw up the required amount of solution into the dropper.
   - Hold the tip of the dropper just above the nostril, and direct the solution laterally toward the midline of the superior concha of the ethmoid bone as the client breathes through the mouth. Do not touch the mucous membrane of the nares. *If the solution is directed toward the base of the nasal cavity, it will run down the eustachian tube. Touching the mucous membrane with the dropper could damage the membrane and cause the client to sneeze.*
   - Repeat for the other nostril if indicated.
   - Ask the client to remain in the position for 5 minutes. *The client remains in the same position to help the solution come in contact with all of the nasal surface or flow into the desired area.*
   - Discard any remaining solution in the dropper, and dispose of soiled supplies appropriately.

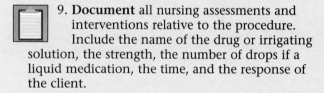

9. **Document** all nursing assessments and interventions relative to the procedure. Include the name of the drug or irrigating solution, the strength, the number of drops if a liquid medication, the time, and the response of the client.

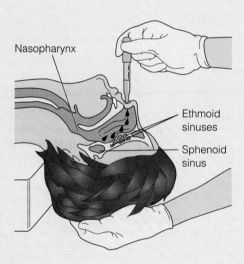

FIGURE 27-9 ◆ Instilling drops into the ethmoid and sphenoid sinuses.

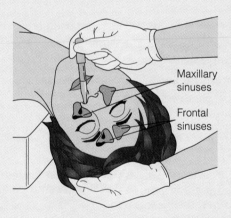

FIGURE 27-10 ◆ Instilling drops into the maxillary and frontal sinuses.

EVALUATION

- Perform follow-up based on findings of the effectiveness of the administration or outcomes that deviated from expected or normal for the client. Relate findings to previous data if available.
- Report significant deviations from normal to the physician.

Vaginal Medications

Vaginal medications, or instillations, are inserted as creams, jellies, foams, or suppositories to relieve infection or to relieve vaginal discomfort (e.g., itching or pain). Medical aseptic technique is usually used. Vaginal creams, jellies, and foams are applied by using a tubular applicator with a plunger. **Suppositories** are inserted with the index finger of a gloved hand. Suppositories are designed to melt at body temperature, so they are generally stored in the refrigerator to keep them firm for insertion.

A vaginal irrigation (douche) is the washing of the vagina by a liquid at a low pressure. Vaginal irrigations are not necessary for ordinary female hygiene but are used to prevent infection by applying an antimicrobial solution that discourages the growth of microorganisms, to remove an offensive or irritating discharge, and to reduce inflammation or prevent hemorrhage by the application of heat or cold.

In hospitals, sterile supplies and equipment are used; in a home, sterility is not usually necessary because people are accustomed to the microorganisms in their environments. Sterile technique is indicated if there is an open wound.

Nursing Process: Vaginal Medications

ASSESSMENT

In addition to the assessment performed by the nurse related to the administration of any medications (see Chapter 26), prior to applying vaginal medications, assess:

- The vaginal orifice for inflammation; amount, character, and odor of vaginal discharge

- For complaints of vaginal discomfort (e.g., burning or itching)

Determine if assessment data influences administration of the medication (i.e., is it appropriate to administer the medication or does the medication need to be held or the physician notified?).

PLANNING

Delegation

Due to the need for assessments and interpretation of client status, vaginal medication administration is not delegated to UAP.

IMPLEMENTATION:
TECHNIQUE 27-5 ADMINISTERING VAGINAL MEDICATIONS

Equipment

- Drape
- Correct vaginal suppository or cream
- Applicator for vaginal cream
- Clean gloves
- Lubricant for a suppository
- Disposable towel
- Clean perineal pad

For an irrigation, add:

- Moistureproof pad
- Vaginal irrigation set (these are often disposable) containing a nozzle, tubing and a clamp, and a container for the solution
- IV pole
- Irrigating solution

Preparation

1. Check the MAR.
   - Check the MAR for the drug name, strength, and prescribed frequency.
   - If the MAR is unclear or pertinent information is missing, compare it with the most recent physician's written order.
   - Report any discrepancies to the charge nurse or physician, as agency policy dictates.

2. Know the reason why the client is receiving the medication, the drug classification, contraindications, usual dose range, side effects, and nursing considerations for administering and evaluating the intended outcomes of the medication.

Performance

1. Compare the label on the medication container with the medication record and check the expiration date.

2. If necessary, calculate the medication dosage.

3. Explain to the client what you are going to do, why it is necessary, and how she can cooperate. Explain to the client that a vaginal instillation is normally a painless procedure, and in fact may bring relief from itching and burning if an infection is present. Many people feel embarrassed about this procedure, and some may prefer to perform the procedure themselves if instruction is provided. Discuss how the results will be used in planning further care or treatments.

4. Wash hands and observe appropriate infection control procedures.

5. Provide for client privacy.

6. Prepare the client.
   - Check the client's identification band, and ask the client's name. *This ensures that the right client receives the medication.*
   - Ask the client to void. *If the bladder is empty, the client will have less discomfort during the treatment, and the possibility of injuring the vaginal lining is decreased.*
   - Assist the client to a back-lying position with the knees flexed and the hips rotated laterally.
   - Drape the client appropriately so that only the perineal area is exposed.

7. Prepare the equipment.

- Unwrap the suppository, and put it on the opened wrapper.

  or

- Fill the applicator with the prescribed cream, jelly, or foam. Directions are provided with the manufacturer's applicator.

8. Assess and clean the perineal area.

- Don gloves. *Gloves prevent contamination of the nurse's hands from vaginal and perineal microorganisms.*

- Inspect the vaginal orifice, note any odor of discharge from the vagina, and ask about any vaginal discomfort.

- Provide perineal care to remove microorganisms. *This decreases the chance of moving microorganisms into the vagina.*

9. Administer the vaginal suppository, cream, foam, jelly, or irrigation.

Suppository

- Lubricate the rounded (smooth) end of the suppository, which is inserted first. *Lubrication facilitates insertion.*

- Lubricate your gloved index finger.

- Expose the vaginal orifice by separating the labia with your nondominant hand.

- Insert the suppository about 8 to 10 cm (3 to 4 in) along the posterior wall of the vagina, or as far as it will go (Figure 27-11 ◆). *The posterior wall of the vagina is about 2.5 cm (1 in) longer than the anterior wall because the cervix protrudes into the uppermost portion of the anterior wall.*

- Ask the client to remain lying in the supine position for 5 to 10 minutes following insertion. The hips may also be elevated on a pillow. *This position allows the medication to flow into the posterior fornix after it has melted.*

Vaginal Cream, Jelly, or Foam

- Gently insert the applicator about 5 cm (2 in).

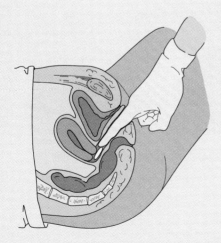

FIGURE 27-11 ◆ Instilling a vaginal suppository.

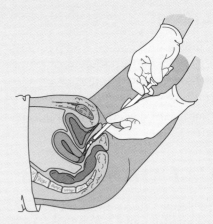

FIGURE 27-12 ◆ Using an applicator to instill a vaginal cream.

- Slowly push the plunger until the applicator is empty (Figure 27-12 ◆).

- Remove the applicator and place it on the towel. *The applicator is put on the towel to prevent the spread of microorganisms.*

- Discard the applicator if disposable or clean it according to the manufacturer's directions.

- Ask the client to remain lying in the supine position for 5 to 10 minutes following the insertion.

Irrigation

- Place the client on a bedpan.

- Clamp the tubing. Hang the irrigating container on the IV pole so that the base is about 30 cm (12 in) above the vagina. *At this height, the pressure of the solution should not be great enough to injure the vaginal lining.*

- Run fluid through the tubing and nozzle into the bedpan. *Fluid is run through the tubing to remove air and to moisten the nozzle.*

- Insert the nozzle carefully into the vagina. Direct the nozzle toward the sacrum, following the direction of the vagina.

- Insert the nozzle about 7 to 10 cm (3 to 4 in), start the flow, and rotate the nozzle several times. *Rotating the nozzle irrigates all parts of the vagina.*

- Use all the irrigating solution, permitting it to flow out freely into the bedpan.

- Remove the nozzle from the vagina.

- Assist the client to a sitting position on the bedpan. *Sitting on the bedpan will help drain the remaining fluid by gravity.*

10. Ensure client comfort.

- Dry the perineum with tissues as required.

- Apply a clean perineal pad if there is excessive drainage.

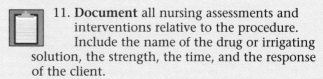 11. **Document** all nursing assessments and interventions relative to the procedure. Include the name of the drug or irrigating solution, the strength, the time, and the response of the client.

- Perform follow-up based on findings of the effectiveness of the administration or outcomes that deviated from expected or normal for the client. Relate findings to previous data if available.

- Report significant deviations from normal to the physician.

Inhaled Medications

Nebulizers deliver most medications administered through the inhaled route. A nebulizer is used to deliver a fine spray (fog or mist) of medication or moisture to a client.

There are two kinds of **nebulization:** atomization and aerosolization. In **atomization,** a device called an *atomizer* produces rather large droplets for inhalation. In *aerosolization,* the droplets are suspended in a gas, such as oxygen. The smaller the droplets, the further they can be inhaled into the respiratory tract. When a medication is intended for the nasal mucosa, it is inhaled through the nose; when it is intended for the trachea, bronchi, and/or lungs, it is inhaled through the mouth.

A *large-volume nebulizer* can provide a heated or cool mist. It is used for long-term therapy, such as that following a tracheostomy. The *ultrasonic nebulizer* (Figure 27-13 ◆) provides 100 percent humidity and can provide particles small enough to be inhaled deeply into the respiratory tract.

The *metered dose (handheld) nebulizer* (Figure 27-14 ◆) is a pressurized container of medication that can be used by the client to release the medication through a nosepiece or mouthpiece. The force with which the air moves through the nebulizer causes the large particles of medicated solution to break up into finer particles, forming a mist or fine spray.

Nursing Process: Inhaled Medications

ASSESSMENT

In addition to the assessment performed by the nurse related to the administration of any medications (see Chapter 26), prior to administering medications with a **metered dose inhaler (MDI)**, assess:

- Lung sounds
- Respiratory rate and depth
- Cough (productive or nonproductive), amount, color, and character of expectorations

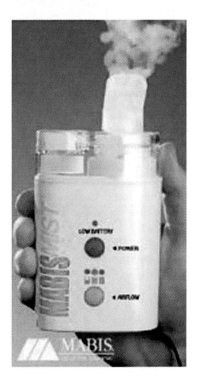

FIGURE 27-13 ◆ Ultrasonic nebulizer.

- Presence of dyspnea
- Vital signs for baseline data

See Chapter 3 for assessment of the chest lung sounds.

Determine if assessment data influences administration of the medication (i.e., is it appropriate to administer the medication or does the medication need to be held or the physician notified?).

PLANNING

Delegation

Due to the need for assessment and interpretation of client status, inhaled medication administration is not delegated to UAP.

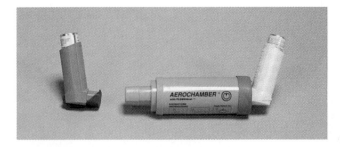

FIGURE 27-14 ◆ Metered dose inhaler.

Equipment

• Metered dose nebulizer with medication canister and extender if indicated

Preparation

1. Check the MAR.
   • Check the MAR for the drug name, strength, and prescribed frequency.
   • If the MAR is unclear or pertinent information is missing, compare it with the most recent physician's written order.
   • Report any discrepancies to the charge nurse or physician, as agency policy dictates.
2. Know the reason why the client is receiving the medication, the drug classification, contraindications, usual dose range, side effects, and nursing considerations for administering and evaluating the intended outcomes of the medication.

Performance

1. Compare the label on the medication container with the medication record and check the expiration date.
2. If necessary, calculate the medication dosage.
3. Explain to the client what you are going to do, why it is necessary, and how he or she can cooperate. Discuss how the results will be used in planning further care or treatments.
4. Wash hands and observe appropriate infection control procedures.
5. Provide for client privacy.
6. Prepare the client.
   • Check the client's identification band, and ask the client's name. *This ensures that the right client receives the medication.*
   • Explain that this nebulizer delivers a measured dose of drug with each push of the medication canister, which fits into the top of the nebulizer.
7. Instruct the client to use the metered dose nebulizer as follows:
   • Check the label to see if the canister should be shaken (most should).
   • Inhale and exhale deeply for several breaths through the nose.
   • Place the mouthpiece of the nebulizer into the mouth with its opening toward the throat or hold the mouthpiece 1 to 2 inches from the open mouth (Figure 27-15 ◆). For a nasal instillation,

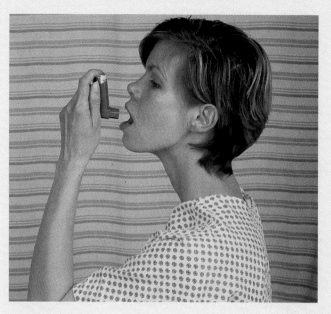

FIGURE 27-15 ◆ Inhaler positioned away from the open mouth.

hold a naris closed and place the nosepiece at the opening of the naris.
   • Then inhale slowly and deeply through the mouth while releasing the dose. The dose is released by pressing down on the medication canister.
   • Hold the breath for 10 seconds. *This allows the aerosol to reach deeper airways.*
   • Exhale slowly through pursed lips. *Controlled exhalation keeps the small airways open during exhalation.*
   • Repeat the inhalation if ordered. Allow 1 minute between inhalations of bronchodilator medications *so the first inhalation has a chance to work and the subsequent dose reaches deeper into the lungs.*
   • Repeat for other naris if administering a nasal instillation.
   • Rinse the mouth to remove any remaining medication.
8. Caution the client about overuse of the nebulizer.
   • Tolerance to the medication and serious side effects (e.g., bronchospasm or adverse cardiac effects) may result.

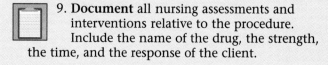

9. **Document** all nursing assessments and interventions relative to the procedure. Include the name of the drug, the strength, the time, and the response of the client.

- Perform follow-up based on findings of the effectiveness of the medication or outcomes that deviated from expected or normal for the client. Relate findings to previous data if available.
- Report significant deviations from normal to the physician.

Rectal Medications

Insertion of medications into the rectum in the form of suppositories is a frequent practice. Rectal administration is a convenient and safe method of giving certain medications. Advantages include the following:

- It avoids irritation of the upper gastrointestinal tract in clients who encounter this problem.
- It is advantageous when the medication has an objectionable taste or odor.
- The drug is released at a slow but steady rate.
- Rectal suppositories are thought to provide higher bloodstream levels (titers) of medication, because the venous blood from the lower rectum is not transported through the liver.

Nursing Process: Rectal Medications

ASSESSMENT

In addition to the assessment performed by the nurse related to the administration of any medications (see Chapter 26), prior to administering rectal medications, assess:

- Client's need for the medication if PRN (e.g., abdominal distention and/or discomfort if the suppository is intended to stimulate defecation)
- Whether the client desires to defecate or time of last defecation (suppositories that are given for a systemic effect should be given when the rectum is free of feces to enhance absorption of the drug)
- Any side effects; any contraindications to the rectal route (e.g., recent rectal surgery or rectal pathology, such as bleeding)

PLANNING

Delegation

Due to the need for assessment and interpretation of client status, rectal medication administration is not delegated to UAP.

IMPLEMENTATION:
TECHNIQUE 27-7 ADMINISTERING RECTAL MEDICATIONS

Equipment

- Correct suppository
- Clean glove
- Lubricant

Preparation

1. Check the MAR.
   - Check the MAR for the drug name, strength, and prescribed frequency.
   - If the MAR is unclear or pertinent information is missing, compare it with the most recent physician's written order.
   - Report any discrepancies to the charge nurse or physician, as agency policy dictates.
2. Know the reason why the client is receiving the medication, the drug classification, contraindications, usual dose range, side effects, and nursing considerations for administering and evaluating the intended outcomes of the medication.

Performance

1. Compare the label on the medication container with the medication record and check the expiration date.

2. If necessary, calculate the medication dosage.

3. Explain to the client what you are going to do, why it is necessary, and how he or she can cooperate. Discuss how the results will be used in planning further care or treatments.

4. Wash hands and observe appropriate infection control procedures.

5. Provide for client privacy.

6. Prepare the client.
   - Check the client's identification band, and ask the client's name. *This ensures that the right client receives the medication.*
   - Assist the client to a left lateral position with the upper leg acutely flexed.
   - Fold back the top bedclothes to expose only the buttocks.

7. Prepare the equipment.
   - Unwrap the suppository, and leave it on the opened wrapper.
   - Don the glove on the hand to be used to insert the suppository. *The glove prevents contamination of the nurse's hand by rectal microorganisms and feces.*
   - Lubricate the smooth, rounded end of the sup-

pository, or see the manufacturer's instructions. *The smooth, rounded end is inserted first. Lubrication prevents anal friction and tissue damage on insertion.*

- Lubricate the gloved index finger.

8. Insert the suppository.

- Ask the client to breathe through the mouth. *This usually relaxes the external anal sphincter.*

- Insert the suppository gently into the anus, rounded end first (or according to the manufacturer's instructions) and along the wall of the rectum with the gloved index finger. For an adult, insert the suppository 10 cm (4 in) (Figure 27-16 ◆). *The rounded end facilitates insertion. The suppository needs to be placed along the wall of the rectum, rather than amid feces, in order to be absorbed effectively.*

- Withdraw the finger. Press the client's buttocks together for a several seconds. *This helps minimize any urge to expel the suppository.*

- Remove the glove by turning it inside out. *Turning the glove inside out contains the rectal microorganisms and prevents their spread.* Wash your hands.

- Ask the client to remain flat or in the left lateral position for at least 5 minutes. *This helps prevent expulsion of the suppository.* The suppository should be retained at least 30 to 40 minutes or according to manufacturer's instructions.

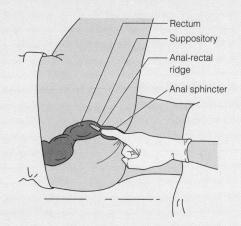

FIGURE 27-16 ◆ Instilling a rectal suppository.

- If the client has been given a laxative suppository, place the call light within easy reach to summon assistance for the bedpan or toilet.

9. **Document** all nursing assessments and interventions relative to the procedure. Include the type of suppository given/name of the drug, the time it was given, the amount of time it was retained if it was expelled, the results or effects, and the response of the client.

AMBULATORY AND COMMUNITY SETTINGS

Topical Medications

- Many topical medications are used by the client at home or applied in the clinic or outpatient setting. The client and family must be taught how to administer the medication and what effects to anticipate. Use diagrams to show techniques such as vaginal medication administration.

- Disinfect equipment such as metered dose inhaler mouthpieces weekly by soaking for 20 minutes in 1 pint of water with 2 ounces of vinegar added.

- Teach clients how to determine the amount of medication remaining in a metered dose inhaler canister:

- Put the canister (without the mouthpiece) in a tub of cold water. If it sinks, it is full. If it floats on the surface, it is empty. If it floats straight up

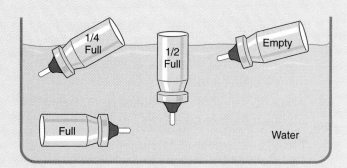

FIGURE 27-17 ◆ Floating an MDI canister to determine the amount remaining.

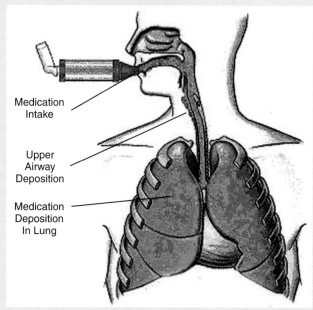

FIGURE 27-18 ◆ Delivery of medication to the lungs using a metered dose inhaler extender.

Topical Medications (continued)

and down with the delivery spout down, it is half full (Figure 27-17 ◆).

- Calculate the number of days' doses in a canister. Divide the number of doses (puffs) in the canister (on the label) by the number of puffs taken per day.

- Review instructions for using an inhaler spacer or chamber. Research shows that these devices assist in delivering the medication deeply into the lungs rather than only to the oropharynx (Figure 27-18 ◆).

AGE-RELATED CONSIDERATIONS

Administering Rectal Medications

Infant/Child

- Obtain assistance to immobilize an infant or young child. This prevents accidental injury due to sudden movement during the procedure.

- For a child or infant, insert a suppository 5 cm (2 in) or less.

EVALUATION

- Perform follow-up based on findings of the effectiveness of the administration or outcomes that deviated from expected or normal for the client. Relate findings to previous data if available.

- Report significant deviations from normal to the physician.

Chapter Summary

TERMINOLOGY

aerosolization
atomization
dermatologic preparation
inhalation

instillation
irrigation
metered dose inhaler (MDI)
nebulization

pruritus
suppository
transdermal patch

FORMING CLINICAL JUDGMENTS

Consider This:

1. The client observes you putting on gloves before applying ordered topical cream. You are asked why you wear them since the client doesn't wear gloves at home when applying the cream. What would be your response?

2. Your client is scheduled for cataract surgery on the right eye. You have an order for antibiotic eye drops OS q1h × 4 before surgery at 10 A.M. Would you question any of these orders? If so, why?

3. Eardrops are administered with the affected ear upward, whereas ear irrigations are performed with the affected ear facing downward. Explain the rationale for this.

4. Would sterile or clean technique be indicated for administration of nose drops? Explain your answer.

5. The client has been using vaginal cream at home for a yeast infection but the infection remains. What questions would you ask to determine if

the client has been performing the cream application properly?

6. The client has just started using a bronchodilator metered dose inhaler for asthma. After a few days, the client reports the inhaler is not providing any relief—just making the client jittery.

What might explain this? What would you suggest?

7. Your client requires a rectal suppository but is unable to lie on the left side. How will you administer the suppository?

RELATED RESEARCH

Foss, S. A., & Keppel, J. W. (1999). In vitro testing of MIDI spacers: A technique for measuring respirable dose-output with actuation in-phase or out-of-phase with inhalation. *Respiratory Care, 44*(12), 1474–1485.

REFERENCES

Blawat, D., & Banks, P. (1997). Comforting touch: Using topical skin preparations. *Nursing, 27*(5), 46–48.

Cochrane, M. G., Bala, M. V., Down, K. E., Mauskopf, J., & Ben-Joseph, R. H. (2000). Inhaled corticosteroids for asthma therapy: Patient compliance, devices, and inhalation technique. *Chest, 117*(2), 542–550.

Gazarian, P. K. (1997). Teaching your patient to use a metered-dose inhaler: The direct route to asthma therapy. *Nursing, 27*(10), 52–54.

McConnell, E. A. (1997). Clinical do's and don'ts: Using transdermal medication patches. *Nursing, 27*(7), 18.

Miller, C. A. (1998). Drug consult: Keeping an eye on the hidden effects of eye drops. *Geriatric Nursing: American Journal of Care for the Aging, 19*, 293–294.

Woodcock, A. (1997). Use of spacers with metered dose inhalers. *Lancet, 349*(9050), 446.

Chapter 28

Administering Parenteral Medications

Techniques

OBJECTIVES

- Identify equipment required for parenteral medications.
- Identify essential aspects of preparing medications from ampules and vials.
- Describe how to mix selected drugs from vials and ampules.
- Identify sites used for subcutaneous, intramuscular, and intradermal injections.
- Describe essential steps for safely administering parenteral medications by intradermal, subcutaneous, intramuscular, and intravenous routes.
- Describe the benefits for using the following analgesic delivery routes: patient-controlled analgesia (PCA), epidural analgesia, and continuous local anesthetics.

Parenteral administration is administration other than through the alimentary tract; that is, by needle. Nurses give parenteral medications intradermally (ID), subcutaneously (SC or SQ), intramuscularly (IM), or intravenously (IV). Because these medications are absorbed more quickly than oral medications and are irretrievable once injected, the nurse must prepare and administer them carefully and accurately. Administering parenteral drugs requires the same nursing knowledge as for oral and topical drugs; however, because injections are invasive procedures, aseptic technique must be used to minimize the risk of infection.

Equipment

Syringes

To administer parenteral medications, nurses use injectable equipment (i.e., syringes, needles, vials, and ampules). Syringes have three parts: the tip, which connects with the needle; the barrel, or outside part, on which the scales are printed; and the plunger, which fits inside the barrel (Figure 28-1 ◆). When handling a syringe, the nurse may touch the outside of the barrel and the handle of the plunger; however, the nurse must *avoid letting any unsterile object contact the tip or inside of the barrel, the shaft of the plunger, or the shaft or tip of the needle.*

There are several kinds of syringes differing in size, shape, and material. The three most commonly used types are the standard hypodermic syringe, the insulin syringe, and the tuberculin syringe (Figure 28-2 ◆). **Hypodermic syringes** come in 2-, 2.5-, and 3-mL sizes. They usually have two scales marked on them: the minim and the milliliter. The milliliter scale is the one normally used; the minim scale is used for very small dosages.

Insulin syringes are similar to hypodermic syringes, but they have a scale specially designed for insulin: a

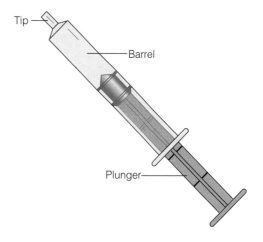

FIGURE 28-1 ◆ The three parts of a syringe.

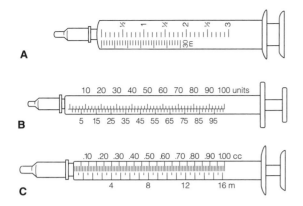

FIGURE 28-2 ◆ Three kinds of syringes: (A) hypodermic syringe marked in tenths (0.1) of milliliters and in minims; (B) insulin syringe marked in 100 units; (C) tuberculin syringe marked in tenths and hundredths (0.01) of cubic millimeters and in minims.

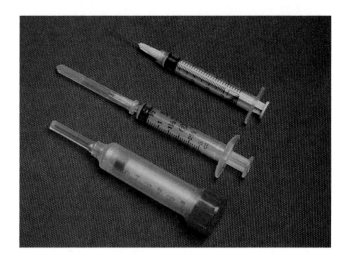

FIGURE 28-3 ◆ Disposable plastic syringes and needles: *top*, with syringe and needle exposed; *middle*, with plastic cap over the needle; *bottom*, with plastic case over the needle and syringe.

100-unit calibrated scale intended for use with U-100 insulin. Several low-dose insulin syringes with a 30- or 50-unit calibrated scale are also available and frequently have a nonremovable needle. All insulin syringes are calibrated on the 100-unit scale in North America. The correct choice of syringe is based on the amount of insulin required.

The **tuberculin syringe** was originally designed to administer tuberculin. It is a narrow syringe, calibrated in tenths and hundredths of a milliliter (up to 1 mL) on one scale and in sixteenths of a minim (up to 1 minim) on the other scale. This type of syringe can also be useful in administering other drugs, particularly when small or precise measurement is indicated (e.g., pediatric dosages).

Syringes are made in other sizes as well (e.g., 5, 10, 20, and 50 mL). These are not generally used to administer drugs directly but can be useful for adding medications to intravenous solutions or for irrigating wounds. The tip of a syringe varies and is classified as either a Luer-Lok or non–Luer-Lok. A Luer-Lok syringe has a tip that requires the needle to be twisted onto it to avoid an accidental removal of the needle. The non–Luer-Lok syringe has a smooth graduated tip and needles slip onto the tip. The non–Luer-Lok syringe is often used for irrigation purposes (e.g., wounds, tubes).

Most syringes used today are made of plastic and are individually packaged for sterility in a paper wrapper or a rigid plastic container (Figure 28-3 ◆). The syringe and needle may be packaged together or separately.

Injectable medications are frequently supplied in disposable **prefilled unit-dose systems**. These are available as (1) prefilled syringes ready for use or (2) prefilled sterile cartridges and needles that require the attachment of a reusable holder (injection system) before use (Figure 28-4 ◆). Examples of the latter system are the Tubex and Carpuject injection systems. The manufacturers provide specific directions for use. Because most prefilled cartridges are overfilled, excess medication must be ejected before the injection to ensure the accurate dosage. Because the needle is fused to the syringe, the nurse cannot change the gauge or length of the needle. The nurse, however, can transfer the medication into a regular syringe if the assessment of the client necessitates a different needle gauge or length.

Needles

Needles are made of stainless steel, and most are disposable. Reusable needles (e.g., for special procedures) need to be sharpened periodically before resterilization because the points become dull with use and are occasionally damaged or acquire burrs on the tips. A dull or damaged needle must *never* be used.

A needle has three discernible parts: the **hub**, which fits onto the syringe; the **cannula**, or **shaft**, which is attached to the hub; and the **bevel**, which is the slanted part at the tip of the needle (Figure 28-5 ◆). A disposable needle has a plastic hub. Needles used for injections have three variable characteristics:

1. *Slant or length of the bevel.* The bevel of the needle may be short or long. Longer bevels provide the sharpest needles and cause less discomfort and are commonly used for subcutaneous and intramuscular injections. Short bevels are used for intradermal and intravenous injections because a long bevel can become occluded if it rests against the side of a blood vessel.

2. *Length of the shaft.* The shaft length of commonly used needles varies from ½ to 2 inches. The appropriate needle length is chosen according to the client's muscle development, the client's weight, and the type of injection.

3. *Gauge (diameter) of the shaft.* The gauge varies from 18 to 28. The larger the gauge number, the

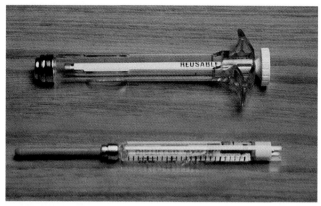

A

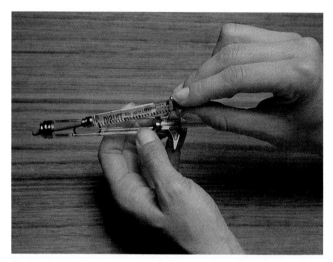

B

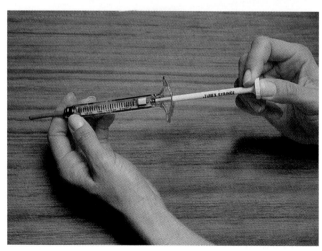

C

FIGURE 28-4 ◆ (A) syringe and prefilled sterile cartridge with needle; (B) assembling the device—the cartridge slides into the syringe barrel, turns, and locks at the needle end; (C) the plunger then screws into the cartridge end.

smaller the diameter of the shaft. Smaller gauges produce less tissue trauma, but larger gauges are necessary for viscous medications, such as penicillin.

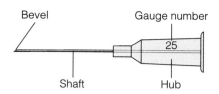

FIGURE 28-5 ◆ The parts of a needle.

For an adult requiring a subcutaneous injection, it is usual to use a needle of 24 to 26 gauge and ⅜ to ⅝ inch long. Obese clients may require a 1-inch needle. For intramuscular injections, a longer needle (e.g., 1 to 1½ inches) with a larger gauge (e.g., 20 to 22 gauge) is used. Slender adults and children usually require a shorter needle. The nurse must assess the client to determine the appropriate needle length.

Preventing Needle-Stick Injuries

One of the most potentially hazardous procedures that health care personnel face is using and disposing of needles and sharps. Needle-stick injuries present a major risk for infection with hepatitis B virus, human immunodeficiency virus (HIV), and many other pathogens. Standards have been set by the Occupational Safety and Health Administration (OSHA) to prevent such injuries. Some of these are summarized in Box 28-1. If an accidental needle-stick injury occurs, the nurse must follow specific steps outlined by the agency.

Safety syringes have been designed to protect health care workers. Safety devices are categorized as either *passive* or *active*. The nurse does not need to activate the passive safety device. For example, for some syringes, after injection, the needle retracts immediately into the barrel (Figure 28-6 ◆). In contrast, the active safety device requires the nurse to manually activate the safety feature. For example, the nurse activates a mechanism to retract the needle into the syringe barrel or the nurse, after injection, manually pulls a plastic sheath or guard over the needle (Figure 28-7 ◆).

Preparing Injectable Medications

Techniques to prepare injectable medications include withdrawing the medication from an ampule or vial into a sterile syringe, using prefilled syringes or using needleless injection systems. See Figure 28-8 ◆ for an example of a needleless system used to access medication from a vial.

Ampules and Vials

Ampules and vials (Figure 28-9 ◆) are frequently used to package sterile parenteral medications. An **ampule**

Box 28-1 *Avoiding Puncture Injuries*

- Use appropriate puncture-proof disposal containers to dispose of *uncapped* needles and sharps. These are provided in all client areas. Never throw sharps in wastebaskets. **Sharps** include any items that can cut or puncture skin such as:

Needles

Surgical blades

Lancets

Razors

Broken glass

Broken capillary pipettes

Exposed dental wires

Reusable items (e.g., large-bore needles, hooks, rasps, drill points)

ANY SHARP INSTRUMENT!

- Never bend or break needles before disposal.
- Never recap used needles except under specified circumstances (e.g., when transporting a syringe to the laboratory for an arterial blood gas or blood culture).
- When recapping a needle:
  - Use a safety mechanical device that firmly grips the needle cap and holds it in place until it is ready to recap.
  - Use a one-handed "scoop" method. This is performed by (1) placing the needle cap and syringe with needle horizontally on a flat surface, (2) inserting the needle into the cap, using one hand, and then (3) using your other hand to pick up the cap and tighten it to the needle hub.

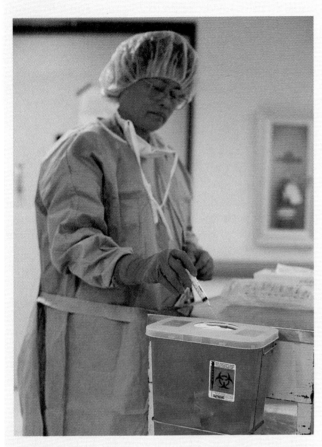

A disposal container for contaminated needles and other sharps.

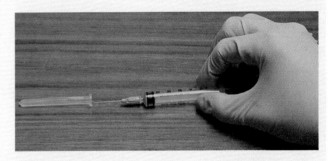

Recapping a used needle using the scoop method.

From *Fundamentals of nursing: Concepts, process, and practice*, 6th ed., by B. Kozier, G. Erb, A. Berman, & K. Burke, 2000, Upper Saddle River, NJ: Prentice Hall Health.

is a glass container usually designed to hold a single dose of a drug. It is made of clear glass and has a distinctive shape with a constricted neck. Ampules vary in size ranging from 1 mL to 10 mL or more. Most ampule necks have colored marks around them, indicating where they are prescored for easy opening.

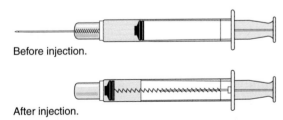

Before injection.

After injection.

FIGURE 28-6 ◆ Passive safety device. The needle retracts immediately into the barrel after injection.

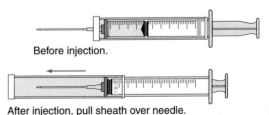

Before injection.

After injection, pull sheath over needle.

FIGURE 28-7 ◆ Active safety device. The nurse manually pulls the sheath or guard over the needle after injection.

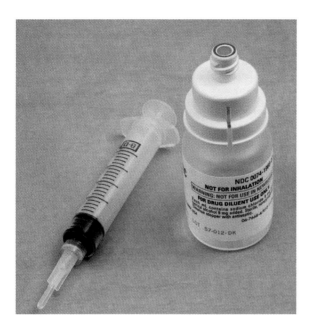

FIGURE 28-8 ◆ A needleless system can extract medicine from a vial.

To access the medication in an ampule, the ampule must be broken at the mark on its constricted neck. Traditionally, a small file is used to score the ampule. Once the ampule is broken, the fluid is aspirated into a syringe.

A **vial** is a small glass bottle with a sealed rubber cap. Vials come in different sizes, from single to multidose vials. They usually have a plastic cap that protects the rubber seal. To access the medication in a vial, the vial must be pierced with a needle or a needleless access system. In addition, air must be injected into a vial before the medication can be withdrawn. Failure to inject air before withdrawing the medication leaves a vacuum within the vial that makes withdrawal difficult.

Several drugs (e.g., penicillin) are dispensed as powders in vials. A liquid (solvent or diluent) must be added to a powdered medication before it can be injected. The technique of adding a **diluent** to a powdered drug to prepare it for administration is called **reconstitution**. Powdered drugs usually have printed instructions (enclosed with each packaged vial) that describe the amount and kind of diluent to be added. Commonly used diluents are sterile water or sterile normal saline. Some preparations are supplied in individual-dose vials; others come in multidose vials. Following are two examples of the preparation of powdered drugs:

1. *Single-dose vial:* Instructions for preparing a single-dose vial direct that 1.5 mL of sterile water be added to the sterile dry powder, thus providing a single dose of 2 mL. The volume of the drug powder was 0.5 mL. Therefore, the 1.5 mL of sterile water plus the 0.5 mL of powder results in 2 mL of solution. In other instances, the addition of a solution does *not* increase the volume. Therefore, it is very important to precisely follow the manufacturer's directions to avoid a medication error.

2. *Multidose vial:* A dose of 750 mg of a certain drug is ordered for a client. On hand is a 10-gram multidose vial. The directions for preparation read: "Add 8.5 mL of sterile water and each milliliter will contain 1.0 gram or 1,000 mg." To determine the amount to inject, the nurse calculates as follows:

1 mL = 1,000 mg

× mL = 750 mg

Cross multiply

× = 0.75

The nurse will give 0.75 mL of the medication.

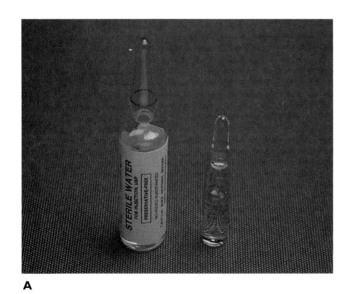

A

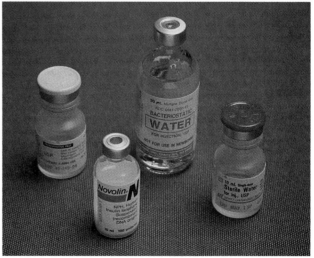

B

FIGURE 28-9 ◆ (A) ampules; (B) vials.

Glass and rubber particulate have been found in medications withdrawn from ampules and vials using a regular needle. As a result, it is strongly recommended that the nurse use a filter needle when withdrawing medications from ampules and vials to prevent withdrawing glass and rubber particles. After drawing the medication into the syringe, the filter needle is replaced with the regular needle for injection. This prevents tracking of the medication through the client's tissues during the insertion of the needle which minimizes discomfort.

Techniques 28-1 and 28-2 describe how to prepare medications from ampules and vials.

Nursing Process: Preparing Injectable Medications

ASSESSMENT

- Assess
  - Client allergies to medication
  - Specific drug action, side effects, interactions, and adverse reactions

- Client's knowledge of and learning needs about the medication
- Intended route of parenteral medication to determine appropriate size of syringe and needle for the client
- Ordered medication for clarity and expiration date
- Perform appropriate assessments (e.g., vital signs, laboratory results) specific to the medication.
- Determine if the assessment data influences administration of the medication (i.e., is it appropriate to administer the medication or does the medication need to be held and/or the physician notified?).

PLANNING

Delegation

Preparing medications from ampules and vials involves knowledge and use of aseptic technique. Therefore, these techniques are not delegated to unlicensed assistive personnel (UAP).

IMPLEMENTATION:
TECHNIQUE 28-1 USING MEDICATION AMPULES

Equipment

- MAR or computer printout
- Ampule of sterile medication
- File (if ampule is not scored) and small gauze square
- Antiseptic swabs
- Needle and syringe
- Filter needle

Preparation

1. Check the medication administration order (MAR).
   - Check the label on the ampule carefully against the MAR to make sure that the correct medication is being prepared.
   - Follow the three checks for administering medications. Read the label on the medication (1) when it is taken from the medication cart, (2) before withdrawing the medication, and (3) after withdrawing the medication.

2. Organize the equipment.

Performance

1. Wash hands and observe other appropriate infection control procedures.

2. Prepare the medication ampule for drug withdrawal.
   - Flick the upper stem of the ampule several times with a fingernail, or, holding the upper stem of the ampule, shake the ampule similar to shaking down a mercury thermometer. *This will bring all the medication down to the main portion of the ampule.*
   - Partially file the neck of the ampule, if necessary, to start a clean break.
   - Place a piece of sterile gauze between your thumb and the ampule neck or around the ampule neck, and break off the top by bending it toward you (Figure 28-10 ◆). *The sterile gauze protects the fin-*

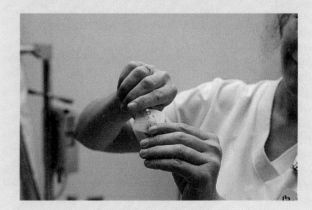

FIGURE 28-10 ◆ Breaking the neck of an ampule.

gers from the broken glass and any glass fragments will spray away from the nurse.

or

- Place the antiseptic wipe packet over the top of the ampule before breaking off the top. *This method ensures that all the glass fragments fall into the packet and reduces the risk of cuts.*

- Dispose of the top of the ampule in the sharps container.

3. Withdraw the medication.

- Place the ampule on a flat surface.

- Using a **filter needle** to withdraw the medication, disconnect the regular needle, leaving its cap on, and attach the filter needle to the syringe. *The filter needle prevents glass particles from being withdrawn with the medication.*

- Remove the cap from the filter needle and insert the needle into the center of the ampule. Do not touch the rim of the ampule with the needle tip or shaft. *This will keep the needle sterile.* Withdraw the amount of drug required for the dosage.

- With a single-dose ampule, hold the ampule slightly on its side, if necessary, to obtain all the medication (Figure 28-11 ◆).

- Replace the filter needle with a regular needle and tighten the cap at the hub of the needle before injecting the client.

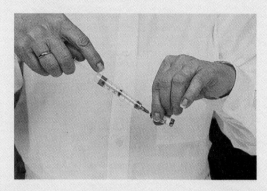

FIGURE 28-11 ◆ Withdrawing a medication from an ampule.

IMPLEMENTATION:
TECHNIQUE 28-2 USING MEDICATION VIALS

Equipment

- MAR or computer printout
- Vial of sterile medication
- Antiseptic swabs
- Needle and syringe
- Filter needle (check agency policy)
- Sterile water or normal saline, if drug is in powdered form

Preparation

Same preparation as described in Technique 28-1.

Performance

1. Wash hands and observe other appropriate infection control procedures.

2. Prepare the medication vial for drug withdrawal.

- Mix the solution, if necessary, by rotating the vial between the palms of the hands, not by shaking. *Some vials contain aqueous suspensions, which settle when they stand. In some instances, shaking is contraindicated because it may cause the mixture to foam.*

- Remove the protective cap, or clean the rubber cap of a previously opened vial with an antiseptic wipe by rubbing in a circular motion. *The antiseptic cleans the cap of dust or grease and reduces the number of microorganisms.*

3. Withdraw the medication.

- Attach a filter needle, as agency practice dictates, to draw up premixed liquid medications from multidose vials. *Using the filter needle prevents any solid particles from being drawn up through the needle.*

- Ensure that the needle is firmly attached to the syringe.

- Remove the cap from the needle, then draw up into the syringe the amount of air equal to the volume of the medication to be withdrawn.

- Carefully insert the needle into the upright vial through the center of the rubber cap, maintaining the sterility of the needle.

- Inject the air into the vial, keeping the bevel of the needle above the surface of the medication (Figure 28-12 ◆). *The air will allow the medication to be drawn out easily because negative pressure will not be created inside the vial. The bevel is kept above the medication to avoid creating bubbles in the medication.*

- Withdraw the prescribed amount of medication using either of the following methods:

  a. Hold the vial down (i.e., with the base lower than the top), move the needle tip so that it is below the fluid level, and withdraw the medication (Figure 28-13 ◆). Avoid drawing up the last drops of the vial. *Proponents of this method say that keeping the vial in the upright position while withdrawing the medication allows particulate matter to precipitate out of the solution.*

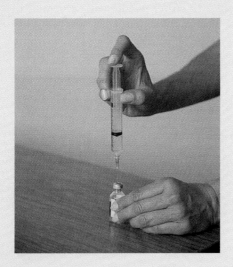

FIGURE 28-12 ◆ Injecting air into a vial.

Leaving the last few drops reduces the chance of withdrawing foreign particles.

or

b. Invert the vial; ensure the needle tip is *below* the fluid level; and gradually withdraw the medication (Figure 28-14 ◆). *Keeping the tip of the needle below the fluid level prevents air from being drawn into the syringe.*

• Hold the syringe and vial at eye level to determine that the correct dosage of drug is drawn into the syringe. Eject air remaining at the top of the syringe into the vial.

• When the correct volume of medication is obtained, withdraw the needle from the vial, and replace the cap over the needle using the scoop method, thus maintaining its sterility.

• If necessary, tap the syringe barrel to dislodge any air bubbles present in the syringe. *The tapping motion will cause the air bubbles to rise to the top of the syringe where they can be ejected out of the syringe.*

• Replace the filter needle, if used, with a regular needle and cover of the correct gauge and length before injecting the client.

Variation: Preparing and Using Multidose Vials

• Read the manufacturer's directions.

• Withdraw an equivalent amount of air from the vial before adding the diluent, unless otherwise indicated by the directions.

• Add the amount of sterile water or saline indicated in the directions.

• If a multidose vial is reconstituted, label the vial with the date and time it was prepared, the amount of drug contained in each milliliter of solution, and your initials. *Time is an important factor to consider in the expiration of these medications.*

• Once the medication is reconstituted, store it in a refrigerator or as recommended by the manufacturer.

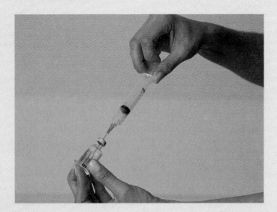

FIGURE 28-13 ◆ Withdrawing a medication from a vial that is held with the base down.

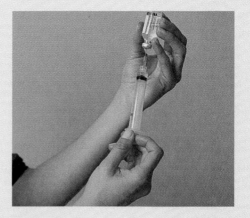

FIGURE 28-14 ◆ Withdrawing a medication from an inverted vial.

Mixing Medications in One Syringe

Frequently, clients need more than one drug injected at the same time. To spare the client the experience of being injected twice, two drugs (if compatible) are often mixed together in one syringe and given as one injection. It is common, for example, to combine two types of insulin in this manner or to combine injectable preoperative medications such as morphine or meperidine (Demerol) with atropine or scopolamine. Drugs can also be mixed in intravenous solutions. When uncertain about drug compatibilities, the nurse should consult a pharmacist or check a compatibility chart before mixing the drugs.

The nurse must also exercise caution when mixing short- and long-acting insulins, because they vary in content. Chemically, insulin is a protein that hydrolyzes in the body to yield a number of amino acids. Some insulin preparations contain an additional modifying protein, such as globulin or protamine, which slows absorption. This fact is particularly relevant to mixing two insulin preparations for injection because many insulin syringes have needles that cannot be changed. A vial of insulin that does not have the added protein (i.e., regular insulin) should *never* be contaminated with insulin that does have the added protein (i.e., Lente or NPH insulin).

Technique 28-3 describes how to mix medications in one syringe. See the variation in Technique 28-3 for an example of mixing insulins.

Nursing Process: Mixing Medications in One Syringe

ASSESSMENT

- Assess
  - Client allergies to medications
  - Specific drug action, side effects, interactions, and adverse reactions
  - Client's knowledge of and learning needs about the medications
  - Intended route of parenteral medication to determine appropriate size of syringe and needle for the client
  - Ordered medications for clarity and expiration date
- Determine that the two medications are compatible.

PLANNING

Delegation

Mixing medications in one syringe involves knowledge and use of aseptic technique. Therefore, this technique is not delegated to unlicensed assistive personnel (UAP).

IMPLEMENTATION:
TECHNIQUE 28-3 MIXING MEDICATIONS IN ONE SYRINGE

Equipment

- MAR or computer printout
- Two vials of medication; one vial and one ampule; two ampules; or one vial or ampule and one cartridge
- Antiseptic swabs
- Sterile hypodermic or insulin syringe and needle (if insulin is being given, use a small-gauge hypodermic needle, e.g., 26 gauge)
- Additional sterile subcutaneous or intramuscular needle (optional)

Preparation

1. Check the MAR.
   - Check the label on the medications carefully against the MAR to make sure that the correct medication is being prepared.
   - Follow the three checks for administering medications. Read the label on the medication (1) when it is taken from the medication cart, (2) before withdrawing the medication, and (3) after withdrawing the medication.
   - Before preparing and combining the medications,

ensure that the total volume of the injection is appropriate for the injection site.

2. Organize the equipment.

Performance

1. Wash hands and observe other appropriate infection control procedures.

2. Prepare the medication ampule or vial for drug withdrawal.
   - See Technique 28-1, step 2, for an ampule.
   - Inspect the appearance of the medication for clarity. Some medications are always cloudy. *Preparations that have changed in appearance should be discarded.*
   - If using insulin, thoroughly mix the solution in each vial prior to administration. Rotate the vials between the palms of the hands and invert the vials. *Mixing ensures an adequate concentration and thus an accurate dose. Shaking insulin vials can make the medication frothy, making precise measurement difficult.*
   - Clean the tops of the vials with antiseptic swabs.

3. Withdraw the medications.

Mixing Medications from Two Vials

- Take the syringe and draw up a volume of air equal to the volume of medications to be withdrawn from both vials A *and* B.

- Inject a volume of air equal to the volume of medication to be withdrawn into vial A. Make sure the needle does not touch the solution. *This prevents cross-contamination of the medications.*

- Withdraw the needle from vial A and inject the remaining air into vial B.

- Withdraw the required amount of medication from vial B. *The same needle is used to inject air into and withdraw medication from the second vial. It must not be contaminated with the medication in vial A.*

- Using a newly attached sterile needle, withdraw the required amount of medication from vial A. Avoid pushing the plunger as that will introduce medication B into vial A. If using a syringe with a fused needle, withdraw the medication from vial A. The syringe now contains a mixture of medications from vials A and B. *With this method, neither vial is contaminated by microorganisms or by medication from the other vial.* Be careful to withdraw only the ordered amount and to not create air bubbles. *The syringe now contains two medications and an excess amount cannot be returned to the vial.*

- See also the Variation later in this procedure.

Mixing Medications from One Vial and One Ampule

- First prepare and withdraw the medication from the vial. *Ampules do not require the addition of air prior to withdrawal of the drug.*

- Then withdraw the required amount of medication from the ampule.

Mixing Medications from One Cartridge and One Vial or Ampule

- First ensure that the correct dose of the medication is in the cartridge. Discard any excess medication and air.

- Draw up the required medication from a vial or ampule into the cartridge. Note that when withdrawing medication from a vial, an equal amount of air must first be injected into the vial.

- If the total volume to be injected exceeds the capacity of the cartridge, use a syringe with sufficient capacity to withdraw the desired amount of med-

ication from the vial or ampule, and transfer the required amount from the cartridge to the syringe.

Variation: Mixing Insulins

The following is an example of mixing 10 units of regular insulin and 30 units of neutral protamine Hagedorn (NPH) insulin, which contains protamine.

- Inject 30 units of air into the NPH vial and withdraw the needle. (There should be no insulin in the needle.) The needle should not touch the insulin (Figure 28-15 ◆, step 1).

- Inject 10 units of air into the regular insulin vial and immediately withdraw 10 units of regular insulin (Figure 28-15, steps 2 and 3). Always withdraw the regular insulin first *to minimize the possibility of contamination.* Remember the saying: clear before cloudy.

- Reinsert the needle into the NPH insulin vial and withdraw 30 units of NPH insulin (Figure 28-15, step 4). (The air was previously injected into the vial.) Be careful to withdraw only the ordered amount and to not create air bubbles. *The syringe now contains two medications, and an excess amount cannot be returned to the vial.*

By using this method, you avoid adding NPH insulin to the regular insulin.

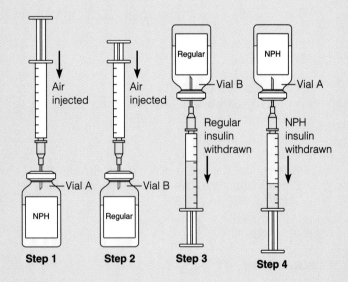

FIGURE 28-15 ◆ Mixing two types of insulin together.

Intradermal Injections

An **intradermal (ID) injection** is the administration of a drug into the dermal layer of the skin just beneath the epidermis. Usually, only a small amount of liquid is used, for example, 0.1 mL. This method of adminis-tration is frequently used for allergy testing and tuberculosis (TB) screening. Common sites for intradermal injections are the inner lower arm, the upper chest, and the back beneath the scapulae (Figure 28-16 ◆). The left arm is commonly used for TB screening and the right arm is used for all other tests.

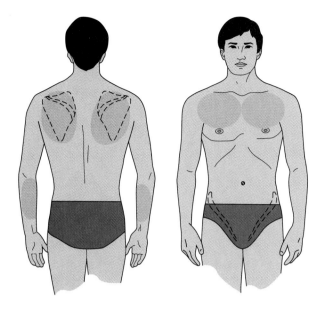

FIGURE 28-16 ◆ Body sites commonly used for intradermal injections.

Nursing Process: Intradermal Injections

ASSESSMENT

Assess:

- Appearance of injection site
- Specific drug action and expected response
- Client's knowledge of drug action and response

Check agency protocol about sites to use for skin tests.

PLANNING

Delegation

The administration of intradermal injections is an invasive technique that involves the application of nursing knowledge, problem solving, and sterile technique. This technique is not delegated to UAP. The nurse, however, can inform the UAP about symptoms of allergic reactions and the necessity to report those observations immediately to the nurse.

IMPLEMENTATION:
TECHNIQUE 28-4 ADMINISTERING INTRADERMAL INJECTIONS

Equipment

- Vial or ampule of the correct medication
- Sterile 1-mL syringe calibrated into hundredths of a milliliter (i.e., tuberculin syringe) and a 25- to 27-gauge needle that is ¼ to ⅝ inch long
- Alcohol swabs
- 2″ × 2″ sterile gauze square (optional)
- Nonsterile gloves (according to agency protocol)
- Band-Aid (optional)
- Epinephrine (a bronchodilator and antihistamine) on hand

Preparation

1. Check the MAR.
   - Check the label on the medication carefully against the MAR to make sure that the correct medication is being prepared.
   - Follow the three checks for administering medications. Read the label on the medication (1) when it is taken from the medication cart, (2) before withdrawing the medication, and (3) after withdrawing the medication.
2. Organize the equipment.

Performance

1. Wash hands and observe other appropriate infection control procedures (e.g., clean gloves).

2. Prepare the medication from the vial or ampule for drug withdrawal.
   - See Techniques 28-1 and 28-2.

3. Prepare the client
   - Check the client's identification band. *This ensures that the right client receives the medication.*

4. Explain to the client that the medication will produce a small bleb, like a blister. The client will feel a slight prick as the needle enters the skin. Some medications are absorbed slowly through the capillaries into the general circulation, and the bleb gradually disappears. Other drugs remain in the area and interact with the body tissues to produce redness and induration (hardening), which will need to be interpreted at a particular time (e.g., in 24 or 48 hours). This reaction will also gradually disappear. *Information facilitates acceptance of and compliance with the therapy.*

5. Provide for client privacy.

6. Select and clean the site.
   - Select a site (e.g., the forearm about a hand's width above the wrist and three or four finger-widths below the antecubital space).
   - Avoid using sites that are tender, inflamed, or swollen and those that have lesions.
   - Put on gloves as indicated by agency policy.
   - Cleanse the skin at the site using a firm circular motion starting at the center and widening the circle outward. Allow the area to dry thoroughly.

7. Prepare the syringe for the injection.

- Remove the needle cap while waiting for the antiseptic to dry.

- Expel any air bubbles from the syringe. Small bubbles that adhere to the plunger are of no consequence. *A small amount of air will not harm the tissues.*

- Grasp the syringe in your dominant hand, holding it between thumb and forefinger. Hold the needle almost parallel to the skin surface, with the bevel of the needle up. *The possibility of the medication entering the subcutaneous tissue increases when using a greater angle than 15 degrees or with the bevel down.*

8. Inject the fluid.

- With the nondominant hand, pull the skin at the site until it is taut. For example, if using the ventral forearm, grasp the client's dorsal forearm and gently pull it to tighten the ventral skin. *Taut skin allows for easier entry of the needle and less discomfort for the client.*

- Insert the tip of the needle far enough to place the bevel through the epidermis into the dermis (Figure 28-17A ◆). The outline of the bevel should be visible under the skin surface.

- Stabilize the syringe and needle, inject the medication carefully and slowly so that it produces a small **wheal** (small raised area like a blister) on the skin (Figure 28-17B). *This verifies that the medication entered the dermis.*

- Withdraw the needle quickly at the same angle that it was inserted. Apply a Band-Aid if indicated.

- Do not massage the area. *Massage can disperse the medication into the tissue or out through the needle insertion site.*

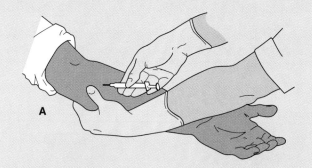

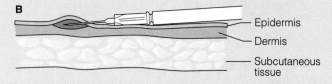

FIGURE 28-17 ◆ For an intradermal injection: (A) the needle enters the skin at a 15-degree or less angle; and (B) the medication forms a bleb under the epidermis.

- Dispose of the syringe and needle safely. *Do not recap the needle in order to prevent needle-stick injuries.*

- Remove gloves.

- Circle the injection site with ink to observe for redness or induration (hardening), per agency policy.

 9. **Document** all relevant information.

- Record the testing material given, the time, dosage, route, site, and nursing assessments.

AMBULATORY AND COMMUNITY SETTINGS

Administering an Intradermal Injection

- Be certain the client understands the need for a follow-up visit to examine the injection site. Set up an appointment for the visit.

- Instruct the client not to wash, rub, or scratch the injection site.

AGE-RELATED CONSIDERATIONS

Administering an Intradermal Injection
Child

- A small child or infant will need to be gently restrained during the procedure. *This prevents injury from sudden movement.*

- Make sure the child understands that the procedure is not a punishment.

- Ask the child not to rub or scratch the injection site. Place a stockinet or gauze dressing over the site if needed. *Rubbing the site can interfere with test results by irritating the underlying tissue.*

- Evaluate the client's response to the testing substance. *Some medications used in testing may cause allergic reactions.* An antidote drug (e.g., epinephrine) may need to be given.
- Evaluate the condition of the site in 24 or 48 hours, depending on the test. Measure the area of redness and induration in millimeters at the largest diameter and document findings.

Subcutaneous Injections

Among the many kinds of drugs administered subcutaneously (just below the skin) are vaccines, preoperative medications, narcotics, insulin, and heparin. Common sites for **subcutaneous (SC or SQ) injections** are the outer aspect of the upper arms and the anterior aspect of the thighs. These areas are convenient and normally have good blood circulation. Other areas that can be used are the abdomen, the scapular areas of the upper back, and the upper ventrogluteal and dorsogluteal areas (Figure 28-18 ◆). Only small

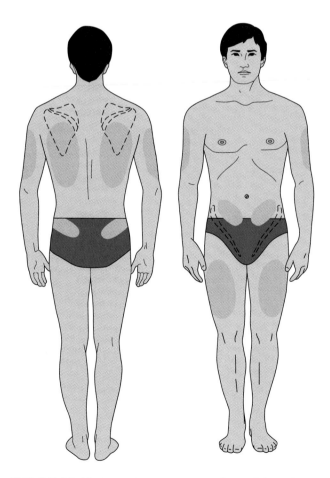

FIGURE 28-18 ◆ Body sites commonly used for subcutaneous injections.

doses (0.5 to 1.0 mL) of medication are usually injected via the subcutaneous route. Check agency policy.

The type of syringe for subcutaneous injections depends on the medication to be given. Generally, a 2-mL syringe is used for most SC injections. However, if insulin is being administered, an insulin syringe is used; and if heparin is being administered, a tuberculin syringe or prefilled cartridge may be used.

Needle sizes and lengths are selected based on the client's body mass, the intended angle of insertion, and the planned site. Generally, a 25-gauge, ⅝-inch needle is used for adults of normal weight and the needle is inserted at a 45 degree angle; a ⅜-inch needle is used at a 90 degree angle.

One method nurses use to determine length of needle is to pinch the tissue at the site and select a needle length that is half the width of the skinfold. To determine the angle of insertion, a general rule to follow relates to the amount of tissue that can be bunched or grasped at the site. A 45-degree angle is used when one inch of tissue can be grasped at the site; a 90-degree angle is used when two inches of tissue can be grasped.

When administering insulin to adults, the current standard needle gauge is 30 gauge and short needles (⅚₆ inch) are now available on 30-, 50-, and 100-unit syringes (Fleming, 1999). Most clients prefer the shorter and thinner needles because they are less painful. The risk of injecting into the muscle is lessened with the shorter needle.

Subcutaneous injection sites need to be rotated in an orderly fashion to minimize tissue damage, aid absorption, and avoid discomfort. This is especially important for the client who must receive repeated injections, such as diabetics. Because insulin is absorbed at different rates at different parts of the body, the diabetic client's blood glucose levels can vary when various sites are used. Insulin is absorbed most quickly when injected into the abdomen and then into the arms, and most slowly when injected into the thighs and buttocks. Current recommendations include rotating injections within an anatomical area (Fleming, 1999).

Nurses have traditionally been taught to aspirate by pulling back on the plunger after inserting the needle and before injecting the medication. The nurse could then determine whether the needle had entered a blood vessel. Absence of blood was believed to indicate that the needle was in subcutaneous tissue and not in the more vascular muscular tissue. Fleming (1999) challenges the traditional practice of aspiration for insulin subcutaneous injections because it "is cumbersome, rarely yields blood, and isn't a reliable indicator of correct needle placement, and there are no clinical studies confirming or rejecting it."

The steps of administering a subcutaneous injection are described in Technique 28-5.

Nursing Process: Subcutaneous Injections

ASSESSMENT

Assess:

- Allergies to medication
- Specific drug action, side effects, and adverse reactions
- Client's knowledge and learning needs about the medication
- Status and appearance of subcutaneous site for lesions, erythema, swelling, ecchymosis, inflammation, and tissue damage from previous injections

- Ability of client to cooperate during the injection
- Previous injection sites used

PLANNING

Delegation

The administration of subcutaneous injections is an invasive technique that involves the application of nursing knowledge, problem solving, and sterile technique. Therefore, this technique is not delegated to UAP. The nurse, however, can inform the UAP of the intended therapeutic effects and/or specific side effects of the medication and direct the UAP to report specific client observations to the nurse for follow-up.

IMPLEMENTATION:
TECHNIQUE 28-5 ADMINISTERING SUBCUTANEOUS INJECTIONS

Equipment

- Client's MAR or computer printout
- Vial or ampule of the correct sterile medication
- Syringe and needle (e.g., 2-mL syringe, 25-gauge needle, ⅝ or ⅝ inch long)
- Antiseptic swabs
- Dry sterile gauze for opening an ampule (optional)
- Disposable gloves

Preparation

1. Check the MAR.
   - Check the label on the medication carefully against the MAR to make sure that the correct medication is being prepared.
   - Follow the three checks for administering medications. Read the label on the medication (1) when it is taken from the medication cart, (2) before withdrawing the medication, and (3) after withdrawing the medication.

2. Organize the equipment.

Performance

1. Wash hands and observe other appropriate infection control procedures (e.g., clean gloves).

2. Prepare the medication from the ampule or vial for drug withdrawal.
   - See Technique 28-1 (ampule) or 28-2 (vial).

3. Provide for client privacy.

4. Prepare the client
   - Check the client's identification band. *This ensures that the right client receives the medication.*
   - Assist the client to a position in which the arm, leg, or abdomen can be relaxed, depending on

the site to be used. *A relaxed position of the site minimizes discomfort.*
   - Obtain assistance in holding an uncooperative client. *This prevents injury due to sudden movement after needle insertion.*

5. Explain the purpose of the medication and how it will help, using language that the client can understand. Include relevant information about effects of the medication. *Information facilitates acceptance of and compliance with the therapy.*

6. Select and clean the site.
   - Select a site free of tenderness, hardness, swelling, scarring, itching, burning, or localized inflammation. Select a site that has not been used frequently. *These conditions could hinder the absorption of the medication and also increase the likelihood of injury and discomfort at the injection site.*
   - Put on clean gloves.
   - As agency protocol indicates, clean the site with an antiseptic swab. Start at the center of the site and clean in a widening circle to about 5 cm (2 in). Allow the area to dry thoroughly. *The mechanical action of swabbing removes skin secretions, which contain microorganisms.*
   - Place and hold the swab between the third and fourth fingers of the nondominant hand, or position the swab on the client's skin above the intended site. *Using this technique keeps the swab readily accessible when the needle is withdrawn.*

7. Prepare the syringe for injection.
   - Remove the needle cap while waiting for the antiseptic to dry. Pull the cap straight off to avoid contaminating the needle by the outside edge of the cap. *The needle will become contaminated if it touches anything but the inside of the cap, which is sterile.*

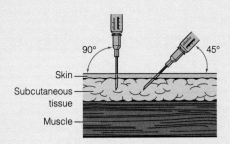

FIGURE 28-19 ◆ Inserting a needle into the subcutaneous tissue using 90- and 45-degree angles.

8. Inject the medication.
   - Grasp the syringe in your dominant hand by holding it between your thumb and fingers. With palm facing to the side or upward for a 45-degree angle insertion, or with the palm downward for a 90-degree angle insertion, prepare to inject (Figure 28-19 ◆).
   - Using the nondominant hand, pinch or spread the skin at the site, and insert the needle using the dominant hand and a firm steady push (Figure 28-20 ◆). Recommendations vary about whether to pinch or spread the skin and at what angle to administer subcutaneous injections. The most important consideration is the depth of the subcutaneous tissue in the area to be injected. If the client has more than ½ inch of adipose tissue in the injection site, it would be safe to administer the injection at a 90-degree angle with the skin spread. If the client is thin or lean and lacks adipose tissue, the subcutaneous injection should be given with the skin pinched and at a 45- to 60-degree angle.
   - When the needle is inserted, move your nondominant hand to the end of the plunger. Some nurses find it easier to move the nondominant hand to the barrel of the syringe and the dominant hand to the end of the plunger.
   - Aspirate by pulling back on the plunger. If blood appears in the syringe, withdraw the needle, discard the syringe, and prepare a new injection. If blood does not appear, continue to administer the medication. *This allows the nurse to determine whether the needle has entered a blood vessel. Subcutaneous medications may be dangerous if placed directly into the bloodstream; they are intended for the subcutaneous tissues, where the absorption time is greater.* See variation for administering a heparin injection.
   - Inject the medication by holding the syringe steady and depressing the plunger with a slow, even pressure. *Holding the syringe steady and injecting the medication at an even pressure minimizes discomfort for the client.*

9. Remove the needle.
   - Remove the needle slowly and smoothly, pulling along the line of insertion while depressing the skin with your nondominant hand. *Depressing the skin places countertraction on it and minimizes the client's discomfort when the needle is withdrawn.*
   - If bleeding occurs, apply pressure to the site with dry sterile gauze until it stops. *Bleeding rarely occurs after subcutaneous injection.*

10. Dispose of supplies appropriately.
   - Discard the uncapped needle and attached syringe into designated receptacles. *Proper disposal protects the nurse and others from injury and contamination. The Centers for Disease Control and Prevention (CDC) recommends not capping the needle before disposal to reduce the risk of needle-stick injuries.*
   - Remove gloves. Wash hands.

11. **Document** all relevant information.
   - Document the medication given, dosage, time, route, and any assessments.
   - Many agencies prefer that medication administration be recorded on the medication record. The nurse's notes are used when PRN medications are given or when there is a special problem.

12. Assess the effectiveness of the medication at the time it is expected to act.

Variation: Administering a Heparin Injection

The subcutaneous administration of heparin requires special precautions because of the drug's anticoagulant properties.

   - Select a site on the abdomen away from the umbilicus and above the level of the iliac crests. Some agencies support the practice of subcutaneous injection of heparin in the thighs or arms as alternate sites to the abdomen.

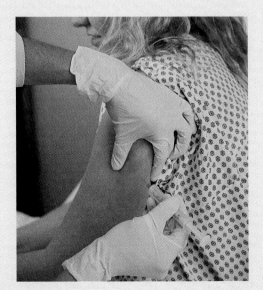

FIGURE 28-20 ◆ Administering a subcutaneous injection into pinched tissue.

- Use a ⅝-inch, 25- or 26-gauge needle, and insert it at a 90-degree angle. If a client is very lean or wasted, use a needle longer than ⅝-inch, and insert it at a 45-degree angle. The arms or thighs may be used as alternate sites.
- Do not aspirate when giving heparin by subcutaneous injection. *Aspiration can possibly damage the surrounding tissue and cause bleeding as well as bruising.*
- Do not massage the site after the injection. *Massaging could cause bleeding and ecchymoses (bruises) and hasten drug absorption.*
- Alternate the sites of subsequent injections.

AMBULATORY AND COMMUNITY SETTINGS

Subcutaneous Injections

- If the client has impaired vision, consider prefilling syringes and storing them in an appropriate environment (e.g., the refrigerator).
- For frequent injections, develop a plan for site rotation with the client.
- For cost-saving measures, teach able clients to safely reuse disposable syringes. Diabetic clients in the home can safely use disposable syringes until the needles become dull which can vary from two to 10 times (Fleming, 1999). Any client reusing syringes should have the ability to safely and correctly recap needles. Clients with poor personal hygiene, acute concurrent illness, open wounds on the hands, or decreased resistance to infection should be discouraged from reusing syringes.
- For insulin-dependent clients, ensure that at least one knowledgeable support person can correctly inject insulin in an emergency situation and recognize and treat hypoglycemia.

EVALUATION

- Conduct appropriate follow up such as desired effect (e.g., relief of pain, sedation, lowered blood sugar, a prothrombin time within preestablished limits), any adverse effects (e.g., nausea, vomiting, skin rash), and clinical signs of side effects.
- Relate to previous findings if available.
- Report deviations from normal to the physician.

Intramuscular Injections

Injections into muscle tissue, or **intramuscular (IM) injections**, are absorbed more quickly than subcutaneous injections because of the greater blood supply to the body muscles. Muscles can also take a larger volume of fluid without discomfort than subcutaneous tissues can, although the amount varies among individuals, chiefly with muscle size and condition and with the site used. An adult with well-developed muscles can usually safely tolerate up to 4 mL of medication in the gluteus medius and gluteus maximus muscles (Figure 28-21 ◆). A volume of 1 to 2 mL is usually recommended for adults with less developed muscles. In the deltoid muscle, volumes of 0.5 to 1 mL are recommended.

Usually, a 2- to 5-mL syringe is needed. The size of syringe used depends on the amount of medication being administered. The standard prepackaged intramuscular needle is 1½ inches and 21 or 22 gauge. Several factors indicate the size and length of the needle to be used:

- The muscle
- The type of medication solution
- The amount of adipose tissue covering the muscle
- The age of the client

For example, a smaller needle such as a 23- or 25-gauge needle 1 inch long is commonly used for the deltoid muscle. More viscous solutions require a larger gauge (e.g., 20 gauge). Very obese clients may require a needle longer than 1½ inches (e.g., 2 inches), and emaciated clients may require a shorter needle (e.g., 1 inch).

A major consideration in the administration of intramuscular injections is the selection of a safe site located away from large blood vessels, nerves, and bone. Several body sites can be used for intramuscular injections. These various sites are discussed in detail next. Contraindications for using a specific site include tissue injury and presence of nodules, lumps, abscesses, tenderness, or other pathology.

Ventrogluteal Site

The **ventrogluteal site** is in the gluteus medius muscle which lies over the gluteus minimus (Figure 28-21). The ventrogluteal site is the *preferred* site for intramuscular injections because the area:

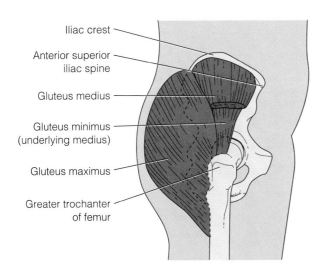

FIGURE 28-21 ◆ Lateral view of the right buttock showing the three gluteal muscles used for intramuscular injections.

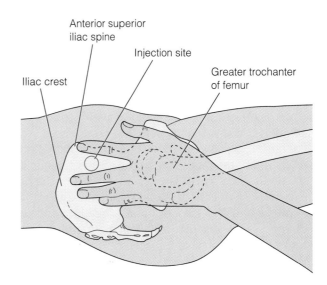

FIGURE 28-22 ◆ The ventrogluteal site for an intramuscular injection.

- Contains no large nerves or blood vessels
- Provides the greatest thickness of gluteal muscle consisting of both the gluteus medius and gluteus minimus
- Is sealed off by bone
- Contains consistently less fat than the buttock area, thus eliminating the need to determine the depth of subcutaneous fat

The site is suitable for children over 7 months and adults. The client position for the injection can be a back, prone, or side-lying position. The side-lying position, however, helps locate the ventrogluteal site more easily. Position the client on his or her side with the knee bent and raised slightly toward the chest. The trochanter will protrude, which facilitates locating the ventrogluteal site. To establish the exact site, the nurse places the heel of the hand on the client's greater trochanter with their fingers pointing toward the client's head. The right hand is used for the left hip and the left hand for the right hip. With the index finger on the client's anterior superior iliac spine, the nurse stretches the middle finger dorsally (toward the buttocks), palpating the crest of the ilium and then pressing below it. The triangle formed by the index finger, the third finger, and the crest of the ileum is the injection site (Figure 28-22 ◆).

Vastus Lateralis Site

The vastus lateralis muscle is usually thick and well developed in both adults and children. The middle third of the muscle is suggested as the **vastus lateralis site.** It is established by dividing the area between the greater trochanter of the femur and the lateral femoral condyle into thirds and selecting the middle third (Figure 28-23 ◆). The client can assume a back-lying or sitting position for an injection into this site.

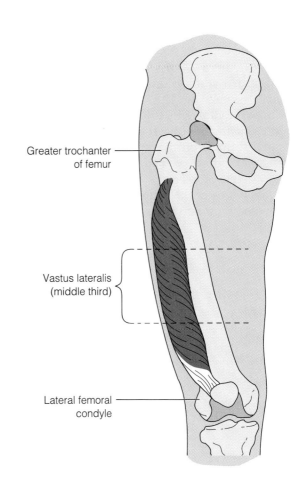

FIGURE 28-23 ◆ The vastus lateralis site of the right thigh, used for an intramuscular injection.

Dorsogluteal Site

The **dorsogluteal site** is composed of the thick gluteal muscles of the buttocks (Figure 28-21). The dorsogluteal site can be used for adults and for children with well-developed gluteal muscles. The nurse must choose the injection site carefully to avoid striking the sciatic nerve, major blood vessels, or bone.

The nurse palpates the posterior superior iliac spine, then draws an imaginary line to the greater trochanter of the femur. This line is lateral and parallel to the sciatic nerve. The injection site is lateral and superior to this line (Figure 28-24 ◆). Palpating the ilium and the trochanter is important; visual calculation alone can result in an injection that is placed too low and injures other structures.

The client needs to assume a prone position with the toes pointed inward or a side-lying position with the upper knee flexed and in front of the lower leg. These positions promote muscle relaxation and therefore minimize discomfort from the injection.

Deltoid Site

The deltoid muscle is found on the lateral aspect of the upper arm. It is not used often for IM injections because it is a relatively small muscle and is very close to the radial nerve and radial artery. It is sometimes considered for use in adults because of rapid absorption from the deltoid area, but no more than 1 mL of solution can be administered. This site is recommended for the administration of hepatitis B vaccine in adults.

The upper landmark for the **deltoid site** is located by the nurse placing four fingers across the deltoid muscle with the first finger on the acromion process. The top of the axilla is the line that marks the lower-border landmark (Figure 28-25 ◆). A triangle within these boundaries indicates the deltoid muscle about 5 cm (2 in) below the acromion process (Figure 28-26 ◆).

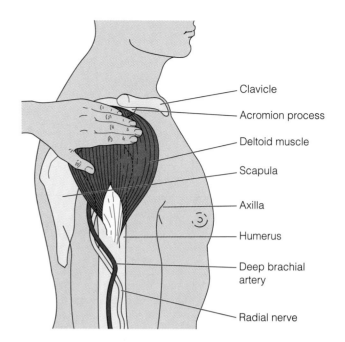

FIGURE 28-25 ◆ A method of establishing the deltoid muscle site for an intramuscular injection.

The use of a pinch–grasp technique can reduce the discomfort of an IM injection into the deltoid muscle. This technique involves grasping the muscle, pulling it about ½ to 1 inch toward the nurse, and applying a pinching pressure hard enough to cause mild discomfort. The injection is given at a 90-degree angle (McCaffery & Pasero, 1999, p. 394). It is important that the nurse informs the client about pinching the skin and explains the purpose.

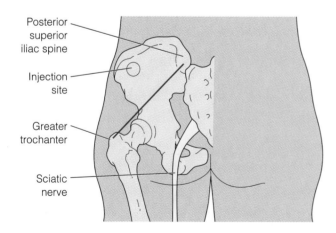

FIGURE 28-24 ◆ The dorsogluteal site for an intramuscular injection.

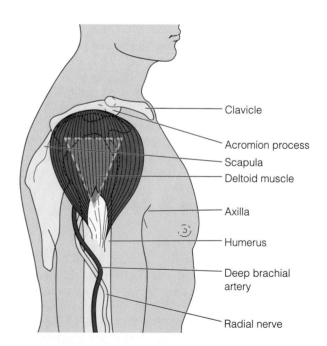

FIGURE 28-26 ◆ The deltoid muscle of the upper arm, used for intramuscular injections.

Rectus Femoris

The rectus femoris muscle, which belongs to the quadriceps muscle group, is used only occasionally for intramuscular injections. It is situated on the anterior aspect of the thigh (Figure 28-27 ◆). Its chief advantage is that clients who administer their own injections can reach the **rectus femoris site** easily. Its main disadvantage is that an injection here may cause considerable discomfort for some people.

Intramuscular Injection Technique

Technique 28-6 describes how to administer an IM injection using the **Z-track technique**, which is recommended for all intramuscular injections. The Z-track method has been found to be less painful than the traditional injection technique (McCaffery & Pasero, 1999).

Nursing Process: Intramuscular Injections

ASSESSMENT

Assess:

- Client allergies to medication(s)
- Specific drug action, side effects, and adverse reactions
- Client's knowledge of and learning needs about the medication
- Tissue integrity of the selected site
- Client's age and weight to determine site and needle size
- Client's ability or willingness to cooperate

Determine whether the size of the muscle is appropriate to the amount of medication to be injected. An average adult's deltoid muscle can usually absorb 0.5 mL of medication, although some authorities believe 1 mL can be absorbed by a well-developed deltoid muscle. The gluteus medius muscle can often absorb 1 to 4 mL, although 4 mL may be very painful.

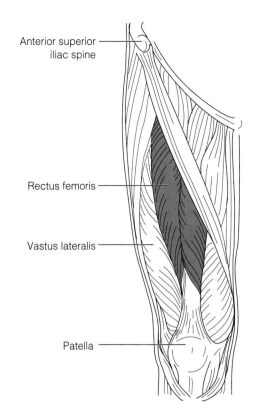

FIGURE 28-27 ◆ The rectus femoris muscle of the upper right thigh, used for intramuscular injections.

PLANNING

Delegation

The administration of IM injections is an invasive technique that involves the application of nursing knowledge, problem solving, and sterile technique. Delegation to UAP would be inappropriate. The nurse, however, can inform the UAP of the intended therapeutic effects and/or specific side effects of the medication and direct the UAP to report specific client observations to the nurse for follow-up.

IMPLEMENTATION:
TECHNIQUE 28-6 ADMINISTERING AN INTRAMUSCULAR INJECTION

Equipment

- MAR or computer printout
- Sterile medication (usually provided in an ampule or vial)
- Syringe and needle of a size appropriate for the amount of solution to be administered

- Antiseptic swabs
- Disposable gloves

Preparation

1. Check the MAR.
   - Check the label on the medication carefully against the MAR to make sure that the correct medication is being prepared.

- Follow the three checks for administering medications. Read the label on the medication (1) when it is taken from the medication cart, (2) before withdrawing the medication, and (3) after withdrawing the medication.
- Confirm that the dose is correct.

2. Organize the equipment.

Performance

1. Wash hands and observe other appropriate infection control procedures (e.g., clean gloves).

2. Prepare the medication from the ampule or vial for drug withdrawal.
   - See Techniques 28-1 (ampule) or 28-2 (vial).
   - Whenever feasible, change the needle on the syringe before the injection. *Because the outside of a new needle is free of medication, it does not irritate subcutaneous tissues as it passes into the muscle.*
   - Invert the syringe needle uppermost and expel all excess air.

3. Provide for client privacy.

4. Prepare the client
   - Check the client's identification band. *This ensures that the right client receives the medication.*
   - Assist the client to a supine, lateral, prone, or sitting position, depending on the chosen site. If the target muscle is the gluteus medius (ventrogluteal site), have the client in the supine position flex the knee(s); in the lateral position, flex the upper leg; and in the prone position, "toe in." *Appropriate positioning promotes relaxation of the target muscle.*
   - Obtain assistance in holding an uncooperative client. *This prevents injury due to sudden movement after needle insertion.*

5. Explain the purpose of the medication and how it will help, using language that the client can understand. Include relevant information about effects of the medication. *Information facilitates acceptance of and compliance with the therapy.*

6. Select, locate, and clean the site.
   - Select a site free of skin lesions, tenderness, swelling, hardness, or localized inflammation and one that has not been used frequently.
   - If injections are to be frequent, alternate sites. Avoid using the same site twice in a row. *This is to reduce the discomfort of intramuscular injections.* If necessary, discuss with the prescribing physician an alternative method of providing the medication.
   - Locate the exact site for the injection. See the discussion of sites earlier in this chapter.

- Put on clean gloves.
- Clean the site with an antiseptic swab. Using a circular motion, start at the center and move outward about 5 cm (2 in).
- Transfer and hold the swab between the third and fourth fingers of your nondominant hand in readiness for needle withdrawal, or position the swab on the client's skin above the intended site. Allow skin to dry prior to injecting medication *as this will help reduce the discomfort of the injection.*

7. Prepare the syringe for injection.
   - Remove the needle cover without contaminating the needle.
   - If using a prefilled unit-dose medication, take caution to avoid dripping medication on the needle prior to injection. If this does occur, wipe the medication off the needle with a sterile gauze. *Medication left on the needle can cause pain when it is tracked through the subcutaneous tissue.*

8. Inject the medication using a Z-track technique.
   - Use the ulnar side of the nondominant hand to pull the skin approximately 2.5 cm (1 inch) to the side (Figure 28-28 ◆). Under some circumstances, such as for an emaciated client or an infant, the muscle may be pinched. *Pulling the skin and subcutaneous tissue or pinching the muscle makes it firmer and facilitates needle insertion.*
   - Holding the syringe between the thumb and forefinger (as if holding a pencil), pierce the skin quickly and smoothly at a 90-degree angle (Figure 28-29 ◆), and insert the needle into the muscle. *Using a quick motion lessens the client's discomfort.*
   - Hold the barrel of the syringe steady with your nondominant hand and aspirate by pulling back on the plunger with your dominant hand. Aspirate for 5 to 10 seconds. *If the needle is in a small blood vessel, it takes time for the blood to appear.* If blood appears in the syringe, withdraw the needle, discard the syringe, and prepare a new injection. *This step determines whether the needle has been inserted into a blood vessel.*
   - If blood does not appear, inject the medication steadily and slowly (approximately 10 seconds per milliliter) while holding the syringe steady. *Injecting medication slowly promotes comfort and allows time for tissue to expand and begin absorption of the medication. Holding the syringe steady minimizes discomfort.*
   - After injection, wait 10 seconds *to permit the medication to disperse into the muscle tissue, thus decreasing the client's discomfort.*

9. Withdraw the needle.
   - Withdraw the needle smoothly at the same angle of insertion. *This minimizes tissue injury.*

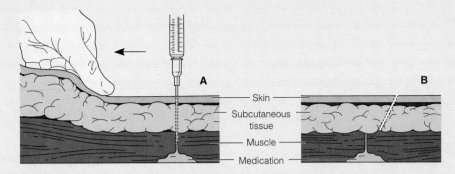

FIGURE 28-28 ◆ Inserting an intramuscular needle at a 90-degree angle using the Z-track method: (A) skin pulled to the side; (B) skin released. *Note:* When the skin returns to its normal position after the needle is withdrawn, a seal is formed over the intramuscular site. This prevents seepage of the medication into the subcutaneous tissues and subsequent discomfort.

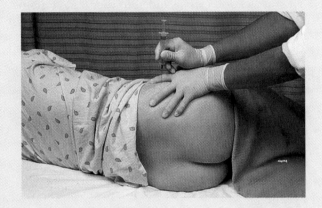

FIGURE 28-29 ◆ Administering an intramuscular injection into the ventrogluteal site.

- Apply gentle pressure at the site with a dry sponge. Do not massage the site. *Massaging the site can increase discomfort of the injection and can result in tissue irritation.*
- If bleeding occurs, apply pressure with a dry sterile gauze until it stops.

10. Discard the uncapped needle and attached syringe into the proper receptacle.

- Remove gloves. Wash hands.

11. **Document** all relevant information.

- Include the time of administration, drug name, dose, route, and the client's reactions.

12. Assess effectiveness of the medication at the time it is expected to act.

AGE-RELATED CONSIDERATIONS

Intramuscular Injections

Infant

- The ventrogluteal site cannot be used for children under 7 months of age.
- The vastus lateralis site is recommended as the site of choice for intramuscular injections for infants 7 months and younger. Because there are no major blood vessels or nerves in the area, it is desirable for infants whose gluteal muscles are poorly developed. It is situated on the anterior lateral aspect of the thigh (see figure).
- Obtain assistance to immobilize an infant or young child. The parent may hold the infant or young child. This prevents accidental injury during the procedure.

Child

- Infants and young children usually require smaller, shorter needles (22 to 25 gauge, ⅝ to 1 inch long) for intramuscular injection.
- The gluteal muscles are developed by walking. Therefore, the dorsogluteal site should not be used for children under 3 years unless the child has been walking for at least 1 year.

Elder

- Older clients may have a decreased muscle mass or muscle atrophy. A shorter needle may be needed. Assessment of appropriate injection site is critical. Absorption of medication may occur more quickly than expected.

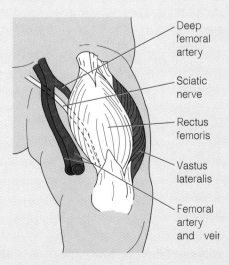

Deep femoral artery

Sciatic nerve

Rectus femoris

Vastus lateralis

Femoral artery and veir

EVALUATION

- Conduct appropriate follow up, such as:
  - Desired effect (e.g., relief of pain or vomiting)
  - Any adverse reactions or side effects
  - Local skin or tissue reactions at injection site (e.g., redness, swelling, pain, or other evidence of tissue damage)
- Relate to previous findings, if available.
- Report significant deviation from normal to physician.

Intravenous Medications

Because **intravenous (IV)** medications enter the client's bloodstream directly by way of a vein, they are appropriate when a rapid effect is required. This route is also appropriate when medications are too irritating to tissues to be given by other routes. When an intravenous line is already established, this route is desirable because it avoids the discomfort of other parenteral routes. Medications are administered intravenously by the following methods:

- Large-volume infusion of IV fluid
- Intermittent intravenous infusion (piggyback setup)
- Volume-controlled infusion
- Intravenous push (IVP) or bolus
- Intermittent injection ports

In all these methods the client has an existing IV line or an IV access site such as a saline or heparin lock. Most agencies have procedures and policies about who may administer an IV medication. Chapter 29 describes the technique for performing a venipuncture and establishing an IV line.

With all IV medication administration, it is very important to observe clients closely for signs of adverse reactions. Because the drug enters the bloodstream directly and acts immediately, there is no way it can be withdrawn or its action terminated. Therefore, the nurse must always take special care to avoid any errors regarding the preparation of the drug and the calculation of the dosage. When the administered drug is particularly potent, an antidote to the drug should be readily available. In addition, the vital signs are assessed before, during, and after the infusion of the drug.

Large-Volume Infusions

Mixing a medication into a large-volume IV container is the safest and easiest way to administer a drug intravenously. The drugs are diluted in volumes of 1,000 mL or 500 mL of compatible fluids. It may be necessary to consult a pharmacist to confirm compatibility. Fluids such as IV normal saline or Ringer's lactate are frequently used. Commonly added drugs are potassium chloride and vitamins. It may also be necessary to ensure the compatibility of some drugs with the plastic IV bag and tubing. A glass IV bottle and special tubing may be used in special situations.

The main danger of infusing a large volume of fluid is circulatory overload (hypervolemia).

The medication can be added to the fluid container that is running or before it is hung and infusing. In some hospitals the pharmacist adds the medication to the container (see Technique 28-7).

Nursing Process: Intravenous Medications

ASSESSMENT

- Inspect and palpate the intravenous insertion site for signs of infection, infiltration, or a dislocated catheter.
- Inspect the surrounding skin for redness, pallor, or swelling.
- Palpate the surrounding tissues for coldness and the presence of edema, which could indicate leakage of the IV fluid into the tissues.
- Take vital signs for baseline data if the medication being administered is particularly potent.
- Determine if the client has allergies to the medication(s).
- Check the compatibility of the medication(s) and IV fluid.

PLANNING

Delegation

Adding medications to IV fluid containers involves the application of nursing knowledge and critical thinking. The nurse does not delegate this technique to UAP. However, the nurse can inform the UAP of the intended therapeutic effects and/or specific side effects of the medication(s) in the IV and direct the UAP to report specific client observations to the nurse for follow-up.

Equipment

- MAR or computer printout
- Correct sterile medication
- Diluent for medication in powdered form (see manufacturer's instructions)
- Correct solution container, if a new one is to be attached
- Antiseptic or alcohol swabs
- Sterile syringe of appropriate size (e.g., 5 or 10 mL) and a 1- to 1½-inch, 20- or 21-gauge sterile needle or equivalent from needleless system
- IV additive label

Preparation

1. Check the MAR.
   - Check the label on the medication carefully against the MAR to make sure that the correct medication is being prepared.
   - Follow the three checks for administering medications. Read the label on the medication (1) when it is taken from the medication cart, (2) before withdrawing the medication, and (3) after withdrawing the medication.
   - Confirm that the dosage and route is correct.
   - Verify which infusion solution is to be used with the medication.
   - Consult a pharmacist, if required, to confirm compatibility of the drugs and solutions being mixed.

2. Organize the equipment.

Performance

1. Wash hands and observe other appropriate infection control procedures.

2. Prepare the medication from the ampule or vial for drug withdrawal.
   - See Technique 28-1 (ampule) or 28-2 (vial).
   - Check the agency's practice for using a filter needle or a needless system to withdraw premixed liquid medications from multidose vials or ampules.

3. Add the medication.

To New IV Container
   - Locate the injection port and carefully remove its cover. Clean the port with the antiseptic or alcohol swab. *This reduces the risk of introducing microorganisms into the container when the needle is inserted.*
   - Remove the needle cap from the syringe, insert the needle through the center of the injection

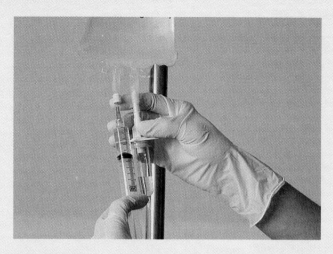

FIGURE 28-30 ◆ Inserting a medication through the injection port of an infusing container.

port, and inject the medication into the bag or bottle (Figure 28-30 ◆).
   - Mix the medication and solution by gently rotating the bag or bottle (Figure 28-31 ◆). *This should disperse the medication throughout the solution.*
   - Complete the IV additive label with name and dose of medication, date, time, and nurse's initials. Attach it upside down on the bag or bottle (Figure 28-32 ◆). *This documents that medication has been added to the solution. When the label is attached upside down, it is easily read when the bag is hanging up.*
   - Clamp the IV tubing. Spike the bag or bottle with IV tubing and hang the IV. *Clamping prevents rapid infusion of the solution.*
   - Regulate infusion rate as ordered.

To an Existing Infusion
   - Determine that the IV solution in the container is sufficient for adding the medication. *Sufficient volume is necessary to dilute the medication adequately.*

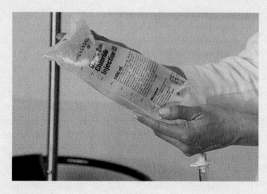

FIGURE 28-31 ◆ Rotating an intravenous bag to distribute a medication.

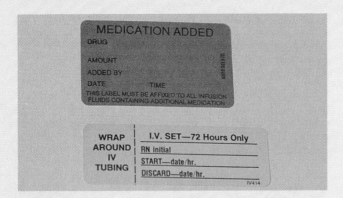

FIGURE 28-32 ◆ *Top*, label indicating a medication added to an IV infusion; *bottom*, label indicating time for IV tubing change.

- Confirm the desired dilution of the medication, that is, the amount of medication per milliliter of solution.
- Close the infusion clamp. *This prevents the medication from infusing directly into the client as it is injected into the bag or bottle.*
- Wipe the medication port with the alcohol or disinfectant swab. *This reduces the risk of introducing microorganisms into the container when the needle is inserted.*
- Remove the needle cover from the medication syringe.
- While supporting and stabilizing the bag with your thumb and forefinger, carefully insert the syringe needle through the port and inject the medication. *The bag is supported during the injection of the medication to avoid punctures.* If the bag or bottle is too high to reach easily, lower it from the IV pole.
- Remove the bag or bottle from the pole and gently rotate the bottle or bag. *This will mix the medication and solution.*
- Rehang the container and regulate the flow rate. *This establishes the correct flow rate.*
- Complete the medication label and apply to the IV container.

4. Dispose of the equipment and supplies according to agency practice. *This prevents inadvertent injury to others and the spread of microorganisms.*

 5. **Document** the medication(s) on the appropriate form in the client's record.

Intermittent Intravenous Infusions

An intermittent infusion is a method of administering a medication mixed in a small amount of IV solution, such as 50 or 100 mL (Figure 28-33 ◆). The drug is administered at regular intervals, such as every 4 hours, with the drug being infused for a short period of time such as 30 to 60 minutes. Two commonly used **additive** or **secondary IV setups** are the tandem and the piggyback.

In a **tandem** setup, a second container is attached to the line of the first container at the lower, secondary port (Figure 28-34A ◆). It permits medications to be administered intermittently or simultaneously with the primary solution.

In the **piggyback** alignment, a second set connects the second container to the tubing of the primary container at the upper port (Figure 28-34B). This setup is used solely for intermittent drug administration. Various manufacturers describe these sets differently, so the nurse must check the manufacturer's labeling and directions carefully.

Traditionally, the tubing of the secondary set has been attached to ports of the primary infusion by inserting a needle through the port and taping it in place. Needleless systems are now available (Figure 28-35 ◆). These needleless systems can use threaded-lock, lever-lock, or needle-lock cannulae to connect the secondary set to the ports of the primary infusion (Figure 28-36 ◆). This design prevents needle-stick injuries and also prevents touch contamination at the

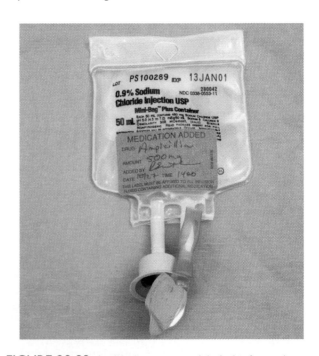

FIGURE 28-33 ◆ Medication in a labeled infusion bag.

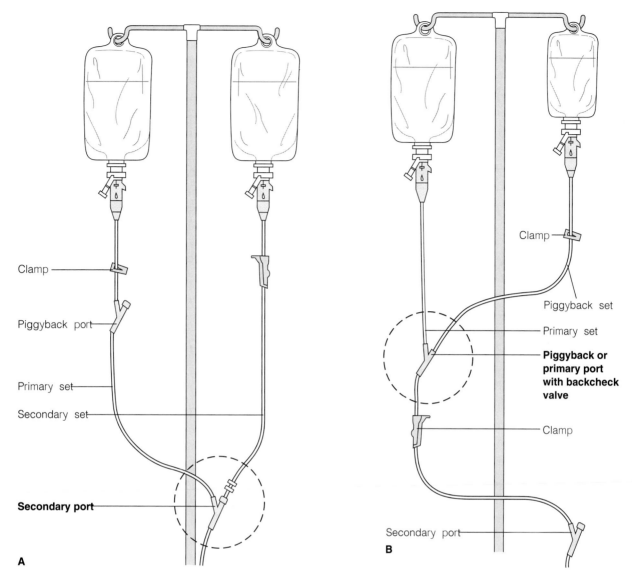

FIGURE 28-34 ◆ Secondary intravenous lines: (A) a tandem intravenous alignment; (B) an intravenous piggyback (IVPB) alignment.

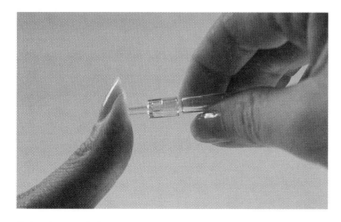

FIGURE 28-35 ◆ A blunt plastic cannula replaces the sharp steel needle.

IV connection site. Technique 28-8 describes the administration of intermittent IV medications using piggyback (IVPB) infusion.

Another method of intermittently administering an IV medication is by a **syringe pump** or mini-infuser. The medication is mixed in a syringe that is connected to the primary IV line via a mini-infuser (see Figure 28-37 ◆).

Intermittent medications may also be administered by **volume-control infusion sets** such as Buretrol, Soluset, Volutrol, and Pediatrol (Figure 28-38 ◆). They are small fluid containers (100 to 150 mL in size) attached below the primary infusion container so that the medication is administered through the client's IV line. Volume-control sets are frequently used to infuse solutions into older clients and children when the volume administered is critical and must be carefully monitored.

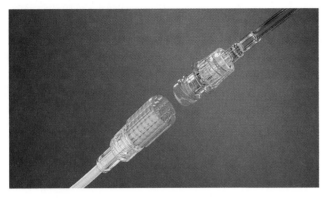

A

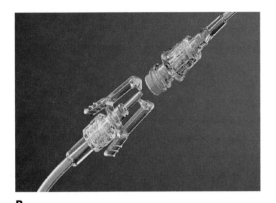

B

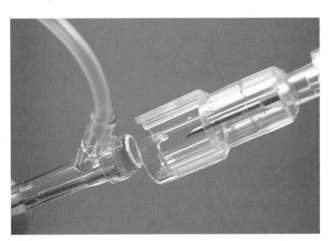

C

FIGURE 28-36 ◆ Needleless cannulae used to connect the tubing of secondary sets to primary infusions: (A) threaded-lock cannula; (B) lever-lock cannula; (C) needle-lock cannula.

Nursing Process: Intermittent Intravenous Infusions

ASSESSMENT

• Inspect and palpate the intravenous insertion site for signs of infection, infiltration, or a dislocated catheter.

FIGURE 28-37 ◆ Syringe pump or mini-infuser for administration of IV medications.

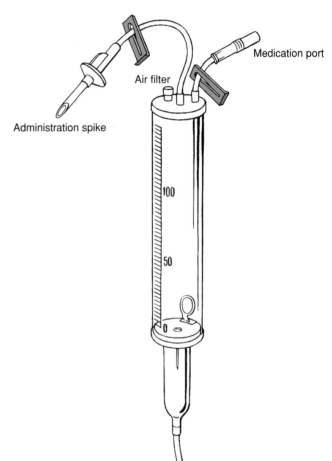

Administration spike

Air filter

Medication port

FIGURE 28-38 ◆ A volume-control set.

- Inspect the surrounding skin for redness, pallor, or swelling.
- Palpate the surrounding tissues for coldness and the presence of edema, which could indicate leakage of the IV fluid into the tissues.
- Take vital signs for baseline data if the medication being administered is particularly potent.
- Determine if the client has allergies to the medication(s).
- Check the compatibility of the medication, primary IV fluid, and any medication(s) in the primary IV bag.
- Determine specific drug action, side effects, normal dosage, recommended administration time, and peak action time.
- Check patency of IV line by assessing flow rate.

PLANNING

Delegation

The administration of intermittent IV medications involves the application of nursing knowledge and critical thinking. Check the state's Nurse Practice Act to verify the scope of practice for the licensed practical nurse/licensed vocational nurse as it relates to IV medication administration. Agency policy also must be checked and followed. This technique is not delegated to UAP. The nurse, however, can inform the UAP of the intended therapeutic effects and/or specific side effects of the medication and direct the UAP to report specific client observations to the nurse for follow-up.

IMPLEMENTATION:
TECHNIQUE 28-8 ADMINISTERING INTERMITTENT INTRAVENOUS MEDICATIONS USING A SECONDARY SET

Equipment

- MAR
- 50- to 250-mL infusion bag with medication (most medication infusion bags are prepared by the pharmacist)
- Secondary administration set
- Antiseptic swabs
- Disposable clean gloves
- Sterile needle if system is not needleless
- Tape
- Sterile needle or needleless adapter, syringe, and saline if medication is incompatible with the primary infusion

Preparation

1. Check the MAR.
   - Check the label on the medication carefully against the MAR to make sure that the correct medication is being prepared.
   - Ensure medication compatibility with primary infusion solution.
2. Organize the equipment.
3. Remove medication bag from the refrigerator 30 minutes before administration, if appropriate.

Performance

1. Wash hands and observe other appropriate infection control procedures.

2. Provide for client privacy.
3. Prepare the client.
   - Check the client's identification band. *This ensures that the right client receives the medication.*
   - If not previously assessed, take the appropriate assessment measures necessary for the medication.
4. Explain the purpose of the medication and how it will help, using language that the client can understand. Include relevant information about the effects of the medication.
5. Assemble the secondary infusion:
   - Close clamp on secondary infusion tubing.
   - Spike the secondary medication infusion bag.
   - Squeeze the drip chamber and fill one-third to one-half full.
   - Hang the secondary container at or above the level of the primary infusion. Use the extension hook to lower the primary infusion if a piggyback setup is required.
   - Attach the sterile needle or needleless cannula to the tubing, open the clamp to prime the tubing and close the clamp when the tubing is filled with solution.
6. Attach the secondary infusion to the primary infusion.
   - Clean the Y-port on the primary IV line with an antiseptic swab. Clean the **primary port** (the port furthest from the client) for a piggyback alignment and the **secondary port** (the port closest to the client) for a tandem setup.

- If the medication is *not* compatible with the primary infusion, temporarily discontinue the primary infusion. Flush the primary line with a sterile saline solution before attaching the secondary set. To flush the line, wipe the port with an antiseptic swab, clamp the primary line, and, using a sterile needleless adapter (or needle) and syringe, instill sufficient sterile saline solution through the port to flush any primary fluid out of the infusion tubing.
- Insert the needleless cannula of the secondary line into the primary tubing port.
- Secure the needle with tape if using a needle system. *Tape prevents needle dislodgement.*
- Attach appropriate label to the secondary tubing. *Secondary tubing is usually changed every 48 hours. Check agency policy.*

7. Administer the medication

Piggyback

- Ensure that the primary line is unclamped if the port has a back-check valve. *The valve automatically stops the flow of the primary infusion while the secondary set infuses and automatically starts it running after the piggyback solution has been administered.*
- Open the clamp on the piggyback line and regulate it in accordance with the recommended rate for the medication. Usually, medications are administered in 30 to 60 minutes.

Tandem Infusion

- Open the clamp on the secondary line and regulate its flow.
- For *continuous* infusion, set the secondary solution to the appropriate drip rate for the medication and then adjust the primary solution to achieve the desired total infusion flow.
- For *intermittent* infusion, clamp the primary line and adjust the primary drip rate after the secondary solution is completed.

8. Check flow rate of primary infusion line when medication is infused.
   - Re-regulate flow rate if needed.
   - Leave the secondary bag and tubing in place for future administration or discard as appropriate.

9. **Document** relevant data.
   - Record the date, time, medication, dose, route, and solution; assessments of the IV site, if appropriate; and the client's response.
   - Record the volume of fluid of medication infusion bag on the client's intake and output record.

Variation: Using a Saline or Heparin Lock

A sterile **injection cap** may be attached to an existing peripheral intravenous catheter or needle to allow medications to be administered intravenously without requiring a continuous intravenous infusion. A port is at one end of the lock and a needleless injection cap at the other end with the extension tubing between the two ends. The device is commonly referred to as a heparin or saline lock because periodic injection with heparin or saline is used to keep blood from coagulating within the tubing.

- Prepare two normal saline prefilled syringes (1 mL each). Some agencies may use a solution of 1 mL of heparin (1,000 units/mL) added to 9 mL normal saline (100 unit/mL solution) for flushing the heparin lock.
- Spike the medication bag with minidrip (60 gtt/mL) IV tubing.
- Attach the needleless adapter to the tubing, prime the tubing, and close the clamp.
- Clean the needleless injection port of the saline/heparin lock with an antiseptic swab.
- Insert first saline syringe into the port and gently aspirate to check for patency. Flush slowly noting any resistance, swelling, pain, or burning. *To ensure placement of IV in vein.*
- Administer the medication regulating the drip rate to allow medication to infuse for appropriate time period.
- When the medication is infused, disconnect the IV tubing maintaining sterility of the end of the IV tubing.
- Insert the second saline (or heparin solution) syringe into the port and gently flush the saline/heparin lock. *This technique clears the tubing and maintains patency.*
- Dispose of syringes in the appropriate container.

Variation: Adding a Medication to a Volume-Control Infusion

- Withdraw the required dose of the medication into a syringe.
- Ensure that there is sufficient fluid in the volume-control fluid chamber to dilute the medication. Generally, at least 50 mL of fluid is used. Check the directions from the drug manufacturer or consult the pharmacist.
- Close the inflow to the fluid chamber by adjusting the upper roller or slide clamp above the fluid chamber; also ensure that the clamp on the air vent of the chamber is open.

- Clean the medication port on the volume-control fluid chamber with an antiseptic swab.
- Inject the medication into the port of the partially filled volume-control set.
- Gently rotate the fluid chamber until the fluid is well mixed.

- Open the line's upper clamp and regulate the flow by adjusting the lower roller or slide clamp below the fluid chamber.
- Attach a medication label to the volume-control fluid chamber.
- Document relevant data and monitor the client and the infusion.

EVALUATION

- Conduct appropriate follow-up, such as desired effect of medication, any adverse reactions or side effects, change in vital signs.
- Reassess status of IV lock site and patency of IV infusion.
- Relate to previous findings, if available.
- Report significant deviations from normal to the physician.

Intravenous Push

Intravenous push (IVP) (bolus) is the intravenous administration of an undiluted drug directly into the systemic circulation. It is used when a medication cannot be diluted or in an emergency. An IV bolus can be introduced directly into a vein by venipuncture or into an existing IV line through an injection port or through an IV lock.

There are two major disadvantages to this method of drug administration: Any error in administration cannot be corrected after the drug has entered the client and the drug may be irritating to the lining of the blood vessels. Before administering a bolus, the nurse should look up the maximum concentration recommended for the particular drug and the rate of administration. The administered medication takes effect immediately (see Technique 28-9).

Nursing Process: Intravenous Push

ASSESSMENT

- Inspect and palpate the IV insertion site for signs of infection, infiltration, or a dislocated catheter.
- Inspect the surrounding skin for redness, pallor, or swelling.
- Palpate the surrounding tissues for coldness and the presence of edema, which could indicate leakage of the IV fluid into the tissues.
- Take vital signs for baseline data if the medication being administered is particularly potent.
- Determine if the client has allergies to the medication(s).
- Check the compatibility of the medication(s) and IV fluid.
- Determine specific drug action, side effects, normal dosage, recommended administration time, and peak action time.
- Check patency of IV line by assessing flow rate.

PLANNING

Delegation

The administration of intravenous medication via IV push involves the application of nursing knowledge and critical thinking. This technique is not delegated to UAP. The nurse, however, can inform the UAP of the intended therapeutic effects and/or specific side effects of the medication and direct the UAP to report specific client observations to the nurse for follow-up.

IMPLEMENTATION:
TECHNIQUE 28-9 ADMINISTERING INTRAVENOUS MEDICATIONS USING IV PUSH

Equipment

IV Push for an Existing Line
- Medication in a vial or ampule
- Sterile syringe (3 to 5 mL) (to prepare the medication)
- Sterile needles 21 to 25 gauge, 2.5 cm (1 in), or equivalent from a needleless system

- Antiseptic swabs
- Watch with a digital readout or second hand
- Disposable gloves

IV Push for an IV Lock
- Medication in a vial or ampule
- Sterile syringe (3 to 5 mL) (to prepare the medication)

- Sterile syringe (3 mL) (for the saline or heparin flush)
- Vial of normal saline to flush the IV catheter or vial of heparin flush solution or both depending on agency practice. *These maintain the patency of the IV lock. Saline is frequently used for peripheral locks.*
- Sterile needles (21 gauge) or equivalent from a needleless system
- Antiseptic swabs
- Watch with a digital readout or second hand
- Disposable gloves

Preparation

1. Check the MAR.
   - Check the label on the medication carefully against the MAR to make sure that the correct medication is being prepared.
   - Follow the three checks for administering medications. Read the label on the medication (1) when it is taken from the medication cart, (2) before withdrawing the medication, and (3) after withdrawing the medication.
   - Calculate medication dosage accurately.
   - Confirm that the route is correct.

2. Organize the equipment.

Performance

1. Wash hands and observe other appropriate infection control procedures.

2. Prepare the medication.

Existing Line

- Prepare the medication according to the manufacturer's direction. *It is important to have the correct dose and the correct dilution.*

IV Lock

   a. Flushing with saline
      - Prepare two syringes, each with 1 mL of sterile normal saline.
   b. Flushing with heparin and saline
      - Prepare one syringe with 1 mL of heparin flush solution.
      - Prepare two syringes with 1 mL each of sterile, normal saline.
      - Draw up the medication into a syringe.

3. Put a small-gauge needle on the syringe if using a needle system.

4. Wash hands and put on clean gloves. *This reduces the transmission of microorganisms and reduces the likelihood of the nurse's hands contacting the client's blood.*

5. Provide for client privacy.

6. Prepare the client.
   - Check the client's identification band. *This ensures that the right client receives the medication.*
   - If not previously assessed, take the appropriate assessment measures necessary for the medication. If any of the findings are above or below the predetermined parameters, consult the physician before administering the medication.

7. Explain the purpose of the medication and how it will help, using language that the client can understand. Include relevant information about the effects of the medication.

8. Administer the medication by IV push.

IV Lock with Needle

- Clean the diaphragm with the antiseptic swab. *This prevents microorganisms from entering the circulatory system during the needle insertion.*
- Insert the needle of the syringe containing normal saline through the center of the diaphragm and aspirate for blood (Figure 28-39 ◆). *The presence of blood confirms that the catheter or needle is in the vein. In some situations, blood will not return even though the lock is patent.*
- Flush the lock by injecting 1 mL of saline slowly. *This removes blood from the needle and the lock.*
- Remove the needle and syringe.
- Clean the lock's diaphragm with an antiseptic swab. *This prevents the transfer of microorganisms.*
- Insert the needle of the syringe containing the prepared medication through the center of the diaphragm.
- Inject the medication slowly at the recommended rate of infusion. Use a watch or digital readout to time the injection. Observe the client closely for adverse reactions. Remove the needle and syringe when all medication is adminis-

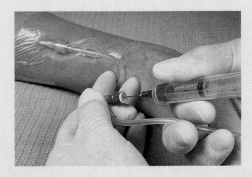

FIGURE 28-39 ◆ Inserting a needle through the diaphragm of an IV lock.

tered. *Injecting the drug too rapidly can have a serious untoward reaction.*

- Withdraw the needle and syringe.
- Clean the diaphragm of the lock.
- Attach the second saline syringe, and inject 1 mL of saline. *The saline injection flushes the medication through the catheter and prepares the lock for heparin if this medication is used. Heparin is incompatible with many medications.*
- If heparin is to be used, insert the heparin syringe and inject the heparin slowly into the lock.

IV Lock with Needleless System

- Remove the protective cap from the needleless port.
- Insert syringe containing normal saline into the lock.
- Flush the lock with 1 mL sterile saline. *This clears the lock of blood.*
- Remove the syringe.
- Insert the syringe containing the medication into the valve (Figure 28-40 ◆).
- Inject the medication following the precautions described previously.
- Withdraw the syringe.
- Repeat injection of 1 mL of saline.
- Place a new sterile cap over the lock.

Existing Line

- Identify the injection port closest to the client. Some ports have a circle indicating the site for the needle insertion. *An injection port must be used because it is self-sealing. Any puncture to the plastic tubing will leak.*
- Clean the port with an antiseptic swab.
- Stop the IV flow by closing the clamp or pinching the tubing above the injection port.
- Connect the syringe to the IV system.
- a. Needle system
  - Hold the port steady.
  - Insert the needle of the syringe that contains the medication through the center of the

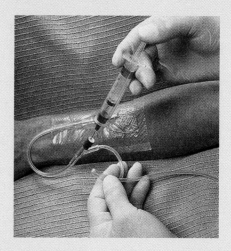

FIGURE 28-41 ◆ Injecting a medication by IV push to an existing IV using a needle system.

port (Figure 28-41 ◆). *This prevents damage to the IV line and to the diaphragm of the port.*
- b. Needleless system
  - Remove the cap from the needleless injection port. Connect the tip of the syringe directly to the port (Figure 28-42 ◆).
  - Pull back on the plunger of the syringe in order to aspirate a small amount of blood. *This confirms that the port is patent and that the medication will enter the bloodstream.*
  - After observing the blood, continue to keep the clamp closed and inject the medication at the ordered rate. Use the watch or digital readout to time the medication administration. *This ensures safe drug administration because a too rapid injection could be dangerous.*

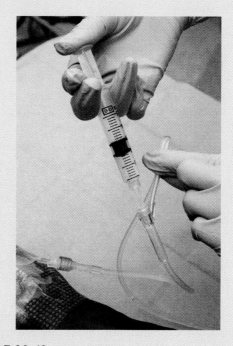

FIGURE 28-42 ◆ Injecting a medication by IV push to an existing IV using a needleless system.

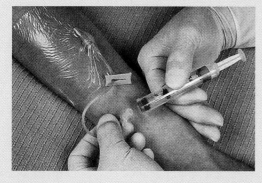

FIGURE 28-40 ◆ Using a needless system to inject a medication into an IV lock.

- Release the clamp or tubing.
- After injecting the medication, withdraw the needle, or for a needleless system, detach the syringe, and attach a new sterile cap to the port.

9. Dispose of equipment according to agency practice. *This reduces needle-stick injuries and spread of microorganisms.*

10. Remove and dispose of gloves. Wash hands.

11. Observe the client closely for adverse reactions.

12. Determine agency practice about recommended times for changing the IV lock. Some agencies advocate a change every 48 to 72 hours for peripheral IV devices.

 13. **Document** all relevant information.
- Record the date, time, drug, dose, and route; client response; and assessments of infusion or heparin lock site if appropriate.

AMBULATORY AND COMMUNITY SETTINGS

Administering IV Push Antibiotics

Shortened hospital stays and the need to cut costs has led to clients or their caregivers being taught to administer IV push antibiotics at home. The antibiotic is delivered IV push directly into a venous access device with pre- and postadministration flushing (Skokal, 2000).

The nurse must:

- Know which antibiotics are unsuitable for IV push administration.
- Know the adverse side effects:
  - Phlebitis (pain and tenderness over the vein, erythema, swelling, and warmth)
  - Speed shock—a systemic reaction when a drug is given too rapidly
  - Venous spasm—cramping and pain above infusion site
  - Infiltration

- Assess caregiver or client's eyesight and manual dexterity. Both are needed for safe administration of the antibiotic.
- Provide thorough teaching about:
  - Venous access device
  - Administration rate (minutes/dose)
  - Schedule for medication administration
  - Flushing technique
  - Adverse reactions
  - Signs that indicate an emergency and to call 911
  - Proper storage of medication
- Inspect appearance of medication and check expiration date

EVALUATION

- Conduct appropriate follow-up such as desired effect of medication; any adverse reactions or side effects, change in vital signs.
- Reassess status of IV lock site and patency of IV infusion, if running.
- Relate to previous findings, if available.
- Report significant deviations from normal to the physician.

Administering Controlled Medications

The nurse has traditionally administered opioids by oral, subcutaneous, intramuscular, and intravenous routes. Newer methods of delivering opiates have been developed and include intraspinal (into the spinal canal) infusion and continuous local anesthetics.

Patient-Controlled Analgesia

Patient-controlled analgesia (PCA) is an interactive method of pain management that permits clients to treat their pain by self-administering doses of analgesics (McCaffery & Pasero, 1999). The oral route for PCA is most common, but the subcutaneous, intravenous, and epidural routes are increasingly being used. The PCA mode of therapy minimizes the rollercoaster effect of peaks of sedation and valleys of pain that occur with the traditional method of PRN dosing. With the parenteral routes, the client administers a predetermined dose of a narcotic by an electronic infusion pump. This allows the client to maintain a more constant level of relief and the tendency for the client to need less medication for pain relief. PCA can be effectively used for clients with acute pain related to a surgical incision, traumatic injury, or labor and delivery, and for chronic pain as with cancer.

PCA pumps are designed with built-in safety mechanisms to prevent client overdosage, abusive use, and narcotic theft. The most significant adverse effects are respiratory depression and hypotension; however, they occur rarely. Although PCA pumps vary in design, they all have the same protective features. The line of the PCA pump, a syringe-type pump, is usually introduced into the injection port of a primary IV fluid line (Figure 28-43 ◆). When clients want a dose of analgesic, they can push a button attached to the infusion pump and the preset dose is delivered. A programmable lockout interval (usually 10 to 15 minutes) follows the dose, when an additional dose cannot be given even if the client activates the button. It is also possible to program the maximum dose that can be delivered over a period of hours (usually four). Many pumps are capable of delivering a low continuous infusion, or **basal rate**, to provide sustained analgesia during times of rest and sleep. Technique 28-10 describes the use of a PCA pump.

Whether in an acute hospital setting, an ambulatory clinic, or with home care, the nurse is responsible for the initial instruction regarding use of the PCA and for the ongoing monitoring of the therapy. The client's pain must be assessed at regular intervals and analgesic use is documented in the client's record.

Nursing Process: Patient-Controlled Analgesia

ASSESSMENT

Assess:

- Pain (intensity, location, presence of radiation, associated factors, precipitating factors, and alleviating factors)
- Client's allergies

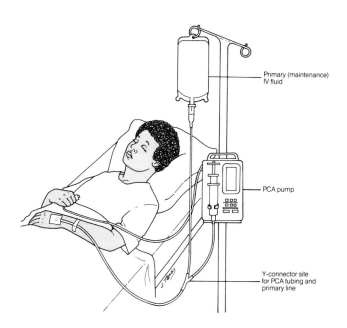

FIGURE 28-43 ◆ PCA line introduced into the injection port of a primary line.

- Baseline vital signs
- Client's understanding of the pump

PLANNING

Delegation

Initiating and maintaining a PCA pump requires application of nursing knowledge, aseptic technique, critical thinking, and administration of a controlled substance and, therefore, is not delegated to UAP. The nurse can inform the UAP of the intended therapeutic effects and specific side effects of the medication and direct the UAP to report specific client observations (e.g., unrelieved pain) to the nurse for follow-up. The UAP must *not* administer a dose (push the button) for the client.

IMPLEMENTATION:

TECHNIQUE 28-10 MANAGING PAIN WITH A PATIENT-CONTROLLED ANALGESIA (PCA) PUMP

Equipment

- Disposable gloves
- IV start kit
- IV catheter
- Primary line IV tubing
- Primary IV fluid (per orders)
- PCA pump and appropriate tubing
- Operational manual for specific pump to be used
- PCA flowsheet

Preparation

Before initiating PCA therapy, determine factors that may contraindicate use (e.g., impaired mental status, impaired respiratory status), the amount of narcotic specified by the order, bolus and continuous infusion dosage parameters, and type of primary fluid. Calculate:

- The initial bolus dose based on the number of milligrams of drug per milliliter of fluid
- The dose per intermittent bolus delivery
- The 4-hour lockout drug limit

Confirm that the drug is premixed with the required amount of diluent.

Performance

1. Explain to the client the purpose and operation of the PCA.

2. Wash hands and observe other appropriate infection control procedures.

3. Provide for client privacy.

4. Prepare the client.
   - Check the client's identification band. *This ensures that the right client receives the medication.*
   - If not previously assessed, take the baseline vital signs. If any of the findings are above or below the predetermined parameters, consult the physician before administering the medication.

5. Set up the primary IV line and fluid.
   - Put on clean gloves.
   - Start the IV line. *This will secure venous access.*

6. Set up the PCA infusion line according to the manufacturer's instructions.
   - Remove the protective caps from the injector (plunger) and premixed drug vial.
   - Connect (screw or twist) the injector into the drug vial.
   - Remove excess air from the vial by pushing the injector into the vial.
   - Connect the PCA tubing to the injector.
   - Prime the PCA tubing up to the point of the Y-connector.
   - Clamp the tubing above the Y-connector. *This prevents accidental bolusing and flushing of the primary line with the narcotic.*
   - Place the injector with attached vial in the PCA machine according to the operational instructions.

7. Connect the PCA infusion line to the primary fluid line.
   - Connect the PCA tubing to the primary fluid line at the Y-connector site. (The clamps should still be closed on the primary IV line and the PCA line).

8. Deliver the loading dose.
   - Set the pump for a lockout time of zero minutes.
   - Set the volume to be delivered based on calculated dosage volume for the loading dose.

   - Inject the loading dose by pressing the loading dose control button.

9. Set the safety parameters for the infusion on the PCA pump according to the manufacturer's instructions. For example:
   - Dose volume limits. *This will limit the amount of drug that the client can receive when the client pushes the control button.*
   - Lockout interval between each dose. The lockout interval is generally between 5 and 12 minutes. *This sets the minimum time that must elapse before the client can receive another dose of the drug. Lockout time is based on the usual onset of the IV narcotic and the assessment of the client.*
   - 4-hour limit. Set the 4-hour dosage limit as specified on the orders. *This is an additional safety feature to limit the amount of medication delivered over 4 hours.*

10. Lock the machine.
    - Close the door on the pump.
    - Look for any digital cues or alarms that may indicate the machine is not set, and make corrections as needed.
    - Lock the machine with the key.

11. Begin the infusion.
    - Release the clamp on the Y-connector, and press the start button to begin the infusion.
    - Place the client control button within reach.

12. Monitor the client.
    - Monitor the status of the client every 2 hours during the first 24 to 36 hours of infusion and regularly thereafter, depending on the client's health and agency protocol.

13. Monitor the infusion.
    - Observe the IV site for signs of infiltration and phlebitis.
    - Inspect the tubing for kinks that may occlude the line.
    - Note the total number of doses and milligrams received.

 14. **Document** all relevant information.
    - Record the initiation of PCA, the dose setting, the doses received, pain intensity, and all assessments. See agency protocol.

PCA Pump

- Monitor for signs and symptoms of oversedation such as excessive drowsiness, slowed respiratory rate, and change in mental status.

- Do not adjust settings without consulting with the appropriate health care provider.

PCA Pump

Children

- Include the parents in teaching.
- Assess the child's ability to use the client control button.

Older Adults

- Carefully monitor for drug side effects.
- Use cautiously for individuals with impaired pulmonary or renal function.
- Assess the client's cognitive and physical ability to use the client control button.

EVALUATION

- Conduct appropriate follow-up:
  - Pain status
  - Respiratory rate and character
  - Amount of medication used
  - Frequency of use
- Relate to previous findings, if available.
- Report significant deviations from normal to the physician.

Patient-Controlled Epidural Analgesia

An increasingly popular method of delivery is the infusion of opiates into the **epidural** or **intrathecal** (subarachnoid) space (Figure 28-44 ◆). Patient-controlled epidural analgesia (PCEA) is often used to manage acute postoperative pain, chronic pain, and intractable cancer pain. The anesthesiologist or nurse anesthetist inserts a needle into the intrathecal or epidural space and threads a catheter through the needle. The catheter is connected to tubing that is then positioned along the spine and over the client's shoulder for the nurse to access. The entire catheter and tubing are taped securely to prevent dislodgement. Nursing care of clients with intraspinal infusions is summarized in Table 28-1.

Temporary catheters, used for short-term acute pain management, are usually placed at the lumbar or thoracic vertebral level and often removed after 2 to 4 days.

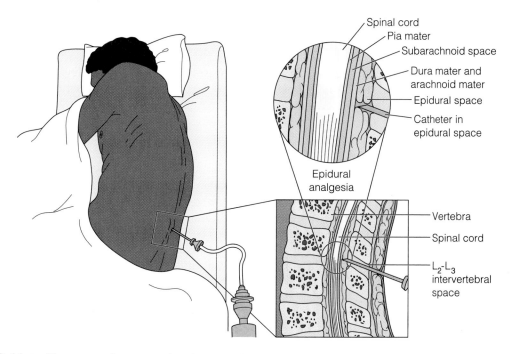

FIGURE 28-44 ◆ Placement of intraspinal catheter in the epidural space.

TABLE 28-1 NURSING INTERVENTIONS FOR CLIENTS RECEIVING ANALGESICS THROUGH AN EPIDURAL CATHETER

Nursing Goals	Interventions
Maintain client safety	• Label the tubing, the infusion bag, and the front of the pump with tape marked EPIDURAL to prevent confusion with similar-looking IV lines.
	• Post sign above client's bed indicating epidural is in place.
	• Secure all connections with tape.
	• If there is no continuous infusion, apply tape over all injection ports on the epidural line to avoid the injection of substances intended for IV administration into the epidural catheter.
	• Do not use alcohol in any care of catheter or insertion site as it can be neurotoxic.
	• Ensure that any solution injected or infused intraspinally is sterile, preservative-free, and safe for intraspinal administration.
Maintain catheter placement	• Secure temporary catheters with tape.
	• When bolus doses are used, gently aspirate prior to medication administration to determine catheter has not migrated into the subarachnoid space. (Expect < 1 mL of fluid return in syringe.)
	• Assist client in repositioning or moving out of bed.
	• Teach client to avoid tugging on the catheter.
	• Assess insertion site for leakage with each bolus dose or at least every 8 to 12 hours.
Prevent infection	• Use strict aseptic techniques with all epidural-related procedures.
	• Maintain sterile occlusive dressing over insertion site.
	• Assess insertion site for signs of infection.
	• Assess for increasing diffuse back pain or tenderness and/or pain and/or paresthesia on intraspinal injection as these are cardinal signs of intraspinal infection (McCaffery & Pasero, 1999, p. 234).
Maintain urinary and bowel function	• Monitor intake and output.
	• Assess for bowel and bladder distention.
Prevent respiratory depression	• Assess sedation level and respiratory status q1h for the first 24 hours and thereafter q4h.
	• Do not administer other opioids or central nervous system depressants unless ordered.
	• Keep an ampule of naloxone hydrochloride (0.4 mg) at the bedside.
	• Notify the clinician in charge if the respiratory rate falls below 8 per minute or if the client is difficult to rouse.

Permanent catheters, for clients with chronic pain, may be tunneled subcutaneously through the skin and exit at the client's side. Tunneling of the catheter reduces the risk of infection and displacement of the catheter. After the catheter is inserted, the nurse is responsible for monitoring the infusion and assessing the client.

A common misconception is that there is a higher incidence of respiratory depression when opioids are administered by the epidural route and, therefore, clients receiving epidural analgesia should be monitored in an intensive care setting. The fact is that respiratory depression occurs less often with epidural analgesia than by the IM route but is closer in comparison to IV PCA (McCaffery & Pasero, 1999, p. 214). Clients who are receiving epidural analgesia do not require intensive care monitoring. The nurse, outside the intensive care setting, can safely monitor the respiratory and sedation status of a client receiving epidural analgesia.

Intraspinal analgesics act directly on opiate receptors in the dorsal horn of the spinal cord. Two commonly used medications are preservative-free morphine sulfate and fentanyl. The major benefit of intraspinal drug therapy is that it exerts a lesser sedative effect than do systemic opiates. The epidural space is most commonly used because the dura mater acts as a protective barrier against infection, including meningitis. Because the epidural catheter is in a space and not a blood vessel, a continuous epidural infusion may be stopped for hours and restarted without concern that the catheter has become occluded (Pasero & McCaffery, 1999, p. 37).

Intraspinal analgesia can be administered by three methods:

1. *Bolus.* For some surgical procedures (e.g., cesarean section), a single bolus may provide sufficient pain control for up to 24 hours. After this time, the client may be given oral or IV analgesics.

Some agencies only allow the anesthesiologist or nurse anesthetist to initiate an epidural infusion or administer a bolus. Check the agency policy.

2. *Continuous infusion administered by pump.* The pump may be external (for acute or chronic pain) or implanted (for chronic pain).

3. *Patient-controlled epidural analgesia.* PCEA is administered by the client using a pump. This is similar to PCA in which a basal rate may meet the client's analgesic needs. If not, the client can push a button to deliver a preset dose.

Continuous Local Anesthetics

Continuous subcutaneous administration of long-acting local anesthetics into or near the surgical site is a new technique being used to provide postoperative pain control. This technique is being used for a variety of surgical procedures including knee arthroplasty, abdominal hysterectomy, hernia repair, and mastectomy (Pasero, 2000, p. 22).

The surgeon inserts a catheter under the subcutaneous tissue and on top of the muscle near or in the surgical wound site. A transparent dressing secures the catheter. The client is given a loading dose of local anesthetic before the continuous infusion is started.

The catheter is connected to an infusion pump that is set at the rate ordered by the physician. The infusion pump may be similar to the type used for IV or epidural analgesia, or it may be a disposable pump if the client will be continuing the treatment at home after discharge from the hospital.

Nursing interventions for the client with infusion of a **continuous local anesthetic** include:

- Conduct pain assessment and documentation every 2 to 4 hours while the client is awake.

- Check the dressing every shift for intactness. The dressing is not usually changed in order to avoid dislodging the catheter. Contact the physician if the dressing becomes loose.

- Check the site of the catheter. It should be clean and dry.

- Assess the client for signs of local anesthetic toxicity (e.g., dizziness; ringing in the ears; a metallic taste; tingling or numbness of the lips, gums, or tongue) (Pasero, 2000, pp. 22–23).

- Notify the physician of signs of local anesthetic toxicity. If detected early, prompt treatment can be initiated and serious complications avoided.

Chapter Summary

TERMINOLOGY

additive IV setup	insulin syringe	secondary IV setup
ampule	intermittent injection ports	secondary port
basal rate	intradermal (ID) injection	shaft
bevel	intramuscular (IM) injection	sharps
cannula	intrathecal	single-dose vial
continuous local anesthetic	intravenous (IV)	subcutaneous (SC or SQ) injection
deltoid site	intravenous push (IVP)	syringe pump
diluent	multidose vial	tandem
dorsogluteal site	parenteral	tuberculin syringe
epidural	patient-controlled analgesia (PCA)	vastus lateralis site
filter needle	piggyback	ventrogluteal site
gauge	prefilled unit-dose system	vial
hub	primary port	volume-control infusion set
hypodermic syringe	reconstitution	wheal
injection cap	rectus femoris site	Z-track technique

FORMING CLINICAL JUDGMENTS

Consider This:

1. What size syringe, needle gauge, and needle length would you consider for the following situations?

   a. Administering a tuberculin test to a 22-year-old male who is 6 feet tall and weighs 180 pounds.

   b. The order is for 5 mL of a medication to be given deep IM. The client is a 40-year-old female who weighs 135 pounds and is 5 feet 7 inches tall.

   c. Administer 0.75 mL subcutaneously in the upper arm to a 50-year-old 300-pound client. The nurse can grasp approximately 2 inches of the client's tissue at the upper arm.

   d. Administer 0.5 mL of a medication by IM injection to an elderly emaciated client.

2. The nurse needs to draw up two compatible medications into one syringe. Describe the process for drawing up the medication and indicate which medication you will draw up first and why.

   a. One medication is a single-dose prefilled sterile cartridge that uses a Tubex syringe and the other is in a multiple-dose vial.

   b. One medication is in a multiple-dose vial and the other is in an ampule.

   c. Each medication is in an ampule.

3. The nurse needs to mix two insulins to equal a total of 24 units. The nurse checks the amount with another nurse, who states that the total indicates 25 units. What would you do if you were the nurse who needed to administer the insulin?

4. No bleb forms when you administer a tuberculin test. What would you do?

5. The physician has ordered a medication to be added to an existing IV solution. You look up the medication in a drug handbook and read that a minimum of 500 mL is required. There is 475 mL remaining in the current IV that is infusing at 100 mL/hr. What do you do?

6. You administered an intermittent IV medication via a saline lock approximately 10 minutes ago. The UAP reports to you that the client is complaining of a burning sensation at the site of the peripheral IV lock. What do you do?

7. The nurse calculates the amount of medication needed for the prescribed order to be 2 mL. The medication is to be given subcutaneously. The nurse checks with the drug handbook and the pharmacist and the amount is within normal parameters. What would you do?

RELATED RESEARCH

Beyea, S. C., & Nicoll, L. H. (1996). Administering IM injections the right way. *American Journal of Nursing, 96*(1), 34–35.

Katsma, D. L., & Katsma, R. (2000). The myth of the 90°-angle intramuscular injection. *Nurse Educator, 25*(1), 34–37.

Klingman, L. (2000). Effects of changing needles prior to administering heparin subcutaneously. *Heart Lung, 29*(1), 70.

REFERENCES

Arnold, L. (1997). My needle stick. *Nursing, 27*(9), 48–50.

Covington, T. P., & Trattler, M. R. (1997). Bull's-eye! Finding the right target for I.M. injections. *Nursing, 27*(1), 62–63.

Fleming, D. R. (1999). Challenging traditional insulin injection practices. *American Journal of Nursing, 99*(2), 72–74.

Martin, D. (1998). Needle-free injection. *Nursing, 28*(7), 52–53.

McCaffery, M., & Pasero, C. (1999). *Pain clinical manual* (2nd ed.). St. Louis: Mosby.

McConnell, E. A. (1998). Clinical do's & don'ts: Admixing drugs in a syringe. *Nursing, 28*(5), 20.

McConnell, E. A. (1998). How to choose and use needle-stick prevention devices. *Nursing, 28*(5), 32-6–32-8.

McConnell, E. A. (1999). Clinical do's & don'ts: Administering a Z-track IM injection. *Nursing, 29*(1), 26.

McConnell, E. A. (1999). Clinical do's & don'ts: Administering an insulin injection. *Nursing, 29*(12), 18.

McConnell, E. A. (2000). Do's & don'ts: Administering an intradermal injection. *Nursing, 30*(3), 17.

Pasero, C. (1999). Using continuous infusion with PCA. *American Journal of Nursing, 99*(2), 22.

Pasero, C. (2000). Continuous local anesthetics. *American Journal of Nursing, 100*(8), 22–23.

Pasero, C., & McCaffery, M. (1999). Providing epidural analgesia. *Nursing, 29*(8), 34–39.

Possanza, C. P. (1997). Special delivery: Using a syringe pump to administer I.V. drugs. *Nursing, 27*(9), 43–45.

Satarawala, R. (2000). Confronting the legal perils of IV therapy. *Nursing, 30*(8), 44–47.

Service Employees International Union. (1998). *SEIU's Guide to Preventing Needlestick injuries* (3rd ed.). Washington: Service Employees International Union.

Skokal, W. (2000). IV push at home? *RN, 63*(10), 26–29.

Wilburn, S. (2000), Preventing needlesticks in your facility. *American Journal of Nursing, 100*(2), 96.

Chapter 29

Administering Intravenous Therapy

Techniques

OBJECTIVES

- Identify common types of intravenous catheters and infusions.
- Identify purposes of intravenous therapy and central venous lines.
- Identify various venipuncture sites.
- Identify relevant assessment data related to intravenous therapy and central venous lines.
- Calculate and regulate infusion rates.
- Differentiate intravenous pumps from controllers.
- Identify interventions required to prevent complications associated with intravenous therapy and central venous catheters.
- Describe essential aspects of administering blood transfusions and total parenteral nutrition (TPN).
- Document essential information related to intravenous therapy and central venous catheters.

Intravenous Infusions

An intravenous (IV) **infusion** is the instillation into a vein of fluid, electrolytes, medications, blood, or nutrient substances. A physician is responsible for ordering the type of solution to be administered, the amount to be given, and the rate at which it is to be infused.

Intravenous therapy can be prescribed for these reasons:

- To supply parenteral fluid, electrolytes, or calories when clients are unable to take in an adequate volume by mouth
- To provide water-soluble vitamins and medications
- To establish a lifeline for rapidly needed medications

Common Types of Solutions

Common solutions administered intravenously include nutrient solutions, electrolyte solutions, and blood volume expanders. *Nutrient solutions* contain some form of carbohydrate (e.g., dextrose or glucose) and water. Water is supplied for fluid requirements, and carbohydrate for calories and energy. For example, 1 liter of 5 percent dextrose in water (D_5W) provides 170 calories.

Electrolyte solutions contain varying amounts of cations and anions. Commonly used solutions are normal saline (0.9 percent sodium chloride solution) and lactated Ringer's solution (which contains sodium, chloride, potassium, calcium, and lactate).

Blood volume expanders are used to increase the volume of blood following severe loss of blood (e.g., from hemorrhage) or plasma (e.g., from severe burns, which draw large amounts of plasma from the bloodstream to the burn site). Common blood volume expanders are dextran, plasma, and human serum albumin.

Solutions such as normal saline are isotonic (similar concentration of solutes as plasma). Half normal saline (0.45 percent sodium chloride) is hypotonic (lesser concentration of solutes than plasma) and will provide extra hydration. Dextrose 5 percent in lactated Ringer's is hypertonic (greater concentration of solutes than plasma) and can draw fluid out of the cells and interstitial spaces into the vascular system.

Peripheral Venipuncture Sites

The site chosen for venipuncture varies with the client's age, the infusion time, the type of solution used, and the condition of veins. For adults, veins in the arm are commonly used. The larger veins of the forearm are preferred to the metacarpal veins of the hand for infusions that need to be given rapidly and for solutions that are hypertonic, are highly acidic or alkaline, or contain irritating medications.

The metacarpal, basilic, and cephalic veins are valuable venipuncture sites (Figure 29-1 ◆A and B). The ulna and radius act as natural splints at these sites, and the client has greater freedom of arm movements for activities such as eating. Although the antecubital basilic and median cubital veins are convenient (Figure 29-1A), use of these veins for prolonged infusions limits arm mobility because a splint is needed to stabilize the elbow joint.

When long-term or caustic IV therapy is needed, a physician may insert a **central venous catheter (CVC)** (Figure 29-2 ◆) or **implanted venous access device (IVAD)** (Figure 29-3 ◆). Specially trained nurses may place a peripherally inserted central catheter (PICC line) into the anticubital space (Figure 29-1A) that is then threaded up into the superior vena cava.

Intravenous Equipment

Because equipment varies according to the manufacturer, the nurse must become familiar with the equipment used in each particular agency.

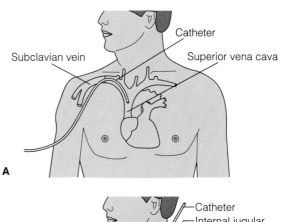

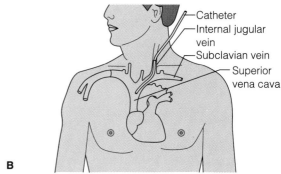

FIGURE 29-2 ◆ Central venous lines with (A) subclavian; and (B) jugular vein insertion.

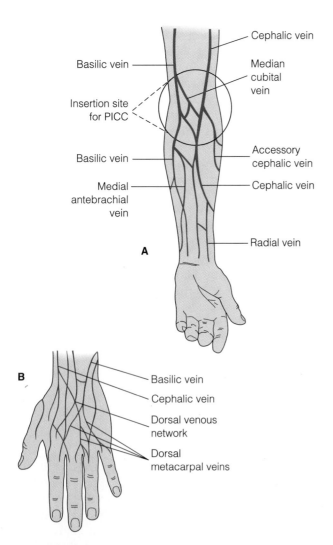

FIGURE 29-1 ◆ Commonly used venipuncture sites of the (A) arm; (B) hand. A also shows the site used for a peripherally inserted central catheter (PICC line).

Solution containers are available in various sizes (e.g., 50, 250, or 1,000 mL) and most are plastic bags (Figure 29-4 ◆). Glass bottles may be required if a medication is incompatible with plastic. Glass solution bottles require an air vent, so that air replaces the solution as it runs out of the bottle. Air vents are not required for plastic solution containers, because the bags collapse under atmospheric pressure when the solution enters the client's vein.

Administration/infusion sets consist of an insertion spike, a drip chamber, a roller valve or screw clamp,

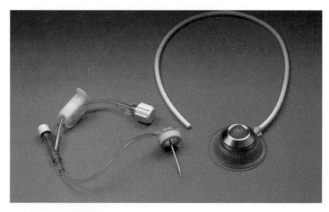

FIGURE 29-3 ◆ An implantable venous access device (right) and a Huber needle with extension tubing.

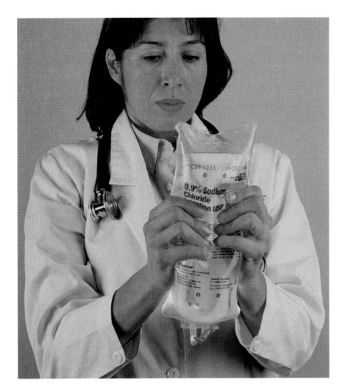

FIGURE 29-4 ◆ A plastic IV bag.

tubing, and a protective cap over the needle adapter (Figure 29-5 ◆). The drip chamber permits a predictable amount of fluid to be delivered. A **macrodrip** drip chamber delivers between 10 and 20 drops per milliliter of solution. The specific amount is written on the

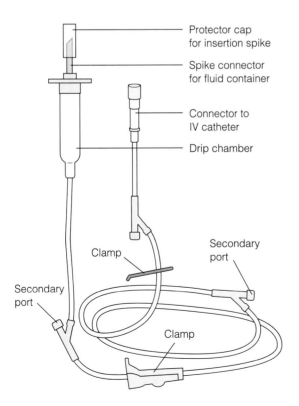

- Protector cap for insertion spike
- Spike connector for fluid container
- Connector to IV catheter
- Drip chamber
- Clamp
- Secondary port
- Secondary port
- Clamp

FIGURE 29-5 ◆ A standard IV infusion set.

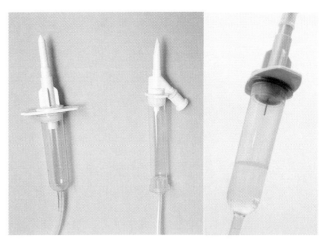

FIGURE 29-6 ◆ Infusion set spikes and drip chambers: nonvented macrodrip, vented macrodrip, nonvented microdrip.

package. **Microdrip** sets deliver 60 drops per milliliter of solution (Figure 29-6 ◆).

Most infusion sets contain one or more injection ports for administering medications or secondary infusions. These ports may be accessed with a needle or, preferably, with needleless connectors to reduce the risk of needle-stick injuries (Figure 29-7 ◆). When

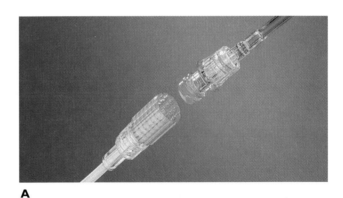

A

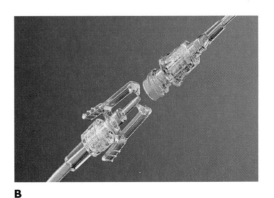

B

FIGURE 29-7 ◆ Needleless cannulae used to connect the tubing of secondary sets to primary tubing: (A) threaded cannula; (B) lever-lock cannula.

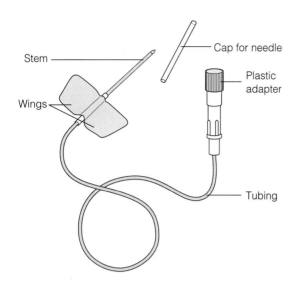

FIGURE 29-8 ◆ Schematic of a butterfly needle with tubing and adapter.

more than one solution needs to be infused at the same time, *secondary sets* such as the **tandem** and the **piggyback IV** setups are used. Another variation is a *volume-control set,* which is used if the volume of fluid or medication administered is to be carefully controlled (see Technique 28-8).

Many kinds of needles and catheters are commonly used for intravenous infusions. A **butterfly (wing-tipped) needle** with plastic flaps attached to the shaft is shown in Figure 29-8 ◆. The flaps are held tightly together to hold the needle securely as it is inserted; after insertion, they are flattened against the skin and secured with tape. They vary in length from 1.5 to 3 cm (½ to 1¼ in), and from 25 gauge (about 0.027 inch outside diameter) to 17 gauge (about 0.055 inch outside diameter). The larger the gauge number, the smaller the diameter of the shaft. Needles of 20 to 22 gauge and short lengths are commonly used for adults. A *catheter* or **angiocatheter** is a plastic tube inserted into the vein. Some catheters fit over a needle/stylet during insertion, whereas others fit inside a

needle (Figure 29-9 ◆). An angiocatheter has a metal stylet that is used to pierce the skin and vein and is then withdrawn, leaving the catheter in place.

IV filters are used to remove air and particulate matter from intravenous infusions and to reduce the risk of complications (e.g., infusion-related phlebitis) associated with routine IV therapies (Figure 29-10 ◆). Most IV filters in current use consist of a membrane (pore size of 0.22 μ, although sizes vary. Some problems associated with filters include (1) clogging of the filter surface, which may stop or slow the flow rate when debris accumulates; and (2) binding of some drugs (e.g., insulin and amphotericin B) to the surface of the filter. When using filters, the nurse remembers that the filter should never be considered a substitute for quality care and meticulous technique.

IV poles (rods) are needed to hang the solution container. Some poles are attached to hospital beds; others stand on the floor or hang from the ceiling. Still others are floor models with casters that can be pushed along when a client is up and walking. The height of most poles is adjustable. The higher the solution container, the greater the force of the solution as it enters the client and the faster the rate of flow.

Rather than using a continuous infusion, an intermittent infusion lock may be created by attaching a sterile injection cap to an existing intravenous catheter. This keeps the venous access available for the administration of intermittent or emergency medications. The device is commonly referred to as a **heparin** or **saline lock** because periodic injection with heparin or saline is used to keep blood from coagulating within the tubing.

Performing Venipuncture

Agency practices vary about which nurses perform venipunctures and start intravenous infusions. In many settings, nurses must be supervised and certified before they are permitted to start infusions on their own. Some agencies have teams of specially prepared nurses who initiate all intravenous infusions.

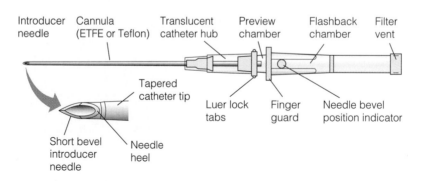

FIGURE 29-9 ◆ Schematic of an over-the-needle catheter.

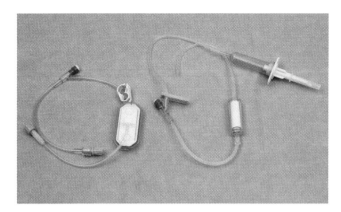

FIGURE 29-10 ◆ Two types of IV filters.

Nursing Process: Performing Venipuncture

ASSESSMENT

Before performing venipuncture, the nurse must determine:

- The physician's exact orders
- Whether the client has any allergies, especially to tape, povidone–iodine, and latex.
- The agency policy about clipping hair in the area before a venipuncture. Shaving is not recommended because of the possibility of nicking the skin and subsequent infection. Examine the available arms and hands for a possible insertion site (see Box 29-1). Avoid sites that have been used recently *since they will be more prone to complications and discomfort.*

PLANNING

Review the client record regarding previous venipuncture. Note any difficulties encountered and how they were resolved.

Delegation

Due to the need for knowledge of anatomy and use of sterile technique, venipuncture is not delegated to unlicensed assistive personnel (UAP). UAP may care for clients with intravenous needles inserted, and the nurse must ensure that the UAP knows how to perform routine tasks such as bathing and positioning without disturbing the IV. The UAP should also know what complications or adverse signs, such as leakage, should be reported to the nurse.

IMPLEMENTATION:
TECHNIQUE 29-1 PERFORMING VENIPUNCTURE

Equipment

Substitute appropriate supplies if the client has tape, antiseptic, or latex allergies.

- Clean or sterile gloves
- Tourniquet or blood pressure cuff
- Antiseptic swabs such as 10 percent povidone–iodine or 2 percent chlorhexidine
- Antiseptic ointment, such as povidone–iodine (optional)
- Intravenous catheter/needle

Choose an IV needle of the appropriate size based on the size of the vein and the purpose of the needle. A 22-gauge needle is indicated for most adults. Always have an extra needle and ones of different sizes available.

- Sterile gauze dressing or transparent occlusive dressing
- Arm splint, if required
- Towel or bed protector
- Local anesthetic (optional)

Preparation

1. If possible, select a time to perform the venipuncture that is convenient for the client. Unless initiating IV therapy is urgent, provide any scheduled care before insertion to minimize excessive movement of the affected limb.

2. Visitors or family members may be asked to leave the room if desired by the nurse or the client.

Performance

1. Explain to the client what you are going to do, why it is necessary, and how he or she can cooperate. Venipuncture can cause discomfort for a few seconds, but there should be no ongoing pain after insertion. If possible, explain how long the needle will need to remain in place and how it will be used.

2. Wash hands and observe appropriate infection control procedures.

3. Prepare the client.
   - Check the client's identification band. *This ensures that the right client receives the venipuncture.*
   - Assist the client to a comfortable position, either sitting or lying. Expose the limb to be used but provide for client privacy.

4. Prepare the final venipuncture site.
   - Check agency protocol about shaving if the site is very hairy.
   - Place a towel or bed protector under the extremity to protect linens (or furniture if in the home).

5. Dilate the vein.
   - Place the extremity in a dependent position (lower than the client's heart). *Gravity slows venous return and distends the veins. Distending the veins makes it easier to insert the needle properly.*
   - Apply a tourniquet firmly 15 to 20 cm (6 to 8 in) above the venipuncture site (Figure 29-11 ◆). Explain that the tourniquet will feel tight. The tourniquet must be tight enough to obstruct venous flow but not so tight that it occludes arterial flow. *Obstructing arterial flow inhibits venous filling.* If a radial pulse can be palpated, the arterial flow is not obstructed. Some practitioners prefer to use a blood pressure cuff. Inflate the cuff to 30 to 40 mm Hg.
   - If the vein is not sufficiently dilated:
     a. Massage or stroke the vein distal to the site and in the direction of venous flow toward the heart. *This action helps fill the vein.*
     b. Encourage the client to clench and unclench the fist. *Contracting the muscles compresses the*

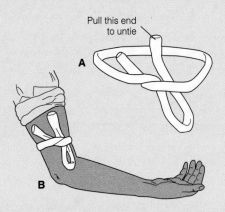

Pull this end
to untie

A

B

FIGURE 29-11 ◆ Applying a tourniquet.

distal veins, forcing blood along the veins and distending them.

   c. Lightly tap the vein with your fingertips. *Tapping may distend the vein.* If the preceding steps fail to distend the vein so that it is palpable, remove the tourniquet and apply heat to the entire extremity for 10 to 15 minutes. *Heat dilates superficial blood vessels, causing them to fill.* Then repeat step 5.

6. Don gloves, and clean the venipuncture site. *Gloves protect the nurse from contamination by the client's blood.*
   - Clean the skin at the site of entry with a topical antiseptic swab (e.g., alcohol), and then an anti-infective solution such as povidone–iodine. In some agencies, 2 percent chlorhexidine is the preferred antiseptic.
   - Use a circular motion, moving from the center outward for several inches. *This motion carries microorganisms away from the site of entry.*
   - Permit the solution to dry on the skin. *The antiseptic should be in contact with the skin for at least 1 minute to be effective.*

7. Insert the catheter, and initiate the infusion.
   - If desired and permitted by policy, inject 0.05 mL 1 percent lidocaine intradermally over the site where you plan to insert the IV needle. Allow 5 to 10 seconds for the anesthetic to take effect. Alternative approaches include injecting normal saline or applying topical anesthetic cream.
   - Use the nondominant hand to pull the skin taut below the entry site. *This stabilizes the vein and can make initial tissue penetration less painful.*
   - Holding the catheter at a 15- to 30-degree angle with bevel up, insert the catheter through the skin and into the vein in one thrust. Sudden lack of resistance is felt as the needle enters the vein.

- Once blood appears in the lumen of the needle or you feel the lack of resistance, reduce the angle of the catheter until it is almost parallel with the skin, and advance the needle and catheter approximately 0.5 to 1 cm (about ¼ in) further. Holding the needle portion steady, advance the catheter until the hub is at the venipuncture site. The exact technique depends on the type of device used. *The catheter is advanced to ensure that it, and not just the metal needle, is in the vein.*

- If there is no blood return, try redirecting the catheter assembly again toward the vein. If the needle has been withdrawn from the catheter even a small distance, or the catheter tip has been pulled out of the skin, the catheter must be discarded and a new one used. *Reinserting the needle into the catheter can result in slicing the catheter apart. A catheter that has been removed from the skin is considered contaminated and cannot be reused.*

- If blood begins to flow out of the vein into the tissues as the needle is inserted, creating a hematoma, the insertion is unsuccessful. This is sometimes referred to as a "blown" vein. Immediately release the tourniquet and remove the needle, applying pressure over the insertion site with dry gauze. Attempt the venipuncture in another site, in the opposite arm if possible. *Placing the tourniquet back on the same arm above the unsuccessful site may cause it to bleed. Placing the IV below the unsuccessful site could result in infusing fluid into the already punctured vein, causing it to leak.*

- Release the tourniquet.

- Stabilize the catheter hub and apply pressure distal to the catheter with your finger. *This prevents excessive blood flow through the catheter.*

- Place the needle directly into a sharps container. If this is not within reach, place the needle into its original package and dispose in sharps container as soon as possible.

- Remove the protective end from the injection cap or the distal end of the tubing, and attach it to the catheter hub.

- Initiate the infusion or flush the catheter with sterile normal saline. *Blood must be removed from the catheter lumen and tubing immediately. Otherwise, the blood will clot inside the lumen.* Watch closely for any signs that the catheter is infiltrated (the tip is outside the vein and the fluid is entering the tissues instead). *Inflammation or infiltration necessitates removal of the IV needle or catheter to avoid further trauma to the tissues.*

8. Tape the catheter.
- Tape the catheter by the "U" method or according to manufacturer's instructions. If using an already opened roll of tape, discard the first rotation of tape around the roll. *The first rotation has been shown to be highly colonized with infec-*

tious organisms (Redelmeier & Livesley, 1999). Using three strips of adhesive tape, each about 7.5 cm (3 in) long:

a. Place one strip, sticky side up, under the catheter's hub.

b. Fold each end over so that the sticky sides are against the skin (Figure 29-12 ◆).

c. Place second strip, sticky side down, over catheter hub.

d. Place third strip, sticky side down, over tubing hub. Do not tape directly over the insertion site. *The tape is not sterile and may contaminate the site.*

Variation: Inserting a Butterfly (Winged-Tip) Needle

- Hold the needle, pointed in the direction of the blood flow, at a 30-degree angle, with the bevel up, and pierce the skin beside the vein about 1 cm (½ in) below the site planned for piercing the vein (Figure 29-13 ◆).

- Once the needle is through the skin, lower the needle so that it is almost parallel with the skin. Lowering the needle reduces the chances of puncturing both sides of the vein. Follow the course of the vein, and pierce one side of the vein. Sudden lack of resistance can be felt as blood enters the needle.

- When blood flows back into the needle tubing, gently advance the needle to its hub.

- Release the tourniquet, attach the infusion or cap, and initiate flow as quickly as possible.

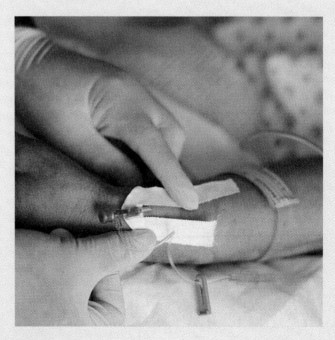

FIGURE 29-12 ◆ Taping an IV catheter using the "U" method.

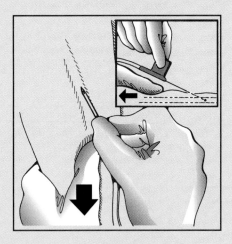

FIGURE 29-13 ◆ Inserting a butterfly needle.

Securing a Butterfly Needle

- Tape the butterfly needle securely by the crisscross (chevron) or "H" method (Figure 29-14 ◆). Place a small gauze square under the hub, if required. *The gauze keeps the needle in position in the vein.* Do not tape directly over the insertion site. *The tape is not sterile and may contaminate the site.*

9. Dress and label the venipuncture site and tubing according to agency policy.

   - In some agencies, the nurse puts a small amount of antiseptic ointment, such as povidone–iodine, over the venipuncture site, then a gauze square or band-aid. In other agencies, a sterile transparent occlusive dressing is applied. *This permits assessment of the site without disturbing the dressing.*

   - Remove soiled gloves and discard appropriately.

   - Loop any tubing, and secure it with tape. *Looping and securing the tubing prevent the weight of the tubing or any movement from pulling on the needle or catheter.*

   - Label the dressing with the date and time of insertion, type and gauge of needle or catheter used, and your initials (Figure 29-15 ◆).

10. Apply a padded arm board to splint the joint, as needed.

11. Discard all used disposable supplies in appropriate receptacles. Cleanse any blood spills according to agency policy. Clean any reusable supplies such as tourniquets.

12. **Document** all assessments and interventions.

    - Record the venipuncture on the client's chart. Some agencies provide a special form for this purpose. Include the date and time of the venipuncture; type and gauge of the needle or catheter; venipuncture site; and the client's general response.

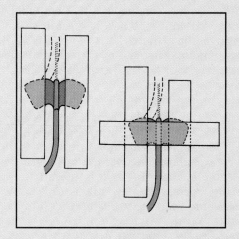

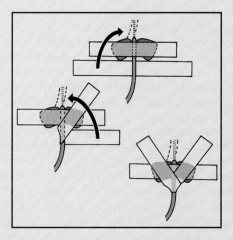

FIGURE 29-14 ◆ Taping the butterfly needle by the "H" and chevron methods.

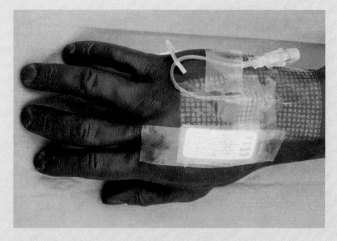

FIGURE 29-15 ◆ A labeled venipuncture site.

Venipuncture

Infant/Child

- For infants, veins in the scalp are used for venipuncture (Figure 29-16 ◆).

- Because infants do not have large veins in the antecubital fossa, blood specimens for examination are usually taken from the external jugular and femoral veins.

- Use a doll to demonstrate venipuncture for children and explain the procedure to the parents.

- Explain the procedure to the young client, encourage questions, and be alert for nonverbal cues. Children may not understand things that seem obvious to adults. For example, a child may think the IV therapy is a punishment.

- A 24-gauge needle is commonly indicated for use with children.

- Apply age-appropriate restraints, arm boards, or other devices to protect the IV site.

Elders

- Skin is often fragile and bruises easily. Select an IV site with adequate healthy tissue to support the needle.

- To distend the vein, tap only lightly to prevent trauma.

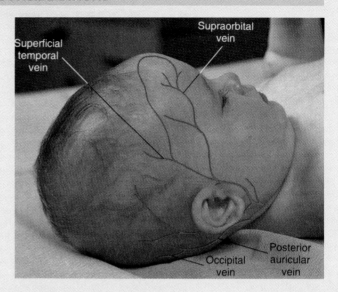

FIGURE 29-16 ◆ Scalp veins on an infant are frequently used for peripheral IV access.

- Consider not using a tourniquet. Elders' superficial veins are often large enough to insert the needle without further distention. Using a tourniquet can cause the vein to burst when the needle enters.

- Minimize the use of alcohol and tape to avoid irritating sensitive skin.

EVALUATION

- Perform follow-up based on findings or outcomes that deviated from expected or normal for the client. Relate findings to previous data if available.

- Regularly check the skin status at IV site (warm temperature and absence of pain, redness, or swelling); status of the dressing; the client's ability to perform self-care activities; and the client's understanding of any mobility limitations.

- Report significant deviations from normal to the physician.

Establishing Intravenous Infusions

An intravenous infusion may be set up before venipuncture so that the infusion can be attached to the needle or catheter immediately after it is inserted.

Nursing Process: Establishing Intravenous Infusions

ASSESSMENT

- Before preparing the infusion, verify the physician's order indicating the type of solution, the

amount to be administered, and the rate of flow of the infusion.

Assess the IV site:

- If the IV needle has already been inserted and is not currently attached to an infusion, ensure that it is patent by aspirating for blood or irrigating with normal saline.

- Inspect the IV site for the presence of **infiltration** or inflammation. *Inflammation or infiltration necessitates removal of the IV needle or catheter to avoid further trauma to the tissues.* Discontinue and relocate the IV site if indicated (see Techniques 29-1, 29-5, and 29-6).

PLANNING

Review the client record regarding previous infusions. Note any complications and how they were managed.

Delegation

Due to the use of sterile technique, intravenous infusion therapy is not delegated to UAP. UAP may care for clients receiving IV therapy, and the nurse must ensure that the UAP knows how to perform routine tasks such as bathing and positioning without disturbing the IV. The UAP should also know what complications or adverse signs, such as leakage, should be reported to the nurse.

Equipment

- Clean gloves
- Infusion set and adapters if needed
- Container of sterile parenteral solution
- Labels for IV tubing and container
- IV pole
- Nonallergenic tape
- Electronic infusion device or pump, as needed

Preparation

1. If possible, select a time to establish the infusion that is convenient for the client. Unless initiating IV therapy is urgent, provide any scheduled care before initiation to minimize excessive movement of the affected limb.

Performance

1. Explain to the client what you are going to do, why it is necessary, and how he or she can cooperate. If possible, explain how long the infusion will need to remain in place.

2. Make sure that the client's clothing or gown can be removed over the IV apparatus if necessary. Some agencies provide special gowns that open over the shoulder and down the sleeve for easy removal.

3. Wash hands and observe appropriate infection control procedures.

4. Prepare the client.
   - Check the client's identification band. *This ensures that the client receives the correct infusion.*
   - Assist the client to a comfortable position, either sitting or lying. Expose the limb to be used but provide for client privacy.

5. Apply a medication label to the solution container if a medication was added. Determine agency policy.
   - In many agencies, medications and labels are applied in the pharmacy; if they are not, apply the label upside down on the container (see Figure 28-33, p. 562). *The label is applied upside down so it can be read easily when the container is hanging up.*

6. Apply a timing strip to the solution container.
   - Mark the strip to indicate the anticipated fluid level at hourly intervals.
   - The timing strip may be applied at the time the infusion is started. Follow agency practice. See discussion of regulating infusion flow rates and Figure 29-20 on page 591.

7. Open and prepare the infusion set.

- Remove tubing from the container, and straighten it out.
- Slide the tubing clamp along the tubing until it is just below the drip chamber to facilitate its access.
- Close the clamp.
- Leave the ends of the tubing covered with the plastic caps until the infusion is started. *This will maintain the sterility of the ends of the tubing.*

8. Spike the solution container.
   - See Technique 28-9 for adding medications to an intravenous fluid container, pages 567–570.
   - Follow manufacturer's instructions to expose the insertion site of the bag or bottle.
   - Remove the cap from the spike, and insert the spike into the insertion site (Figure 29-17 ◆).

9. Hang the solution container on the pole.
   - Adjust the pole so that the container is suspended about 1 m (3 ft) above the client's head. *This height is needed to enable gravity to overcome venous pressure and facilitate flow of the solution into the vein.*

10. Partially fill the drip chamber with solution. (*Note:* This step may be performed outside of the client's room and then the system transported to the client's bedside.)
    - Squeeze the chamber gently until it is half full of solution (Figure 29-18 ◆). *The drip chamber is partly filled with solution to prevent air from moving down the tubing.*

11. Prime the tubing.
    - Remove the protective cap, and hold the tubing over a container. Maintain the sterility of the end of the tubing and the cap.
    - Release the clamp, and let the fluid run through the tubing until all bubbles are removed. Tap the tubing if necessary with your fingers to help the bubbles move. *The tubing is primed to prevent the introduction of air into the client. Air bubbles smaller than 0.5 mL usually do not cause problems in peripheral lines.*

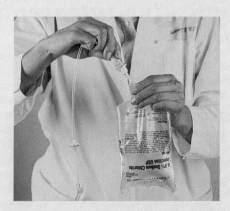

FIGURE 29-17 ◆ Inserting the spike.

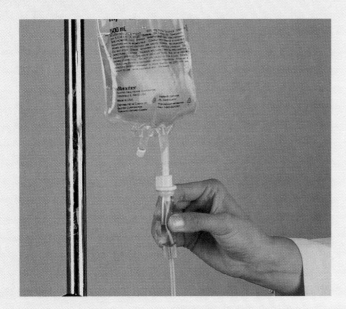

FIGURE 29-18 ◆ Squeezing the drip chamber.

- Reclamp the tubing, and replace the tubing cap, maintaining sterile technique.
- For caps with air vents, do not remove the cap when priming this tubing. *The flow of solution through the tubing will cease when the cap is moist with one drop of solution.*
- If an infusion control pump, electronic device, or controller is being used, follow the manufacturer's directions for inserting the tubing and setting the infusion rate (see Technique 29-3).

12. Disconnect the used tubing or remove the cap on an intermittent device.
- Don clean gloves.
- Place a sterile swab under the hub of the catheter. *This absorbs any leakage that might occur when the tubing is disconnected.*
- Clamp the tubing.
- Holding the hub of the catheter with the non-dominant hand, remove the tubing or cap with the dominant hand, using a twisting, pulling motion. *Holding the catheter firmly but gently maintains its position in the vein.*
- Place the end of the used tubing or cap in a basin or other receptacle.

Variation: Starting an Infusion on a Central Line (See Also Techniques 29-8 and 29-9)
- Don clean gloves and mask.
- Clean the junction of the catheter and tubing or cap with antiseptic, as required by agency protocol. *This prevents the transfer of microorganisms from the client's skin to the open CVC catheter hub when it is detached; it also decreases the number of microorganisms at the catheter-tubing junction.*
- Ask the client to perform Valsalva's maneuver (that is, to take a deep breath and bear down) and to turn the head away while you detach the IV tubing or cap by rotating it out of the hub.

Performance of Valsalva's maneuver reduces the risk of air embolism, and turning the head to the side reduces the chances of contaminating the equipment.

13. Connect the new tubing, and establish the infusion.
- Continue to hold the catheter and grasp the new tubing with the dominant hand.

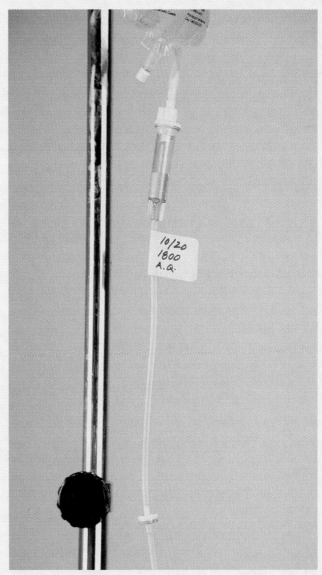

FIGURE 29-19 ◆ (A) Tubing labeled with date, time, and nurse's initials. (B) Also shown is a preprinted label.

- Remove the protective tubing cap, and maintaining sterility, insert the tubing end securely into the needle hub.
- Open the clamp to start the solution flowing.

14. Ensure appropriate infusion flow.
    - Remove gloves.
    - Apply a padded arm board to splint the joint, as needed.
    - Adjust the infusion rate of flow according to the order.

15. Label the IV tubing.
    - Label the tubing with the date and time of attachment and your initials (Figure 29-19 ◆). This labeling may also be done when the container is set up. *The tubing is labeled to ensure*

that it is changed at regular intervals (i.e., every 24 to 72 hours according to agency policy).

16. Loop the tubing and secure it with tape. *Looping and securing the tubing prevent the weight of the tubing or any movement from pulling on the needle or catheter.*

17. **Document** all assessments and interventions.
    - Record the infusion on the client's chart. Some agencies provide a special form for this purpose (See Figure 29-24 pages 597–598). Include the date and time of beginning the infusion; amount and type of solution used, including any additives (e.g., kind and amount of medications); container number; flow rate; and the client's general response.

EVALUATION

- Perform follow-up based on findings or outcomes that deviated from expected or normal for the client. Relate findings to previous data if available.

- Regularly check the client for intended and adverse effects of the infusion.

- Examine the IV site at regular intervals.

- Report significant deviations from normal to the physician.

Regulating Intravenous Flow Rates

An important nursing function is to regulate the flow rate of an intravenous infusion. The physician may describe in the order how long an infusion should last (e.g., 1,000 mL over 8 hours). It is then a nursing responsibility to calculate the correct flow rate and regulate the infusion. Problems that can result from incorrectly regulated infusions include hypervolemia and hypovolemia. Unless a regulating device (i.e., an **infusion controller**, **infusion pump**, or in-line manual adjuster) is being used, the nurse administering the intravenous solution must regulate the drops per minute manually by using the roller clamp to ensure that the prescribed amount of solution will be infused in the correct time span.

Infusion sets each have their own type of drip chamber; so, it is important to know the number of drops per milliliter of solution for a particular set before calculating a drip rate. This rate, called the **drop or drip factor**, is printed on the tubing package. Common drop factors are 10, 12, 15, and 20 for **macrodrips** (regular/macro infusion sets) and 60 for **microdrips** (minidrip infusion sets).

Two methods of indicating flow rates are designating the number of milliliters or cubic centimeters to be administered in 1 hour (mL/hr or cc/hr) and the number of drops to be given in 1 minute (gtts/min).

Occasionally, the IV rate order will read "keep vein open" (KVO) or "to keep open" (TKO). This order does not provide adequate direction for the nurse unless agency policy specifies the milliliters per hour equivalent for this order. Some IV pumps have a "keep open" rate choice built in. If the IV is not on this type of pump and no policy exists, contact the physician for clarification.

Milliliters per Hour

Hourly rates of infusion can be calculated by dividing the total infusion volume by the total infusion time in hours. For example, if 3,000 mL is infused in 24 hours, the number of milliliters per hour is:

$$\frac{3,000 \text{ mL (total infusion volume)}}{24 \text{ hr (total infusion time)}} = 125 \text{ mL/hr}$$

Nurses need to check infusions at least every hour to ensure that the indicated milliliters per hour have infused. A strip of adhesive marking the exact time and/or amount to be infused should be taped to the solution container. Some agencies make premarked labels available (Figure 29-20 ◆). Do not write directly on the IV bag or the strip with a felt-tip open. *Ink from felt-tip pens can leach through the bag into the fluid.*

Drops per Minute

The nurse who begins an infusion must regulate the drops per minute to ensure that the prescribed amount of solution will infuse. Drops per minute are calculated by the following formula:

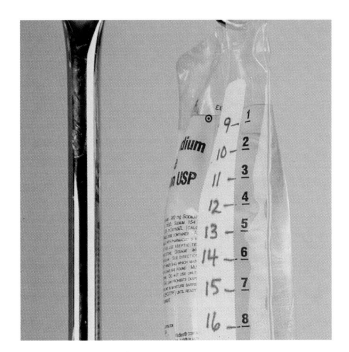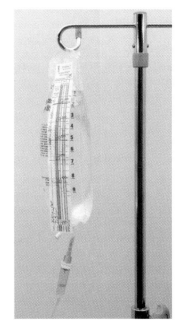

FIGURE 29-20 ◆ Timing label on an IV container.

Drops per minute =

$$\frac{\text{Total infusion volume} \times \text{drop/mL (or drop factor)}}{\text{Total time of infusion in } \textit{minutes}}$$

If the requirements are 1,000 mL in 8 hours (480 minutes) and the drip factor is 20 drops/mL, the drops per minute should be:

$$\frac{1,000 \text{ mL} \times 20 \text{ drops /mL}}{480 \text{ min}} = 41 \text{ drops/min}$$

Approximating this rate as 40 drops/min, the nurse must then regulate the drops per minute by tightening or releasing the intravenous tubing clamp and counting the drops the same way a pulse is counted.

Devices such as battery-operated controllers and infusion pumps with alarm systems facilitate a regulated flow. Newer systems are programmable and include drug libraries with dose rate calculators, automatic flushing between medications, dual or triple simultaneous line control, memory, multiple alarm settings (air in line, pressure/resistance, battery), schedule reminders, volume settings down to 0.1 mL, panel locks, and digital displays (Figure 29-21 ◆).

Nursing Process: Using an Infusion Controller or Pump

ASSESSMENT

Before preparing the infusion device, the nurse first verifies the physician's order indicating the type of

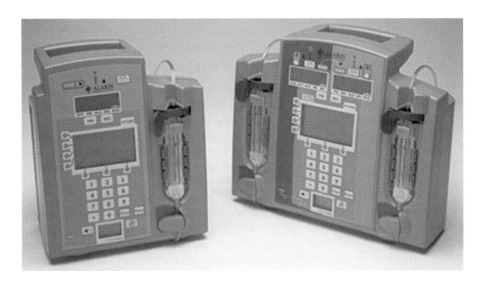

FIGURE 29-21 ◆ Programmable infusion pumps.

solution, the amount to be administered, and the rate of flow of the infusion.

PLANNING

Review the client record regarding previous infusions and use of infusion devices. Note any complications and how they were managed.

Delegation

Due to the need for sterile technique and technical complexity, use of infusion devices is not delegated to UAP. UAP may care for clients with such devices, and the nurse must ensure that the UAP knows how to perform routine tasks such as positioning and changing gowns when a device is in place. The UAP should also know what complications or adverse signs, such as alarms, should be reported to the nurse.

IMPLEMENTATION:

TECHNIQUE 29-3 USING AN INFUSION PUMP OR CONTROLLER

Equipment

- Infusion controller or pump
- The IV solution or medication
- An IV pole
- An IV administration set with compatible IV tubing
- Alcohol swabs and tape
- Label for tubing
- Time strip for container

Preparation

1. Review the use of the pump outside of the client's room. Read all appropriate materials and confirm how to set the device.

Performance

1. Explain to the client what you are going to do, why it is necessary, and how he or she can cooperate. Explain what the device sounds like during normal use, the various alarms, and to notify the nurse if an alarm sounds.

2. Make sure that the client's clothing or gown can be removed over the IV apparatus if necessary. Some agencies provide special gowns that open over the shoulder and down the sleeve for easy removal.

3. Wash hands and observe appropriate infection control procedures.

4. Prepare the client.
   - Check the client's identification band. *This ensures that the right client receives the infusion.*
   - Assist the client to a comfortable position, either sitting or lying. Expose the limb as needed but provide for client privacy.

Infusion Controller

1. Attach the controller to the IV pole.
   - Attach the controller to the IV pole so that it will be below and in line with the IV container.

- Plug the machine into the electric outlet, unless battery power is used.

2. Set up the IV infusion.
   - Open the IV container, maintaining the sterility of the port, and spike the container with the administration set.
   - Place the IV container on the IV pole, and position the drip chamber 76 cm (30 in) above the venipuncture site. *This provides sufficient gravitational pressure for the fluid to flow into the client.*
   - Fill the drip chamber of the IV tubing one-third full. *If the drip chamber is filled more than halfway, the drops may be miscounted.*
   - Prime the tubing, and close the clamp. *Nonvolumetric controllers (regulators that measure the infusion in drops/minute) use tubing that is gravity-primed. Priming expels all the air from the tubing.*

3. Attach the IV drop sensor, and insert the IV tubing into the controller.
   - Attach the IV drop sensor (electronic eye) to the drip chamber so that it is below the drip orifice and above the fluid level in the drip chamber (Figure 29-22 ◆). *This placement ensures an accurate drop count. If the sensor is placed too high, it can miss drops; if placed too low it may mistake splashes for drops.*
   - Make sure the sensor is plugged into the controller.
   - Insert the tubing into the controller according to the manufacturer's instructions.

4. Initiate the infusion.
   - Perform a venipuncture or connect the tubing to the existing IV catheter.

5. Set volume control for the appropriate volume per hour.
   - Press the power button.
   - Close the door to the controller, and ensure that all tubing clamps are wide open. *This enables the controller to regulate the fluid flow.*
   - Set the controls on the front of the controller to

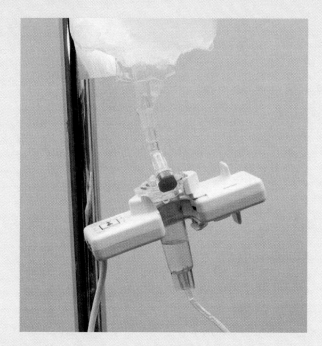

FIGURE 29-22 ◆ An IV controller.

the appropriate infusion rate and volume. Set the volume at 50 mL less than the required amount if the controller counts the volume infused. *This will give you time to attach a new container before the present one runs out completely.*

• Press the start button.

• Count the drops for 15 seconds, and multiply the result by 4. *This verifies that the rate has been correctly set and the controller is operating accurately.*

6. Set the alarm. *The alarm notifies the nurse when a set volume of fluid has been infused or indicates malfunctioning of the equipment.*

7. Monitor the infusion.

• Check the volume of fluid infused every hour, and compare it with the time tape on the IV container. This confirms the actual volume of fluid infused.

• If the volume infused does not coincide with the time tape or the alarm sounds, check that:

a. The time tape is accurate.

b. The rate/volume settings are accurate.

c. The drip chamber is correctly filled.

d. The IV tubing clamp is fully open.

e. The container still has solution.

f. The drop sensor is correctly placed.

g. The IV container is correctly placed.

h. The tubing is not pinched or kinked.

i. The IV has not infiltrated or clotted at the insertion site.

Infusion Pump

1. Attach the pump to the IV pole.

• Attach the pump at eye level on the IV pole. *Because the pump does not depend on gravity pressure, it can be placed at any level. Eye level is convenient for checking its functioning.*

• Plug the machine into the electric outlet, unless battery power is used.

2. Set up the infusion.

• Check the manufacturer's directions before using an IV filter or before infusing blood. *Infusion pump pressures may damage filters or cause rate inaccuracies. Certain models may also cause hemolysis of red blood cells.*

• Open the IV container, maintaining the sterility of the port, and spike the container with the administration set.

• Place the IV container on the IV pole above the pump.

• Fill the drip chamber, and rotate it as described in step 2 above.

• Prime the tubing, and close the clamp. Some pumps have a cassette that must also be primed. Manufacturers give instructions for doing this. Often, the cassette must be tilted to be filled with fluid. Some pumps must have the power on, the tubing and cassette in place in order to perform priming.

3. Insert the IV tubing into the pump.

• Press the power button to the "on" position.

• Load the machine according to the manufacturer's instructions.

4. Initiate the infusion (Figure 29-23 ◆).

• Perform venipuncture or connect the tubing to the IV needle.

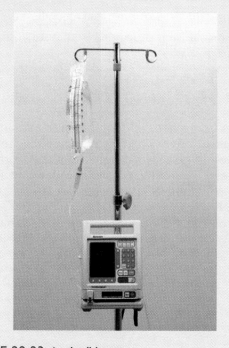

FIGURE 29-23 ◆ An IV pump.

- Set dials for the required drops per minute or milliliters per hour.
- Press the start button.

5. Set the alarms, and monitor the infusion.
- See steps 6 and 7 above.

 6. **Document** relevant information.
- Record the date and time of starting the infusion, the type and amount of fluid being infused, the rate at which it is being infused, the infusion device used, the status of the IV insertion site, and any adverse responses of the client.

AGE-RELATED CONSIDERATIONS

Regulating Intravenous Flow Rates

Infant/Child

- Emphasize to children that the IV controller or pump is not a toy and shouldn't be touched unless an adult is present. Children are naturally curious and will want to examine the equipment.
- Use a volume control chamber (Buretrol or Soluset) with the pump/controller for pediatric clients (see Figure 28-38, p. 564).
- Explain the procedure to the young client, encourage questions, and be alert for nonverbal cues.

Children may not understand things that seem obvious to adults. For example, a child may think the IV therapy is a punishment.

Elders

- Check the IV flow rate frequently for older adult clients. Elders are at increased risk to develop fluid overload if IV fluid is infused too rapidly.
- For older clients, check the IV site often for signs of infiltration. Veins become more fragile with aging.

EVALUATION

- Perform follow-up based on findings or outcomes that deviated from expected or normal for the client. Relate findings to previous data if available.
- Regularly check the client for intended and adverse effects of the infusion.
- Examine the IV site at regular intervals.
- Report significant deviations from normal to the physician.

Maintaining Infusions

Once an intravenous infusion has been established, it is the nurse's responsibility to maintain the prescribed flow rate and to prevent complications associated with IV therapy. Current research indicates that routine change of peripheral IV catheters/needles and IV tubing can be performed every 72 hours (or according to agency policy). Dressings should be changed on the IV site only when soiled, wet, or dislodged (see Technique 29-1).

Nursing Process: Maintaining Infusions

ASSESSMENT

In maintaining the infusion, the nurse will examine the appearance of infusion site; patency of system; type of fluid being infused and rate of flow; and the response of the client.

Gather the pertinent data:

- From the physician's order, determine the type and sequence of solutions to be infused.
- Determine the rate of flow and infusion schedule.

PLANNING

Review the client record regarding previous infusions and use of infusion devices. Note any complications and how they were managed.

Delegation

Due to the need for sterile technique and technical complexity, inspection of IV sites and regulation of IV rates is not delegated to UAP. UAP may care for clients with such devices, and the nurse must ensure that the UAP knows what complications or adverse signs should be reported to the nurse.

Performance

1. Explain to the client what you are going to do, why it is necessary, and how he or she can cooperate.

2. Provide for client privacy and prepare the client.

   • Check the client's identification band. *This ensures that the right client is receiving the infusion.*

   • Assist the client to a comfortable position, either sitting or lying. Expose the IV site but provide for client privacy.

3. Wash hands and observe appropriate infection control procedures.

4. Ensure that the correct solution is being infused.

   • Compare the label on the container (including added medications) to the order. If the solution in incorrect, slow the rate of flow to a minimum to maintain the patency of the catheter. *Stopping the infusion may allow a thrombus to form in the IV catheter. If this occurs, the catheter must be removed and another venipuncture performed before the infusion can be resumed.*

   • Change the solution to the correct one. Document and report the error according to agency protocol.

5. Observe the rate of flow every hour.

   • Compare the rate of flow at least hourly against the infusion schedule. *Infusions that are off schedule can be harmful to a client.* To read the volume in an IV bag, pull the edges of the bag apart at the level of the fluid and read the volume remaining. *Stretching the bag allows the fluid meniscus to fall to the proper level.*

   • Observe the position of the solution container. If it is less than 1 m (3 ft) above the IV site, readjust it to the correct height of the pole. *If the container is too low, the solution may not flow into the vein because there is insufficient gravitational pressure to overcome the pressure of the blood within the vein.*

   • If the rate is too fast, check agency policy. The physician may need to be notified.

     • In some agencies, you will slow the infusion so that it will be completed at the planned time. *Solution administered too quickly may cause fluid overload.* If the client has received significantly more fluid than planned, assess for manifestations of hypervolemia: dyspnea; rapid, labored breathing; cough; crackles (rales); tachycardia; and bounding pulses.

     • In other agencies, if the order is for a specified amount of fluid per hour, the IV may be adjusted to the correct rate and the client monitored for signs of fluid overload. In this case, make the appropriate revisions on the container time strip.

   • If the rate is too slow, adjust the IV to the prescribed rate. Also, check agency policy. Some agencies permit nursing personnel to adjust an IV that is behind time by an additional 10 percent. Adjustments above 10 percent may require a physician's order. *Solution that is administered too slowly can supply insufficient fluid, electrolytes, or medication for a client's needs.*

   • If the prescribed rate of flow is 150 mL/hr or more, check the rate of flow more frequently, for example, every 30 minutes.

6. Inspect the patency of the IV tubing and needle.

   • Observe the drip chamber. If it is less than half full, squeeze the chamber to allow the correct amount of fluid to flow in.

   • Inspect the tubing for pinches, kinks, or obstructions to flow. Arrange the tubing so that it is lightly coiled and under no pressure. Sometimes the tubing becomes caught under the client's arm and the weight of the arm blocks the flow.

   • Observe the position of the tubing. If it is dangling below the venipuncture, coil it carefully on the surface of the bed. *The solution may not flow upward into the vein against the force of gravity.*

   • If the infusion is dripping at less than the prescribed rate even when adjusted, lower the solution container below the level of the infusion site, and observe for a return flow of blood from the vein. *A return flow of blood indicates that the needle is patent and in the vein. Blood returns because venous pressure is greater than the fluid pressure in the IV tubing (siphoning). Absence of blood return may indicate that the needle is no longer in the vein or that the tip of the catheter is partially obstructed by a thrombus, the vein wall, or a valve in the vein. (Note: With some catheters, no blood may appear even with patency because the soft catheter walls collapse during siphoning.)*

   • If the infusion is dripping at less than the prescribed rate even when adjusted, determine whether the bevel of the catheter is against the wall of the vein. Carefully raise or lower the hub of the needle. If the flow rate improves, tape a sterile gauze pad under or over the hub to secure the modified position of the catheter bevel.

   • If there is leakage, locate the source. If the leak is at the catheter connection, tighten the tubing into the catheter. If the leak is elsewhere in the tubing, slow the infusion and replace the tubing. Estimate the amount of solution lost, if it was substantial. If fluid is leaking at the insertion site, the needle may be blocked. Check agency policy regarding irrigating potentially clotted needles.

7. Inspect the insertion site for fluid infiltration.

   • When an IV needle becomes dislodged from the vein, fluid flows into interstitial tissues, causing swelling. This is known as infiltration and is manifested by localized swelling, coolness, pallor, and discomfort at the IV site.

   • If infiltration is present, stop the infusion and remove the catheter. Restart the infusion at another site.

   • Apply a warm compress to the site of the infiltration. *Warmth promotes comfort and vasodilation, facilitating absorption of the fluid from interstitial tissues.*

8. Inspect the insertion site for **phlebitis** (inflammation of a vein).

   • Inspect the site at least every 8 hours. Phlebitis can occur as a result of mechanical trauma or chemical irritation (such as from intravenous electrolytes, especially potassium and magnesium, and medications). Signs of phlebitis are redness, warmth, and swelling at the intravenous site and burning pain along the course of the vein.

   • If phlebitis is detected, discontinue the infusion, and apply warm compresses to the venipuncture site. Do not use this injured vein for further infusions.

9. Inspect the intravenous site for bleeding.

   • Oozing or bleeding into the surrounding tissues can occur while the infusion is freely flowing

but is more likely to occur after the needle has been removed from the vein.

   • Observation of the venipuncture site is extremely important for clients who bleed readily, such as those receiving anticoagulants.

10. Teach the client ways to help maintain the infusion system, for example:

    • Avoid sudden twisting or turning movements of the arm with the needle or catheter.

    • Avoid stretching or placing tension on the tubing.

    • Try to keep the tubing from dangling below the level of the needle.

    • Notify a nurse if:

      a. The flow rate suddenly changes or the solution stops dripping.

      b. The client notices the solution container is nearly empty.

      c. There is blood in the IV tubing.

      d. Discomfort or swelling is experienced at the IV site.

      e. The pump or controller alarm sounds.

 11. **Document** relevant information.

   • Record the status of the IV insertion site and any adverse responses of the client.

• Document the client's IV fluid intake at least every 8 hours according to agency policy. Include the date and time; amount and type of solution used; container number; flow rate; and the client's general response. In most agencies, the amount remaining in each IV container is also recorded at the end of the shift (Figure 29-24 ◆).

AMBULATORY AND COMMUNITY SETTINGS

Intravenous Infusions

• In the home, plant hangers, robe hooks, or over-the-door S hooks may be used to hang an IV container.

• Evaluate the client or caregiver's ability to operate the infusion device at home.

• Emphasize the need for handwashing and clean technique when handling IV equipment. Set aside a clean area in the home to store the IV equipment.

• Demonstrate the device, and ask for a return demonstration from the client or caregiver.

• Discuss complications, such as infiltration, power failure, or equipment problems, and the measures to take when they arise.

• Make certain the client knows how and where to obtain supplies.

VENIPUNCTURE

DATE	TIME	SITE CODE	TYPE / GAUGE NEEDLE	INIT.	DC DATE	INIT.

CODES

SITE LOCATION:

RH	HAND		LH	HAND
RF	FOREARM		LF	FOREARM
RA	ANTECUBITAL		LA	ANTECUBITAL
RU	UPPER ARM		LU	UPPER ARM
RS	SUBCLAVIAN		LS	SUBCLAVIAN
RJ	JUGULAR		LJ	JUGULAR
RL	LEG		LL	LEG
VA	VASCULAR ACCESS			

SITE CONDITION:
A. PATENT WITHOUT REDNESS OR SWELLING OCCLUSIVE DRESSING INTACT
B. PATENT WITH MILD REDNESS AND/OR SWELLING OCCLUSIVE DRESSING INTACT
C. DRAINAGE (SEE NOTE)
D. DISLODGED / OCCLUDED
E. INFILTRATED
F. OCCLUSIVE DRESSING CHANGED

Division of Nursing
Oakland, California 94609

I.V. ORDERS

DATE ORDERED	INITIALS TRANS.	INITIALS CHECK	SOLUTION / ADDITIVE(S)	INFUSION RATE	DURATION

I.V.'s ADMINISTERED

DATE	TIME	INIT.	SITE LOC.	BOTTLE NUMBER	SOLUTION / ADDITIVE(S)	SHIFT	AMOUNT ABSORBED	AMOUNT REMAINING	TIME TUBING CHANGE	SITE COND.	TOTAL INFUSED
						0600					
						1400					
						2200					
						0600					
						1400					
						2200					
						0600					
						1400					
						2200					
						0600					
						1400					
						2200					
						0600					
						1400					
						2200					
						0600					
						1400					
						2200					

SUMMIT
MEDICAL CENTER

SIGN.

INIT.	SIGNATURE / TITLE	INIT.	SIGNATURE / TITLE	INIT.	SIGNATURE / TITLE

Intravenous Therapy Record

AFFIX PATIENT
I.D. LABEL HERE

MPN-105 86-6105-0

FIGURE 29-24 ◆ IV flow record.

CODES

SITE LOCATION:

RH	HAND	LH	HAND
RF	FOREARM	LF	FOREARM
RA	ANTECUBITAL	LA	ANTECUBITAL
RU	UPPER ARM	LU	UPPER ARM
RS	SUBCLAVIAN	LS	SUBCLAVIAN
RJ	JUGULAR	LJ	JUGULAR
RL	LEG	LL	LEG
VA	VASCULAR ACCESS		

SITE CONDITION:

A. PATENT WITHOUT REDNESS OR SWELLING
   OCCLUSIVE DRESSING INTACT
B. PATENT WITH MILD REDNESS AND/OR SWELLING
   OCCLUSIVE DRESSING INTACT
C. DRAINAGE (SEE NOTE)
D. DISLODGED / OCCLUDED
E. INFILTRATED
F. OCCLUSIVE DRESSING CHANGED

I.V.'s ADMINISTERED

DATE	TIME	INIT.	SITE LOC.	BOTTLE NUMBER	SOLUTION / ADDITIVE(S)	SHIFT	AMOUNT ABSORBED	AMOUNT REMAINING	TIME TUBING CHANGE	SITE COND.	TOTAL INFUSED
						0600					
						1400					
						2200					
						0600					
						1400					
						2200					
						0600					
						1400					
						2200					
						0600					
						1400					
						2200					
						0600					
						1400					
						2200					
						0600					
						1400					
						2200					
						0600					
						1400					
						2200					
						0600					
						1400					
						2200					
						0600					
						1400					
						2200					
						0600					
						1400					
						2200					
						0600					
						1400					
						2200					
						0600					
						1400					
						2200					

SIGN.

INIT.	SIGNATURE / TITLE	INIT.	SIGNATURE / TITLE	INIT.	SIGNATURE / TITLE

FIGURE 29-24 ◆ IV flow record. (*continued*)

EVALUATION

- Perform follow-up based on findings or outcomes that deviated from expected or normal for the client. Consider urinary output compared to intake; tissue turgor; specific gravity of urine; vital signs and lung sounds compared to baseline data.
- Regularly check the client for intended and adverse effects of the infusion.
- Report significant deviations from normal to the physician.

Intermittent Infusion Devices

The purpose of intermittent infusion devices is to provide venous access when IV administration of medications or fluids is needed only on a discontinuous basis. The nurse may establish the IV catheter initially as an intermittent device (see Technique 29-1) or convert a continuous IV to intermittent.

Nursing Process: Intermittent Infusion Devices

ASSESSMENT

Gather the pertinent data:

- A specific order may be written to insert or convert intravenous access to a heparin or saline lock. The order also may be implied. For example, IV fluids are to be discontinued but the client has orders for an IV antibiotic every 6 hours or is receiving analgesics intravenously.
- From the physician's order, determine the type and sequence of intermittent infusions.

PLANNING

Review the client record regarding previous infusions and use of infusion devices. Note any complications and how they were managed.

Delegation

Due to the need for sterile technique and technical complexity, use of IV devices is not delegated to UAP. UAP may care for clients with such devices, and the nurse must ensure that the UAP knows what complications or adverse signs should be reported to the nurse.

IMPLEMENTATION:
TECHNIQUE 29-5 MAINTAINING INTERMITTENT INFUSION DEVICES

Equipment

- Intermittent infusion cap or device (Figure 29-25 ◆)
- Clean gloves
- Sterile 2″ × 2″ or 4″ × 4″ gauze
- Sterile saline for injection (without preservative) or heparin flush solution (10 units/mL or 100 units/mL) in a prefilled syringe, a 3-mL syringe with a 25-gauge needle, or a needleless infusion device
- Isopropyl alcohol wipes

- Tape
- Clean emesis basin

Performance

1. Explain to the client what you are going to do, why it is necessary, and how he or she can cooperate. Explain the reason for leaving the intermittent device. Changing an IV to a heparin or saline lock should cause no discomfort other than that associated with removing tape from the IV tubing.

2. Provide for client privacy and prepare the client.
   - Check the client's identification band. *This ensures that the right client is receiving the IV therapy.*
   - Assist the client to a comfortable position, either sitting or lying. Expose the IV site but provide for client privacy.

3. Wash hands and observe appropriate infection control procedures.

4. Assess the IV site and determine the patency of the catheter (see Technique 29-3). If the catheter is not fully patent or there is evidence of phlebitis or infiltration, discontinue the catheter and establish a new IV site.

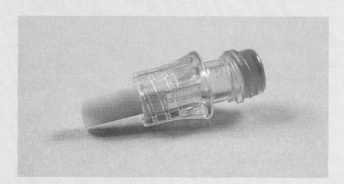

FIGURE 29-25 ◆ Intermittent infusion device with injection port.

- Expose the IV catheter hub and loosen any tape that is holding the IV tubing in place or that will interfere with insertion of the intermittent infusion plug into the catheter.
- Open the gauze pad and place it under the IV catheter hub.
- Open the alcohol wipe and intermittent infusion cap, leaving the plug in its sterile package.
- Clamp the IV tubing to stop the flow of IV fluid.

5. Remove the IV tubing and insert the intermittent infusion plug into the IV catheter.
   - Don clean gloves.
   - Stabilize the IV catheter with your nondominant hand and use the little finger to place slight pressure on the vein above the end of the catheter. Twist the IV tubing adapter to loosen it from the IV catheter and remove it, placing the end of the tubing in a clean emesis basin (Figure 29-26 ◆).
   - Pick up the intermittent infusion plug from its package and remove the protective sleeve from the male adapter (blue in Figure 29-25), maintaining its sterility. Insert the plug into the IV catheter, twisting it to seat it firmly or engage the Luer-Lok.

6. Instill saline or heparin solution per agency policy. *Saline or heparin is used to maintain patency of the IV catheter when fluids are not infusing through the catheter.*

7. Tape the intermittent infusion plug in place using a chevron or "U" method (Figure 29-12). *Tape provides added security to prevent the infusion plug from coming out of the intravenous catheter. It also promotes comfort, preventing the plug from catching on clothing or bedding.*

8. Teach the client how to maintain the lock.
   - Avoid manipulating the catheter or infusion

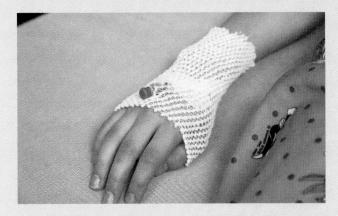

FIGURE 29-27 ◆ Intermittent infusion device in place.

plug and protect it from catching on clothing or bedding. A gauze bandage such as Kerlix or Kling may be wrapped over the plug to protect it when it is not in use (Figure 29-27 ◆).
   - Cover the site with an occlusive dressing when showering; avoid immersing the site.
   - Flush the catheter with saline or heparin solution as directed.
   - Notify the primary care provider if the plug or catheter comes out, if the site becomes red, inflamed, or painful, or if any drainage or bleeding occurs at the site.

9. Accessing the device to infuse fluids or medication:
   - Cleanse the cap with povidone–iodine or alcohol according to agency policy.
   - Use a threaded lock needleless or needle connector for infusions (Figure 29-28 ◆).

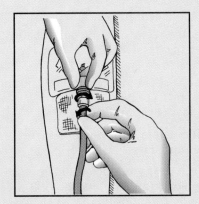

FIGURE 29-26 ◆ Separating the IV catheter from the infusion tubing.

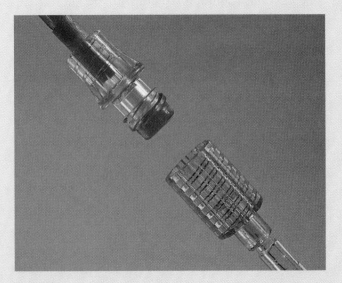

FIGURE 29-28 ◆ Threaded lock intermittent infusion connector.

10. Flush the device with prescribed solution after each use or every 8 hours if not in use.

 11. **Document** relevant information.
  • Record the date and time of converting the infusion device, the status of the IV insertion site, and any adverse responses of the client.

EVALUATION

• Perform follow-up based on findings or outcomes that deviated from expected or normal for the client. Relate findings to previous data if available.

• Examine the IV site at regular intervals.

• Report significant deviations from normal to the physician.

Discontinuing Infusions

When the intravenous access is no longer required, the nurse removes the IV catheter or needle.

Nursing Process: Discontinuing Infusions

ASSESSMENT

Gather the pertinent data. A specific order may be written to discontinue intravenous therapy. Ensure that it is not necessary to maintain an intermittent device.

PLANNING

Review the client record regarding previous infusions. Note any complications and how they were managed.

Delegation

Due to the need for sterile technique and technical complexity, removal of IV devices is not delegated to UAP. The nurse must ensure that the UAP knows what complications or adverse signs following removal should be reported to the nurse.

IMPLEMENTATION:
TECHNIQUE 29-6 DISCONTINUING INFUSION DEVICES

Equipment

• Clean gloves
• Small sterile dressing and tape
• Dry or antiseptic-soaked swabs, according to agency practice

Performance

1. Explain to the client what you are going to do, why it is necessary, and how he or she can cooperate. Explain the reason for removing the IV.

2. Provide for client privacy and prepare the client.
   • Check the client's identification band. *This ensures that the right client is having the IV therapy discontinued.*
   • Assist the client to a comfortable position, either sitting or lying. Expose the IV site but provide for client privacy.

3. Wash hands and observe appropriate infection control procedures.

4. Prepare the equipment.
   • Clamp the infusion tubing. *Clamping the tubing prevents the fluid from flowing out of the needle onto the client or bed.*
   • Loosen the tape at the venipuncture site while

holding the needle firmly and applying countertraction to the skin. *Movement of the needle can injure the vein and cause discomfort to the client. Countertraction prevents pulling the skin and causing discomfort.*
   • Don clean gloves, and hold a sterile gauze above the venipuncture site.

5. Withdraw the needle or catheter from the vein.
   • Withdraw the needle or catheter by pulling it out along the line of the vein. *Pulling it out in line with the vein avoids pain and injury to the vein.*
   • Immediately apply firm pressure to the site, using sterile gauze, for 2 to 3 minutes. *Pressure helps stop the bleeding and prevents hematoma formation.*
   • Hold the client's arm or leg above heart level if any bleeding persists. *Raising the limb decreases blood flow to the area.*
   • Teach the client to inform the nurse if the site begins to bleed at any time or the client notes any other abnormalities in the area.

6. Examine the catheter removed from the client.
   • Check the catheter to make sure it is intact. *If a piece of tubing remains in the client's vein, it could move centrally (toward the heart or lungs) and cause serious problems.*

- Report a broken catheter to the nurse in charge or physician immediately.
- If the broken piece can be palpated, apply a tourniquet above the insertion site. *Application of a tourniquet decreases the possibility of the piece moving until a physician is notified.*

7. Cover the venipuncture site.
- Apply the sterile dressing. *The dressing continues the pressure and covers the open area in the skin, preventing infection.*

8. Read the amount remaining in the IV solution container, if infusions are being discontinued, and discard the used supplies appropriately.

9. **Document** all relevant information.
- Record the amount of fluid infused on the intake and output record and on the chart, according to agency practice. Include the container number, type of solution used, time of discontinuing the infusion, and the client's response.

EVALUATION

- Perform follow-up based on findings or outcomes that deviated from expected or normal for the client. Relate findings to previous data if available.
- Report significant deviations from normal to the physician.

Blood Transfusions

A blood **transfusion** is the introduction of whole blood or components of the blood (e.g., plasma or erythrocytes) into the venous circulation (see Table 29-1).

Blood Groups

Human blood is classified into four main groups (A, B, AB, and O) on the basis of antigens on the erythrocyte surface. These antigens can cause antibody reactions when in contact with mismatched blood. Blood transfusions must be matched to the client's blood type in terms of compatible antigens. Mismatched blood will cause a hemolytic reaction.

Rh antigens, also on the surface of erythrocytes, are present in about 85 percent of the population and can cause hemolytic reactions in persons with antibody to that antigen. Persons who possess the **Rh factor** are referred to as *Rh positive;* those who do not are referred to as *Rh negative.* Unlike the A and B antigens, the Rh factor cannot cause a hemolytic reaction on the first exposure to mismatched blood, because the Rh antibody is *not* normally present in the plasma of Rh-negative persons.

Transfusion Reactions

In order to avoid hemolytic transfusion reactions, blood from the donor and from the recipient are tested for compatibility. This is referred to as a *type and crossmatch.* Nonhemolytic transfusion reactions are febrile, allergic, fluid overload, and sepsis (see Table 29-2). The

TABLE 29-1	BLOOD PRODUCTS FOR TRANSFUSION
Product	**Use**
Whole blood	Primarily used for cardiac surgery or acute hemorrhage. Replaces blood volume and all blood products: RBCs, plasma, plasma proteins, fresh platelets, and other clotting factors.
Red blood cells	Used to increase the oxygen-carrying capacity of blood in anemias, surgery, disorders with slow bleeding. One unit raises hematocrit by approximately 4%.
Autologous red blood cells	Used for blood replacement following planned elective surgery. Client donates blood for autologous transfusion 4–5 weeks prior to surgery.
Platelets	Replaces platelets in clients with bleeding disorders or platelet deficiency. Fresh platelets most effective.
Plasma	Expands blood volume and provides clotting factors. Does not need to be typed and crossmatched (contains no RBCs).
Albumin	Blood volume expander; provides plasma proteins.
Clotting factors and cryoprecipitate	Used for clients with clotting factor deficiencies. Each provides different factors involved in the clotting pathway; cryoprecipitate also contains fibrinogen.

From *Fundamentals of nursing: Concepts, process, and practice,* 6th ed., by B. Kozier, G. Erb, A. Berman, & K. Burke, 2000, Upper Saddle River, NJ: Prentice Hall Health.

TABLE 29-2 **TRANSFUSION REACTIONS**

Reaction: Cause	Clinical Signs	Nursing Intervention*
Hemolytic reaction: incompatibility between client's blood and donor's blood	Chills, fever, headache, backache, dyspnea, cyanosis, chest pain, tachycardia, hypotension	1. Discontinue the transfusion immediately. 2. Keep the vein open with normal saline, or according to agency protocol. 3. Send the remaining blood, a sample of the client's blood, and a urine sample to the laboratory. 4. Notify the physician immediately. 5. Monitor vital signs. 6. Monitor fluid intake and output.
Febrile reaction: sensitivity of the client's blood to white blood cells, platelets, or plasma proteins	Fever; chills; warm, flushed skin; headache; anxiety, muscle pain	1. Discontinue the transfusion immediately. 2. Give antipyretics as ordered. 3. Notify the physician.
Allergic reaction (mild): sensitivity to infused plasma proteins	Flushing, itching, urticaria, bronchial wheezing	1. Stop or slow the transfusion, depending on agency protocol. 2. Notify the physician. 3. Administer medication (antihistamines) as ordered.
Allergic reaction (severe): antibody-antigen reaction	Dyspnea, chest pain, circulatory collapse, cardiac arrest	1. Stop the transfusion. 2. Keep the vein open with normal saline. 3. Notify the physician immediately. 4. Monitor vital signs. Administer cardiopulmonary resuscitation (CPR) if needed. 5. Administer medications and/or oxygen as ordered.
Circulatory overload: blood administered faster than the circulation can accomodate	Cough, dyspnea, crackles (rales), distended neck veins, tachycardia, hypertension	1. Place the client upright, with feet dependent. 2. Administer diuretics and oxygen as ordered. 3. Notify the physician. 4. Stop or slow the transfusion.
Sepsis: contaminated blood administered	High fever, chills, vomiting, diarrhea, hypotension	1. Stop the transfusion. 2. Send the remaining blood to laboratory. 3. Notify the physician. 4. Obtain a blood specimen from the client for culture. 5. Administer IV fluids, antibiotics.

*Nurses should follow agency's protocol regarding interventions. These may vary among agencies.

From *Fundamentals of nursing: Concepts, process, and practice*, 6th ed., by B. Kozier, G. Erb, A. Berman, & K. Burke, 2000, Upper Saddle River, NJ: Prentice Hall Health.

nurse must assess a client closely for transfusion reactions. Signs of an acute reaction include sudden chills or fever, low back pain, a drop in blood pressure, nausea, flushing, agitation, or respiratory disorders. Signs of less severe allergic reactions include hives and itching but no fever.

Blood Administration

The nurse or other personnel obtain blood in plastic bags from the blood bank. One unit of whole blood is 500 mL; a unit of packed red blood cells (RBCs) is 200 to 250 mL.

Blood administration sets (Y-sets) are used to keep the vein open while starting the transfusion, to flush the line with saline before the blood enters the tubing (e.g., when running an intravenous infusion that is not saline), and to use if any adverse effects arise from the transfusion (Figure 29-29 ◆). The infusion tubing has a filter inside the drip chamber.

Blood transfusions are commonly administered through a 20-gauge needle or catheter. Smaller needles may slow the infusion and could damage blood cells.

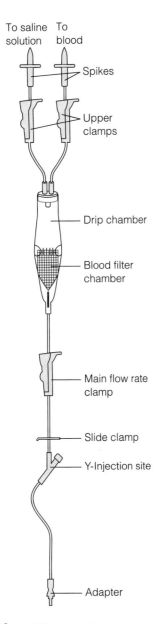

To saline solution   To blood

Spikes

Upper clamps

Drip chamber

Blood filter chamber

Main flow rate clamp

Slide clamp

Y-Injection site

Adapter

FIGURE 29-29 ◆ Y blood tubing.

Nursing Process: Blood Transfusions

ASSESSMENT

Gather the pertinent data. Know the purpose of the transfusion:

- To restore blood volume after severe hemorrhage
- To restore the capacity of the blood to carry oxygen
- To provide plasma factors, such as antihemophilic factor (AHF) or factor VIII, or platelet concentrates, which prevent or treat bleeding

Confirm the physician's order for the number and type of units and the desired speed of infusion.

PLANNING

Review the client record regarding previous transfusions. Note any complications and how they were managed.

Type and crossmatch procedures can take several hours. Plan to begin the transfusion as soon as notified that the component is ready. Note any premedication ordered by the physician (e.g., acetaminophen or diphenhydramine). Schedule their administration (usually 30 minutes prior to the transfusion).

Delegation

Due to the need for sterile technique and technical complexity, blood transfusion is not delegated to UAP. The nurse must ensure that the UAP knows what complications or adverse signs can occur and should be reported to the nurse.

IMPLEMENTATION:
TECHNIQUE 29-7 ADMINISTERING BLOOD TRANSFUSIONS

Equipment

- Unit of whole blood, packed RBCs, or other component
- Blood administration set with 170- to 260-μ filter
- Supplemental blood filter, if needed
- IV pump, if needed
- 250 mL normal saline for infusion
- IV pole
- Venipuncture start kit containing a 20-gauge needle or catheter (if one is not already in place)
- Alcohol swabs
- Tape
- Clean gloves

Preparation

1. Verify client consent and obtain baseline data before the transfusion.
   - If required by policy, verify that a signed consent form was obtained.
   - Assess vital signs for baseline data, including blood pressure, pulse, respiratory rate and depth, and temperature. Many agencies use the transfusion form that comes with the unit from the blood bank to record these values.

- Determine any known allergies or previous adverse reactions to blood.
- Note specific signs related to the client's pathology and the reason for the transfusion. For example, for an anemic client, note the hemoglobin and hematocrit levels.

2. Establish the intravenous line.
- If the client has an intravenous solution infusing, check whether the needle is appropriate to administer blood (20 gauge or larger).
- If the client does not have an IV solution infusing, check agency policies. In some agencies an infusion must be running before the blood is obtained from the blood bank. In this case, you will need to perform a venipuncture on a suitable vein (see Technique 29-1) and start an IV infusion of normal saline.

Performance

1. Explain to the client what you are going to do, why it is necessary, and how he or she can cooperate. Explain the reason for the transfusion. Instruct the client to report promptly any sudden chills, nausea, itching, rash, dyspnea, back pain, or other unusual symptoms.

2. Provide for client privacy and prepare the client.
- Check the client's identification band. Do not administer blood to a client without an arm band. *This ensures that the right client is receiving the transfusion.*
- Assist the client to a comfortable position, either sitting or lying. Expose the IV site but provide for client privacy.

3. Wash hands and observe appropriate infection control procedures.

4. Prepare the infusion equipment.
- Ensure that the blood filter inside the drip chamber is suitable for the blood components to be transfused. Attach the blood tubing to the blood filter, if necessary. *Blood filters have a surface area large enough to allow the blood components through easily but are designed to trap clots.*
- Put on gloves.
- Close all the clamps on the Y-set: the main flow rate clamp and both Y-line clamps.
- Insert the piercing pin (spike) into the saline solution.
- Hang the container on the IV pole about 1 m (36 in) above the venipuncture site.

5. Prime the tubing.
- Open the upper clamp on the normal saline tubing, and squeeze the drip chamber until it covers the filter and one-third of the drip chamber above the filter.
- Tap the filter chamber to expel any residual air in the filter.

- Open the main flow rate clamp, and prime the tubing with saline.
- Close both clamps.

6. Start the saline solution.
- If an IV solution incompatible with blood is infusing, stop the infusion and discard the solution and tubing according to agency policy.
- Attach the blood tubing primed with normal saline to the intravenous catheter.
- Open the saline and main flow rate clamps and adjust the flow rate. Use only the main flow rate clamp to adjust the rate.
- Allow a small amount of solution to infuse to make sure there are no problems with the flow or with the venipuncture site. *Infusing normal saline before initiating the transfusion also clears the IV catheter of incompatible solutions or medications.*

7. Obtain the correct blood component for the client.
- Check the physician's order with the requisition.
- Check the requisition form and the blood bag label with a laboratory technician or according to agency policy. Specifically, check the client's name, identification number, blood type and Rh group, the blood donor number, and the expiration date of the blood. Observe the blood for abnormal color, clumping, gas bubbles, and extraneous material. Return outdated or abnormal blood to the blood bank.
- With another nurse (the agency may require a registered nurse), compare the laboratory blood record with:
  a. The client's name and identification number
  b. The number on the blood bag label
  c. The blood type and Rh group on the blood bag label
- If any of the information does not match *exactly*, notify the charge nurse and the blood bank. Do not administer blood until discrepancies are corrected or clarified.
- Sign the appropriate form with the other nurse according to agency policy.
- Make sure that red blood cells are left at room temperature for no more than 30 minutes before starting the transfusion. *RBCs deteriorate and lose their effectiveness after 2 hours at room temperature. Lysis of RBCs releases potassium into the bloodstream, causing hyperkalemia.* Agencies may designate different times at which the blood must be returned to the blood bank if it has not been started. *As blood components warm, the risk of bacterial growth also increases.* If the start of the transfusion is unexpectedly delayed, return the blood to the blood bank. Do not store blood in the unit refrigerator. *The temperature of unit refrigerators is not precisely regulated and the blood may be damaged.*

Variation: Infusing Other Blood Components

- *Platelets:* Pooled platelets usually contain 200 to 400 mL (4 to 6 units). Do not refrigerate platelets and keep them agitated at all times. Do not use microaggregate filters. Infuse at 10 mL/min.
- *Fresh frozen plasma:* 200 to 250 mL/unit. Infuse within 24 hours of thawing, at 5 to 10 mL/minute.

8. Prepare the blood bag.
   - Invert the blood bag gently several times to mix the cells with the plasma. Rough handling can damage the cells.
   - Expose the port on the blood bag by pulling back the tabs (Figure 29-30 ◆).
   - Insert the remaining Y-set spike into the blood bag.
   - Suspend the blood bag.

9. Establish the blood transfusion.
   - Close the upper clamp below the IV saline solution container.
   - Open the upper clamp below the blood bag. The blood will run into the saline-filled drip chamber. If necessary, squeeze the drip chamber to reestablish the liquid level with drip chamber one-third full. (Tap the filter to expel any residual air within the filter.)
   - Readjust the flow rate with the main clamp.

10. Observe the client closely for the first 15 minutes.
    - Run the blood slowly for the first 15 minutes at 20 drops/min.

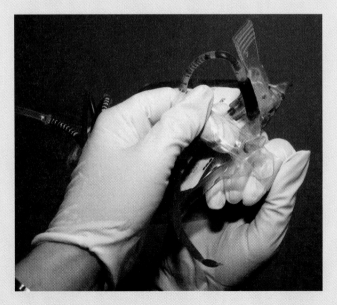

FIGURE 29-30 ◆ Exposing the port on the blood bag by pulling back the tabs.

- Note adverse reactions, such as chilling, nausea, vomiting, skin rash, or tachycardia. *The earlier a transfusion reaction occurs, the more severe it tends to be. Promptly identifying such reactions helps to minimize the consequences.*
- Remind the client to call a nurse immediately if any unusual symptoms are felt during the transfusion.
- If any of these reactions occur, report these to the nurse in charge, and take appropriate nursing action. See Table 29-2 on page 603.

11. **Document** relevant data.
    - Record starting the blood, including vital signs, type of blood, blood unit number, sequence number (e.g., #1 of three ordered units), site of the venipuncture, size of the needle, and drip rate.

12. Monitor the client.
    - Fifteen minutes after initiating the transfusion (or according to agency policy), check the vital signs of the client. If there are no signs of a reaction, establish the required flow rate. Most adults can tolerate receiving one unit of blood in 1½ to 2 hours. Do not transfuse a unit of blood for longer than 4 hours.
    - Assess the client including vital signs every 30 minutes or more often, depending on the health status and agency policy. If the client has a reaction and the blood is discontinued, send the blood bag to the laboratory for investigation of the blood.

13. Terminate the transfusion.
    - Don clean gloves.
    - If no infusion is to follow, clamp the blood tubing and remove the needle (See Technique 29-6).
    - If the primary IV is to be continued, flush the maintenance line with saline solution. Disconnect the blood tubing system and reestablish the intravenous infusion using new tubing. Adjust the drip to the desired rate.
    - Discard the administration set according to agency practice. Needles should be placed in a sharps container. Administration sets may be bagged and labeled before being discarded. See agency policy.
    - Remove gloves.
    - Again monitor vital signs.

14. Follow agency protocol for appropriate disposition of the blood bag.
    - On the requisition attached to the blood unit, fill in the time the transfusion was completed and the amount transfused.

- Attach one copy of the requisition to the client's record.
- If required, return the blood bag and requisition to the blood bank.

15. **Document** relevant data.
   - Record completion of the transfusion, the amount of blood absorbed, the

blood unit number, and the vital signs. If the primary intravenous infusion was continued, record connecting it. Also record the transfusion on the IV flow sheet and intake and output record.

EVALUATION

- Perform follow-up based on findings or outcomes that deviated from expected or normal for the client. Relate findings to previous data if available.
- Report significant deviations from normal to the physician.

Central Venous Access

Sometimes, access to the vascular system through peripheral intravenous lines is not possible or not desirable. In these cases, central venous access may be used. A central venous line is a catheter inserted into a large vein located centrally in the body. The tip of the catheter may terminate in the vein, the superior vena cava, or in the right atrium of the heart. X-ray confirms correct placement of the catheter.

Physicians usually insert central venous lines, although nurses who are specially prepared may insert certain types. Central venous lines are inserted primarily to:

- Spare the client numerous venipunctures associated with short-term peripheral IV catheters (especially those with phobias against needles)
- Administer solutions that are highly irritating to smaller veins
- Provide access for frequent blood sampling
- Monitor central venous pressure (CVP)

Types of Central Venous Lines

Standard central venous lines are catheters of variable length, usually made of polyurethane or silicone rubber. There are four major types of central lines: (1) percutaneous central catheters, (2) peripherally inserted central catheters, (3) central venous tunneled catheters, and (4) implanted ports. Percutaneous central catheters are commonly inserted through the chest wall into the subclavian vein and through the neck into the internal jugular vein (Figure 29-2, page 580). A peripherally inserted central catheter (PICC) is a long venous catheter 50 to 60 cm (20 to 24 in) in length, extending into the distal third of the superior vena cava (Figure 29-31 ◆). PICC lines can remain in place for 6 months

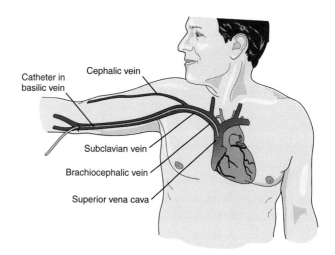

FIGURE 29-31 ◆ Placement of a PICC line.

Catheter in basilic vein
Cephalic vein
Subclavian vein
Brachiocephalic vein
Superior vena cava

or more. A variation of the PICC, peripherally inserted midline catheters are 8 to 20 cm (3 to 8 in) long and are used for therapy lasting 3 to 4 weeks. Both catheters are used for inpatient and outpatient settings.

For percutaneous insertion, the practitioner inserts a catheter with stylet to penetrate the vein. Once the vein is entered and the needle placed correctly, the catheter is advanced over or through the needle to the desired length and sutured or secured in place. When the catheter is in place, the stylet is withdrawn.

Catheters may also be inserted surgically. Because these catheters are implanted through a subcutaneous tunnel, they are often referred to as central venous tunneled catheters (CVTCs). Examples are the *Hickman, Broviac,* and *Groshong* catheters (Figure 29-32 ◆). These catheters may remain in place for many years.

Multilumen catheters are designed with each lumen having a separate port. These allow simultaneous infusion of **total parenteral nutrition (TPN)** therapy, central venous pressure readings, blood transfusions, antibiotics, blood drawing, and any other needed uses. With percutaneous or tunneled catheters, the nurse should be consistent and always use the same port for the same purpose.

Implanted ports are single or multiple lumen subclavian vein catheters attached to a reservoir that is surgically placed completely under the skin, usually in the client's upper chest (see Figure 29-3).

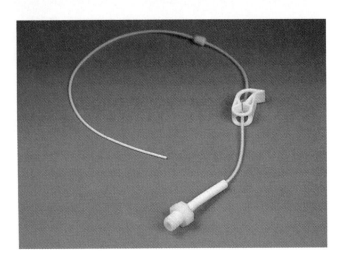

FIGURE 29-32 ◆ Broviac catheter.

Complications Associated with Central Venous Lines

Many of the sepsis problems associated with conventional IV therapy are also associated with central venous lines. Moreover, the problems are magnified because (1) clients with central venous lines are often critically ill, may be malnourished, and are sometimes immunosuppressed; (2) the catheters are left in place for long periods of time; and (3) the intralipids used in TPN therapy support the growth of a wide variety of microorganisms. Infection control is therefore of utmost importance during central venous catheter therapy.

Nursing Process: Caring for the Client with a Central Venous Access Device

ASSESSMENT

In maintaining the central venous catheter device, the nurse will examine the appearance of the infusion site, patency of the system, type of fluid being infused and rate of flow, and the response of the client.
  Gather the pertinent data:

- From the client record, determine the purpose of the central line, how and when it was inserted, and the type of catheter used.
- Determine the type of infusion, rate of flow, and infusion schedule.

PLANNING

Review the client record regarding the insertion of the central line and previous infusions. Note any complications and how they were managed.

Delegation

Due to the need for sterile technique and technical complexity, maintaining and monitoring central venous lines are not delegated to UAP. UAP may care for clients with central lines, and the nurse must ensure that the UAP knows what complications or adverse signs should be reported to the nurse.

IMPLEMENTATION:
TECHNIQUE 29-8 MANAGING CENTRAL LINES

Equipment

- Soft-tipped clamp without teeth
- Alcohol or povidone–iodine wipes
- 10-mL syringe
- Sterile normal saline
- Heparin flush solution (e.g., 100 units heparin per 1 mL of saline)

Performance

1. Explain to the client what you are going to do, why it is necessary, and how he or she can cooperate.

2. Provide for client privacy and prepare the client.
   - Check the client's identification band. *This ensures that the right client is receiving the infusion.*
   - Assist the client to a comfortable position, either sitting or lying. Expose the IV site but provide for client privacy.

3. Wash hands and observe appropriate infection control procedures.

4. Label each lumen of multilumen catheters.
   - Mark each lumen or port of the tubing with a description of its purpose (e.g., the distal lumen for CVP monitoring and infusing blood; the middle lumen for TPN; and the proximal lumen for other IV solutions or for blood samples).
   or
   - Use a color code established by the agency to label the proximal, middle, and distal lumens. *Labeling prevents mixing of incompatible medications or infusions and reserves each lumen for specific therapies.*

5. Monitor tubing connections.
   - Ensure that all tubing connections are taped or secured according to agency protocol.
   - Check the connections every 2 hours.
   - Tape cap ends if agency protocol indicates.

6. Change tubing according to agency policy.
   - See Technique 29-2.
   - Some agencies advocate changing TPN tubing every 24 hours and tubing for other infusions every 48 to 72 hours.

7. Change the catheter site dressing according to agency policy.
   - See Technique 29-9.
   - Most agencies recommend that the dressing be changed every 48 to 72 hours.

8. Administer all infusions as ordered.
   - Use a controller or pump for all fluids (see Technique 29-3).
   - Maintain the fluid flow at the prescribed rate.
   - Whenever the line is interrupted for any reason, instruct the client to perform Valsalva's maneuver. If the client is unable to perform Valsalva's maneuver, place the client in a supine position, and clamp the lumen of the catheter with a soft-tipped clamp. Place a strip of tape (about 3 inches from the end) over the catheter before applying the clamp. *The clamp is placed over the taped area to prevent damage to the tubing. A clamp without teeth prevents piercing.*

9. Cap lumens without continuous infusions, and flush them regularly.
   - Close lumens not in use with an intermittent infusion cap to seal the end of a catheter.
   - Clean the adapter caps with alcohol or povidone–iodine swab before penetration.
   - Flush noninfusing lumens with heparin flush solution every 8 hours or according to agency protocol. *Flushing prevents obstruction of the catheter by a blood clot. The exact amount and frequency of flush depends on the catheter type and agency practice.* Some agencies use normal saline solution instead of heparin solution to flush catheters. *Research indicates that heparin isn't always necessary to keep IV lines open.*
   - Use a 10-mL or larger syringe to flush. *Smaller syringes can exert too much pressure that can damage the catheter.* Create turbulent flow with the flush by pushing, then pausing, and then pushing again. *Turbulent flow helps keep the catheter free of residue.* Keep pressure on the syringe plunger as the syringe is disconnected. *Positive pressure prevents back flow of blood into the catheter.*
   - Always aspirate for blood before flushing (or infusing medications). *This validates that the catheter is appropriately placed in the vein.*

10. Administer medications as ordered.
    - If a capped lumen used for medication has been flushed with heparin solution, aspirate and dis-

card or flush the line with 5 to 10 mL of normal saline according to agency protocol before giving the medication. *Many medications are incompatible with heparin.*
    - After the medication is instilled through the lumen, inject normal saline first and then the heparin flush solution if indicated by agency protocol. *The saline solution flushes the line of the medication. The heparin maintains the patency of the catheter by preventing blood clotting.*

11. Monitor the client for complications.
    - Assess the client's vital signs, skin color, mental alertness, appearance of the catheter site, and presence of adverse symptoms at least every 4 hours.
    - If air embolism is suspected, give the client 100 percent oxygen by mask, place the client in a left Trendelenburg position, and notify the physician. *Lowering the head increases intrathoracic pressure, decreasing the flow of air into the vein during inhalation. A left side-lying position helps prevent the air from moving to the pulmonary artery.*
    - If sepsis is suspected, replace a TPN, blood, or other infusion with 5 percent or 10 percent dextrose solution, change the IV tubing and dressing, save the remaining solution for lab analysis, record the lot number of the solution and any additives, and notify the physician immediately. When changing the dressing, take a culture of the catheter site as ordered by the physician or according to agency protocol.
    - If a lumen appears to be occluded, the cause could be thrombus, precipitate, or mechanical. An x-ray is done first to determine if the catheter is properly located. Fluoroscopy can demonstrate the presence of a thrombus by indicating the fluid path through the catheter. If a thrombus is found, thrombolytic therapy using an enzyme such as streptokinase is indicated. Follow agency guidelines for use of these agents. If drugs infused into the lumen may have created a precipitate, the pharmacist can assist in determining whether an acidic, alkaline, or lipid precipitate is likely and the appropriate solution to dissolve it. If the occlusion is mechanical, consult policy to determine if the nurse may reposition the catheter or the physician must be notified.

12. **Document** all relevant information.
    - Record the date and time of any infusion started; type of solution, drip rate, and number of milliliters infusing per hour; dressing or tubing changes; appearance of insertion site; and all other nursing assessments.

AMBULATORY AND COMMUNITY SETTINGS

Managing Central Lines

- When caring for a central catheter in the home, place equipment on a clean towel or nonsterile drape.
- Assess the home environment and help the client choose a clean, dry place to store the IV supplies.
- Evaluate the client or caregiver's ability and willingness to perform catheter care at home. Ask for a return demonstration of all teaching.

- Emphasize the need for handwashing and clean technique when working with the central catheter.
- Ensure that the client knows how and where to obtain supplies.
- Discuss possible complications of a central line, such as phlebitis, sepsis, or thrombus formation, and explain when to notify the health care provider.

AGE-RELATED CONSIDERATIONS

Managing Central Lines

Child

- Explain all procedures to the young client beforehand, using play therapy to demonstrate. Encourage questions, and be alert for nonverbal cues. Children may not understand things that seem obvious to adults. For example, a child may think the IV therapy is a punishment.

- Young clients can help with catheter care procedures by holding nonsterile supplies and handing them to the nurse. Participating gives the child a sense of control.
- Tell the young client not to play with the IV tubing, flow clamp, or any other part of the equipment. Encourage the child to decorate the IV tubing with colorful stickers.

EVALUATION

- Perform follow-up based on findings or outcomes that deviated from expected or normal for the client. Relate findings to previous data if available.
- Report significant deviations from normal to the physician.

Changing Central Line Dressings

For tunneled catheters that have healed, no dressing is indicated. The Intravenous Nurses Society recommends changing transparent dressings without gauze at regular intervals (no interval specified) unless wet, loose, or soiled. Many agencies recommend changing the dressing 24 hours after insertion and then every 7 days. No antibacterial ointment should be applied to the site. Caps placed on central lines when not in use should be changed every 3 to 7 days (Sansivero, 1997). If the infusion tubing also requires changing, it may be desirable to do this at the same time as the dressing change (see Technique 29-2).

Nursing Process: Changing Central Line Dressings

ASSESSMENT

Gather the pertinent data. Know the purpose of the central line. Confirm the physician's order for the central line (i.e., whether it is to have an infusion or be capped).

Determine:

- Any allergy to tape, iodine, or components of fluids infused.
- Any bleeding tendency. Such clients, especially those receiving anticoagulants, require special observation.
- Client's ability to understand instructions during the procedure and to perform Valsalva's maneuver.

PLANNING

Review the client record regarding previous care of central lines. Note any complications and how they were managed.

Delegation

Due to the need for sterile technique and technical complexity, changing a central line dressing is not delegated to UAP. UAP may care for clients with central lines, and the nurse must ensure that the UAP knows what complications or adverse signs should be reported to the nurse.

Equipment

- Central line dressing set

  or

- Two face masks (one for the nurse and one for the client)
- Three 70 percent isopropyl alcohol swabs
- Three antiseptic swabs (e.g., 2 percent chlorhexidine, 1 percent iodine tincture, or povidone–iodine solutions)
- Clean gloves
- Sterile gloves
- 4" × 4" gauze sponges
- Precut sterile drain gauze or 2" × 2" gauze and sterile scissors
- Tincture of benzoin or other skin prep
- Cotton-tipped applicators
- Occlusive tape or transparent semipermeable polyurethane dressing such as Op-Site or Tegaderm
- Nonallergenic 2.5-cm (1-in) tape

Performance

1. Explain to the client what you are going to do, why it is necessary, and how he or she can cooperate.

2. Provide for client privacy and prepare the client.

   - Check the client's identification band. *This ensures that the right client is receiving care.*
   - Assist the client to a comfortable position, either sitting or lying. Expose the central line site but provide for client privacy.

3. Wash hands and observe appropriate infection control procedures.

4. Prepare the client.

   - Don a mask, and have the client don a mask (if tolerated or as agency protocol indicates), and/or ask the client to turn the head away from the insertion site. *This helps protect the insertion site from the nurse's and client's nasal and oral microorganisms. Turning the client's head also makes the site more accessible.*

5. Prepare the equipment.

   - Open the sterile supplies.

6. Cleanse the site.

   - Don clean gloves. Remove the soiled dressing by pulling the tape or transparent dressing slowly and gently from the skin. *This prevents catheter displacement and skin irritation.*

   - Inspect the skin for signs of irritation or infection. Inspect the catheter for signs of leakage or other problems. If infection is suspected, take a swab of the drainage for culture, label it, send it to the laboratory, and notify the physician.

   - Don sterile gloves.

   - Clean the catheter insertion site with three alcohol swabs and let the skin dry. Repeat the procedure with three antiseptic swabs and let the skin dry at least 2 minutes.

   - Clean in a circular motion, moving from the insertion site outward to the edge of the adhesive border. If possible, use one hand to lift the catheter so you can clean under it. *Cleaning from the insertion site outward and discarding the sponges after each wipe avoids introducing contaminants from the uncleaned area to the site.*

7. Apply the new dressing.

   - Secure the catheter to the skin with tape or steri-strips.

   - Apply sterile drain gauze around the catheter. *This protects the catheter and skin surrounding the insertion site from airborne contaminants. Gauze is recommended for the first 24 hours after initial central line insertion to absorb exudate.*

   - Apply tincture of benzoin to the skin surrounding the gauze, and allow it to air dry about 1 minute. *This protects the skin when adhesive is applied and promotes adhesion of the cover dressing. Appropriate drying time is essential to prevent skin breakdown when the dressing is removed.* Secure the dressing to the skin with occlusive tape or bandage.

   - Cover with 1 or 2 4" × 4" gauze dressings

     or

   - Apply a transparent semipermeable polyurethane dressing. *This type of dressing allows gas exchange but is impermeable to liquids and microorganisms. It also allows visualization of the site.*

8. Secure the tubing.

   - Loop and tape the catheter tubing. *Looping prevents tension on the catheter and its inadvertent detachment if the tubing is pulled.*

   - Label the dressing with the date, time, and your initials.

9. **Document** all relevant information.

   - Record the appearance of catheter insertion site; presence of drainage, the type of dressing applied, client complaints or concerns, and patency of tubing (if evaluated).

- Perform follow-up based on findings or outcomes that deviated from expected or normal for the client. Relate findings to previous data if available.
- Report significant deviations from normal to the physician.

Implanted Vascular Access Devices

As noted above, implanted venous access devices (IVADs) or ports are surgically placed completely under the skin. Thus, they have the advantages of not being visible and not requiring dressing changes or other care associated with central lines that have an external component. However, IVADs must be accessed using a needle inserted through the client's skin. This needle must be a noncoring **Huber needle** so that pieces of the port septum are not removed each time the needle is inserted through the septum and into the port reservoir (see Figure 29-3 and Figure 29-33 ◆).

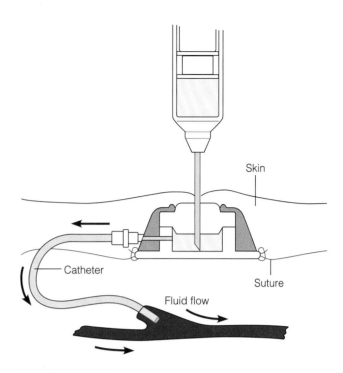

FIGURE 29-33 ◆ A needle inserted into an implanted port.

Nursing Process: Implanted Vascular Access Devices

ASSESSMENT

Gather the pertinent data. Know the purpose of the IVAD. Confirm the physician's order for the IVAD (i.e., whether it is to have an infusion or be irrigated).

PLANNING

Review the client record regarding previous care of the IVAD. Note any complications and how they were managed.

Delegation

Due to the need for sterile technique and technical complexity, accessing an IVAD is not delegated to UAP. UAP may care for clients with such devices and the nurse must ensure that the UAP knows what complications or adverse signs should be reported to the nurse.

IMPLEMENTATION:
TECHNIQUE 29-10 WORKING WITH IMPLANTED VASCULAR ACCESS DEVICES

Equipment

- IV solution container and administration set

  or
- Blood or blood product with transfusion set and priming saline

  or
- Blood specimen tubes and syringe and needle
- Sterile gloves
- 5-mL syringes of normal saline flush and heparinized saline (100 U/mL of heparin)
- 2 percent lidocaine with subcutaneous syringe and needle (optional)
- Povidone–iodine and alcohol solution and swabs
- 22-gauge Huber needle (with extension tubing if indicated)

- Adhesive or nonallergenic tape
- Occlusive dressing materials (e.g., 2″ x 2″ gauze, semipermeable transparent dressing)

Preparation

1. Assemble the equipment.
   - Attach the IV tubing to the infusion or transfusion container.
   - Prime the infusion tubing with fluid.
   - Prepare syringes of normal saline and heparinized saline. Saline followed by heparinized saline is used to flush the device before and after medications or periodically if not in use (check agency policy). *Heparinized saline may help prevent clotting.*

Performance

1. Explain to the client what you are going to do, why it is necessary, and how he or she can cooperate.

2. Provide for client privacy and prepare the client.
   - Check the client's identification band. *This ensures that the right client is receiving the infusion.*
   - Assist the client to a comfortable position, either sitting or lying. Expose the IVAD site but provide for client privacy.

3. Wash hands and observe appropriate infection control procedures.

4. Prepare the site.
   - Locate the IVAD device, and grasp it between two fingers of your nondominant hand to stabilize it. IVADs may have top entry or side entry ports, depending on the design. Palpate and locate the septum, the disc at the center of the port where the needle will be inserted.
   - Apply sterile gloves.
   - *Optional:* Inject 2 percent lidocaine subcutaneously over the needle insertion site. *This anesthetizes the area for injection.* It may be ordered during the first few weeks after the implant surgery, when the area is tender and swollen and more pain from the needle puncture is felt. Other topical anesthetics may be used.
   - An ice pack may be placed over the site for several minutes to reduce discomfort from the needle puncture.
   - Prepare the skin in accordance with agency policy and let the area dry after applying such solutions as povidone–iodine and alcohol.

5. Insert the Huber needle.
   - Connect the needle to a flushing syringe.
   - Grasp both sides of the septum, again anchoring the port with the nondominant hand.
   - Insert the needle at a 90-degree angle to the septum, and push it firmly through the skin and septum until it contacts the base of the IVAD chamber.
   - Avoid tilting or moving the needle when the septum is punctured. *Needle movement can damage the septum and cause fluid leakage.*
   - When the needle contacts the base of the septum, aspirate for blood to determine correct placement. If no blood is obtained, remove the needle and repeat the procedure after having the client move the arms and change position. *Movement can free the catheter from the vessel wall, where it may be lodged.*

   - Infuse the saline flush. There should be no sign of subcutaneous infiltration after infusion of the flush.

6. Prevent manipulation or dislodgement of the needle.
   - If the needle will remain in place for longer than needed to withdraw a blood sample or flush an unused port, secure the needle.
   - Support the Huber needle with 2" x 2" dressings and apply an occlusive transparent dressing to the needle site.
   - Loop and tape the tubing. *Looping prevents tension on the needle.*

7. Attach infusion tubing or an intermittent infusion access cap to the Huber needle.
   - A Huber needle can remain in place for 1 week before it needs to be changed. *The lock allows for infusion of medications or fluid without repeated puncturing of the skin.*

8. After use, perform a final flush with heparinized saline.
   - When flushing, maintain positive pressure, and clamp the tubing immediately before the flush is finished. *These actions avoid reflux of the heparinized saline.*

Variation: Obtaining a Blood Specimen

To obtain a blood specimen:
- Withdraw 10 mL of blood and discard it. *This initial specimen may be diluted with saline and heparin from previous flushes.*
- Draw up the required amount of blood and transfer it to the appropriate containers.
- Slowly instill 5 to 20 mL of normal saline, according to agency policy, over a 5-minute period. *This thoroughly flushes the catheter and avoids excess pressure.*
- Inject 5 mL of heparin flush solution (100 U/mL) to prevent clotting.

9. **Document** all relevant information.
   - Record the appearance of the IVAD site; any difficulty accessing the port and interventions used; presence of drainage; the type of dressing applied; infusions given; and client complaints or concerns. Note any clinical signs indicating venous thrombosis (pain in the neck, arm, and/or shoulder on the side of the insertion site; neck and/or supraclavicular swelling); infection (redness and swelling at the site); and dislodgement of the needle or catheter (shortness of breath, chest pain, coolness in the chest).

AGE-RELATED CONSIDERATIONS

Working with Implanted Vascular Access Devices

Child

- Explain all procedures to the young client beforehand, using play therapy to demonstrate. Encourage questions, and be alert for nonverbal cues. Children may not understand things that seem obvious to adults. For example, a child may think the IV therapy is a punishment.

- Implanted ports have less impact on self-image than tunneled CVCs since they are not readily visible and require no daily care. As with ports in adults, the IVAD may be used for infusions or for drawing blood (Figure 29-34 ◆).

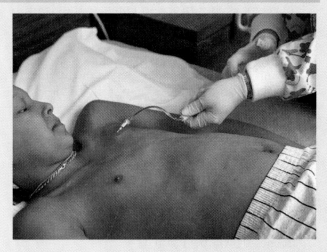

FIGURE 29-34 ◆ Drawing blood from an implanted port (child).

EVALUATION

- Perform follow-up based on findings or outcomes that deviated from expected or normal for the client. Relate findings to previous data if available.

- Report significant deviations from normal to the physician.

Parenteral Nutrition

Parenteral nutrition has two forms: total (TPN) and peripheral (PPN). TPN, also referred to as **hyperalimentation**, is the intravenous infusion of water, protein, carbohydrates, electrolytes, minerals, and vitamins through a central vein. **Peripheral parenteral nutrition (PPN)**, delivered into the smaller peripheral veins, cannot handle as concentrated a solution as central lines (maximum 10 percent dextrose) but can accommodate lipids. For example, a 20 percent lipid emulsion can provide nearly 2,000 kilocalories (Kcal) per day by a peripheral vein. PPN is considered to be a safe and convenient form of therapy over central venous TPN. It does not have the metabolic problems associated with highly concentrated dextrose solutions or the septic complications associated with CVCs. One major disadvantage, however, is the frequent incidence of phlebitis associated with PPN. PPN is administered to clients whose needs for intravenous nutrition will last only a short time or in whom placement of a CVC is contraindicated. It is a form of therapy used more frequently to *prevent* nutritional deficits than to correct them.

A description of the components of parenteral nutrition is provided in Table 29-3. TPN formulas provide all of the known essential nutrients in quantities that promote weight maintenance or gain and wound healing. The proportion of nutrients and total calories delivered vary with the individual's nutritional needs. Thus, a thorough nutritional assessment is required to determine the appropriate TPN regimen. TPN is indicated for clients who are unable to ingest or absorb food via the gastrointestinal tract.

Dextrose, amino acids, electrolytes, vitamins, and minerals are mixed together in one container and infused as the primary TPN solution. Lipid emulsions containing primarily essential fatty acids are administered from a separate container through a Y-connector into the TPN intravenous line or are combined with the TPN solution.

The client receiving TPN is at risk for the same complications as are clients with a CVC plus metabolic complications. Significant changes occur in the client's fluid, electrolyte, glucose, amino acid, vitamin, and mineral levels. Hyperglycemia, hypoglycemia, acidosis, and electrolyte deficiency or excesses such as hyperkalemia, hyponatremia, and hypocalcemia, are potential complications that require meticulous monitoring during therapy.

Nursing Process: Parenteral Nutrition

ASSESSMENT

- Gather the pertinent data. Know the purpose of the TPN.

TABLE 29-3 — COMPONENTS OF PARENTERAL NUTRITION

Component	Description
Protein	Supplied as crystalline synthetic amino acids; contains essential and nonessential amino acids (4 calories/gram of protein; 1 gram nitrogen/6 grams protein)
Carbohydrate	Supplied as dextrose at 4 calories/gram. Peripheral administration 0 to 10% dextrose; central administration up to 50%, although usual is 20 to 25%
Electrolytes	Added to formula; can include sodium, potassium, chloride, acetate, calcium, phosphorus, magnesium; administered according to need
Minerals	Added to formula; can include zinc, chromium, manganese, and copper; administered according to need
Vitamins	Recommended allowances of vitamins A, thiamine, riboflavin, B_6, B_{12}, C, D, E, folic acid, niacin, biotin, and pantothenic acid
Fat/Lipids	Contains primarily essential fatty acids; 9 calories/gram

From *Fundamentals of nursing: Concepts, process, and practice,* 6th ed., by B. Kozier, G. Erb, A. Berman, & K. Burke, 2000, Upper Saddle River, NJ: Prentice Hall Health.

- Confirm the physician's order for the TPN
- Obtain vital signs, including recent body temperature; client's weight; fluid balance; and any allergy to contents of the TPN solution.

PLANNING

Review the client record regarding previous TPN. Note any complications and how they were managed.

Delegation

Due to the need for sterile technique and technical complexity, administration of TPN is not delegated to UAP. UAP may care for clients receiving TPN, and the nurse must ensure that the UAP knows what complications or adverse signs should be reported to the nurse.

IMPLEMENTATION:
TECHNIQUE 29-11 PROVIDING TOTAL PARENTERAL NUTRITION

Equipment

- TPN solution
- Timing tape
- Infusion pump
- Tubing with filter

Preparation

1. Inspect and prepare the solution.
   - Remove the ordered TPN solution from the refrigerator 1 hour before use, and check each ingredient and the proposed rate against the order on the chart. *Infusion of a cold solution can cause pain, hypothermia, and venous spasm and constriction.*
   - Inspect the solution for cloudiness or presence of particles, and ensure that the container is free from cracks.
   - Before administering any TPN solution, check its expiration date. Most solutions must be used within 24 hours of preparation, unless they are refrigerated.
   - Apply a timing tape on the solution container.

Performance

1. Explain to the client what you are going to do, why it is necessary, and how he or she can cooperate.

2. Provide for client privacy and prepare the client.
   - Check the client's identification band. *This ensures that the right client is receiving the TPN.*
   - Assist the client to a comfortable position, either sitting or lying. If necessary, expose the central line site but provide for client privacy.

3. Wash hands and observe appropriate infection control procedures.

4. Change the solution container to the TPN solution ordered.
   - Ensure that correct placement of the central line catheter has been confirmed by x-ray examination.
   - Ensure that the tubing has an in-line filter connected at the end of the TPN tubing. For plain TPN, use a 0.22-micron filter (Figure 29-35A ◆). For TPN with lipids, the filter must be 1.2 microns (Figure 29-35B). Plain lipids are infused without a filter. *The filter traps bacteria and particles that can form in the TPN solution.*
   - Attach and connect the tubing to an infusion pump, if not present. See Technique 29-3 on pages 592–594. *A pump eliminates the changes in flow rate that occur with alterations in the client's activity and position.*

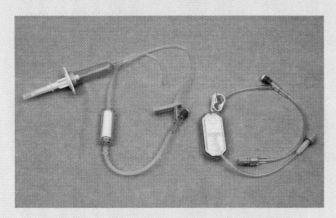

FIGURE 29-35 ◆ (A) 0.22 μ filter used for TPN; (B) 1.22 μ filter for use with TPN containing lipids.

- Attach the TPN solution to the IV administration tubing. If a multiple-lumen tube is in place, attach the infusion to the appropriate lumen.
- If lipids are being infused separately from the TPN, connect the lipid tubing to the injection port closest to the IV catheter.

5. Regulate and monitor the flow rate.
- Establish the prescribed rate of flow and monitor the infusion at least every 30 minutes.
- Never accelerate an infusion that has fallen behind schedule. *Wide fluctuations in blood glucose can occur if the rate of TPN infusion is irregular.*
- Never interrupt or discontinue the infusion abruptly. If TPN solution is temporarily unavailable, infuse a solution containing at least 5 percent dextrose. *This prevents rebound hypoglycemia.*
- During the initial stage of a lipid infusion (i.e., the first hour), closely monitor vital signs, and signs of any side effects (e.g., fever, flushing, diaphoresis, dyspnea, cyanosis, headache, nausea, or vomiting).
- Start lipid infusions very slowly according to the physician's orders, the manufacturer's directions, and agency policy. For a 10 percent emulsion, start at 1 mL/min for the first 5 minutes then up to 4 mL/min for the next 25 minutes. If well tolerated, set ordered rate thereafter.

6. Monitor the client for complications.
- Change the administration set and filter every 24 hours.
- Monitor the vital signs every 4 hours. If fever or abnormal vital signs occur, notify the physician. *An elevated temperature is one of the earliest indications of catheter-related sepsis.*
- Collect double-voided urine specimens in accordance with agency policy, and test the urine for specific gravity. If the specific gravity is abnormal, notify the physician, who may alter the constituents of the TPN solution.
- Assess fingerstick blood glucose levels every 6 hours according to agency protocol (see Technique 4-2). *Blood glucose is tested to make certain the infusion is not running too rapidly for the body to metabolize glucose or too slowly for caloric needs to be met.* Notify the physician of abnormal glucose levels. For hyperglycemia, supplementary insulin may be ordered SQ or added directly to the TPN solution. For hypoglycemia the infusion rate may need to be increased.
- Measure the daily fluid intake and output and calorie intake. *Precise replacement for fluid and electrolyte deficits can then be more readily determined.*
- Monitor the results of laboratory tests (e.g., serum electrolytes and blood urea nitrogen) and report abnormal findings to the physician.

7. Assess weight and anthropometric measurements.
- Weigh the client daily, at the same time and in the same garments. A gain of more than 0.5 kg (1.1 lb) per day indicates fluid excess and should be reported.
- Measure arm circumference and triceps skinfold thickness weekly or in accordance with agency protocol to assess the physical changes.

8. **Document** all relevant information.
- Record the type and amount of infusion, rate of infusion, vital signs q4h, fingerstick blood glucose levels as ordered, client's weight daily, and anthropometric measurements.

EVALUATION

- Perform follow-up based on findings or outcomes that deviated from expected or normal for the client. Relate findings to previous data if available.

- Report significant deviations from normal to the physician.

Chapter Summary

TERMINOLOGY

angiocatheter
butterfly (wing-tipped) needles
central venous catheter (CVC)
drop or drip factor
heparin lock
hyperalimentation
Huber needle
implanted port
implanted venous access device
(IVAD)

infiltration
infusion
infusion controller
infusion pump
macrodrip
microdrip
peripheral parenteral nutrition
(PPN)
phlebitis

piggyback IV
Rh factor
saline lock
tandem
total parenteral nutrition (TPN)
transfusion

FORMING CLINICAL JUDGMENTS

Consider This:

1. Your client has had surgery on the left arm and now requires IV antibiotics. The client is right-handed. Where would you place the IV and why?

2. You have plugged new IV tubing into the peripheral catheter when you notice that there are several inches of air in the tubing. How would you handle this situation?

3. One hour after starting a new IV on a pump/controller 125 mL was supposed to have been infused. You check the amount infused but find that slightly less than 100 mL have gone in. What steps would you follow?

4. At shift report, the offgoing nurse states that there is 300 mL left in an IV of D_5W with 40 mEq of KCl running at 100 mL per hour. When you check the IV about 30 minutes later, it is empty and the client is complaining of stinging at the site. There is redness at the site extending about 2 inches along the vein. What would you do?

5. It is now time to irrigate an intermittent infusion device for patency. The catheter has been in place 48 hours. The transparent membrane dressing shows dried blood. You are unable to aspirate a blood return. What would you do?

6. In discontinuing an IV needle, you have put pressure on the site after removing the needle. What other steps should you take?

7. Proper technique for beginning a blood transfusion requires the nurse to close the upper clamp on the priming saline before opening the clamp to the blood. What would happen if the nurse fails to close the saline clamp?

8. Your client will be receiving chemotherapy for cancer for 6 months. The client requests your input on the physician's statement that either an implanted port or a tunneled central catheter would be advisable. How would you respond regarding the advantages and disadvantages of each?

9. Your client with a central IV catheter is unable to perform Valsalva's maneuver. What would you do when disconnecting the tubing to attach a new infusion set?

10. Upon assessing your restless client, you find that the Huber needle has been pulled out of the client's implanted port. What would be your next steps?

11. How must TPN be infused differently if it has lipids combined in the same infusion bag?

Related Research

Breier S. J. (1999). Home intravenous therapy down under: Consumer perspectives. *Journal of Intravenous Nursing, 22,* 187–193.

Campbell, L. (1999). IV-related phlebitis, complications and length of hospital stay: 2. *British Journal of Nursing, 7*(22), 1364, 1366, 1368–1370.

Cobett, S., & LeBlanc, A. (1999). IV site infection: A prospective, randomized clinical trial comparing the efficacy of three methods of skin antisepsis: CINA conference '99. *CINA: Official Journal of the Canadian Intravenous Nurses Association, 15,* 48–49.

Redelmeier, D., & Livesley, N. J. (1999). Adhesive tape and intravascular-catheter-associated infections. *Journal of General Internal Medicine, 14,* 373–375.

Sheppard, K., LeDesma, M., Morris, N. L., & O'Connor, K. (1999). A prospective study of two intravenous catheter securement techniques in a skilled nursing facility. *Journal of Intravenous Nursing, 22,* 151–156.

References

Angeles, T. (1997). IV rounds: Catheter selection: Choosing the right size. *Nursing, 27*(2), 18.

Carlson, K. R. (1999). Correct utilization and management of peripherally inserted central catheters and midline catheters in the alternate care setting. *Journal of Intravenous Nursing, 22*(6 Suppl.): S46–50.

Carroll, P. L. (1998). Reducing the risk of needlestick injury associated with implanted ports. *Home Healthcare Nurse, 16,* 225–235.

Cook, N. (1999). Central venous catheters: Preventing infection and occlusion. *British Journal of Nursing, 8,* 980, 982, 984, 986–988.

Dougherty, L. (2000). Central venous access devices. *Nursing Standard, 14*(43), 45–50, 53–54.

Drewett, S. R. (2000). Complications of central venous catheters: Nursing care. *British Journal of Nursing, 9,* 466, 468, 470–478.

Fitzpatrick, L., & Fitzpatrick, T. (1997). Blood transfusion: Keeping your patient safe. *Nursing, 27*(8), 34–42.

Frey, A. M. (1997). Tips for pediatric IV insertion. *Nursing, 27*(9), 32.

Hadaway, L. C. (1999). Vascular access devices: Meeting patients' needs. *MEDSURG Nursing, 8,* 296–298, 300–303.

Hadaway, L. C. (1999). IV Rounds: Choosing the right vascular access device, Part I. *Nursing, 29*(2), 18.

Hadaway, L. C. (1999). IV Rounds: Choosing the right vascular access device, Part II. *Nursing, 29*(7), 28–29.

Hadaway, L. C. (2000). IV Rounds: Managing vascular access device occlusions, Part I. *Nursing, 30*(7), 20.

Hadaway, L. C. (2000). IV Rounds: Managing vascular access device occlusions, Part 2. *Nursing, 30*(8), 14.

Hood, B. (1999). Physical assessment of the older adult receiving IV therapy at home: CINA conference '99. *CINA: Official Journal of the Canadian Intravenous Nurses Association, 15,* 27–30.

LaRue, G. D., & Farnsworth, P. A. (2000). Silicone catheter fracture secondary to stress events and a dressing technique to reduce those events. *Journal of Intravenous Nursing, 23*(2), 89–98.

Macklin, D. (2000). Removing PICC: Handling such complications as phlebitis and catheter fracture. *American Journal of Nursing, 100*(1), 52–54.

Masoorli, S. (1997). IV rounds: Central lines—Controversies in care. *Nursing, 27*(3), 72.

Masoorli, S. (1997). Managing complications of central venous access devices. *Nursing, 27*(8), 59–64.

McConnell, E. A. (1998). Clinical do's and don'ts: Administering parenteral nutrition. *Nursing, 28*(7), 18.

McConnell, E. A. (2000). Clinical do's and don'ts: Changing a central venous catheter dressing. *Nursing, 30*(4), 24.

McConnell, E. A. (2000). Clinical do's and don'ts: Infusing packed RBC's. *Nursing, 30*(2), 17.

McConnell, E. A. (1997). Clinical do's and don'ts: Safely administering a blood transfusion. *Nursing, 27*(6), 30.

McConnell, E. A. (2000). Infusion perfusion: IV pumps for every need. *Nursing Management, 31*(4), 53–55.

Milliam, D. A., & Hadaway, L. C. (2000). On the road to successful IV starts. *Nursing, 30*(4), 34–48.

Parker, L. (1999). IV devices and related infections: Causes and complications. *British Journal of Nursing, 8,* 1491, 1493, 1495, 1497–1498.

Plumer, A. (1997). *Principles and practices of intravenous therapy* (6th ed.). Boston: Little Brown.

Roth, D. (1997). IV rounds: Venipuncture tips for geriatric patients. *Nursing, 27*(10), 69.

Safer needle devices: Part 2. *RN, 63*(2), 59–60.

Sansivero, G. E. (1997). IV rounds: Maintaining a PICC line: What you should know. *Nursing, 27*(4), 14.

Schulmeister, L., & Camp-Sorrell, D. (2000). Chemotherapy extravasation from implanted ports. *Oncology Nursing Forum, 27,* 531–538.

Todd, J. (1999). Peripherally inserted central catheters and their use in IV therapy. *British Journal of Nursing, 8,* 140, 142, 144, 146–148.

Workman, B. (1999). Peripheral intravenous therapy management. *Nursing Standard 14*(4), 53–60, 62.

Chapter 30

Performing Wound and Pressure Ulcer Care

Techniques

OBJECTIVES

- Identify assessment data pertinent to skin integrity, pressure sites, and wounds.
- Describe purposes of commonly used dressing materials.
- Describe wound irrigation.
- Identify essential aspects of securing a dressing.
- Identify purposes and essential aspects of transparent wound barrier, hydrocolloid, wet-to-damp, and alginate dressings.
- State purposes of bandages and binders.
- Identify common types of bandages.
- Identify basic turns in bandaging.
- Identify essential guidelines for bandaging.

Types of Wounds

The skin serves a variety of functions, including protecting the individual from injury. Impaired skin integrity is not a frequent problem for most healthy people but is a threat to elders and clients with restricted mobility, chronic illness, trauma, and those undergoing invasive procedures. When the skin is penetrated, the inflammatory process of the individual's immune response acts to eliminate the foreign material, if possible, and prepare the injured body area for healing. This injured body area is called a **wound.**

Body wounds are either intentional or unintentional. *Intentional* traumas occur during therapy. Examples are operations, venipunctures, or radiation burns. Although removing a tumor is therapeutic, the surgeon must cut into body tissues, thus traumatizing them. *Unintentional* wounds are accidental; for example, a person may fracture an arm in an automobile collision. If the tissues are traumatized without a break in the skin, the wound is *closed.* The wound is *open* when the skin or mucous membrane surface is broken.

Wounds are frequently described according to how they are acquired (see Table 30-1). Wounds can also be described according to the likelihood and degree of wound contamination.

- *Clean wounds* are uninfected wounds that have minimal inflammation and do not enter the respiratory, gastrointestinal, genital, or urinary tracts.

- *Clean-contaminated wounds* are surgical wounds in which the respiratory, gastrointestinal, genital, or urinary tract has been entered. Such wounds show no evidence of infection.

- *Contaminated wounds* include open, accidental wounds and surgical wounds involving a major break in sterile technique or a large amount of spillage from the gastrointestinal tract. Contaminated wounds show evidence of inflammation.

- *Dirty or infected wounds* include wounds containing dead tissue and wounds with evidence of a clinical infection (e.g., purulent drainage).

Pressure Ulcers

Pressure ulcers, also called decubitus ulcers or bedsores, are reddened areas, sores, or ulcers of the skin over bony prominences (see Figure 30-1 ◆). They are due to interruption of the blood circulation to the tissue, resulting in a localized ischemia. The tissue is caught between two hard surfaces, usually the surface of the bed and the bony skeleton. The localized ischemia means that the cells are deprived of oxygen and nutrients, and the waste products of metabolism accumulate in the cells. The tissue dies because of the resulting anoxia. Prolonged, unrelieved pressure also damages the small blood vessels.

Preventing Pressure Ulcers

Preventive measures to reduce the risks of developing pressure ulcers include manipulation of the environment, ongoing assessment, proper positioning and nutrition, meticulous hygiene, and instruction in preventing pressure areas. The nurse manipulates the environment when making the client's bed, providing a smooth, firm, wrinkle-free foundation on which the client can lie. Some clients may require a special mattress, such as an alternating pressure, egg crate, or flotation mattress (available for beds and wheelchairs), to decrease pressure on body parts.

TABLE 30-1	TYPES OF WOUNDS	
Type	**Cause**	**Description and Characteristics**
Incision	Sharp instrument (e.g., knife or scalpel)	Open wound; painful; deep or shallow
Contusion	Blow from a blunt instrument	Closed wound, skin appears ecchymotic (bruised) because of damaged blood vessels
Abrasion	Surface scrape, either unintentional (e.g., scraped knee from a fall) or intentional (e.g., dermal abrasion to remove pockmarks)	Open wound involving the skin; painful
Puncture	Penetration of the skin and often the underlying tissues by a sharp instrument, either intentional or unintentional	Open wound
Laceration	Tissues torn apart, often from accidents (e.g., with machinery)	Open wound; edges are often jagged
Penetrating wound	Penetration of the skin and the underlying tissues, usually unintentional (e.g., from a bullet or metal fragments)	Open wound

From *Fundamentals of nursing: Concepts, process, and practice,* 6th ed., by B. Kozier, G. Erb, A. Berman, & K. Burke, 2000, Upper Saddle River, NJ: Prentice Hall Health.

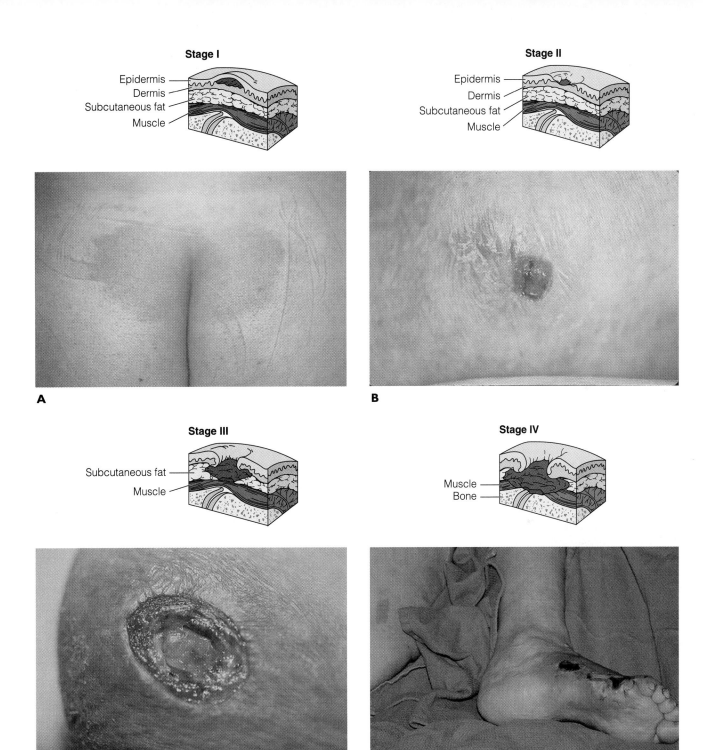

FIGURE 30-1 ◆ Four stages of pressure ulcers.

Nursing Process: Assessing Wounds and Pressure Ulcers

PLANNING

Before assessing the wound, review the client record for information regarding the cause of the wound, the length of time the wound has been present, and previous treatment and response to treatment.

Determine factors that may hinder wound healing:

• *Malnutrition.* A poorly nourished person often has insufficient amounts of the vitamins and trace substances needed to synthesize wound-healing elements and have resistance to infection.

- *Obesity.* Adipose tissue has a limited blood supply; thus, an obese client is more likely to acquire an infection and have poor wound healing.

- *Medications.* Some medications may retard healing. Corticosteroids can suppress the inflammatory reaction. In addition, the prolonged use of antibiotics can increase the likelihood of infection from resistant organisms.

- *Smoking.* Smoking reduces the amount of functional hemoglobin and causes peripheral vasoconstriction.

- *Compromised host.* A compromised host is a person at unusual risk for infection. For example, clients who have diabetes mellitus or cancer may be at increased risk for getting an infection.

Determine results of laboratory data pertinent to healing (e.g., leukocyte count and blood coagulation studies).

Delegation

Assessment is a technique not delegated to unlicensed assistive personnel (UAP). However, UAP may observe the wound during usual care and must report abnormal findings to the nurse. Abnormal findings must be validated and interpreted by the nurse.

IMPLEMENTATION:
TECHNIQUE 30-1 ASSESSING WOUNDS AND PRESSURE ULCERS

Equipment

- Clean gloves
- Sterile gloves
- Disposable millimeter ruler
- Paper or plastic for tracing the wound (optional)
- Sterile cotton tip applicator swab
- Adequate lighting

Preparation

If the wound is dressed or will be dressed after assessment, gather the appropriate additional supplies before beginning assessment.

Performance

1. Explain to the client what you are going to do, why it is necessary, and how he or she can cooperate. Discuss how the results will be used in planning further care or treatments.

2. Wash hands and observe appropriate infection control procedures.

3. Provide for client privacy.

4. Apply clean gloves.

5. If necessary, remove the existing dressing (see Technique 30-2).

6. Assess the wound for:

   - *Appearance.* Inspect the wound itself for signs of healing and approximation of the wound edges.

   - *Drainage.* Observe the location, color, consistency, odor, and degree of saturation of dressings. Note the number of gauzes saturated or the diameter of drainage on gauze.

   - *Size.* To determine the width and length of the wound's surface area or its circumference, use a disposable measuring guide. For irregularly shaped wounds, use paper or a transparent wound dressing, and trace and date the margins of the wounds.

   - *Depth.* To determine wound depth, probe the deepest part of the wound with a sterile swab. Place your forefinger on the swab at surface level, and then measure the distance with a disposable measuring guide.

   - *Swelling.* Wearing sterile gloves, palpate wound edges for tension and tautness of tissues; minimal to moderate swelling is normal in early stages of wound healing.

   - *Pain.* Expect severe to moderate pain for 3 to 5 days after surgery; persistent or increasing pain, or sudden onset of severe pain may indicate internal hemorrhaging or infection.

   - *Drains or tubes.* Inspect drain security and placement, amount and character of drainage, and functioning of collecting apparatus, if present.

7. Determine the stage of a pressure ulcer.

   - Use the stages described by the Panel for Predication and Prevention of Pressure Ulcers in Adults (Figure 30-1).

   - Request a consultation from a Wound-Ostomy-Continence nurse if appropriate. *Initial staging of pressure ulcers can be difficult. The surface evidence may not be truly indicative of underlying tissue damage. Necrotic tissue on the surface (eschar) of the ulcer may require removal for complete assessment.*

8. **Document** the assessment and the client's response in the client record using forms or checklists supplemented by narrative notes when appropriate. Many agencies use a designated wound/skin documentation sheet (Figure 30-2 ◆).

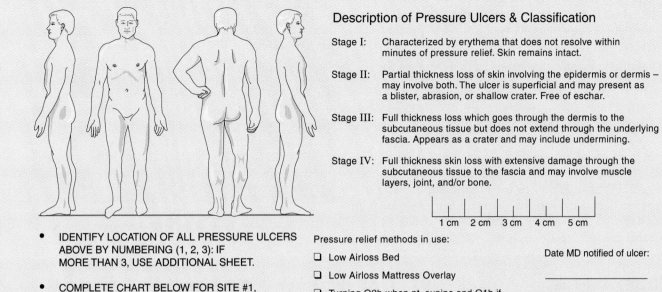

Description of Pressure Ulcers & Classification

Stage I: Characterized by erythema that does not resolve within minutes of pressure relief. Skin remains intact.

Stage II: Partial thickness loss of skin involving the epidermis or dermis – may involve both. The ulcer is superficial and may present as a blister, abrasion, or shallow crater. Free of eschar.

Stage III: Full thickness loss which goes through the dermis to the subcutaneous tissue but does not extend through the underlying fascia. Appears as a crater and may include undermining.

Stage IV: Full thickness skin loss with extensive damage through the subcutaneous tissue to the fascia and may involve muscle layers, joint, and/or bone.

1 cm 2 cm 3 cm 4 cm 5 cm

- • IDENTIFY LOCATION OF ALL PRESSURE ULCERS ABOVE BY NUMBERING (1, 2, 3): IF MORE THAN 3, USE ADDITIONAL SHEET.

- • COMPLETE CHART BELOW FOR SITE #1, USE REVERSE SIDE FOR SITES 2 & 3.

Patient Admitted On: _____

Date Sheet Initiated: _____

Pressure relief methods in use:

❑ Low Airloss Bed

❑ Low Airloss Mattress Overlay

❑ Turning Q2h when pt. supine and Q1h if HOB↑

❑ Pressure Reducing Mattress Overlay

❑ Other _____

Date MD notified of ulcer:

_____

DOCUMENT WEEKLY AND P.R.N. SIGNIFICANT CHANGE IN ULCER'S APPEARANCE

SITE #1: LOCATION	DESCRIBE TREATMENT:				FREQUENCY:
DATE / TIME					
DIMENSIONS: LENGTH (in. cm.)					
WIDTH					
DEPTH					
ODOR (None or Foul)					
DESCRIBE DRAINAGE (Purulent, Serous, Serosanguinous) & AMOUNT (Scant, Moderate, Copious)					
STAGE (See Above)					
COMMENTARY: ie: Describe tissue surrounding ulcer: is there undermining? % necrotic vs % granular, etc.					
NURSE					

WOUND/SKIN DOCUMENTATION SHEET

FIGURE 30-2 ◆ Wound/skin documentation sheet.

- Perform follow-up assessments and interventions based on findings that deviate from expected or normal for the client. Relate findings to previous assessment data if available.

- Report significant deviations from normal to the physician.

Dressing Wounds

The purpose of the wound **dressing** must be determined before the proper type of dressing can be selected. Dressings may be used to protect the wound, provide humidity to the wound surface, absorb drainage, prevent bleeding, immobilize, and hide the wound from view. In addition, the dressing is influenced by the location, size, and type of wound.

Dressing Materials

Gauze, with or without absorbent padding, is commonly used to cover wounds (Figure 30-3 ◆). Plain gauze can be applied to wounds in several modes (Table 30-2 ◆).

Telfa gauze is a special type. It has a shiny, nonadherent surface on one or both sides and is applied with the shiny surface on the wound. Exudate seeps through this surface and collects on the absorbent material on the other side or is sandwiched between the two nonadherent surfaces. Since the dressing does not adhere, it does not cause injury to the wound when removed. *Petrolatum* gauze, another nonadherent type, is impregnated with petroleum jelly. It is placed against the wound and usually covered with 4" × 4" gauze. Nonadherent dressings should not be used when wound **debridement** (removal of infected and necrotic material) is desired.

Larger and thicker gauze dressings, referred to as

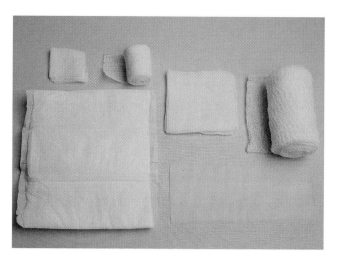

FIGURE 30-3 ◆ Frequently used dressing materials.

composite dressings, *surgipads,* or *abdominal pads,* may be used to cover plain gauze. They not only hold the other gauzes in place but also absorb and collect excess drainage. Surgipads are more absorbent on one side, and this side is placed toward the wound; the less absorbent, more protective side is placed outward to protect the wound from external contamination. The outer side is often indicated with a blue stripe.

More specialized types of wound dressings are described in Table 30-3. Use of these dressings for pressure ulcers is found in Table 30-4.

Dressing Changes

Nursing Process: Dressing Wounds

ASSESSMENT

Before changing a dressing, review the client record for information regarding the cause of the wound, the

TABLE 30-2	MODES OF APPLYING GAUZE DRESSINGS	
Dressing	**Description**	**Purpose**
Dry-to-dry		Protect the wound. If the wound is open or draining, necrotic debris and exudates are trapped in the interstices of the gauze layer and are removed when the dressing is removed.
Wet-to-damp	A layer of wide mesh gauze saturated with saline or antimicrobial solution lies packed into the wound surface. A second layer of dry absorbent cotton or Dacron is on top.	Debride the wound. Necrotic debris is softened by the solution and then adheres to the mesh gauze as it dries. It is removed when the dressing is removed. Also, moisture helps dilute viscous exudates.
Wet-to-wet or **Wet-to-dry**	These dressings are no longer used due to the tissue damage caused. Dressings that remain saturated at all times do not promote debridement and can cause maceration of healthy tissue. Dressings that have dried completely and are then removed without soaking disrupt granulation tissue and are very painful for the client.	

TABLE 30-3 **SELECTED TYPES OF WOUND DRESSINGS**

Dressing	Description	Purpose	Examples
Transparent adhesive films/wound barriers	Adhesive plastic semipermeable *nonabsorbent* dressings that allow exchange of oxygen between the atmosphere and wound bed. They are impermeable to bacteria and water.	To provide protection against contamination and friction; to maintain a clean moist surface that facilitates cellular migration; to provide insulation by preventing fluid evaporation; and to facilitate wound assessment	Op-Site, Tegaderm, Bio-occlusive, ACU-derm
Impregnated nonadherent dressings	Woven or nonwoven cotton or synthetic materials that are impregnated with petrolatum, saline, zinc-saline, antimicrobials, or other agents. Require secondary dressings to secure them in place, retain moisture, and provide wound protection.	To cover, soothe, and protect partial- and full-thickness wounds without exudate	Vaseline gauze, Carragauze, Dermagran Wet Dressing, Xeroform
Hydrocolloids	Waterproof adhesive wafers, pastes, or powders. Wafers, designed to be worn for up to 7 days, consist of two layers. The inner adhesive layer has particles that absorb exudate and form a hydrated gel over the wound; the outer film provides a seal.	To absorb exudate; to produce a moist environment that facilitates healing but does not cause maceration of surrounding skin; to protect the wound from bacterial contamination, foreign debris, and urine or feces; and to prevent shearing	DuoDERM, Comfeel, Tegasorb, Restore, Replicare
Hydrogels	Glycerin or water-based *nonadhesive* jellylike sheets, granules, or gels that are oxygen permeable, unless covered by a plastic film. May require secondary occlusive dressing.	To liquefy necrotic tissue or slough, rehydrate the wound bed, and fill in dead space	Aquasorb, ClearSite, Elasto-Gel, Intrasite, Vigilon
Polyurethane foams	*Nonadherent* hydrocolloid dressings that need to have their edges taped down or sealed. Require secondary dressings to obtain an occlusive environment. Surrounding skin must be protected to prevent maceration.	To absorb light to moderate amounts of exudate; to debride wounds	Lyofoam, Allevyn, Nuderm, Flexan
Exudate absorbers	Nonadherent dressings of powder, beads or granules, or paste that conform to the wound surface and absorb up to 20 times their weight in exudate; require a secondary dressing.	To provide a moist wound surface by interacting with exudate; to form a gelatinous mass; to absorb exudate; to eliminate dead space or pack wounds; and to support debridement	Debrisan, Triad paste, Sorbsan

From *Fundamentals of nursing: Concepts, process, and practice*, 6th ed., by B. Kozier, G. Erb, A. Berman, & K. Burke, 2000, Upper Saddle River, NJ: Prentice Hall Health.

length of time the wound has been present, and previous treatment and response to treatment.

Determine allergies to wound cleaning agents, dressings, or tape; complaints of discomfort; the time of the last pain medication; and signs of systemic infection (e.g., elevated body temperature, diaphoresis, malaise; leukocytosis).

PLANNING

If possible, schedule the dressing change at a time convenient for the client. Some dressing changes

TABLE 30-4 DRESSINGS FOR PRESSURE ULCERS

Dressing	Mechanism of Action	Stage I	II	III	IV
Dry gauze	Wicks drainage away from wound surface			✓	✓
Wet-to-damp gauze	Maintains moist wound environment, wicks drainage away from wound surface			✓	✓
Transparent barrier	Retains wound moisture, allows gas exchange, does not stick to wound surface	✓	✓		
Hydrocolloid	Occlusive, repels moisture and dirt, maintains moist wound environment	✓	✓	✓	
Hydrogel	Maintains moist wound environment			✓	✓
Alginate	Maintains moist wound environment, absorbs exudate			✓	✓

require only a few minutes and others can take much longer. Dressing changes necessitated by a change in the wound or dressing condition may not be scheduled.

Delegation

Due to the need for aseptic technique and assessment skills, most dressing changes are not delegated to UAP. In some states, UAP may apply dry dressings to clean, chronic wounds. UAP should observe an exposed wound or dressing during usual care and must report abnormal findings to the nurse. In some agencies, UAP may be permitted to reinforce the dressing (apply additional dry dressings over a saturated bandage) but this must be reported to the nurse as soon as possible. Assessment of the wound and abnormal findings must be validated and interpreted by the nurse.

IMPLEMENTATION:
TECHNIQUE 30-2 PERFORMING A DRY DRESSING CHANGE

Equipment

- Clean gloves
- Sterile gloves
- 4" × 4" gauze
- Hypoallergenic tape, tie tapes, or binder
- Bath blanket (if necessary)
- Moistureproof bag
- Mask (optional)
- Acetone or another solution (if necessary to loosen adhesive)
- Sterile dressing set; if none is available, gather the following sterile items:
  - Drape or towel
  - Gauze squares
  - Container for the cleaning solution
  - Antimicrobial solution
  - Forceps
- Additional supplies required for the particular dressing (e.g., extra gauze dressings and ointment or powder, if ordered)

Preparation

- Acquire assistance for changing a dressing on a restless or confused adult. *The person might move and contaminate the sterile field or the wound.*
- Make a cuff on the moistureproof bag for disposal of the soiled dressings, and place the bag within reach. It can be taped to the bedclothes or bedside table. *Making a cuff keeps the outside of the bag free from contamination by the soiled dressings and prevents subsequent contamination of the nurse's hands or of sterile instrument tips when discarding dressings or sponges. Placement of the bag within reach prevents the nurse from reaching across the sterile field and the wound and potentially contaminating these areas.*

Performance

1. Explain to the client what you are going to do, why it is necessary, and how he or she can coop-

erate. Discuss how the results will be used in planning further care or treatments.

2. Wash hands and observe appropriate infection control procedures.

3. Provide for client privacy. Assist the client to a comfortable position in which the wound can be readily exposed. Expose only the wound area, using a bath blanket to cover the client, if necessary. *Undue exposure is physically and psychologically distressing to most people.*

4. Don a facemask, as indicated. *A mask may be worn for surgical dressing changes to prevent contamination of the wound by droplet spray from the nurse's respiratory tract.*

5. Remove outer dressings.
   • Remove binders, if used, and place them aside. Untie tie tapes, if used.
   • If adhesive tape was used, remove it by holding down the skin and pulling the tape gently but firmly toward the wound. *Pressing down on the skin provides countertraction against the pulling motion. Tape is pulled toward the incision to prevent strain on the sutures or wound.*
   • Use a solvent to loosen tape, if required. *Moistening the tape with acetone or a similar solvent lessens the discomfort of removal, particularly from hairy surfaces.*
   • Don disposable gloves, and remove the outer dressing.
   • Lift the dressing so that the underside is away from the client's face. *The appearance and odor of the drainage may be upsetting to the client.*

6. Dispose of soiled dressings appropriately.
   • Place the soiled dressing in the moistureproof bag without touching the outside of the bag. *Contamination of the outside of the bag is avoided to prevent the spread of microorganisms to the nurse and subsequently to others.*
   • Remove gloves, dispose of them in the moistureproof bag, and wash your hands.

7. Remove inner dressings.
   • Open the sterile dressing set, using surgical aseptic technique.
   • Place the sterile drape beside the wound, and don sterile gloves (optional).
   • Remove the underdressings with forceps or sterile gloves. *Forceps or gloves are used to prevent contamination of the wound by the nurse's hands and contamination of the nurse's hands by wound drainage.*
   • Assess the location, type (color, consistency), and odor of wound drainage, and the number of gauzes saturated or the diameter of drainage collected on the dressings.
   • Discard the soiled dressings in the bag. To avoid contaminating the forceps tips on the edge of the paper bag, hold the dressings 10 to 15 cm (4 to 6 in) above the bag, and drop the dressings into it.
   • After the dressings are removed, discard the forceps, or set them aside from the sterile field. *These forceps are now contaminated by the wound drainage.*

8. Clean the wound if indicated (see also Box 30-1).
   • Clean the wound, using a new pair of forceps and moistened swabs.
   • Keep the forceps tips lower than the handles at all times. *This prevents their contamination by fluid traveling up to the handle and nurse's wrist and back to the tips.*
   • Clean with strokes from the top to the bottom, starting at the center and continuing to the outside (Figure 30-4 ◆).

Box 30-1 *Guidelines for Cleaning Wounds*

• Use physiologic solutions, such as isotonic saline or lactated Ringer's solution, to clean or irrigate wounds. If antimicrobial solutions are used, make sure they are well diluted.

• When possible, warm the solution to body temperature before use. This prevents lowering of the wound temperature, which slows the healing process.

• If a wound is grossly contaminated by foreign material, bacteria, slough, or necrotic tissue, clean the wound at every dressing change. Foreign bodies and devitalized tissue act as a focus for infection and can delay healing.

• If a wound is clean, has little exudate, and reveals healthy granulation tissue, avoid repeated cleaning. Unnecessary cleaning can delay wound healing by traumatizing newly produced, delicate tissues, reducing the surface temperature of the wound, and removing exudate which itself may have bactericidal properties.

• Use gauze squares. Avoid using cotton balls and other products that shed fibers onto the wound surface. The fibers become embedded in granulation tissue and can act as foci for infection. They may also stimulate "foreign body" reactions, prolonging the inflammatory phase of healing and delaying the healing process.

• Clean superficial noninfected wounds by irrigating them with normal saline. The hydraulic pressure of an irrigating stream of fluid dislodges contaminating debris and reduces bacterial colonization.

• To retain wound moisture, avoid drying a wound after cleaning it.

From *Fundamentals of nursing: Concepts, process, and practice*, 6th ed., by B. Kozier, G. Erb, A. Berman, & K. Burke, 2000, Upper Saddle River, NJ: Prentice Hall Health.

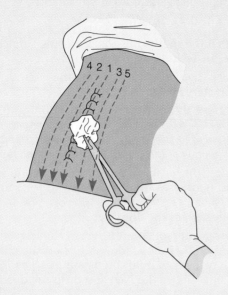

FIGURE 30-4 ◆ Cleaning a wound from top to bottom.

or

- Clean outward from the wound (Figure 30-5 ◆). *The wound is cleaned from the least to the most contaminated area, for example, from the top of the incision, which is drier, to the bottom of the incision, where any drainage will collect and which is considered more contaminated, or from the center outward.*

- Use a separate swab for each stroke, and discard each swab after use. *This prevents the introduction of microorganisms to other wound areas.*

- Repeat the cleaning process until all drainage is removed.

9. Assess the overall appearance of the wound (See Technique 30-1).

10. Apply sterile dressings.

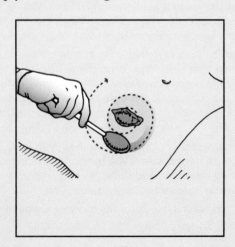

FIGURE 30-5 ◆ Cleaning a wound from the center outward.

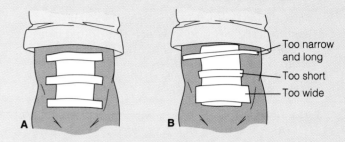

FIGURE 30-6 ◆ Taping the dressing.

Too narrow and long
Too short
Too wide

- Apply sterile dressings one at a time over the wound, using sterile forceps or sterile gloves. Start at the center of the wound and move progressively outward. The final surgipad can be picked up by hand, touching only the outside, which is often marked by a blue line down the center.

- Remove and discard gloves, wash hands.

11. Secure the dressing with tape, tie tapes, or a binder.

- Place the tape so that the dressing cannot be folded back to expose the wound. Place strips at the ends of the dressing, and space tapes evenly in the middle (Figure 30-6 ◆).

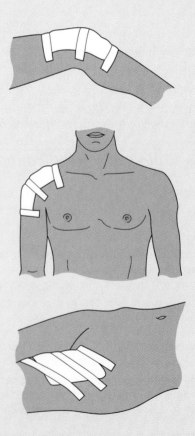

FIGURE 30-7 ◆ Dressings over moving parts taped at right angle to the joint movement.

- Ensure that the tape is long and wide enough to adhere to the skin but not so long or wide that it loosens with activity.
- Place the tape in the opposite direction from the body action, for example, across a body joint or crease, not lengthwise (Figure 30-7 ◆).
- *Montgomery straps (tie tapes) are commonly used for wounds requiring frequent dressing changes. These straps prevent skin irritation and discomfort caused by removing the adhesive each time the dressing is changed.*

12. **Document** the dressing change and the client's response in the client record using forms or checklists supplemented by narrative notes when appropriate. Many agencies use a designated wound/skin documentation sheet (Figure 30-2).

EVALUATION

- Perform follow-up based on findings that deviate from expected or normal for the client. Relate findings to previous assessment data if available.
- Report significant deviations from normal to the physician.

Transparent Wound Barriers

Transparent semipermeable membrane dressings help retain wound moisture while allowing gases (oxygen, carbon dioxide) to pass into and away from the wound. They are occlusive in that they allow bathing without removing or changing the dressing and microorganisms are repelled. **Transparent wound barriers** do not adhere to wound surfaces.

IMPLEMENTATION:
TECHNIQUE 30-3 APPLYING A TRANSPARENT WOUND BARRIER

Equipment

- Clean gloves
- Sterile gloves (optional)
- Hair scissors or clippers
- Alcohol or acetone
- Moistureproof bag
- Sterile gauze and the wound-cleaning agents specified by the physician or agency (e.g., sterile saline)
- Wound barrier dressing
- Scissors
- Paper tape

Preparation

Review the order regarding frequency and type of dressing change, and determine agency protocol about solutions used to clean the wound and whether clean or sterile technique is to be used. Many agencies recommend clean rather than sterile technique for chronic wounds such as a pressure ulcer.

If possible, schedule the dressing change at a time convenient for the client. Some dressing changes require only a few minutes and others can take much longer.

Performance

1. Explain to the client what you are going to do, why it is necessary, and how he or she can cooperate. Discuss how the results will be used in planning further care or treatments.

2. Wash hands and observe appropriate infection control procedures.

3. Provide for client privacy. Assist the client to a comfortable position in which the wound can be readily exposed. Expose only the wound area, using a bath blanket to cover the client, if necessary. *Undue exposure is physically and psychologically distressing to most people.*

4. Remove the existing dressing (see Technique 30-2, steps 5 through 7).

5. Thoroughly clean the skin area around the wound.
   - Put on disposable gloves.
   - Clean the skin well with normal saline or a mild cleansing agent. Always rinse the adjacent skin well before applying a dressing.
   - Clip the hair about 5 cm (2 in) around the wound area if indicated.
   - Remove gloves, and dispose of them in the moistureproof bag.

6. Clean the wound if indicated.
   - Put on clean or sterile gloves in accordance with agency practice.
   - Clean the wound with the prescribed solution.
   - Dry the surrounding skin with dry gauze.

7. Assess the wound.
   - See Technique 30-1.

8. Apply the wound barrier.
   - Review the instructions on the barrier package.

Remove part of the paper backing on the dressing (Figure 30-8 ◆).

- Apply the dressing at one edge of the wound site, allowing at least 2.5-cm (1-in) coverage of the skin surrounding the wound.

- Gently lay or press the barrier over the wound. Keep it free of wrinkles, but avoid stretching it too tightly. *A stretched dressing restricts mobility.*

- Remove and dispose of gloves appropriately.

9. Reinforce the dressing only if absolutely needed.

- Apply paper or other porous tape to "window frame" the edges of the dressing.

10. Assess the wound at least daily.

- Determine the extent of serous fluid accumulation under the dressing, wound healing, and the need to repair the dressing.

- If excessive serum has accumulated, consider replacing the transparent wound barrier with a more absorbent type of dressing, such as hydrocolloid.

- If the dressing is leaking, remove it and apply another dressing.

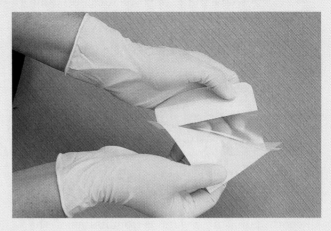

FIGURE 30-8 ◆ Transparent wound dressing.

11. **Document** the dressing change and the client's response in the client record using forms or checklists supplemented by narrative notes when appropriate. Many agencies use a designated wound/skin documentation sheet (see Figure 30-2).

EVALUATION

- Perform follow-up based on findings that deviate from expected or normal for the client. Relate findings to previous assessment data if available.

- Report significant deviations from normal to the physician.

Hydrocolloid Dressing

Hydrocolloid dressings are frequently used for stasis and pressure ulcers. They are occlusive, allow bathing without removing or changing the dressing, and repel external microorganisms. They do not adhere to wound surfaces. They can remain in place for up to 1 week and are easily molded to fit the wound and body location. However, they are also opaque and do not allow easy examination of the wound. If microorganisms are present in the wound, the dressing can facilitate their growth. Therefore, they are not used on infected wounds.

Equipment

- Clean gloves
- Sterile gloves (optional)
- Dressing set, including scissors and paper tape
- Moistureproof bag
- Sterile gauze and the wound-cleaning agents specified by the physician or agency (e.g., sterile saline)

- Hydrocolloid dressing at least 3 to 4 cm (1.5 in) larger than wound on all four sides (Figure 30-9 ◆)

Preparation

- Review the order regarding frequency and type of dressing change, and determine agency protocol about solutions used to clean the wound and whether clean or sterile technique is to be used. Many agencies recommend clean rather than

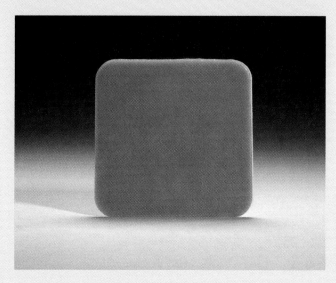

FIGURE 30-9 ◆ Hydrocolloid dressing.

sterile technique for chronic wounds such as a pressure ulcer.

- Change the dressing if it leaks, is dislodged, or develops an odor. Otherwise, it may remain in place up to 1 week.
- If possible, schedule the dressing change at a time convenient for the client. Some dressing changes require only a few minutes and others can take much longer.

Performance

1. Explain to the client what you are going to do, why it is necessary, and how he or she can cooperate. Discuss how the results will be used in planning further care or treatments.

2. Wash hands and observe appropriate infection control procedures.

3. Provide for client privacy. Assist the client to a comfortable position in which the wound can be readily exposed. Expose only the wound area, using a bath blanket to cover the client, if necessary. *Undue exposure is physically and psychologically distressing to most people.*

4. Remove the existing dressing (see Technique 30-2, steps 5 through 7).

5. Thoroughly clean the skin area around the wound.
   - Put on disposable gloves.
   - Clean the skin well but gently with normal saline or a mild cleansing agent. Always rinse the adjacent skin well before applying a dressing.
   - Clip the hair about 5 cm (2 in) around the wound area if indicated.
   - Leave the residue that is difficult to remove on the skin. It will wear off in time. Attempts to remove residue can irritate the surrounding skin.
   - Remove gloves, and dispose of them in the moistureproof bag.

6. Clean the wound if indicated.
   - Put on clean disposable or sterile gloves in accordance with agency practice.
   - Clean the wound with the prescribed solution.
   - Dry the surrounding skin with dry gauze.

7. Assess the wound.
   - See Technique 30-1.

8. Apply the dressing.
   - Follow the manufacturer's instructions.
   - Remove and dispose of the gloves.
   - Optional: Apply tape to "window frame" the edges of the dressing or according to agency protocol. *Taping prevents the dressing from sticking to bed linens and the edges from lifting.*

9. Assess and change the dressing as indicated.
   - Inspect the dressing at least daily for leakage, dislodgement, odor, and wrinkling.
   - Change the dressing if any of these signs are present.

10. **Document** the dressing change and the client's response in the client record using forms or checklists supplemented by narrative notes when appropriate. Many agencies use a designated wound/skin documentation sheet (see Figure 30-2).

EVALUATION

- Perform follow-up based on findings that deviate from expected or normal for the client. Relate findings to previous assessment data if available.
- Report significant deviations from normal to the physician.

Treating Wounds

Sometimes, simply applying a dressing over a wound is not adequate to promote healing. If this is the case, the wound may need more aggressive cleaning such as can be done through irrigating or packing the wound with various materials.

Irrigating a Wound

An irrigation is the washing or flushing out of an area. Wound irrigation is performed using sterile technique and normal saline or antiseptic solution.

Nursing Process: Irrigating a Wound

ASSESSMENT

Review the client's record to determine:

- Previous appearance and size of the wound

- Character of the exudate
- Presence of pain and the time of the last pain medication
- Clinical signs of systemic infection
- Allergies to the wound irrigation agent or tape

PLANNING

Before irrigating a wound, determine (1) the type of irrigating solution to be used, (2) the frequency of irrigations, and (3) the temperature of the solution.

If possible, schedule the irrigation at a time convenient for the client. Some irrigations require only a few minutes, and others can take much longer.

Delegation

Due to the need for aseptic technique and assessment skills, wound irrigations are not delegated to UAP. However, UAP may observe the wound and dressing during usual care and must report abnormal findings to the nurse. Abnormal findings must be validated and interpreted by the nurse.

IMPLEMENTATION:
TECHNIQUE 30-5 IRRIGATING A WOUND

Equipment

- Sterile dressing equipment and dressing materials
- Sterile syringes (e.g., a 30- to 60-mL syringe) with a catheter of an appropriate size (e.g., 18 or 19 gauge) or an irrigating (catheter) tip syringe
- Sterile basin for the irrigating solution
- Moistureproof bag
- Basin to receive the irrigation returns
- Irrigating solution, usually 200 mL (6.5 oz) of solution warmed to body temperature, according to the agency's or physician's choice
- Clean gloves
- Sterile gloves
- Moistureproof sterile drape

Performance

1. Explain to the client what you are going to do, why it is necessary, and how he or she can cooperate. Discuss how the results will be used in planning further care or treatments.

2. Wash hands and observe appropriate infection control procedures.

Provide for Client Privacy

3. Prepare the client.
   - Assist the client to a position in which the irrigating solution will flow by gravity from the upper end of the wound to the lower end and then into the basin.
   - Place the waterproof drape over the client and the bed.
   - Put on clean gloves and remove and discard the old dressing.
   - If indicated, clean the wound from the center of the wound outward, using circular strokes.
   - Use a separate swab for each stroke, and discard each swab after use. *This prevents the introduction of microorganisms to other wound areas.*

   - Assess the wound and drainage (see Technique 30-1).
   - Remove and discard disposable gloves.

4. Prepare the equipment.
   - Open the sterile dressing set and supplies.
   - Pour the ordered solution into the solution container.
   - Position the basin below the wound to receive the irrigating fluid.
   - Put on sterile gloves.

5. Irrigate the wound.
   - Instill a steady stream of irrigating solution into the wound (see Figure 30-10 ◆). Make sure all areas of the wound are irrigated.
   - Use either a syringe with a catheter attached or with irrigating tip to flush the wound. *Effective irrigation requires 4 to 15 pounds per square inch of pressure. These devices provide this pressure; bulb syringes do not.*

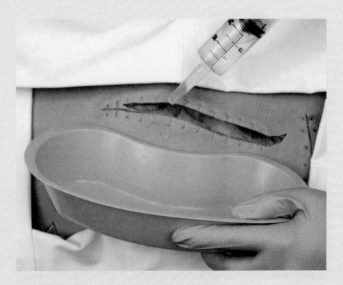

FIGURE 30-10 ◆ Irrigating a wound.

- If you are using a catheter to reach tracks or crevices, insert the catheter into the wound until resistance is met. Do not force the catheter. *Forcing the catheter can cause tissue damage.*
- Continue irrigating until the solution becomes clear (no exudate is present). *The irrigation washes away tissue debris and drainage so that later returns are clearer.*
- Dry the area around the wound. *Moisture left on the skin promotes the growth of microorganisms and can cause skin irritation and breakdown.*

6. Assess and dress the wound.
   - Assess the appearance of the wound again, noting in particular the type and amount of exudate

still present and the presence and extent of granulation tissue.
   - Apply a sterile dressing to the wound based on the amount of drainage expected (see Table 30-3).

7. **Document** the irrigation and the client's response in the client record using forms or checklists supplemented by narrative notes when appropriate. Many agencies use a designated wound/skin documentation sheet (see Figure 30-2).

EVALUATION

- Perform follow-up based on findings that deviate from expected or normal for the client. Relate findings to previous assessment data if available.
- Report significant deviations from normal to the physician.

Packing a Wound

Gauze may be placed in a wound to facilitate formation of granulation tissue, removal of necrotic material, and healing by secondary intention. Generally, continuous-thread, moistened 4″ × 4″ gauze, without filling, is used, although medicated gauze and narrow packing gauze may be ordered.

Nursing Process: Packing a Wound

ASSESSMENT

Review the client's record to determine:

- Previous appearance, size, and treatment of the wound

- Character of any exudate
- Presence of pain and the time of the last pain medication
- Clinical signs of systemic infection
- Allergies to the medications or tape

PLANNING

Before packing a wound, determine the type of packing to be used and the frequency of dressing changes.

If possible, schedule the dressing change at a time convenient for the client. Some packings require only a few minutes and others can take much longer.

Delegation

Due to the need for aseptic technique and assessment skills, wound packing is not delegated to UAP. However, UAP may observe the wound and dressing during usual care and must report abnormal findings to the nurse. Abnormal findings must be validated and interpreted by the nurse.

IMPLEMENTATION:
TECHNIQUE 30-6 PERFORMING A WET-TO-DAMP DRESSING CHANGE

Equipment

- Sterile packing gauze
- Sterile dressing equipment and dressing materials
- Solution for wetting gauze (e.g., sterile saline)
- Sterile bowl
- Forceps or cotton-tipped applicators (optional)
- Moistureproof bag
- Clean gloves
- Sterile gloves

Performance

1. Explain to the client what you are going to do, why it is necessary, and how he or she can cooperate. Discuss how the results will be used in planning further care or treatments.

2. Wash hands and observe appropriate infection control procedures.

Provide for Client Privacy

3. Prepare the client. Assist the client to a comfortable position in which the wound can be readily

exposed. Expose only the wound area, using a bath blanket to cover the client, if necessary. *Undue exposure is physically and psychologically distressing to most people.*

4. Remove the existing dressing and clean the wound if indicated (see Technique 30-2, steps 5 through 8).
   - If the previous gauze dressing adheres to any tissue during removal, soak it with sterile normal saline. *This facilitates removal and prevents disruption of new granulation tissue.*

5. Prepare the supplies.
   - Open the packages of the sterile dressing set, gauze, and bowl.
   - Pour the ordered solution into the bowl.
   - Put on sterile gloves.
   - Place the gauze into the bowl and thoroughly saturate them with solution.
   - Wring out the packing gauze until it is slightly moist. Avoid packing that is too wet. *Excessively wet gauze increases the risk for bacterial growth, may macerate the surrounding skin, and does not dry out sufficiently before the next dressing change.*

6. Pack the wound with the damp gauze.
   - Using your sterile gloved fingers, forceps, or an applicator, pack the gauze into all depressions and grooves of the wound (Figure 30-11 ◆). Cover all exposed surfaces. *Necrotic material is usually more prevalent in depressed wound areas and needs to be covered with gauze.*
   - Do not pack too tightly. *Too tight application inhibits wound edges from contracting and compresses capillaries.*

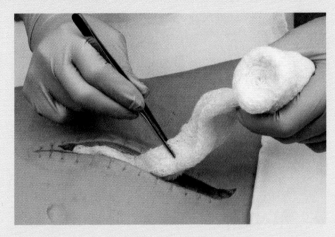

FIGURE 30-11 ◆ Packing a wound with roller gauze.

   - Pack only to the edge of the wound. *Overlapping the skin with moist gauze can cause maceration.*

7. Dress the wound.
   - If indicated, protect the surrounding skin with skin sealant or hydrocolloid dressing.
   - Apply 4″ × 4″ gauze or other absorbent dressings to protect the wound and take up excess drainage.

8. **Document** the dressing change and the client's response in the client record using forms or checklists supplemented by narrative notes when appropriate. Many agencies use a designated wound/skin documentation sheet (Figure 30-2).

EVALUATION

- Perform follow-up based on findings that deviate from expected or normal for the client. Relate findings to previous assessment data if available.
- Report significant deviations from normal to the physician.

Using Alginates

Alginate dressings (Kaltostat, Seasorb) are made from a type of seaweed and are capable of absorbing up to 20 times their weight in fluid. They come in both rope and sheet forms that conform to the wound shape and become gel-like when activated. They can be used in both clean and infected draining wounds.

Nursing Process: Using Alginates

ASSESSMENT

Review the client's record to determine:

- Previous appearance, size, and treatment of the wound
- Character of exudate
- Presence of pain and the time of the last pain medication
- Clinical signs of systemic infection
- Allergies to the alginate or tape

PLANNING

If possible, schedule the dressing change at a time convenient for the client. Some packings require only a few minutes, and others can take much longer.

Delegation

Due to the need for aseptic technique and assessment skills, alginate dressing changes are not delegated to UAP. However, UAP may observe the dressing during usual care and must report abnormal findings to the nurse. Abnormal findings must be validated and interpreted by the nurse.

IMPLEMENTATION:

TECHNIQUE 30-7 USING ALGINATES ON WOUNDS

Equipment

- Alginate dressing
- Sterile dressing equipment and secondary dressing materials
- Solution for irrigation (e.g., sterile saline or water)
- Irrigating syringe
- Bowl
- Basin to collect irrigation
- Forceps or cotton-tipped applicators (optional)
- Moistureproof bag
- Clean gloves
- Sterile gloves

Performance

1. Explain to the client what you are going to do, why it is necessary, and how he or she can cooperate. Discuss how the results will be used in planning further care or treatments.

2. Wash hands and observe appropriate infection control procedures.

Provide for Client Privacy

3. Prepare the client. Assist the client to a comfortable position in which the wound can be readily exposed. Expose only the wound area, using a bath blanket to cover the client, if necessary. *Undue exposure is physically and psychologically distressing to most people.*

4. Prepare the supplies.
   - Open the sterile dressing set and supplies.

   - Pour the ordered solution into the solution container.
   - Position the basin below the wound to receive the irrigating fluid.

5. Remove the existing dressing and clean the wound.
   - Apply clean gloves, remove and discard the outer secondary dressing in the moistureproof bag.
   - If the previous alginate dressing has absorbed drainage, it will be in gel form. Irrigate the wound with the prescribed solution until all of the dressing has been removed.
   - If the dressing does not appear in gel form or does not remove easily with irrigation, either the secondary dressing is not maintaining a moist environment or the wound is no longer producing enough exudate to warrant alginate dressing.

6. Pack the wound with the alginate.
   - Apply sterile gloves.
   - Pack the alginate into all depressions and grooves of the wound. Cover all exposed surfaces.

7. Dress the wound.
   - Cover the alginate with petrolatum gauze, foam, or other secondary dressing that will keep with alginate in place and provide a moist wound environment.

8. **Document** the dressing change and the client's response in the client record using forms or checklists supplemented by narrative notes when appropriate. Many agencies use a designated wound/skin documentation sheet (Figure 30-2).

AMBULATORY AND COMMUNITY SETTINGS

Wound Care

- Perform appropriate client teaching for promoting wound healing and maintenance of healthy skin.

Maintaining Intact Skin

- Discuss relationship between adequate nutrition (especially fluids, protein, vitamins B and C, iron, and calories) and healthy skin.
- Demonstrate appropriate positions for pressure relief.

- Establish a turning or repositioning schedule.
- Demonstrate application of appropriate skin protection agents and devices.
- Instruct to report persistent reddened areas.
- Identify potential sources of skin trauma and means of avoidance.

Promoting Wound Healing

- Discuss importance of adequate nutrition (especially fluids, protein, vitamins B and C, iron, and calories).

Wound Care (*continued*)

- Instruct in wound assessment and provide mechanism for documenting.
- Emphasize principles of asepsis, especially handwashing and proper methods of handling used dressings.
- Provide information about signs of wound infection and other complications to report.
- Reinforce appropriate aspects of pressure ulcer prevention.
- Demonstrate wound care techniques such as wound cleansing, dressing change.

- Discuss pain control measures, if needed.
- Instruct the client and family where to obtain needed supplies. Be sensitive to the cost of dressings (e.g., transparent barriers are costly) and suggest less expensive alternatives if necessary. Be creative in the use of household items for padding pressure areas.
- Instruct the client and family in proper disposal of contaminated dressings. All contaminated items should be double-bagged in moistureproof bags.
- Verify how the client may bathe with the wound (i.e., does the wound need to be covered with a waterproof barrier or should it be cleansed in the shower?).

AGE-RELATED CONSIDERATIONS

Wound Care

Child

- Remind the child not to touch the wound, drains, or dressing. Cover with an appropriate bandage that will remain intact during the child's usual activities. Cover a transparent dressing with opaque material if viewing the site is distressing to the child. Restrain only when all alternatives have been tried and absolutely necessary.
- Demonstrate wound care on a doll. Reassure the child that the wound will not be permanent and does not mean anything will fall out of their body.

Elders

- Hold wrinkled skin taut during application of a transparent dressing. Obtain assistance if needed.
- Skin is more fragile and can easily tear with removal of tape (especially adhesive tape). Use paper tape and tape remover as indicated, keeping tape use to the minimum required. Use extreme caution during tape removal.
- Elders who are immobilized are at increased risk for skin breakdown and pressure ulcers.
- Wound healing may be slower in elders than in younger clients.

EVALUATION

- Perform follow-up based on findings that deviate from expected or normal for the client. Relate findings to previous assessment data if available.
- Report significant deviations from normal to the physician.

Bandages and Binders

A **bandage** is a strip of cloth used to wrap some part of the body. Bandages are available in various widths, most commonly 1.5 to 7.5 cm (0.5 to 3 in), and are usually supplied in rolls for easy application to a body part.

Many types of materials are used for bandages. Gauze is one of the most commonly used; it is light and porous and readily molds to the body. It is also relatively inexpensive, so it is generally discarded when soiled. Gauze is frequently used to retain dressings on wounds and to

bandage the fingers, hands, toes, and feet. It supports dressings and at the same time permits air to circulate; it can also be impregnated with petroleum jelly or other medications for application to wounds.

Many kinds of elasticized bandages are applied to provide pressure to an area. They are commonly used to provide support and improve the venous circulation in the legs.

Before applying a bandage, the nurse needs to know its purpose and to assess the area requiring support. General guidelines for bandaging are in Box 30-2.

Applying bandages to various parts of the body involves one or more of five basic bandaging turns: circular, spiral, spiral reverse, recurrent, and figure eight. *Circular* turns are used to anchor bandages and to terminate them. Circular turns usually are not applied directly over a wound because of the discomfort the bandage would cause.

Spiral turns are used to bandage parts of the body that are fairly uniform in circumference (e.g., the upper arm or upper leg). *Spiral reverse* turns are used to

Box 30-2 *Guidelines for Bandaging*

• Whenever possible, bandage the part in its normal position, with the joint slightly flexed to avoid putting strain on the ligaments and the muscles of the joint.

• Pad between skin surfaces and over bony prominences to prevent friction from the bandage and consequent abrasion of the skin.

• Always bandage body parts by working from the distal to the proximal end to aid the return flow of venous blood.

• Bandage with even pressure to prevent interference with blood circulation.

• Whenever possible, leave the end of the body part (e.g., the toe) exposed so that you will be able to determine the adequacy of the blood circulation to the extremity.

• Cover dressings with bandages at least 5 cm (2 in) beyond the edges of the dressing to prevent the dressing and wound from becoming contaminated.

• Face the client when applying a bandage to maintain uniform tension and the appropriate direction of the bandage.

bandage cylindrical parts of the body that are not uniform in circumference (e.g., the lower leg or forearm). *Recurrent* turns are used to cover distal parts of the body (e.g., the end of a finger, the skull, or the stump of an amputation). *Figure-eight* turns are used to bandage an elbow, knee, or ankle, because they permit some movement after application.

A **binder** bandage is designed for a specific body part; for example, the triangular binder **(sling)** fits the arm. Binders are used to support large areas of the body, such as the abdomen, arm, or chest. Most binders are made of muslin (plain-woven cotton fabric), flannel, or synthetic material that may or may not be elasticized. Some abdominal binders are made of an elasticized netlike material that fits the body contours and allows air to circulate around the body part.

• *Triangular arm binder (sling):* Usually applied as a full triangle to support the arm, elbow, and forearm of the client or to reduce or prevent swelling of a hand.

• *T-binder (single or double T):* To retain pads, dressings, or packs in the perineal area. Single T-binders

are often used for females, and double T-binders for males to prevent undue pressure on the penis. The double T-binder can also provide greater support for large dressings on both males and females.

• *Straight abdominal binder:* To provide support to the abdomen. This binder is a rectangular piece of material long enough to encircle the client's abdomen with some overlap. It can be made from any material (e.g., a towel).

Nursing Process: Bandages and Binders

ASSESSMENT

Assess the area to be bandaged or to which a binder is to be applied for:

• Swelling

• Presence of and status of wounds (open wounds will require a dressing before a bandage or binder is applied)

• Presence of drainage (amount, color, odor, and viscosity)

• Adequacy of circulation (skin temperature, color, and sensation). Pale or cyanotic skin, cool temperature, tingling, and numbness can indicate impaired circulation.

• Presence of pain (location, intensity, onset, and quality)

Determine:

• The client's ability to reapply the bandage or binder when needed

• The client's ability to carry out activities of daily living (e.g., eat, dress, write, comb hair, bathe, and drive).

PLANNING

If possible, schedule the bandaging at a time convenient for the client. Some bandages or bindings require only a few minutes to apply, and others can take much longer.

Delegation

Application of binders can be delegated to UAP or family members/caregivers after the nurse has performed initial assessment that the UAP can perform this skill safely. Application of bandages over wounds is not delegated to UAP but may be taught to clients or family members/caregivers for home care purposes.

IMPLEMENTATION:
TECHNIQUE 30-8 APPLYING BANDAGES AND BINDERS

Equipment

• Clean bandage or binder of the appropriate material and width

• Padding, such as abdominal (ABD) pads or gauze squares

- Tape or safety pins
- Clean gloves, if an open wound is present

Performance

1. Explain to the client what you are going to do, why it is necessary, and how he or she can cooperate. Discuss how the results will be used in planning further care or treatments.

2. Wash hands and observe appropriate infection control procedures.

3. Provide for client privacy.

4. Position and prepare the client appropriately.

   - Provide the client with a chair or bed, and arrange support for the area to be bandaged. For example, if a hand needs to be bandaged, ask the client to place the elbow on a table, so that the hand does not have to be held up unsupported. *Because bandaging takes a little time, holding up a body part without support can fatigue the client.*

   - Make sure that the area to be bandaged is clean and dry. Wash and dry the area if necessary. *Washing and drying remove microorganisms, which flourish in dark, warm, moist areas.*

   - Align the part to be bandaged with slight flexion of the joints, unless this is contraindicated. *Slight flexion places less strain on the ligaments and muscles of the joint.*

5. Apply the bandage.

Circular Turns

   - Hold the bandage in your dominant hand, keeping the roll uppermost, and unroll the bandage about 8 cm (3 in). This length of unrolled bandage allows good control for placement and tension.

- Apply the end of the bandage to the part of the body to be bandaged. Hold the end down with the thumb of the other hand (Figure 30-12 ◆).

- Encircle the body part a few times or as often as needed, making sure that each layer overlaps one-half to two-thirds of the previous layer. This provides even support to the area.

- The bandage should be firm, but not too tight. Ask the client if the bandage feels comfortable. A tight bandage can interfere with blood circulation, while a loose bandage does not provide adequate protection.

- Secure the end of the bandage with tape or a safety pin over an uninjured area. Pins can cause discomfort when situated over an injured area.

Spiral Turns

- Make two circular turns. *Two circular turns anchor the bandage.*

- Continue spiral turns at about a 30-degree angle, each turn overlapping the preceding one by two-thirds the width of the bandage (Figure 30-13 ◆).

- Terminate the bandage with two circular turns, and secure the end as described for circular turns.

Spiral Reverse Turns

- Anchor the bandage with two circular turns, and

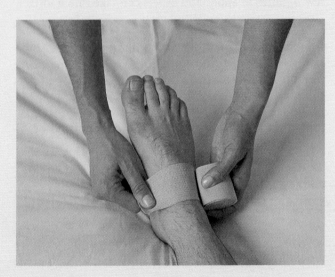

FIGURE 30-12 ◆ Starting a bandage with circular turns.

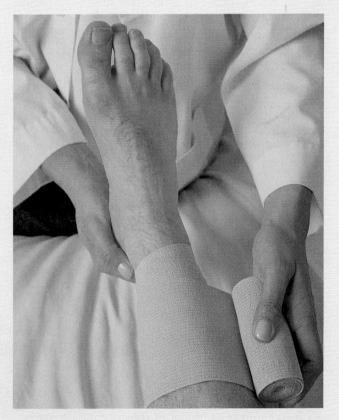

FIGURE 30-13 ◆ Applying spiral turns.

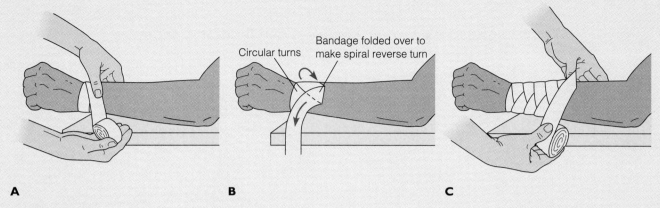

A **B** **C**

FIGURE 30-14 ◆ Applying spiral reverse turns.

bring the bandage upward at about a 30-degree angle.

- Place the thumb of your free hand on the upper edge of the bandage (Figure 30-14 ◆A). *The thumb will hold the bandage while it is folded on itself.*
- Unroll the bandage about 15 cm (6 in), and then turn your hand so that the bandage falls over itself (Figure 30-14B).
- Continue the bandage around the limb, overlapping each previous turn by two-thirds the width of the bandage. Make each bandage turn at the same position on the limb so that the turns of the bandage will be aligned (Figure 30-14C).
- Terminate the bandage with two circular turns, and secure the end as described for circular turns.

Recurrent Turns

- Anchor the bandage with two circular turns.
- Fold the bandage back on itself, and bring it centrally over the distal end to be bandaged (Figure 30-15 ◆).
- Holding it with the other hand, bring the bandage back over the end to the right of the center bandage but overlapping it by two-thirds the width of the bandage.

- Bring the bandage back on the left side, also overlapping the first turn by two-thirds the width of the bandage.
- Continue this pattern of alternating right and left until the area is covered. Overlap the preceding turn by two-thirds the bandage width each time.
- Terminate the bandage with two circular turns (Figure 30-16 ◆). Secure the end appropriately.

Figure-Eight Turns

- Anchor the bandage with two circular turns.
- Carry the bandage above the joint, around it, and then below it, making a figure eight (Figure 30-17 ◆).
- Continue above and below the joint, overlapping the previous turn by two-thirds the width of the bandage.
- Terminate the bandage above the joint with two circular turns, and then secure the end appropriately.

Triangular Arm Sling

- Ask the client to flex the elbow to an 80-degree angle or less, depending on the purpose. The thumb should be facing upward or inward toward the body. *An 80-degree angle is sufficient to support the forearm, to prevent swelling of the hand, and to relieve pressure on the shoulder joint (e.g., to*

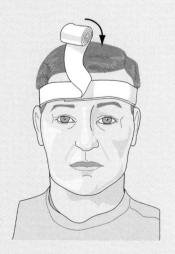

FIGURE 30-15 ◆ Starting recurrent bandage.

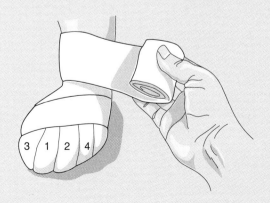

FIGURE 30-16 ◆ Completing a recurrent bandage.

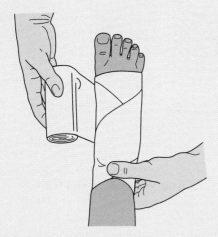

FIGURE 30-17 ◆ Applying a figure-eight bandage.

support the paralyzed arm of a stroke client whose shoulder might otherwise become dislocated). A more acute angle is preferred if there is swelling of the hand (see how to apply a sling for maximum hand elevation, below).

- Place one end of the unfolded triangular binder over the shoulder of the uninjured side so that the binder falls down the front of the chest of the client with the point of the triangle (apex) under the elbow of the injured side.
- Take the upper corner, and carry it around the neck until it hangs over the shoulder on the injured side.
- Bring the lower corner of the binder up over the arm to the shoulder of the injured side. Using a square knot, secure this corner to the upper corner at the side of the neck on the injured side (Figure 30-18A ◆). *A square knot will not slip. Tying the knot at the side of the neck prevents pressure on the bony prominences of the vertebral column at the back of the neck.*

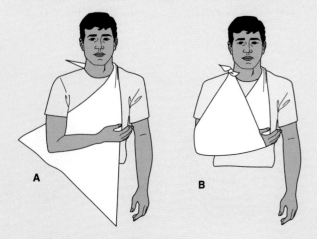

FIGURE 30-18 ◆ Large arm sling.

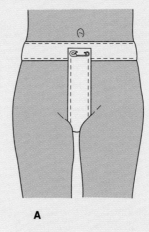

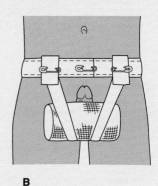

FIGURE 30-19 ◆ T-Binders: (A) single tail; (B) two tails.

- Make sure the wrist is supported, *to maintain alignment.*
- Fold the sling neatly at the elbow, and secure it with safety pins or tape. It may be folded and fastened at the front (Figure 30-18B).
- Remove the sling periodically to inspect the skin for indications of irritation, especially around the site of the knot.

T-Binder

- Select the appropriate binder for the client, and place it smoothly under the person with the waistband at waist level.
- Bring the waist tails around the client, overlap them, and secure them with a pin placed horizontally. *The pins placed horizontally allow comfort when bending at the waist and moving.*
- Bring the center tail up between the legs (Figure 30-19A ◆). The two tails of the double T-binder are brought up on either side of the penis (Figure 30-19B). When dressings are in place, take care to touch only the outside of the dressings to prevent contamination of the wound or yourself.

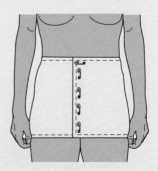

FIGURE 30-20 ◆ A straight abdominal binder.

- Fasten the ties at the waist with a safety pin placed horizontally.

Straight Abdominal Binder

- With the client in a supine position, place the binder smoothly under the body, with the upper border of the binder at the waist and the lower border at the level of the gluteal fold. *A binder placed over the waist interferes with respiration; one placed too low interferes with elimination and walking.*

- Apply padding over the iliac crests if the client is thin.

- Bring the ends around the client, overlap them, and secure them with pins or Velcro (Figure 30-20 ◆). Place the top pin horizontally at the waist to allow for comfort when moving.

6. **Document** the application of the bandage or binder and the client's response in the client record using forms or checklists supplemented by narrative notes when appropriate.

AMBULATORY AND COMMUNITY SETTINGS

Applying Bandages and Binders

- Assess the client or caregiver's ability and willingness to perform the bandaging procedure.

- Ensure that the client has the proper supplies and knows how to obtain replacement supplies.

- The client should have two binders so that there is one to wear while the other is being washed. Bandages and binders should be washed inside a mesh laundry bag to keep them from becoming twisted and to prevent Velcro or hooks from catching on other laundry.

- Instruct the client's caregiver to:
  a. Wash hands thoroughly before handling dressing supplies and applying the bandage.
  b. Report skin breakdown, redness, pain, or pallor of the affected area.
  c. Check for adequate peripheral circulation after applying the bandage.

AGE-RELATED CONSIDERATIONS

Applying Bandages and Binders
Child

- Allow the child to help with the procedure by holding supplies, opening boxes, counting turns, and so on.

- If a young client is apprehensive, demonstrate the procedure on a doll or stuffed animal.

- Encourage the child to decorate his bandage.

- Teach the caregivers to apply bandages and binders safely.

Elders

- Older clients may need extra support during the procedure, especially if arthritis, contractures, or tremors are present.

- Avoid constricting the client's circulation with a tight bandage or binder. Observe skin and bony prominences frequently for signs of impaired circulation. The risk for skin breakdown increases with age.

EVALUATION

- Perform follow-up based on findings that deviate from expected or normal for the client. Relate findings to previous assessment data if available.

- Report significant deviations from normal to the physician.

Chapter Summary

TERMINOLOGY

alginate	eschar	wet-to-damp dressing
bandage	hydrocolloid	wet-to-dry dressing
binder	pressure ulcer	wound
debridement	sling	
dressing	transparent wound barrier	

FORMING CLINICAL JUDGMENTS

Consider This:

1. Your client has several different wounds of varying shapes and sizes. How would you document these in the client record?

2. You are in the client's home to change a dressing over a healing surgical wound that has significant drainage. How would you dispose of the soiled dressings?

3. What would be one appropriate use of a transparent semipermeable membrane dressing? Why?

4. Many practitioners apply paper tape around the four edges of a hydrocolloid dressing. Why would they do this?

5. You observe a colleague irrigating a wound using a 30-mL syringe with an 18-gauge needle attached. Why would this be correct or incorrect technique?

6. In preparing to perform a wet-to-damp dressing, the client record reveals that the dressings have been changed every 12 hours and that the client experiences significant pain during removal of the previous dressing. How would you proceed?

7. The client has a stage 3 pressure ulcer over the right trochanter. A recent journal article suggests you dress this with alginate. Assuming the physician agrees, do you believe this would make an appropriate dressing? Why or why not?

8. What are four assessments that should be made for a client with a bandage or binder?

RELATED RESEARCH

Campbell, K., Woodbury, M. G., Whittle, H., Labate, T., & Hoskin, A. (2000). A clinical evaluation of 3M No Sting Barrier Film. *Ostomy Wound Management, 46*(1), 24–26, 28–30.

Walsh, J. (1999). The four-layer bandage system from a nursing perspective. *British Journal of Nursing, 8,* 381–382, 384–386.

REFERENCES

Benbow, M. (1999). The challenge of managing heavily exuding wounds. *Community Nurse, 5*(9), 47–48, 50.

Casey, G. (2000). Three steps to effective wound care. *Nursing Standard, 14*(40), 58, 61.

Foster, L., & Moore, P. (1999). Acute surgical wound care 3: Fitting the dressing to the wound. *British Journal of Nursing, 8,* 200, 202, 204, 206–209.

Fowler, E. (1998). Wound infection: A nurse's perspective. *Ostomy Wound Management, 44*(8), 44–52.

Hampton, S. (1999). Dressing for the occasion. *Nursing Times, 95*(47), 58, 60.

Hess, C. T. (1998). Keeping tabs on a pressure ulcer. *Nursing, 28*(1), 18.

Hess, C. T. (2000). Wound care. When to use alginate dressings. *Nursing 30*(2), 26.

Hess, C. T. (2000). Wound care. When to use composite dressings. *Nursing 30*(5), 26.

Krasner, D. L., & Sibbal, R. G. (1999). Nursing management of chronic wounds: Best practices across the continuum of care. *Nursing Clinics of North America, 34,* 933–953.

Nesselroth, S. M., & Gahtan, V. (2000). Management of pressure ulcers in the home care setting. *Home Health Care Consultant, 7*(4), 34–42.

Pompeo, M., & Baxter, C. (2000). Sacral and ischial pressure ulcers: Evaluation, treatment, and differentiation. *Ostomy Wound Management, 46*(1), 18–20, 22–23.

Pontieri-Lewis, V. (1999). Focus on wound care. Principles for selecting the right wound dressing. *MEDSURG Nursing, 8,* 267–270.

Rolstad, B. S. (1997). Wound dressings: Making the right match. *Nursing, 27*(6), 32-1–32-3.

Russell, L. (2000). Understanding physiology of wound healing and how dressings help. *British Journal of Nursing, 9,* 10, 12, 14, 16.

Thompson, J. (2000). A practical guide to wound care. *RN, 63*(1), 48–53.

Waldrop, J. D. (2000). Principles of wound management and topical therapies. *Home Health Care Consultant, 7*(4), 29–33.

Chapter 31

Cast Care

Techniques

OBJECTIVES

- Describe ways a plaster cast is supported, elevated, and handled before it is dry.
- Differentiate care of plaster and synthetic casts.
- List actions required for detecting and preventing neurovascular impairments and skin irritation due to casts.
- Outline interventions required to keep a cast clean and dry.
- Identify essential considerations for positioning clients with casts.
- Discuss appropriate teaching for clients with casts.

Casts

Casts are generally applied to immobilize a body part so that healing can take place without further injury. The degree of immobilization of the person varies with the type of cast. Some people are confined to bed for weeks or even months, whereas others are able to resume most daily activities with only slight inconvenience from the cast. Although casts are applied for reasons other than fractures, this chapter focuses on clients who have fractures.

Cast Materials

In addition to the traditional **plaster of paris** cast material, several synthetic materials are now available: polyester and cotton, fiberglass, fiberglass-free/latex-free, and thermoplastics. See Table 31-1. These materials come in a roll of casting tape that is soaked in water to begin activation and soften it and then molded around the affected body part.

Padding Materials

Before the cast is applied, the affected area must be padded. **Stockinette**, a soft, flexible, tubular, cloth material, is placed over the body part before the cast material is applied. The distal end of the stockinette is

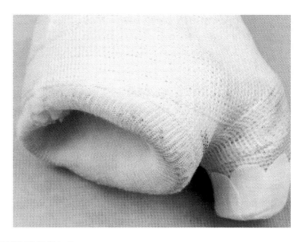

FIGURE 31-1 ◆ Stockinette folded back over the cast to form a smooth edge.

folded back over the edge of the cast material to provide a smooth border (Figure 31-1 ◆). *Cotton sheet wadding* or padding is often applied directly over stockinette to pad bony prominences or between skin surfaces. Sheet wadding clings and molds to the contours of the limb. *Felt padding* may be needed over bony prominences or joints that are vulnerable to skin breakdown. If the synthetic cast will be placed in water for bathing, polypropylene stockinette and polyester padding must be used because they dry eas-

TABLE 31-1	CAST MATERIALS		
Type of Material	**Description**	**Application**	**Setting Time and Weight-Bearing Restrictions**
Plaster of paris	Open-weave cotton rolls or strips saturated with powdered calcium sulfate crystals (gypsum)	Applied after being soaked in tepid water for a few seconds until bubbling stops	Dries in 48 hours, no weight bearing allowed until dry
Synthetics Polyester and cotton (e.g., Cutter Cast)	Open-weave polyester and cotton tape permeated with water-activated polyurethane resin	Applied after being soaked in cool water, 26°C (80°F); used within 2 to 3 minutes of soaking	Sets in 7 minutes, weight bearing allowed in 15 minutes
Fiberglass; water-activated (e.g., Scotchcast, Delta-lite) or light-cured (e.g., Lightcast II); Fiberglass-free/Latex-free (e.g., Delta-cast, Flashcast)	Open-weave fiberglass tape impregnated with water-activated polyurethane resin (Scotchcast) or photosensitive polyurethane resin (Lightcast II)	Applied after being immersed in tepid water for 10 to 15 seconds (Scotchcast); applied with silicone type hand cream to keep it from sticking (Lightcast II)	Sets in 15 minutes, weight bearing allowed in 30 minutes (Scotchcast); sets after being exposed for 3 minutes to a special ultraviolet lamp, weight bearing allowed immediately (Lightcast II)
Thermoplastic (e.g., Hexcelite)	Knitted thermoplastic polyester fabric in rigid rolls	Applied after being heated in water at 76 to 82°C (170 to 180°F) for 3 to 4 minutes to make the rolls soft and pliable. Remove excess water by squeezing between towels before applying	Sets in 5 minutes, weight bearing allowed in 20 minutes

ily. Waterproof linings have been used in some cases in which contact with urine may occur.

Types of Casts

The *long arm cast* (Figure 31-2A ◆) extends from the axilla to the fingers of the hand, allowing for elbow flexion. It immobilizes the wrist, the radius, the ulna, and the humerus. The *short arm cast* (Figure 31-2B) extends from below the elbow to the fingers. It immobilizes the wrist, the radius, and the ulna. The *shoulder*

spica cast (Figure 31-2C) extends around the chest and the entire arm to the fingers. The arm is usually abducted to immobilize the shoulder bones (e.g., the clavicle).

The *long,* or *full, leg cast* (Figure 31-2D) extends from above the knee to the toes. The *short leg cast* (Figure 31-2E) begins just below the knee and extends to the toes. The *hip spica cast* (Figure 31-2F) begins at waist level or above. It immobilizes the hip joint and the femur, extends down one entire leg, and may cover all or part of the second leg. A single spica covers one leg

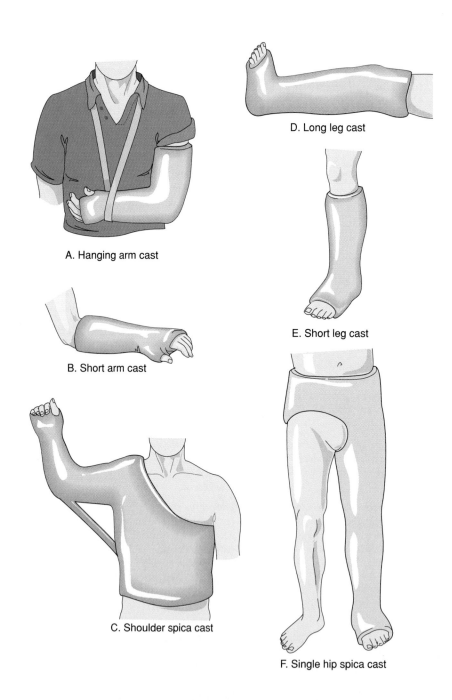

A. Hanging arm cast

B. Short arm cast

C. Shoulder spica cast

D. Long leg cast

E. Short leg cast

F. Single hip spica cast

FIGURE 31-2 ◆ Types of casts: (A) long arm cast; (B) short arm cast; (C) shoulder spica cast; (D) long, or full, leg cast; (E) short leg cast; (F) single hip spica cast.

only. A double hip spica covers both legs to the toes. The *body cast* extends from the axillae to encompass the entire trunk. It is often used to immobilize the spine.

Care for Clients with Casts

Essential nursing for clients who have casts includes continual assessment and intervention to prevent pressure on underlying blood vessels, nerves, and the skin; to maintain the integrity of the cast itself; and to prevent problems associated with immobility. Common cast pressure areas are shown in Table 31-2. A finger width should fit between the cast and the client's skin.

Because a plaster cast is porous and will absorb water or urine, every effort is made to keep the cast dry. Casts that become wet soften, and their function is impaired; thus, tub baths and showers are contraindicated. Casts that become soiled with feces develop an irremovable odor. Elimination presents a particular problem for people with long leg, body, and hip spica casts. There is no effective way to keep a plaster cast clean other than wiping it with a damp cloth. The best approach is to prevent soils and stains, especially those from food spills, urine, and feces.

Synthetic casts can be cleaned readily and may, with the physician's agreement, be immersed in water if polypropylene stockinette and padding were applied.

Nursing Process: Care for Clients with Casts

ASSESSMENT

- Assess vital signs to establish the client's status both before and after cast application.
- Examine all extremities for edema, peripheral pulses, pain, and other signs of injury.
- Determine if the client has underlying diseases or conditions that would predispose to poor wound healing or create additional risks for complications from casts (e.g., diabetes, immune disorders,

TABLE 31-2	COMMON CAST PRESSURE AREAS
Type of Cast	**Common Pressure Areas**
Short arm cast	Radial styloid
	Ulnar styloid
	Joint at base of thumb
Hanging arm cast	Radial styloid
	Ulnar styloid
	Olecranon
	Lateral epicondyle
Short leg cast	Heel
	Achilles tendon
	Malleolus
Long leg cast	Heel
	Achilles tendon
	Malleolus
	Popliteal artery behind knee
	Peroneal nerve at side of knee
Hip spica	As above for long leg cast
	Sacrum
	Iliac crests

impaired mental status, diabetes, or peripheral vascular disease).

PLANNING

Delegation

The nurse should perform baseline assessment of all new casts. Care of clients with stable casts may be delegated to unlicensed assistive personnel (UAP). The status of the cast is observed during usual care and may be recorded by persons other than the nurse. However, assessment of complications from the cast requires the expertise of a nurse. Abnormal findings detected by UAP must be validated and interpreted by the nurse.

IMPLEMENTATION:
TECHNIQUE 31-1 INITIAL CAST CARE

Equipment

- Pillows to support the casted areas

Preparation

Review the client record to determine the reason for the cast and the initial status of the client's extremity. Examine the record regarding pain assessment findings and interventions.

Performance

1. Explain to the client what you are going to do, why it is necessary, and how he or she can cooper-

ate. Discuss how the results will be used in planning further care or treatments.

2. Wash your hands and observe appropriate infection control procedures.

3. Provide for client privacy as indicated.

4. Assess the neurovascular status of the affected limbs.

• Assess the toes or fingers for nerve and circulatory impairments every 30 minutes for 4 hours following cast application, and then every 3 hours for the first 24 to 48 hours or until all signs and symptoms of impairment are negative. *Rapid swelling under a cast can cause neurovascular problems, necessitating frequent neurovascular assessments by the nurse.* Increase the frequency of neurovascular assessments in accordance with the client's condition (e.g., presence of circulatory impairment).

5. Support and handle the cast appropriately.

• Immediately after the cast is applied, place it on pillows. Avoid using plastic or rubber pillows. *The pillows provide even pressure and support the curves of the cast and promote venous blood return, thereby decreasing the possibility of swelling. Plastic or rubber pillows do not allow the heat of a drying cast to dissipate and so cause discomfort.*

• Until a cast has set or hardened (10 to 20 minutes), support the cast in the palms of your hands rather than with the fingertips, and extend your fingers so that your fingertips do not touch the plaster. *Fingertip pressure can cause dents in unset plaster and subsequent skin pressure areas.*

• When the cast is set, continue to handle the cast in your palms, but you may then wrap your fingers around the contour of the cast.

6. Implement measures to reduce swelling.

• Control swelling by elevating arms or legs on pillows or, for a leg fracture, by elevating the foot of the bed. Immediately after injury and surgery, elevate the limb above the level of the client's heart. Generally, three pillows are needed to achieve high elevation of a leg. As circulation improves and healing progresses, the elevation can be gradually reduced to two pillows (moderate elevation) and then to one pillow (low elevation). *Swelling can cause neurovascular impairment.*

• Apply ice packs to control perineal edema associated with a hip spica cast. Although ice packs are a less effective method of control, elevation of the area is obviously difficult.

• Report excessive swelling and indications of neurovascular impairment to the physician or nurse in charge. The physician may **bivalve** a cast if it appears to be too tight. Bivalving a cast is cutting

the cast partially or completely (Figure 31-3 ◆). *This relieves the pressure of the cast but still provides support.*

7. Use appropriate means to dry the plaster cast thoroughly.

• Extremity plaster casts usually take 24 to 48 hours to dry completely; spica or body casts require 48 to 72 hours. Drying time depends on the temperature, humidity, size of the cast, and method used for drying. The cast is dry when it no longer feels damp. A dry cast feels dry, looks white and shiny, and is odorless, hard, and resonant when tapped. Synthetic casts take only 10 to 15 minutes to harden completely.

• Expose the cast to the circulating air. Place sheets and blankets only over areas that do not have the cast.

• Check agency policy about the recommended turning frequency for clients with different kinds of casts. *Frequent turning promotes even drying of the cast.*

• Turn the client with an extremity cast or body spica every 2 to 4 hours.

• Use regular pillows. *Plastic or rubber pillows hinder drying and do not allow the heat of a drying cast to dissipate.*

• Avoid the use of artificial means to facilitate drying. These means include fans, hair dryers, infrared lamps, and electric heaters. *Artificial methods dry the outer surface of the cast while the inner portion remains soft and spongy. Such a cast cracks readily at points of strain. Natural methods dry the cast evenly.*

8. Monitor bleeding if an open reduction was done or if the injury was a compound fracture.

• Monitor bloodstains or other drainage on the cast for 24 to 72 hours after surgery or injury or longer if necessary.

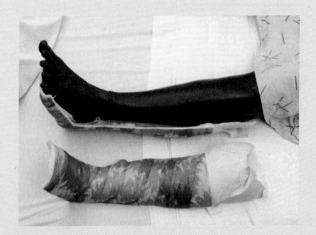

FIGURE 31-3 ◆ Bivalved cast.

- Outline the stained area with a pen at least every 8 hours if it is changing, and note the time and date, so that any further bleeding can be determined.

9. Assess pain and pressure areas.

- Never ignore any complaints of pain, burning, or pressure. If a client is unable to communicate, be alert to changes in temperament, restlessness, or fussiness.

- Determine particularly whether the pain is persistent and if it occurs over a bony prominence or joint. See Table 31-2 for common pressure points associated with various casts.

- Do not disregard the cessation of persistent pain or discomfort complaints. *Cessation of complaints can indicate a skin slough. When a skin slough occurs, superficial skin sensation is lost and the client no longer feels pain.*

- When a pressure area under the cast is suspected, the physician may either bivalve the cast so that all of the skin beneath the cast can be inspected or cut a **window** in the cast over only the area of concern. When a cast is windowed:

a. Retain the piece (cast and padding) that was cut out. Some physicians order that it be taped back if there is no skin problem present but that it be left out if there is a pressure area present. *Putting back the piece prevents window edema, which occurs when skin pressure at the window is not equal to that from the remainder of the cast.*

b. Inspect the skin under the window at scheduled time intervals.

10. **Document** findings in the client record using forms or checklists supplemented by narrative notes when appropriate. Record each assessment (whether or not there are problems). Examples of documentation include: "Toes warm to touch, color pink," "Blanching satisfactory," "Moves toes readily; states no numbness or tingling; states leg painful." Record specific nerve function assessments such as "Able to hyperextend R thumb," "Sensation felt at web space between R thumb and index finger."

AMBULATORY AND COMMUNITY SETTINGS

Cast Care

- For itching, suggest that the client use a hair dryer on cool, a vacuum cleaner on reverse, or an ice bag over the outside of the itching area. *These are safer ways to resolve itching and less irritating to the skin than inserting an object into the cast.*

- Before discharge from the hospital, instruct the client to:

a. Observe for indications of nerve or circulatory impairment, such as extreme coldness or blueness of toes or fingers; extreme continuous swelling of casted toes or fingers; numbness or tingling ("pins and needles" sensation) in casted toes or fingers; continuous complaints of pain; or inability to move the toes or fingers.

b. Keep the plaster cast dry.

c. Avoid strenuous activity and follow medical advice about exercises.

d. Elevate the arm or leg frequently to prevent dependent edema.

e. Move the toes or fingers frequently.

f. Observe the skin around the cast edges frequently, and keep it clean and dry.

g. Report any increase in pain; unexplained fever; foul odor from within the cast; decreased circulation; numbness; inability to move the fingers or toes; or a weakened, cracked, loose, or tight cast.

- Review modifications that may be necessary in clothing, toileting, sleeping, and other activities of daily living.

AGE-RELATED CONSIDERATIONS

Cast Care

Child

- Teach parents of young children ways to prevent the child from placing small items under the cast. Parents also need to ensure that the top of a body cast is covered during meals so that food does not fall inside the cast.

- If possible, allow the child to choose the color of the synthetic cast.

- Reassure the child that the saw used for windowing, bivalving, and removing the cast is not painful. Have an adult present to support the child during these procedures. Let the child keep the cast pieces when removed.

Elders

- Elders who are immobilized are at increased risk for skin breakdown and decubitus ulcers.

- Wound healing may be slower in elders than in younger clients.

- Elders may be less able to manage the additional weight and imbalance caused by the cast. Take appropriate steps in planning for use of crutches or other mobility aids.

- Perform detailed follow-up based on findings that deviated from expected or normal for the client. Relate findings to previous assessment data if available.
- Report significant deviations from normal to the physician.

Nursing Process: Ongoing Cast Care

ASSESSMENT

- Perform a general head-to-toe assessment of the client.
- Determine if the client has underlying diseases or conditions that would predispose to poor wound healing or create additional risks for complications from casts (e.g., diabetes, immune disorders, impaired mental status, or peripheral vascular disease).

PLANNING

Delegation

Care of clients with stable casts may be delegated to UAP. The status of the cast is observed during usual care and may be recorded by persons other than the nurse. However, assessment of complications from the cast requires the expertise of a nurse. Abnormal findings detected by UAP must be validated and interpreted by the nurse.

IMPLEMENTATION:
TECHNIQUE 31-2 ONGOING CAST CARE

Equipment

- Pillows to support the casted areas.

Preparation

Review the client record to determine previous status of the cast and the client's extremities. Examine the record regarding pain assessment findings and interventions.

Performance

1. Explain to the client what you are going to do, why it is necessary, and how he or she can cooperate. Discuss how the results will be used in planning further care or treatments.

2. Wash your hands and observe appropriate infection control procedures.

3. Provide for client privacy as indicated.

4. Continue to assess the client for problems.
   - Assess the neurovascular status of the affected limb at regular intervals in accordance with agency protocol.
   - Inspect the skin near and under the cast edges whenever neurovascular assessments are made and/or whenever the client is turned.
   - Check the cast daily for a foul odor. *This kind of odor may indicate skin excoriation from pressure or an infected area beneath the cast.*

5. Implement measures to prevent skin irritation at the edges of the cast.
   - Wash crumbs of plaster from the skin with a damp cloth and feel along the cast edges to check for rough edges or areas that press into the client's skin. *As a plaster cast dries, small bits of plaster frequently break off from its rough edges. If they fall inside the cast, they can cause discomfort and irritation.*
   - Remove the resin of synthetic casting materials with a swab moistened with alcohol, acetone, or nail polish remover. Check the manufacturer's directions.
   - When it is dry, cover any rough edges and protect areas of the cast that may come in contact with urine. "**Petal**" the edges with small strips of waterproof tape as follows (Figure 31-4 ◆):
     a. Cut several strips of 2.5-cm (1-in) adhesive, 5 to 7.5 cm (2 to 3 in) long. Then curve all corners of each strip. *Square or pointed ends tend to curl.*
     b. Insert one end of each strip as far as possible inside the cast, and bring the other end out over the cast edge.

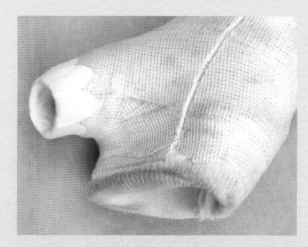

FIGURE 31-4 ◆ Completed petalled cast.

c. Press the petals firmly against the plaster.

d. Overlap successive petals slightly.

6. Provide skin care to all areas vulnerable to pressure.

- Examine all areas vulnerable to pressure and breakdown at least every 4 hours. For clients with sensitive skin or potential skin problems, provide care every 2 hours during the day and every 3 hours at night.

  a. Reach under the cast edges as far as possible and massage the area.

  b. Also provide skin care over all bony prominences not under the cast (e.g., the sacrum, heels, ankles, wrists, elbows, and feet). *These are potential pressure areas if the client is confined to bed.*

7. Keep the cast clean and dry.

Plaster Cast

- Place a bib or towel over a body cast to catch spills. If a spill does wet the cast, allow the area to air dry.

- Use a slipper (fracture) bedpan for people with long leg, hip spica, or body casts. *The flat end placed correctly under the client's buttocks lessens the chance of spillage and minimizes the amount of lifting required by the client and/or nurse.*

- Before placing the client on the bedpan, tuck plastic or other waterproof material around the top of a long leg cast or in around the perineal cutout. For a perineal cutout, funnel one end of the plastic into the bedpan.

- Remove the plastic when elimination is completed. *If left in place, waterproof material makes the cast edge airtight and prevents evaporation of perspiration, which is irritating to the skin.*

- For people with long leg casts, keep the cast supported on pillows while the client is on the bedpan. *If the cast dangles, urine may run down the cast.*

- For clients with hip spica casts, support both extremities and the back on pillows so that they are as high as the buttocks. *This prevents urine from running back into the cast.*

- When removing the bedpan, hold it securely while the client is turning or lifting the buttocks. *This prevents dripping and spilling.*

- After removing the bedpan, thoroughly clean and dry the perineal area.

Synthetic Cast

- Wash the soiled area with warm water and a mild soap.

- Thoroughly rinse the soap from the cast.

- Dry thoroughly to prevent skin maceration and ulceration under the cast.

- If the cast is immersed in water, dry the cast and underlying padding and stockinette thoroughly.

First, blot excess water from the cast with a towel. Then, use a handheld blow dryer on the cool or warm setting, directing the air stream in a sweeping motion over the exterior of the cast for about 1 hour or until the client no longer feels a cold clammy sensation like that produced by a wet bathing suit. *This drying procedure is essential to prevent skin maceration and ulceration.*

8. Turn and position the client in correct alignment to prevent the formation of pressure areas.

- Place pillows in such a way that:

  a. Body parts press against the edges of the cast as little as possible.

  b. Toes, heels, elbows, and so on, are protected from pressure against the bed surface.

  c. Body alignment is maintained.

- Plan and implement a turning schedule that will incorporate all the possible positions. *Repositioning prevents pressure areas.* Generally, clients can be placed in lateral, prone, and supine positions unless surgical procedures or any other factors contraindicate them. Attach a trapeze to the Balkan frame to enable the client to assist with moving.

- Turn people with large casts or those unable to turn themselves at least once every 4 hours. If the person is at risk for skin breakdown, turn every 1 to 3 hours as needed.

- When turning the client in a long leg cast to the unaffected side, place a pillow between the legs to support the cast.

- Use at least three persons to turn a person in a *damp* hip spica cast. When the cast is dry, the individual can usually turn with the assistance of one nurse. To turn a client from the supine to prone position, follow these steps:

  a. Remove the support pillows only when an assistant is supporting the cast.

  b. Move the client to one side of the bed.

  c. Ask the client to place the arms above the head or along the sides.

  d. Have two assistants go to the other side of the bed while you remain to provide security for the person who is at the edge of the bed.

  e. Place pillows along the bed surface to receive the cast when the client turns.

  f. Roll the client toward the two assistants onto the pillows.

  g. Adjust the pillows as needed so that they provide proper support and comfort, and prevent pressure areas.

9. Encourage range-of-motion (ROM) and isometric exercises.

- Unless contraindicated, encourage active ROM exercises for all joints on the unaffected extremities, as well as on the joints proximal and distal to the cast. If active exercises are contraindicated, implement active–assistive or passive exercises, depending on the client's abilities and disabilities. (See Technique 8-1.) *Exercise helps prevent joint stiffness and muscle atrophy.*

- Encourage the client to move toes and/or fingers of the casted extremity as frequently as possible. *Moving these extremities enhances peripheral circulation and decreases swelling and pain.*

- Teach isometric (muscle-setting) exercises for extremities in a cast. *Isometric exercise will minimize muscle atrophy in the affected limb.*

  a. Teach the isometric exercises on the client's unaffected limb before the person applies it to the affected limb.

  b. Demonstrate muscle palpation while the client is carrying out the exercise. *Palpation enables the person to feel the changes that occur with muscle contraction and relaxation.*

10. Provide client teaching to promote self-care, comfort, and safety.

- Teach people immobilized in bed with large body casts ways to turn and to move safely by using a trapeze, the side rails, and other such devices.

- Instruct clients with leg casts about ways to walk effectively with crutches (see Technique 6-5).

- Instruct people with arm casts how to apply slings (see Technique 30-8).

- Teach clients how to resolve itching under the cast safely. Discourage the person from using long sharp objects to scratch under the cast. *These objects can break the skin and cause an infection, because bacteria flourish in the warm, dark, moist environment under the cast.*

- When healing is complete and the cast is removed, the underlying skin is usually dry, flaky, and encrusted, since layers of dead skin have accumulated. Instruct clients to remove this debris gently and gradually.

  a. Apply oil (e.g., mineral, olive, or baby oil).

  b. Soak the skin in warm water and dry it.

  c. Caution the client not to rub the area too vigorously. *Vigorous rubbing can cause bleeding or excoriation.*

  d. Repeat steps a and b for several days. *Gradual removal of skin exudate avoids skin irritation.*

11. **Document** findings in the client record using forms or checklists supplemented by narrative notes when appropriate. Record each assessment (whether or not there are problems). Examples of documentation include: "Toes warm to touch, color pink," "Blanching satisfactory," "Moves toes readily; states no numbness or tingling; states leg painful." Record specific nerve function assessments such as "Able to hyperextend R thumb," "Sensation felt at web space between R thumb and index finger."

EVALUATION

- Perform detailed follow-up based on findings that deviated from expected or normal for the client. Relate findings to previous assessment data if available.

- Report significant deviations from normal to the physician.

Chapter Summary

TERMINOLOGY

bivalve

petal

plaster of paris

stockinette

spica

synthetic casts

window

FORMING CLINICAL JUDGMENTS

Consider This:

1. A teenager is to be casted for a severe fracture of the elbow with significant tissue swelling and a break in the skin. The physician plans to cast the elbow in a 45-degree flexed position for several days and then recast in a 90-degree flexed position. When told that a plaster cast will be used, the client is upset, insisting that a colorful syn-

thetic cast will be easier to care for and allow showering. What data will you use to explain the choice of plaster to the client?

2. Your elderly client is being visited in the home to check on a casted Colles' fracture of the wrist. The fingers appear swollen, somewhat dusky in color, and cool. What further assessments are indicated, and what actions would you take?

REFERENCES

Adkins, L. M. (1997). Cast changes: Synthetic versus plaster. *Pediatric Nursing, 23,* 422, 425–427.

Baxter, P. (2000). Splints for all seasons. *Advance for Providers of Post-Acute Care, 3*(3), 18–19.

Capper, C. (1998). Synthetic casting tapes: Ben-efits and uses of Delta-Cast Conformable. *British Journal of Nursing, 7,* 1162–1166.

Maher, A. B., Salmond, S. W., & Pellion, T. A. (1998). *Orthopaedic nursing* (2nd ed.). Philadelphia: W. B. Saunders.

McConnell, E.W.A. (1997). Clinical do's and don'ts: Assisting with cast application. *Nursing, 27*(12), 28.

Prior, M., & Miles, S. (1999). Casting: Part one. *Emergency Nursing, 7*(2), 33–39.

Prior, M., & Miles, S. (1999). Casting: Part two. *Emergency Nursing, 7*(3), 32–39.

Prior, M., & Miles, S. (1999). Principles of casting. *Journal of Orthopaedic Nursing, 3,* 162–170.

Chapter 32

Performing Perioperative Care

Techniques

OBJECTIVES

- Describe the phases of the perioperative period.
- Describe essential preoperative teaching, including moving, performing leg exercises, and coughing and deep-breathing exercises.
- Discuss ongoing nursing assessments required for the postoperative client.
- Identify the clinical signs of potential postoperative complications and describe nursing interventions to prevent them.
- Establish and manage gastrointestinal suction.
- Identify purposes of wound drains.
- Describe various methods of suturing.
- Perform appropriate wound care for a postoperative client.

S urgery is a unique experience of a planned physical alteration encompassing three phases: preoperative, intraoperative, and postoperative. These three phases are together referred to as the **perioperative period.**

The **preoperative phase** begins when the decision to have surgery is made and ends when the client is transferred to the operating table. The nursing activities associated with this phase include assessing the client, identifying potential or actual health problems, planning specific care based on the individual's needs, and providing preoperative teaching for the client and support people.

The **intraoperative phase** begins when the client is transferred to the operating table and ends when the client is admitted to the **postanesthesia care unit (PACU)**, also called the **postanesthetic room (PAR)** or **recovery room (RR).** The nursing activities related to this phase include a variety of specialized procedures designed to create and maintain a safe therapeutic environment for the client and the health care personnel.

The **postoperative phase** begins with the admission of the client to the postanesthesia area and ends when healing is complete. During the postoperative phase, nursing activities include assessing the client's response (physiologic and psychological) to surgery, performing interventions to facilitate healing and prevent complications, teaching and providing support to the client and support people, and planning for home care. The goal is to assist the client to achieve the most optimal health status possible.

Today, more than 70 percent of all elective surgeries are performed in an outpatient setting (Brockway, 1997, p. 388). The client comes to the hospital the day of surgery, has the operation, and leaves the same day. In these instances, the three phases of the perioperative period are significantly shortened and the postoperative phase continues at home. The nurse's role in assessing, teaching, and following up is vital to successful outcomes for the client who undergoes day surgery.

Preoperative Teaching

Preoperative teaching is a vital part of nursing care. Studies have shown that preoperative teaching reduces clients' anxiety and postoperative complications as well as increasing their satisfaction with the surgical experience. Good preoperative teaching also facilitates the client's return to work and other activities of daily living. Four dimensions of preoperative teaching have been identified as important to clients:

1. Information, including what will happen to the client, when and what the client will experience, such as expected sensations and discomfort. The nurse needs to listen carefully and attentively to the client to identify specific concerns and fears.

2. Psychosocial support to reduce anxiety. The nurse provides support by actively listening and providing accurate information. It is important to rectify any misperceptions the client may have.

3. The roles of the client and support people in preoperative preparation, the surgical procedure, and during the postoperative phase. Understanding his or her role during the perioperative experience increases the client's sense of control and reduces anxiety. This includes what will be expected of the client, desired behaviors, self-care activities, and what the client can do to facilitate recovery.

4. Skills training, for example, moving, deep breathing, coughing, splinting incisions with the hands or a pillow, and using an incentive spirometer.

If the client is scheduled for same-day surgery, preoperative teaching is often provided before the day of surgery using some combination of videos and verbal and written instructions. The client may have an appointment with day-surgery staff (usually scheduled to coincide with preoperative diagnostic testing) to discuss preoperative concerns, or a nurse working with the surgeon may complete teaching. Written instructions are provided, especially when surgery is scheduled several days or weeks hence. Teaching is then reinforced on admission to the surgery unit and immediate or continuing concerns are addressed.

Preoperative instructions for all clients are summarized in Box 32-1. Technique 32-1 provides guidelines for teaching clients about moving, leg exercises, deep breathing, and coughing.

The purposes for teaching about the importance of each of these activities include:

Moving

- To maintain blood circulation
- To stimulate respiratory function
- To decrease stasis of gas in the intestine
- To facilitate early ambulation

Leg Exercises

- To stimulate blood circulation, thereby preventing thrombophlebitis and thrombus formation

Deep Breathing and Coughing

- To facilitate lung aeration, thereby preventing atelectasis and pneumonia

Nursing Process: Preoperative Teaching

ASSESSMENT

Assess:

- Vital signs
- Discomfort
- Temperature and color of feet and legs

Box 32-1 *Preoperative Instructions*

Preoperative Regimen

- Explain the need for preoperative tests (e.g., laboratory, x-ray, electrocardiogram).
- Discuss bowel preparation, if required.
- Discuss skin preparation, including operative area and preoperative bath or shower.
- Discuss preoperative medications, if ordered.
- Explain individual therapies ordered by the physician, such as intravenous therapy, the insertion of a urinary catheter or nasogastric tube, use of a spirometer, or antiemboli stockings.
- Discuss the visit by the anesthetist.
- Explain the need to restrict food and oral fluids at least 8 hours before surgery.
- Provide a general timetable for perioperative events, including the time of surgery.
- Discuss the need to remove jewelry, make-up, and all prostheses (e.g., eyeglasses, hearing aids, complete or partial dentures, wig) immediately before surgery.
- Inform client about the preoperative holding area, and give the location of the waiting room for support people.
- Teach deep-breathing and coughing exercises, leg exercises, ways to turn and move, and splinting techniques.
- Complete the preoperative checklist.

Postoperative Regimen

- Discuss the postanesthesia recovery room's routines and emergency equipment.
- Review type and frequency of assessment activities.

- Discuss pain management.
- Explain usual activity restrictions and precautions related to getting up for the first time postoperatively.
- Describe usual dietary alterations.
- Discuss postoperative dressings and drains.
- Provide an explanation and tour of intensive care unit if client is to be transferred there postoperatively.

Day-Surgery Clients

- Confirm place and time of surgery, including when to arrive (e.g., 1 to 1½ hours before scheduled surgery) and where to register (e.g., reception desk).
- Discuss what to wear (e.g., clients having hand surgery should wear a garment with large sleeve openings to fit over a bulky dressing; all clients need to leave valuables at home).
- Explain the need for a responsible adult to drive or accompany the client home, and arrange a place for them to meet.
- Discuss medications including specific preoperative medications and the client's current medication regimen.
- Review with the client any tests ordered and the need for a urine specimen the morning of surgery.
- Communicate by telephone the evening before surgery to confirm time of surgery and arrival time, and call again the evening after surgery to assess progress.

From *Fundamentals of nursing: Concepts, process, and practice*, 6th ed., by B. Kozier, G. Erb, A. Berman, & K. Burke, 2000, Upper Saddle River, NJ: Prentice Hall Health.

- Breath sounds
- Presence of dyspnea or cough
- Learning needs of the client
- Anxiety level of the client
- Client experience with previous surgeries and anesthesia

PLANNING

Before commencing to teach moving, leg exercises, deep-breathing exercises, and coughing, determine (1) the type of surgery, (2) the time of the surgery, (3) the name of the surgeon, (4) the preoperative orders, and (5) the agency's practices for preoperative care. Also, verify that the physician has completed the medical

history and physical examination and that the client or the family has signed the consent form.

Delegation

Assessment of the learning needs of the client and their support people and determining the teaching content and appropriate strategies for teaching requires application of professional knowledge and critical thinking. Preoperative teaching is conducted by the nurse and is not delegated to unlicensed assistive personnel (UAP). The UAP, however, can reinforce teaching, assist the client with the exercises, and report to the nurse if the client is unable to perform the exercises.

Equipment

- Pillow
- Teaching materials (e.g., videotape, written materials) if available at the agency

Preparation

Check that potential distracters (e.g., pain, TV, visitors) to teaching are not present. Include the family in the teaching, if appropriate.

Performance

1. Explain to the client what you are going to do, why it is necessary, and how he or she can cooperate. Discuss how the client's participation in the exercises he or she is going to be taught preoperatively will be helpful during the postoperative recovery.

2. Wash hands and observe appropriate infection control procedures.

3. Provide for client privacy.

4. Show the client ways to turn in bed and to get out of bed.

   - Instruct a client who will have a right abdominal incision or a right-sided chest incision to turn to the left side of the bed and sit up as follows:

     a. Flex the knees.

     b. Splint the wound by holding the left arm and hand or a small pillow against the incision.

     c. Turn to the left while pushing with the right foot and grasping a partial side rail on the left side of the bed with the right hand.

     d. Come to a sitting position on the side of the bed by using the right arm and hand to push down against the mattress and swinging the feet over the edge of the bed.

   - Teach a client with left abdominal or left-sided chest incision to perform the same procedure but splint with the right arm and turn to the right.

   - For clients with orthopedic surgery (e.g., hip surgery), use special aids, such as a trapeze, to assist with movement.

5. Teach the client the following three leg exercises:

   - Alternate dorsiflexion and plantar flexion of the feet (see Chapter 8, Figure 8-28). *This exercise is sometimes referred to as calf pumping, because it alternately contracts and relaxes the calf muscles, including the gastrocnemius muscles (see Figure 32-1 ◆).*

   - Flex and extend the knees, and press the backs of the knees into the bed while dorsiflexing the

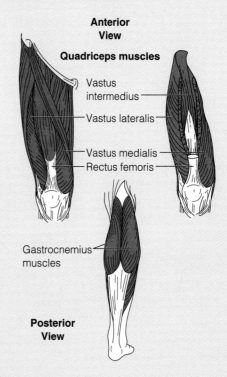

Anterior View

FIGURE 32-1 ◆ Leg muscles: anterior and posterior views.

feet (Figure 32-2 ◆). Instruct clients who cannot raise their legs to do isometric exercises that contract and relax the muscles.

- Raise and lower the legs alternately from the surface of the bed. Flex the knee of the stable

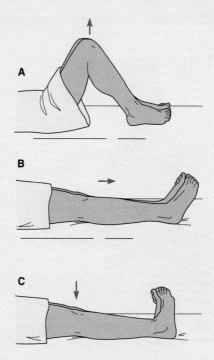

FIGURE 32-2 ◆ Flexing and extending the knees.

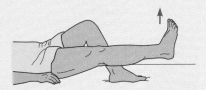

FIGURE 32-3 ◆ Raising and lowering the legs.

leg and extend the knee of the moving leg (Figure 32-3 ◆). *This exercise contracts and relaxes the quadriceps muscles.*

6. Demonstrate deep-breathing (diaphragmatic) exercises as follows.

• Place your hands palms down on the border of your rib cage, and inhale slowly and evenly through the nose until the greatest chest expansion is achieved (Figure 32-4 ◆).

• Hold your breath for 2 to 3 seconds.

• Then exhale slowly through the mouth.

• Continue exhalation until maximum chest contraction has been achieved.

7. Help the client perform deep-breathing exercises.

• Ask the client to assume a sitting position.

• Place the palms of your hands on the border of the client's rib cage to assess respiratory depth.

• Ask the client to perform deep breathing, as described in step 6.

8. Instruct the client to cough voluntarily after a few deep inhalations.

• Ask the client to inhale deeply, hold the breath

for a few seconds, and then cough once or twice.

• Ensure that the client coughs deeply and does not just clear the throat.

9. Demonstrate ways to splint the abdomen when coughing, if the incision will be painful when the client coughs.

• Show the client how to support the incision by placing the palms of the hands on either side of the incision site or directly over the incision site, holding the palm of one hand over the other. *Coughing uses the abdominal and other accessory respiratory muscles. Splinting the incision may reduce pain while coughing if the incision is near any of these muscles.*

• Show the client how to splint the abdomen with clasped hands and a firmly rolled pillow held against the client's abdomen (Figure 32-5 ◆).

10. Inform the client about the expected frequency of these exercises.

• Instruct the client to start the exercises as soon after surgery as possible.

• Encourage clients with abdominal or chest surgery to carry out deep breathing and coughing at least every 2 hours, taking a minimum of five breaths at each session. Note, however, that the number of breaths and frequency of deep breathing varies with the client's condition. People who are susceptible to pulmonary problems may need deep-breathing exercises every hour. People with chronic respiratory disease may need special breathing exercises (e.g., pursed-lip breathing), abdominal breathing, exercises using various kinds of incentive spirometers). See Chapter 20.

 11. **Document** the teaching and all assessments. Some agencies may have a preoperative teaching flow sheet. Check agency policy.

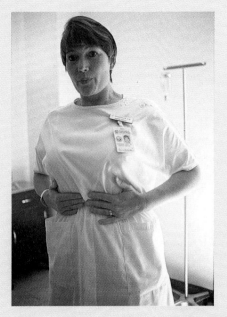

FIGURE 32-4 ◆ Demonstrating deep breathing exercise.

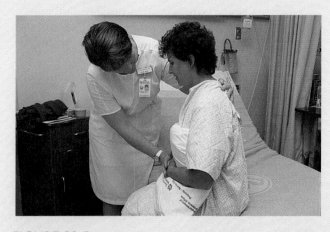

FIGURE 32-5 ◆ Splinting an incision with a pillow while coughing.

Postoperative Teaching

Adults want information about activities they normally perform while they are recovering at home. This is important information for all surgical clients and particularly clients having the surgery at a same-day surgery center. Discuss the following areas:

- *Food.* Eat small portions at first as anesthesia and pain medications slow gastric emptying.
- *Bowel movements.* Constipation occurs frequently as a result of decreased gastrointestinal mobility due to many causes (e.g., anesthesia, decreased activity, pain medications). Discuss strategies to prevent constipation.
- *Sexual activity.* Intimacy such as gentle hugging and kissing is allowed for clients when they feel like it. Full sexual intercourse takes longer. By the time the wound soreness and tenderness is gone (2 to 4 weeks), the strength of the incision is adequate for sexual intercourse (Fox, 1998).
- *Wound care.* Discuss questions related to wound strength, pain, and infection.

- *Lifting.* Be specific about weight limits, if appropriate. Relate the weight limit to everyday items (e.g., a gallon of milk weighs approximately 8 pounds).
- *Pain.* Provide information about the client's pain medications. Ask the client to describe his or her daily activities and discuss ways to avoid or reduce painful activities.
- *Bathing.* Check with the surgeon as some want the wound to be kept dry. There is no evidence that water on a closed wound is harmful or interferes with wound healing. If allowed, inform the client to shower, letting the water wash over the incision for a short time (2 to 3 minutes) and gently pat the incision dry (Fox, 1998).
- *Infection.* Discuss the signs and symptoms of wound infection and when the client should call the physician.
- *Activities.* Advise the client that they will tire easily and to plan short activities with frequent rest breaks.

Preoperative Teaching

Children

- Parents need to know what to expect and to be able to express their concerns.
- Separation from parents often is the child's greatest fear; the time of separation should be minimized and parents allowed to interact with the child both immediately preceding and following the surgery.
- Teaching of the child (both timing and content) should be geared to the child's developmental level and cognitive abilities.
- Use simple terms to help the child understand (e.g., "You will have a sore tummy").

- Play is an effective teaching tool with children; the child can put a bandage on an "incision" on a doll.

Elders

- Assess hearing ability to ensure the older client hears the necessary information.
- Assess short-term memory. Presenting one focused idea at a time and repeating or reinforcing information may be necessary.
- Older adults are at greater risk for postoperative complications, such as pneumonia. Reinforce moving and deep breathing and coughing exercises.

EVALUATION

Conduct appropriate follow up such as:

- Client's demonstrated ability to perform moving, leg exercises, deep-breathing, and coughing exercises
- Client's verbalization of key information presented

Preparing for the Postoperative Client

While the client is in the operating room, the client's bed and room are prepared for the postoperative phase. In some agencies, the client is brought back to the unit on a stretcher and transferred to the bed in the room. (See Chapter 11 for information on making a surgical bed.) In other agencies, the client's bed is brought to the surgery suite, and the client is transferred there. In the latter situation, the bed needs to be made with clean linens as soon as the client goes to surgery so that it can be taken to the operating room when needed. In addition, the nurse must obtain and set up any special equipment, such as an intravenous (IV) pole, suction, oxygen equipment, and orthopedic appliances (e.g., traction). If these are not requested on the client's record, the nurse should consult with the perioperative nurse or surgeon.

Postoperative Phase

Immediate Postanesthetic Care

Immediate postanesthetic care is usually provided in a PAR or RR. Recovery room nurses have specialized skills to care for clients recovering from anesthesia and surgery (Figure 32-6 ◆). Assessment of the client in the immediate postanesthetic period is summarized in Box 32-2. Once the health status has stabilized, the client is returned to the nursing unit or, in the case of a day-surgery client, to the day-surgery area before discharge.

Ongoing Postoperative Nursing Care

As soon as the client returns to the nursing unit, the nurse conducts an initial assessment. The sequence of these activities varies with the situation. For example, the nurse may need to check the physician's "stat" orders before conducting the initial assessment; in such a case, nursing interventions to implement the orders can be carried out at the same time as assessment.

Many hospitals have postoperative protocols for regular assessment of clients. In some agencies, assessments are made every 15 minutes until vital signs stabilize, every hour for the next 4 hours, then every 4 hours for the next 2 days. It is important that the assessments be made as often as the client's condition requires.

Assessment continues throughout the postoperative period. See Box 32-3 for postoperative assessment guidelines and Table 32-1 regarding potential postoperative problems. Nursing interventions designed to prevent these problems include early ambulation, deep breathing and coughing exercises, adequate

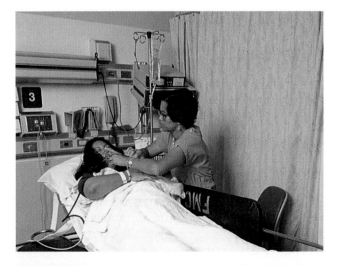

FIGURE 32-6 ◆ Recovery room nurse provides constant assessment and care for clients recovering from anesthesia and surgery.

Box 32-2 *Immediate Postanesthetic Phase*

- Adequacy of airway
- Oxygen saturation
- Adequacy of ventilation
  - Respiratory rate, rhythm, and depth
  - Use of accessory muscles
  - Breath sounds
- Cardiovascular status
  - Heart rate and rhythm
  - Peripheral pulse amplitude and equality
  - Blood pressure
  - Capillary filling
- Level of consciousness
  - Not responding
  - Arousable with verbal stimuli
  - Fully awake
  - Oriented to time, person, and place
- Presence of protective reflexes (e.g., gag, cough)
- Activity, ability to move extremities
- Skin color (pink, pale, dusky, blotchy, cyanotic, jaundiced)
- Fluid status
  - Intake and output
  - Status of IV infusions (type of fluid, rate, amount in container, patency of tubing)
  - Signs of dehydration or fluid overload
- Condition of operative site
  - Status of dressing
  - Drainage (amount, type, and color)
- Patency of and character and amount of drainage from catheters, tubes, and drains
- Discomfort (i.e., pain) (type, location, and severity), nausea, vomiting
- Safety (i.e., necessity for side rails, call bell within reach)

From *Fundamentals of nursing: Concepts, process, and practice*, 6th ed., by B. Kozier, G. Erb, A. Berman, & K. Burke, 2000, Upper Saddle River, NJ: Prentice Hall Health.

hydration, leg exercises, monitoring fluid intake and output, and early recognition of signs of complications.

Techniques commonly implemented in the postoperative period are discussed elsewhere in this book. For example, intravenous therapy techniques are discussed in Chapter 29; parenteral medications in Chapter 28; pain management in Chapter 14; assisting clients to move and ambulate in Chapter 6; promoting circulation in Chapter 19; and breathing exercises in

Box 32-3 *Postoperative Assessment Guidelines*

Assess:

- *Level of consciousness.* Assess orientation to time, place, and person. Most clients are fully conscious but drowsy when returned to their room or area. Assess reaction to verbal stimuli and ability to move extremities.

- *Vital signs.* Take the client's vital signs (pulse, respiration, blood pressure, and oxygen saturation level) every 15 minutes until stable or in accordance with agency protocol. Compare initial findings with PACU data.

- *Skin temperature and temperature,* particularly that of the lips and nail beds. The color of the lips and nail beds are indicators of tissue perfusion (passage of blood through the vessels). Pale, cyanotic, cool, and moist skin may be a sign of circulatory problems.

- *Comfort.* Assess pain with the client's vital signs and as needed between vital sign measurements. Assess the location and intensity of the pain. Do not assume that reported pain is incisional; other causes may include muscle strains, flatus, and angina. Evaluate the client for objective indicators of pain: pallor, perspiration, muscle tension, and reluctance to cough, move, or ambulate. Determine when and what analgesics were last administered and assess the client for any side effects of medication such as nausea and vomiting.

- *Fluid balance.* Assess the type and amount of intravenous fluids, flow rate, and infusion site. Monitor the client's fluid intake and output. In addition to watching for shock, assess the client for signs of circulatory overload and monitor serum electrolytes.

- *Dressing and bedclothes.* Inspect the client's dressings and bedclothes underneath the client. Excessive bloody drainage on dressings or on bedclothes, often appearing underneath the client, can indicate hemorrhage. The amount of drainage on dressings is recorded by describing the diameter of the stains or by denoting the number and type of dressings saturated with drainage. Later, when dressings are changed, inspect the wound for signs of localized infection.

- *Any difficulties with voiding and/or bladder distention.*

- *Return of peristalsis.* Auscultate the client's abdomen to confirm the return of peristalsis. Note the passage of flatus and stool.

- *Tolerance of food and fluids ingested.*

- *Drains and tubes.* Determine color, consistency, and amount of drainage from all tubes and drains. All tubes should be patent and tubes and suction equipment should be functioning. Drainage bags must be hanging properly.

Chapter 20. This chapter includes the techniques of managing gastrointestinal suction and surgical wound care.

Suction

Some clients return from surgery with a gastric or intestinal tube in place and orders to connect the tube to suction. The suction ordered can be continuous or intermittent. Intermittent suction is applied when a single-lumen gastric tube (Levin tube) is used to reduce the risk of damaging the mucous membrane near the distal port of the tube. Continuous suction may be applied if a double-lumen tube (Salem sump tube) is in place (Figure 32-7 ◆). Fluids and electrolytes must be replaced intravenously when gastric suction or continuous drainage is ordered. Nasogastric tubes may be irrigated if the lumen becomes clogged. They are generally irrigated before and after tube feedings or the instillation of medications. Nasogastric irrigation may require a physician's order, particularly following gastrointestinal surgery. Technique 32-2 describes the management of gastrointestinal suction.

Suction may also be applied to other drainage tubes such as chest tubes or a wound drain. The physician orders the type and amount of suction. Most agencies have wall suction units available (Figure 32-8 ◆). A suction regulator with a drainage receptacle connects to a wall outlet that provides negative pressure. Check the receptacle frequently to prevent excess drainage from interfering with the suction apparatus; empty or change the receptacle according to agency policy. Portable electric suction units or pumps (e.g., the Gomco pump) may be used in the home or when wall suction is not available.

Nursing Process: Postoperative Phase

ASSESSMENT

Assess:

- Presence of abdominal distention on palpation
- Auscultated bowel sounds
- Abdominal discomfort
- Vital signs for baseline data

PLANNING

Before initiating gastric suction, determine (1) whether the suction is continuous or intermittent; (2) the ordered suction pressure (a low suction pressure is between 80 and 100 mm Hg, and a high pressure is between 100 and 120 mm Hg); and (3) whether there is an order to irrigate the gastrointestinal tube, and if so, the type of solution to use.

TABLE 32-1   POTENTIAL POSTOPERATIVE PROBLEMS

Problem	Clinical Signs	Preventive Interventions
Pneumonia	Elevated temperature, cough, expectoration of blood-tinged or purulent sputum, dyspnea, chest pain	Deep-breathing exercises and coughing, moving in bed, early ambulation
Atelectasis	Dyspnea, tachypnea, tachycardia; diaphoresis, anxiety; pleural pain, decreased chest wall movement; dull or absent breath sounds; decreased oxygen saturation (SaO_2)	Deep-breathing exercises and coughing, moving in bed, early ambulation
Pulmonary embolism	Sudden chest pain, shortness of breath, cyanosis, shock (tachycardia, low blood pressure)	Turning, ambulation, antiemboli stockings, sequential compression devices (SCDs)
Hypovolemia	Tachycardia, decreased urine output, decreased blood pressure	Early detection of signs; fluid and/or blood replacement
Hemorrhage	Overt bleeding (dressings saturated with bright blood; bright, free-flowing blood in drains or chest tubes), increased pain, increasing abdominal girth, swelling or bruising around incision	Early detection of signs; fluid and/or blood replacement
Thrombophlebitis	Aching, cramping pain; affected area is swollen, red, and hot to touch; vein feels hard; discomfort in calf when foot is dorsiflexed or when client walks (Homans' sign)	Early ambulation, leg exercises, antiemboli stockings, SCDs, adequate fluid intake
Thrombus	Venous: same as thrombophlebitis Arterial: pain and pallor of affected extremity; decreased or absent peripheral pulses	Venous: same as thrombophlebitis Arterial: maintaining prescribed position; early detection of signs
Embolus	In venous system, usually becomes a pulmonary embolus (see pulmonary embolism); signs of arterial emboli may depend on the location	As for thrombophlebitis or thrombus; careful maintenance of IV catheters
Urinary retention	Fluid intake larger than output; inability to void or frequent voiding of small amounts, bladder distention, suprapubic discomfort, restlessness	Monitoring of fluid intake and output, interventions to facilitate voiding, urinary catheterization as needed
Urinary tract infection	Burning sensation when voiding, urgency, cloudy urine, lower abdominal pain	Adequate fluid intake, early ambulation, aseptic straight catheterization only as necessary, good perineal hygiene
Nausea and vomiting	Complains of feeling sick to the stomach, retching or gagging	IV fluids until peristalsis returns; then clear fluids, full fluids, and regular diet; antiemetic drugs if ordered; analgesics for pain
Constipation	Absence of stool elimination, abdominal distention, and discomfort	Adequate fluid intake, high-fiber diet, early ambulation
Tympanites	Obvious abdominal distention, abdominal discomfort (gas pains), absence of bowel sounds	Early ambulation; avoid using a straw, provide water at room temperature
Postoperative ileus	Abdominal pain and distention; constipation; absent bowel sounds; vomiting	IV fluids until peristalsis returns; gradual reintroduction of oral feeding; early ambulation
Wound infection	Purulent exudates, redness, tenderness, elevated body temperature, wound odor	Keeping wound clean and dry, surgical aseptic technique when changing dressings
Wound dehiscence (separation of a suture line before the incision heals)	Increased incision drainage, tissues underlying skin become visible along parts of the incision	Adequate nutrition, appropriate incisional support, and avoidance of strain
Wound evisceration (extrusion of internal organs and tissues through the incision)	Opening of incision and visible protrusion of organs	Same as for wound dehiscence
Postoperative depression	Anorexia, tearfulness, loss of ambition, withdrawal, rejection of others, feelings of dejection, sleep disturbances (insomnia, excessive sleeping)	Adequate rest, physical activity, opportunity to express anger and other negative feelings

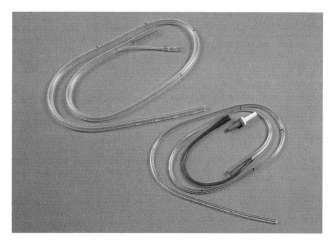

FIGURE 32-7 ◆ Nasogastric tubes used for gastric decompression. Top left: Levin (single-lumen) tube. Lower right: Salem sump (double-lumen) tube with antireflux valve.

Delegation

Managing gastrointestinal suction requires application of knowledge and problem solving and is not delegated to UAP. The UAP, however, can assist with emptying the drainage receptacle and reporting changes in amount and/or color of the drainage to the nurse.

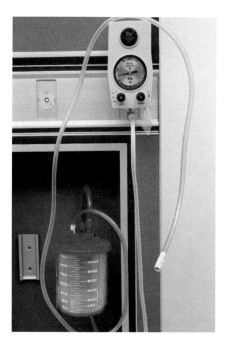

FIGURE 32-8 ◆ Wall suction unit for generating negative pressure for nasogastric suction.

IMPLEMENTATION:
TECHNIQUE 32-2 MANAGING GASTROINTESTINAL (GI) SUCTION

Equipment

Initiating Suction

- Gastrointestinal tube in place in the client
- Basin
- 50-mL syringe with an adapter
- Stethoscope
- Suction device for either continuous or intermittent suction
- Connector and connecting tubing
- Disposable gloves

Maintaining Suction

- Graduated container as required to measure gastric drainage
- Basin of water
- Cotton-tipped applicators
- Ointment or lubricant
- Disposable gloves

Irrigation

- Disposable gloves
- Stethoscope

- Disposable irrigating set containing a sterile 50-mL syringe, moisture-resistant pad, basin, and graduated container
- Sterile normal saline (500 mL) or the ordered solution

Performance

1. Explain to the client what you are going to do, why it is necessary, and how he or she can cooperate. Discuss the purpose(s) for the gastrointestinal suction.

2. Wash hands and observe other appropriate infection control procedures (e.g., clean gloves).

3. Provide for client privacy.

Initiating Suction

4. Position the client appropriately.
   - Assist the client to a semi-Fowler's position if it is not contraindicated. *In semi-Fowler's position, the tube is not as likely to lie against the wall of the stomach and will therefore suction most efficiently. Semi-Fowler's position also prevents reflux of gastric contents, which could lead to aspiration.*

5. Confirm that the tube is in the stomach.

- Put on clean gloves.
- Aspirate stomach contents and check the acidity using a pH test strip.
- Insert air into the tube with the syringe and listen with a stethoscope over the stomach (just below the xiphoid process) for a swish of air.
- Use other methods in accordance with agency protocol. See Chapter 15, Technique 15-2.

6. Set and check the suction.

- Connect the appropriate suction regulator to the wall suction outlet and the collection device to the regulator. **Intermittent suction regulators** generally are used with single-lumen tubes and apply suction for a set interval (15 to 60 seconds), followed by an interval of no suction. Intermittent suction is set at 80 to 100 mm Hg or as ordered by the physician. Check the suction level by occluding the drainage tube and observing the regulator dial during a suction cycle. **Continuous suction regulators** are used with double-lumen (e.g., Salem sump) nasogastric tubes. Set continuous suction as ordered by the physician, or at 60 to 120 mm Hg.
- If using a portable suction machine, turn on the machine and regulate the suction as above. The Gomco pump has two settings: low intermittent for single-lumen tubes, and high for double-lumen tubes.
- Test for proper suctioning by holding the open end of the suction tube to the ear and listening for a sucking noise or by occluding the end of the tube with a thumb.

7. Establish gastric suction.

- Connect the gastrointestinal tube to the tubing from the suction by using the connector.
- If a Salem sump tube is in place, connect the larger lumen to the suction equipment. This double-lumen tube has a smaller tube running inside the primary suction tube. *The smaller tube provides a continuous flow of atmospheric air through the drainage tube at its distal end and prevents excessive suction force on the gastric mucosa at the drainage outlets. Damage to the gastric mucosa is thus avoided.*
- Always keep the air vent tube of a Salem sump tube open and above the level of the stomach when suction is applied. *Closing the vent would stop the sump action and cause mucosal damage. Keeping the end of the air vent tube higher than the stomach prevents reflux of gastric contents into the air lumen of the tube.*
- After suction is applied, watch the tubing for a few minutes until the gastric contents appear to be running through the tubing into the recepta-

cle. A Salem sump tube makes a soft, hissing sound when it is functioning correctly.

- If the suction is not working properly, check that all connections are tight and that the tubing is not kinked.
- Coil and pin the tubing on the bed so that it does not loop below the suction bottle. *If the tubing falls below the suction bottle, the suction may be obstructed because of the pressure required to push the fluid against gravity.*

8. Assess the drainage.

- Observe the amount, color, odor, and consistency of the drainage. Normal gastric drainage has a mucoid (resembling mucus) consistency and is either colorless or yellow-green because of the presence of bile. A coffee-ground color and consistency may indicate bleeding.
- Test the gastric drainage for pH and blood (by using Hematest) when indicated. A person who has had gastrointestinal surgery can be expected to have some blood in the drainage.

Maintaining Suction

9. Assess the client and the suction system regularly.

- Assess the client every 30 minutes until the system is running effectively and then every 2 hours, or as the client's health indicates, to ensure that the suction is functioning properly. If the client complains of fullness, nausea, or epigastric pain or if the flow of gastric secretions is absent in the tubing or in the collection bottle, ineffective suctioning or blockage of the nasogastric tube is likely.
- Inspect the suction system for patency of the system (e.g., kinks or blockages in the tubing) and tightness of the connections. *Loose connections can permit air to enter and thus decrease the effectiveness of the suction by decreasing the negative pressure.*

10. Relieve blockages if present.

- Put on clean gloves.
- Check the suction equipment. To do this, disconnect the nasogastric tube from the suction over a collecting basin (to collect gastric drainage), and then, with the suction on, place the end of the suction tubing in a basin of water. If water is drawn into the drainage bottle, the suction equipment is functioning properly, but the nasogastric tube is either blocked or positioned incorrectly.
- Reposition the client (e.g., to the other side) if permitted. *This may facilitate drainage.*
- Rotate the nasogastric tube, and reposition it. This step is contraindicated for clients with gastric surgery. *Moving the tube may interfere with gastric sutures.*

- Irrigate the nasogastric tube as agency protocol states or on the order of the physician (see steps 14 to 16).

11. Prevent reflux into the vent lumen of a Salem sump tube. *Reflux of gastric contents into the vent lumen may occur when stomach pressure exceeds atmospheric pressure. In this situation, gastric contents follow the path of least resistance and flow out the vent lumen rather than the drainage lumen.* To prevent reflux:

- Place the vent tubing higher than the client's stomach.

- Keep the drainage collection container below the level of the client's stomach and do not allow it to become too full. A collection device placed above the level of fluid in the stomach or that is too full may interfere with drainage, allowing reflux of gastric contents into the air lumen.

- Keep the drainage lumen free of particulate matter that may obstruct the lumen (see steps 14 to 16 for irrigating a nasogastric tube).

12. Ensure client comfort.

- Clean the client's nostrils as needed, using the cotton-tipped applicators and water. Apply a water-soluble lubricant or ointment.

- Provide mouth care every 2 to 4 hours and as needed. Some postoperative clients are permitted to suck ice chips or a moist cloth to maintain the moisture of the oral mucous membranes.

13. Empty the drainage receptacle according to agency policy or physician's order.

- Clamp the nasogastric tube, and turn off the suction.

- Put on clean gloves.

- If the receptacle is graduated, determine the amount of drainage.

- Disconnect the receptacle.

- If the receptacle is not graduated, empty the contents into a graduated container and measure.

- Inspect the drainage carefully for color, consistency, and presence of substances (e.g., blood clots).

- Discard and replace a full receptacle or rinse the receptacle with warm water and reattach it to the suction. Check agency policy.

- Turn on the suction and unclamp the nasogastric tube.

- Observe the system for several minutes to make sure function is reestablished.

- Go to step 17.

Irrigating a Gastrointestinal Tube

14. Prepare the client and the equipment.

- Place the moisture-resistant pad under the end of the gastrointestinal tube.

- Turn off the suction.

- Put on clean gloves.

- Disconnect the gastrointestinal tube from the connector.

- Determine that the tube is in the stomach. See step 5 above and Technique 15-2. *This ensures that the irrigating solution enters the client's stomach.*

15. Irrigate the tube.

- Draw up the ordered volume of irrigating solution in the syringe; 30 mL of solution per instillation is usual, but up to 60 mL may be given per instillation if ordered.

- Attach the syringe to the nasogastric tube, and slowly inject the solution.

- Gently aspirate the solution. *Forceful withdrawal could damage the gastric mucosa.*

- If you encounter difficulty in withdrawing the solution, inject 20 mL of air and aspirate again, and/or reposition the client or the nasogastric tube. *Air and repositioning may move the end of the tube away from the stomach wall.* If aspirating difficulty continues, reattach the tube in intermittent low suction, and notify the nurse in charge or physician.

- Repeat the preceding steps until the ordered amount of solution is used.

- Note: A Salem sump tube can also be irrigated through the vent lumen without interrupting suction. However, only small quantities of irrigant can be injected via this lumen compared to the drainage lumen.

- After irrigating a Salem sump tube, inject 10 to 20 mL of air into the vent lumen while applying suction to the drainage lumen. *This tests the patency of the vent and ensures sump functioning.*

16. Reestablish suction.

- Reconnect the nasogastric tube to suction.

- If a Salem sump tube is used, inject the air vent lumen with 10 mL of air after reconnecting the tube to suction.

- Observe the system for several minutes to make sure it is functioning.

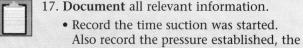 17. **Document** all relevant information.

- Record the time suction was started. Also record the pressure established, the color and consistency of the drainage, and nursing assessments.

- During maintenance, record assessments, supportive nursing measures, and data about the suction system.

- When irrigating the tube, record verification of tube placement; the time of the irrigation; the amount and type of irrigating solution used; the amount, color, and consistency of the returns; the patency of the system following the irrigation; and nursing assessments.

EVALUATION

- Conduct appropriate follow-up such as: relief of abdominal distention or discomfort; bowel sounds; character and amount of gastric drainage; integrity of nares; hydration of oral mucous membranes; patency of tube; system functioning.
- Relate to previous findings if available.
- Report significant deviations from normal to the physician.

Wound Care and Surgical Dressings

Most clients return from surgery with a sutured wound covered by a dressing, although in some cases the wound may be left unsutured. Dressings are inspected regularly to ensure that they are clean, dry, and intact. Excessive drainage may indicate hemorrhage, infection, or an open wound.

When dressings are changed, the nurse assesses the wound for appearance, size, drainage, swelling, pain, and the status of a drain or tubes. Details about these assessments are outlined in Box 32-4.

Not all surgical dressings require changing. Sometimes, surgeons in the operating room apply a dressing that remains in place until the sutures are removed and no further dressings are required. In many situations, however, surgical dressings are changed regularly to prevent the growth of microorganisms.

In some instances a client may have a **Penrose drain** (flat, thin rubber tube) inserted. The Penrose drain allows for fluid to flow from the wound. As there is no collection device, be prepared to change the dressing more often. In this situation, the main surgical incision is considered cleaner than the surgical stab wound made for the Penrose drain insertion because there is usually considerable drainage. The main incision is therefore cleaned *first,* and under no circumstances are materials that were used to clean the stab wound used subsequently to clean the main incision. In this way, the main incision is kept free of the microorganisms around the stab wound. Cleaning a wound and applying a sterile dressing are detailed in Technique 32-3.

Nursing Process: Wound Care and Surgical Dressings

ASSESSMENT

Assess:

- Client allergies to wound cleaning agents
- The appearance and size of the wound

BOX 32-4 *Assessing Surgical Wounds*

Appearance

- Inspect color of wound and surrounding area and approximation of wound edges.

Size

- Note size and location of dehiscence, if present.

Drainage

- Observe location, color, consistency, odor, and degree of saturation of dressings. Note number of gauzes saturated or diameter of drainage on gauze.

Swelling

- Observe the amount of swelling; minimal to moderate swelling is normal in early stages of wound healing.

Pain

- Expect severe to moderate postoperative pain for 3 to 5 days; persistent severe pain or sudden onset of severe pain may indicate internal hemorrhaging or infection.

Drains or Tubes

- Inspect drain security and placement, amount and character of drainage, and functioning of collecting apparatus, if present.

- The amount and character of exudates
- Client complaints of discomfort
- The time of the last pain medication
- Signs of systemic infection (e.g., elevated body temperature, diaphoresis, malaise, leukocytosis)

PLANNING

Before changing a dressing, determine any specific orders about the wound or dressing.

Delegation

Cleaning a newly sutured wound, especially one with a drain, requires application of knowledge, problem solving, and aseptic technique. As a result, this procedure is not delegated to UAP. The nurse can ask the UAP to report soiled dressings that need to be changed or if a dressing has become loose and needs to be reinforced. The nurse is responsible for the assessment and evaluation of the wound.

TECHNIQUE 32-3 CLEANING A SUTURED WOUND AND CHANGING A DRESSING ON A WOUND WITH A DRAIN

Equipment

- Bath blanket (if necessary)
- Moistureproof bag
- Mask (optional)
- Acetone or another solution (if necessary to loosen adhesive)
- Disposable gloves
- Sterile gloves
- Sterile dressing set; if none is available, gather the following sterile items:
  - Drape or towel
  - Gauze squares
  - Container for the cleaning solution
  - Cleaning solution (e.g., normal saline)
  - Two pairs of forceps
  - Gauze dressings and surgipads
  - Applicators or tongue blades to apply ointments
- Additional supplies required for the particular dressing (e.g., extra gauze dressings and ointment, if ordered)
- Tape, tie tapes, or binder

Preparation

Prepare the client and assemble the equipment.

- Acquire assistance for changing a dressing on a restless or confused adult. *The person might move and contaminate the sterile field or the wound.*
- Assist the client to a comfortable position in which the wound can be readily exposed. Expose only the wound area, using a bath blanket to cover the client, if necessary. *Undue exposure is physically and psychologically distressing to most people.*
- Make a cuff on the moistureproof bag for disposal of the soiled dressings, and place the bag within reach. It can be taped to the bedclothes or bedside table. *Making a cuff helps keep the outside of the bag free from contamination by the soiled dressings and prevents subsequent contamination of the nurse's hands or of sterile instrument tips when discarding dressing or sponges. Placement of the bag within reach prevents the nurse from reaching across the sterile field and the wound and potentially contaminating these areas.*
- Put on a face mask, if required. *Some agencies require that a mask be worn for surgical dressing changes to prevent contamination of the wound by droplet spray from the nurse's respiratory tract.*

Performance

1. Explain to the client what you are going to do, why it is necessary, and how he or she can cooperate. Discuss how the results will be used in planning further care or treatments.

2. Wash hands and observe other appropriate infection control procedures.

3. Provide for client privacy.

4. Remove binders and tape.
   - Remove binders, if used, and place them aside. Untie tie tapes, if used. Montgomery straps (tie tapes) are commonly used for wounds requiring frequent dressing changes (Figure 32-9 ◆). *These straps prevent skin irritation and discomfort caused by removing the adhesive each time the dressing is changed.*
   - If adhesive tape was used, remove it by holding down the skin and pulling the tape gently but firmly toward the wound. *Pressing down on the skin provides countertraction against the pulling motion. Tape is pulled toward the incision to prevent strain on the sutures or wound.*
   - Use a solvent to loosen tape, if required. *Moistening the tape with acetone or a similar solvent lessens the discomfort of removal, particularly from hairy surfaces.*

5. Remove and dispose of soiled dressings appropriately.
   - Put on clean disposable gloves, and remove the outer abdominal dressing or surgipad.
   - Lift the outer dressing so that the underside is *away* from the client's face. *The appearance and odor of the drainage may be upsetting to the client.*

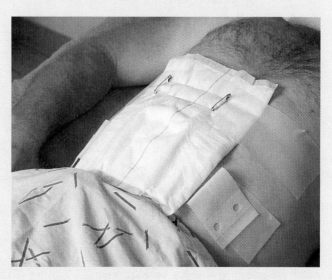

FIGURE 32-9 ◆ Montgomery straps with dressing.

- Place the soiled dressing in the moistureproof bag without touching the outside of the bag. *Contamination of the outside of the bag is avoided to prevent the spread of microorganisms to the nurse and subsequently to others.*

- Remove the under dressings, taking care not to dislodge any drains. If the gauze sticks to the drain, support the drain with one hand and remove the gauze with the other.

- Assess the location, type (color, consistency), and odor of wound drainage, and the number of gauzes saturated or the diameter of drainage collected on the dressings.

- Discard the soiled dressings in the bag as before.

- Remove gloves, dispose of them in the moisture-proof bag, and wash hands.

6. Set up the sterile supplies.

- Open the sterile dressing set, using surgical aseptic technique.

- Place the sterile drape beside the wound.

- Open the sterile cleaning solution, and pour it over the gauze sponges in the plastic container.

- Put on sterile gloves.

7. Clean the wound, if indicated.

- Clean the wound, using your gloved hands or forceps and gauze swabs moistened with cleaning solution.

- If using forceps, keep the forceps tips lower than the handles at all times. *This prevents their contamination by fluid traveling up to the handle and nurse's wrist and back to the tips.*

- Use the cleaning methods illustrated and described in Figure 32-10 ◆ or one recommended by agency protocol.

- Use a separate swab for each stroke, and discard each swab after use. *This prevents the introduction of microorganisms to other wound areas.*

- If a drain is present, clean it next, taking care to avoid reaching across the cleaned incision. Clean the skin around the drain site by swabbing in half or full circles from around the drain site outward, using separate swabs for each wipe (Figure 32-10C).

- Support and hold the drain erect while cleaning around it. Clean as many times as necessary to remove the drainage.

- Dry the surrounding skin with dry gauze swabs as required. Do not dry the incision or wound itself. Moisture facilitates wound healing.

8. Apply dressings to the drain site and the incision.

- Place a precut 4″ × 4″ gauze snugly around the drain (Figure 32-11 ◆), or open a 4″ × 4″ gauze to 4″ × 8″, fold it lengthwise to 2″ × 8″, and place the 2″ × 8″ gauze around the drain so that the ends overlap. *This dressing absorbs the drainage and helps prevent it from excoriating the skin. Using*

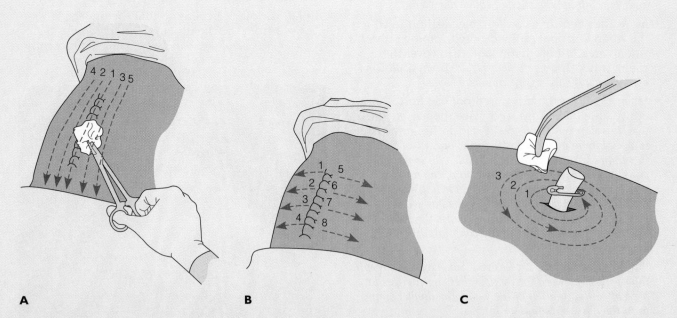

A **B** **C**

FIGURE 32-10 ◆ Methods of cleaning surgical wounds: (A) cleaning the wound from top to bottom, starting at the center; (B) cleaning a wound outward from the incision; (C) cleaning around a Penrose drain site. For all methods, a clean sterile swab is used for each stroke.

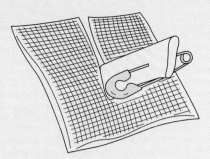

FIGURE 32-11 ◆ Precut gauze in place around a drain.

precut gauze or folding it as described, instead of cutting the gauze, prevents any threads from coming

loose and getting into the wound, where they could cause inflammation and provide a site for infection.

- Apply the sterile dressings one at a time over the drain and the incision. Place the bulk of the dressings over the drain area and below the drain, depending on the client's usual position. *Layers of dressings are placed for best absorption of drainage, which flows by gravity.*

- Apply the final surgipad, remove gloves, and dispose of them. Secure the dressing with tape or ties.

9. **Document** the procedure and all nursing assessments.

EVALUATION

- Conduct appropriate follow-up, such as amount of granulation tissue or degree of healing; amount of drainage and its color, consistency, and odor; presence of inflammation; degree of discomfort associated with the incision or drain site.

- Relate to previous findings, if available.

- Report significant deviations from normal to the physician.

Wound Drains and Suction

Surgical drains are inserted to permit the drainage of excessive serosanguineous fluid and purulent material and to promote healing of underlying tissues. These drains may be inserted and sutured through the incision line, but they are most commonly inserted through stab wounds a few centimeters away from the incision line so that the incision itself may be kept dry. Without a drain, some wounds would heal on the surface and trap the discharge inside. Then, the tissues under the skin could not heal because of the discharge and an abscess might form. These drains (e.g., the Penrose drain) have an open end that drains onto a dressing.

Drains vary in length and width. The length can be 25 to 35 cm (10 to 14 in), and the width 1.2 to 4 cm (0.5 to 1.5 in). To facilitate drainage and healing of tissues from the inside to the outside, the physician may order that the drain be pulled out or shortened 2 to 5 cm (1 to 2 in) each day. When a drain is completely removed, the remaining stab wound usually heals within a day or two. In some agencies, this shortening procedure is performed only by physicians; in others, it is ordered by the physician and performed by nurses. When changing a dressing of a draining wound, the nurse should be careful not to dislodge the drain. Shortening the drain is usually

done when the dressing is changed. Steps involved in shortening a drain are shown in Box 32-5.

A **closed wound drainage system** consists of a drain connected to either an electric suction or a portable drainage suction, such as a **Hemovac** (Figure 32-12 ◆) or **Jackson–Pratt** (Figure 32-13 ◆). The closed system reduces the possible entry of microorganisms into the wound through the drain. The drainage tubes are sutured in place and connected to a reservoir. For example, the Jackson–Pratt drainage tube is connected to a reservoir that maintains constant low suction. These portable wound suctions also provide for accurate measurement of the drainage.

The surgeon inserts the wound drainage tube during surgery. Generally, the suction is discontinued from 3 to 5 days postoperatively or when the drainage is minimal. Nurses are responsible for maintaining the wound suction, which hastens the healing process by draining excess exudates that might otherwise interfere with the formation of granulation tissue.

Closed wound drainage systems have directions for use printed on the drainage container. When emptying the container, the nurse should wear gloves and avoid touching the drainage port. Technique 32-4 describes how to maintain a closed wound drainage system.

Nursing Process: Wound Drains and Suction

ASSESSMENT

Assess:

- Amount, color, consistency, clarity, and odor of the drainage

- Discomfort around the area of the drain

- Clinical signs of infection (e.g., elevated body temperature)

- Tube patency (e.g., movement of drainage through tube to collection device; connection sites intact)

Box 32-5 *Shortening a Penrose Drain*

- Remove dressings, put on sterile gloves, and clean the incision (Technique 32-3).
- Clean the drain site appropriately (Figure 32-10C). Assess the amount and character of drainage, including odor, thickness, and color.
- If the drain has *not* been shortened before, cut and remove the suture holding it in place. *The drain is sutured to the skin during surgery to keep it from slipping into the body cavity.*
- Firmly grasp the drain by its full width at the level of the skin and pull the drain out the required length. *Grasping the full width of the drain ensures even traction.*

- Insert a sterile safety pin through the base of the drain as close to the skin as possible by holding the drain tightly against the skin edge and inserting the pin above your fingers (see figure). *The pin keeps the drain from falling back into the incision. Holding the drain securely in place at the skin level and inserting the pin above the fingers prevents the nurse from pulling the drain further out or pricking the client during this step.*
- With the sterile scissors, cut off the excess drain so that about 2.5 cm (1 in) remains above the skin (see figure). Discard the excess in the waste bag.
- Apply dressings to the drain site and the incision.

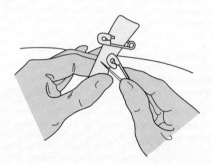

Pinning a drain.

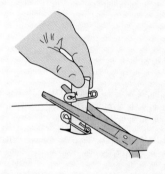

Shortening a drain.

PLANNING

Delegation

Assessment of the wound, wound drainage, and patency of the wound suction requires application of knowledge and problem solving and is the responsibility of the nurse and is not delegated to UAP. The UAP, however, can empty the drainage unit, measure the drainage, and record the amount on the intake and output record. The nurse must ensure that the UAP knows how to empty the unit without contaminating it.

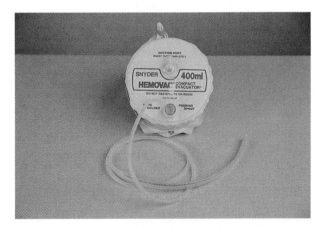

FIGURE 32-12 ◆ Hemovac closed wound drainage system.

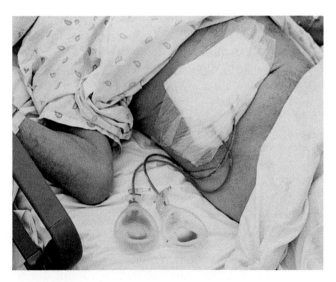

FIGURE 32-13 ◆ Two Jackson–Pratt devices compressed to facilitate collection of exudates.

Equipment

- Disposable gloves
- Calibrated drainage receptacle
- Moistureproof pad
- Alcohol sponge
- Closed wound drainage system (e.g., Hemovac or Jackson–Pratt)

Preparation

Determine the type and placement of the client's closed wound drainage.

Performance

1. Explain to the client what you are going to do, why it is necessary, and how he or she can cooperate.

2. Wash hands and observe other appropriate infection control procedures.

3. Provide for client privacy.

4. Empty the drainage unit.
   - Put on clean gloves.
   - Place the Hemovac or Jackson–Pratt unit on the waterproof pad.
   - Open the plug of the drainage unit.
   - Invert the unit and empty it into the collecting receptacle (Figure 32-14 ◆).

5. Reestablish suction.

Hemovac
- Place the unit on a solid, flat surface with port open.
- Place palm of hand on unit and press the top and the bottom together.
- While holding the top and bottom together, cleanse the opening and plug with alcohol swab (Figure 32-15 ◆).
- Replace the drainage plug before releasing hand pressure. *This reestablishes the vacuum necessary for the closed drainage system to work.*

Jackson–Pratt
- Compress the bulb with the port open.
- While maintaining tight compression on the bulb, cleanse the ends of the emptying port.
- Insert the plug into the emptying port. *This reestablishes the vacuum necessary for the closed drainage system to work.*

6. Secure the unit to the client's gown or position suction unit on the bed.
   - Ensure that the unit is below the level of the wound *as this facilitates drainage.*

7. **Document** all relevant information.
   - Record the emptying of the drainage unit and the nursing assessments.
   - Record the amount and type of drainage on the intake and output record.

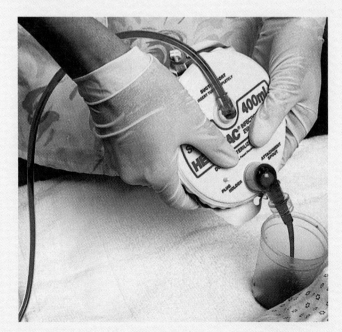

FIGURE 32-14 ◆ Emptying drainage from Hemovac drainage system.

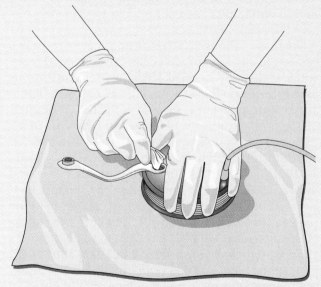

FIGURE 32-15 ◆ With one hand, press the top and bottom together. With the other hand, clean the opening and plug with an alcohol swab. Replace the plug before releasing hand.

AMBULATORY AND COMMUNITY SETTINGS

Closed Wound Drainage System

- Schedule regular nursing visits to teach wound care and to observe the drainage site.
- Teach the client or a caregiver to empty, measure, and record the drainage at least once daily.
- Instruct the caregiver to observe the wound daily for signs of infection, such as redness, edema, tenderness or purulent drainage. The client's temperature should be measured twice daily. *Elevated temperature can indicate infection.*
- Ensure that the client has the proper supplies and knows how to obtain new items as needed.
- Notify the physician of excess drainage, signs of infection, or occlusion of the tube.
- Determine when the physician plans to remove the drain and help the client keep the appointment.

EVALUATION

- Conduct appropriate follow-up, such as amount of drainage and its color, clarity, consistency, and odor; increased or decreased discomfort; and clinical signs of infection.
- Relate to previous findings if available.
- Report significant deviations from normal to the physician.

Sutures

Sutures are threads used to sew body tissues together. Sutures used to attach tissues beneath the skin are often made of an absorbable material that disappears in several days. Skin sutures, by contrast, are made of a variety of nonabsorbable materials, such as silk, cotton, linen, wire, nylon, and Dacron (polyester fiber). Silver wire clips or **staples** are also available. Usually, sutures and staples are removed 7 to 10 days after surgery if healing is adequate.

There are various methods of suturing. Skin sutures can be broadly categorized as either **interrupted** (each stitch is tied and knotted separately) or **continuous** (one thread runs in a series of stitches and is tied only at the beginning and at the end of the run). Common methods of suturing are illustrated in Figure 32-16 ◆.

Retention sutures are very large sutures used in addition to skin sutures for some incisions (Figure 32-17 ◆). They attach underlying tissues of fat and muscle as well as skin and are used to support incisions in obese individuals or when healing may be prolonged. They are frequently left in place longer than skin sutures (14 to 21 days) but in some instances are removed at the same time as the skin sutures. To prevent these large sutures from irritating the incision, the surgeon may place rubber tubing over them.

The physician orders the removal of sutures. In some agencies, only physicians remove sutures; in others, registered nurses and nursing students with appropriate supervision may do so. Agency policies about removal of retention sutures vary. The nurse should verify whether they are to be removed and who may remove them.

Sterile technique and special suture scissors are used in suture removal. The scissors have a short, curved cutting tip that readily slides under the suture (Figure 32-18 ◆). Wire clips or staples are removed

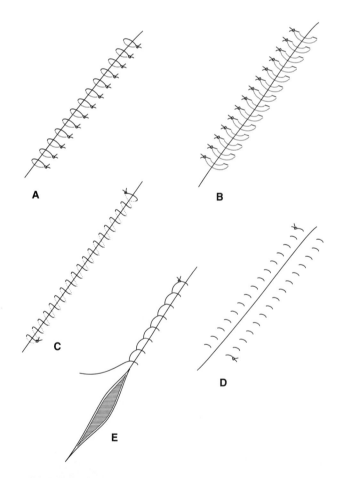

FIGURE 32-16 ◆ Common sutures: (A) plain interrupted; (B) mattress interrupted; (C) plain continuous; (D) mattress continuous; (E) blanket continuous.

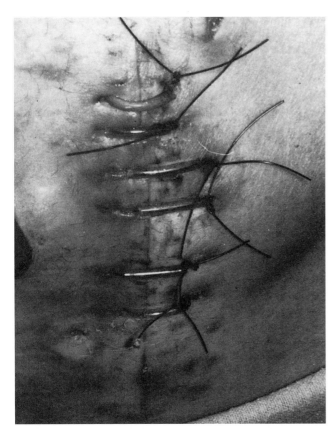

FIGURE 32-17 ◆ A surgical incision with retention sutures.

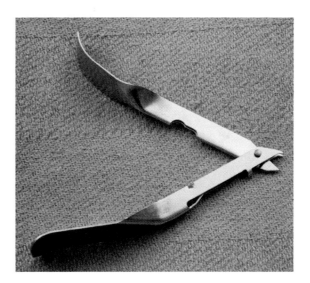

FIGURE 32-19 ◆ Staple remover.

with a special instrument that squeezes the center of the clip to remove it from the skin (Figures 32-19 ◆ and 32-20 ◆).

Nursing Process: Sutures

ASSESSMENT

Assess:

• Appearance of suture line

• Factors contraindicating suture removal (e.g., nonuniformity of closure, inflammation, presence of drainage)

PLANNING

Before removing skin sutures, verify (1) the orders for suture removal (many times only alternate interrupted sutures or staples are removed one day and the remaining sutures or staples are removed a day or two later); (2) whether a dressing is to be applied following the suture removal; and (3) when the client may bathe or shower. Some physicians prefer no dressing; others prefer a small, light gauze dressing to prevent friction by clothing.

Delegation

Removal of sutures or staples requires application of knowledge and problem solving and is not delegated to UAP.

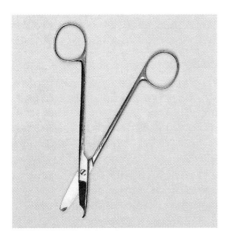

FIGURE 32-18 ◆ Suture scissors.

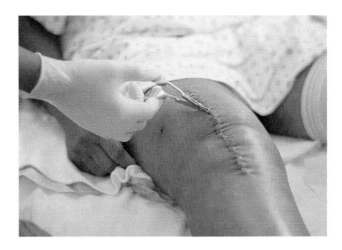

FIGURE 32-20 ◆ Removing surgical clips or staples.

Equipment

- Waterproof bag
- Sterile gloves
- Nonsterile gloves
- Sterile dressing equipment including:
  - Sterile suture scissors
  - Sterile hemostat or forceps
  - Sterile butterfly tape or Steri-Strips (optional)
- Tape (if a dressing is to be applied)

Performance

1. Explain to the client what you are going to do, why it is necessary, and how he or she can cooperate. Inform the client that suture removal may produce slight discomfort, such as a pulling or stinging sensation, but should not be painful.

2. Wash hands and observe other appropriate infection control procedures.

3. Provide for client privacy.

4. Remove dressings and clean the incision.
   - Put on sterile gloves.
   - Clean the suture line with an antimicrobial solution before and after suture removal. *This is generally done as a prophylactic measure to prevent infection.*

5. Remove the sutures.

Plain Interrupted Sutures
- Grasp the suture at the knot with a pair of forceps.
- Place the curved tip of the suture scissors under the suture as close to the skin as possible, either on the side opposite the knot (Figure 32-21 ◆) or directly under the knot. Cut the suture. *Sutures are cut as close to the skin as possible on one side of the visible part because the visible suture material is contaminated with skin bacteria and must not be pulled beneath the skin during removal. Suture material that is beneath the skin is considered free from bacteria.*
- With the forceps or hemostat, pull the suture out in one piece. Inspect carefully to make sure that all suture material is removed. *Suture material left beneath the skin acts as a foreign body and causes inflammation.*
- Discard the suture onto a piece of sterile gauze or into the moistureproof bag, being careful not to contaminate the forceps tips. Sometimes, the suture sticks to the forceps and needs to be removed by wiping the tips on a sterile gauze.
- Continue to remove *alternate* sutures, such as the

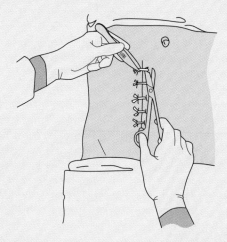

FIGURE 32-21 ◆ Removing a plain interrupted skin suture.

third, fifth, seventh, and so forth. *Alternate sutures are removed first so that remaining sutures keep the skin edges in close approximation and prevent any dehiscence from becoming large.*
- If no dehiscence occurs, remove the remaining sutures. If dehiscence does occur, do not remove the remaining sutures, and report the dehiscence to the nurse in charge.
- If Steri-Strips are ordered by the physician or a little **wound dehiscence** occurs, apply a sterile Steri-Strip over the wound or gap:
  a. Attach the Steri-Strip to one side of the incision.
  b. Press the wound edges together.
  c. Attach the Steri-Strip to the other side of the incision. *The Steri-Strip (a thin strip of sterile, nonwoven, porous fabric tape) holds the wound edges as close together as possible and promotes healing. Some physicians order Steri-Strip application to provide additional support to the healing wound.*
- If a large dehiscence occurs, cover the wound with sterile gauze and report the problem immediately to the nurse in charge or physician.

Mattress Interrupted Sutures
- When possible, cut the visible part of the suture close to the skin, at A and B in Figure 32-22 ◆, opposite the knot and remove this small visible piece. Discard it as described above. In some sutures, the visible part opposite the knot may be so small that it can be cut only once.
- Grasp the knot (C) with forceps. Remove the remainder of the suture beneath the skin by pulling out in the direction of the knot.

Plain Continuous Sutures
- Cut the thread of the first suture opposite the

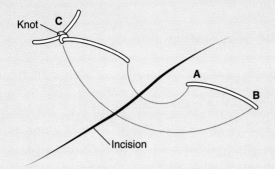

FIGURE 32-22 ◆ Mattress interrupted sutures.

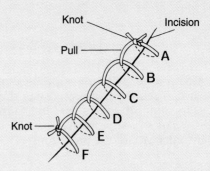

FIGURE 32-24 ◆ Blanket continuous sutures.

knot at A in Figure 32-23 ◆. Then cut the thread of the second suture on the same side at B.

- Grasp the knot (C) with the forceps and pull. *This removes the first stitch and the piece of thread beneath the skin, which is attached to the second stitch.* Discard the suture.
- Cut off the visible part of the second suture at D, and discard it.
- Grasp the suture at E and pull out the underlying loop between D and E.
- Cut the visible part at F and remove it.
- Repeat the above two steps at G through J, until the last knot is reached. Note that after the first stitch is removed, each thread is cut down the same side, below the original knot.
- Cut the last suture at L and pull out the last suture at K.

Blanket Continuous Sutures

- Cut the threads that are opposite the looped blanket edge; for example, cut at A through F in Figure 32-24 ◆.
- Pull each stitch out at the looped edge.

Mattress Continuous Sutures

- Cut the visible suture at both skin edges opposite the knot (at A and B in Figure 32-25 ◆) and the next suture opposite the knot (at C and D). Remove and discard the visible portions as described above.
- Pull the first suture out by the knot at E.

- Lift the second suture between F and G to pull out the underlying suture between G and C. Cut off the visible part at F as close to the skin edge as possible.
- Go to the opposite side between H and I. Lift out the suture between F and I and cut off all the visible part close to the skin at H.
- Lift the suture between J and K to pull out the suture between H and K and cut the suture close to the skin at J.
- Repeat the above two steps, working from side to side of the incision until the last suture is reached.
- Cut the visible suture opposite the knot at L and M. Pull out all remaining pieces of suture at O.

6. Clean and cover the incision.
   - Clean the incision again with antimicrobial solution.
   - Apply small, light, sterile gauze dressing if any small dehiscence has occurred or if this is agency practice.

7. Instruct the client about follow-up wound care.
   - Generally, if a wound is dry and healing well, the person can take showers in a day or two.
   - Instruct the client to contact the physician if increased redness, drainage, or open areas are observed.

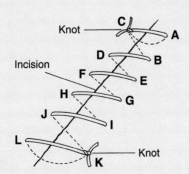

FIGURE 32-23 ◆ Plain continuous sutures.

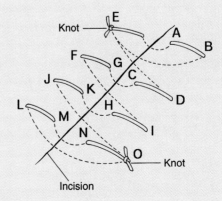

FIGURE 32-25 ◆ Mattress continuous sutures.

8. **Document** the suture removal, number of sutures removed, appearance of the incision, application of a dressing, Steri-Strips or butterfly tapes (if appropriate), client teaching, and client tolerance of the procedure.

Variation: Removing Staples

- Repeat steps 1 through 4.
- Place lower tips of sterile staple remover under the staple.

- Squeeze the handles together until they are completely closed. *Pressing the handles together causes the staple to bend in the middle and pulls the edges of the staple out of the skin.* Do not lift the staple remover when squeezing the handles.
- When both ends of the staple are visible, gently move the staple away from the incision site.
- Hold the staple remover over a disposable container, release the staple remover handles and release the staple.
- Repeat steps 6 through 8.

AMBULATORY AND COMMUNITY SETTINGS

Removing Sutures or Staples

- Perform the procedure in a well-lighted, private area of the home.
- Instruct the client to observe the incision daily and call the health care provider if increased redness, drainage, or open areas are observed.

- Provide instructions and supplies for care of the incision, and tell the client when to shower for the first time.
- Assess the client's ability to keep the incision clean and protected at home.

EVALUATION

- Conduct appropriate follow-up, such as: status of suture line, any wound separation, or discharge.

- Relate to previous findings, if available.
- Report significant deviations from normal to the physician.

Chapter Summary

TERMINOLOGY

closed wound drainage system
continuous suction regulators
continuous sutures
drains
Hemovac
intermittent suction regulators
interrupted sutures

intraoperative phase
Jackson–Pratt
Penrose drain
perioperative period
postanesthesia care unit (PACU)
postanesthetic room (PAR)
postoperative phase

preoperative phase
recovery room (RR)
retention sutures
staples
sutures
wound dehiscence
Wound evisceration

FORMING CLINICAL JUDGMENTS

Consider This:

1. The client does not understand English and preoperative teaching needs to be done. What would you do?

2. The client returned from surgery with a Salem sump tube in place and connected to suction. The nurse notes that gastric contents are coming out of the blue air vent of the tube. What would you do?

3. What action would you take if the postop client has diminished breath sounds in the right base and a respiratory rate of 24/min?

4. The UAP informs you that a client, who had major abdominal surgery 4 days ago, said that "something gave way" and the client felt a "popping" sensation in his incision. What would you do?

RELATED RESEARCH

Lookinland, S., & Pool, M. (1998). Study on effect of methods of preoperative education in women. *AORN Journal, 67*(1), 203–213.

Mimnaugh, L. Winegar, M., Mabrey, Y., & Davis, J. E. (1999). Sensations experienced during removal of tubes in acute postoperative patients. *Applied Nursing Research, 12*(2), 78–85.

REFERENCES

Ben-Hamida, A., & Meyrick-Thomas, J. (1998). Postoperative wound drainage. *Care of the Critically Ill, 14*(2), insert 4p.

Brenner, Z. R. (1999). Preventing postoperative complications: What's old, what's new, what's tried-and-true. *Nursing, 29*(10), 34–39.

Brockway, P. M. (1997). The ambulatory surgical nurse: Evolution, competency, and vision. *Nursing Clinics of North America, 32*(2), 387–394.

Castille, K. (1998). Suturing. *Nursing Standard, 12*(41), 41–48.

DeFazio-Quinn, D. M. (1997). Ambulatory surgery: An evolution. *Nursing Clinics of North America, 32*(2), 377–386.

Dunn, D. (1998). Preoperative assessment criteria and patient teaching for ambulatory surgery patients. *Journal of PeriAnesthesia Nursing, 13*(5), 274–291.

Ennis, D. (1999). Reducing the risk of surgical site infection. *Nursing, 29*(6), 32-1–32.2.

Fox, V. J. (1998). Postoperative education that works. *AORN Journal, 67*(5), 1010–1017.

Hrouda, B. S. (2000). How to remove surgical sutures and staples. *Nursing, 30*(2), 54–55.

Kost, M. (1999). Conscious sedation: Guarding your patient against complications. *Nursing, 29*(4), 34–39.

McConnell, E. A. (1999). Clinical do's & don'ts: Using a closed-wound drainage system. *Nursing, 29*(6), 32.

McConnell, E. A. (1998). Clinical do's & don'ts: Managing wound dehiscence and evisceration. *Nursing, 28*(9), 26.

Shaheen, K. W. (1998). Jackson–Pratt drains: Patient discharge instructions. *Plastic Surgical Nursing, 18*(1), 50.

Van Keuren, K., & Eland, J. A. (1997). Perioperative pain management in children. *Nursing Clinics of North America, 32*(1), 31–43.

Appendix A   Root Words, Prefixes, and Suffixes

Word element	Meaning
Root Words	
Circulatory System	
angio, vaso	vessel
arteria	artery
cardio	heart
embolus	moving clot
hem, hema, hemato	blood
lympho	lymph
thrombo	clot (of blood)
vena, phlebo	vein
Digestive System	
ano, procto	anus
appendeco	appendix
bucca	cheek
caeco	cecum
cholecyst	gallbladder
colo	colon
duodeno	duodenum
entero	intestines
esophago	esophagus
gastro	stomach
gingiva	gum
glossa	tongue
hepato	liver
ileo	ileum
jejuno	jejunum
os, stomato	mouth
pancreas	pancreas
pharyngo	pharynx
recto	rectum
Skeletal System	
skeleto	skeleton
Respiratory System	
bronchus, broncho	bronchus (pl. bronchi)
laryngo	larynx
naso, rhino	nose
pulmo, pneuma, pneum	lung (sac with air)
tonsillo	tonsil
tracheo	trachea
Nervous System	
cerebrum	brain
neuro	nerve
oculo, ophthalmo	eye
oto	ear
psych, psycho	mind
Urinary System	
cysto	bladder
pyelo	pelvis of kidney
reni, reno, nephro	kidney
uretero	ureter

Word element	Meaning
urethro	urethra
uro	urine
Female Reproductive System	
cervico	cervix
labio	labium (pl. labia)
ovario, oophoro	ovary
perineo	perineum
tubo, salpingo	fallopian tube
utero	womb; uterus
vagino, colpo	vagina
vulvo	vulva
Male Reproductive System	
orchido	testes
Regions of the Body	
abdomino	abdomen
cervico, tracheo	neck
crani, cephalo	head
dorsum	back
thoraco	chest
Tissues	
chondro	cartilage
cutis, dermato	skin
lipo	fat
musculo, myo	muscle
myelo	marrow
osteo	bone
Miscellaneous	
cyto	cell
genetic	formation, origin
gram	tracing or mark
graph	writing, description
kinesis	motion
lapar	flank; through the abdominal wall
meter	measure
oligo	small, few
phobia	fear
photo	light
pyo	pus
roentgen	x-ray
scope	instrument for visual examination
Prefixes	
a, an, ar	without or not
ab	away from
acro	extremities
ad	toward, to
adeno	glandular
aero	air
ambi	around, on both sides
amyl	starch
ante	before, forward

Word element	Meaning	Word element	Meaning
anti	against, counteracting	mono	single
bi	double	multi	many
bili	bile	myelo	bone marrow, spinal cord
bio	life	myo	muscle
bis	two	neo	new
brachio	arm	nephro	kidney
brady	slow	neuro	nerve
broncho	bronchus (pl. bronchi)	nitro	nitrogen
cardio	heart	noct	night
cervico	neck	non	not
chole	gall or bile	ob	against, in front of
cholecysto	gallbladder	oculo	eye
circum	around	odonto	tooth
co	together	ophthalmo	eye
contra	against, opposite	ortho	straight, normal
costo	ribs	os	mouth, opening
cyto	cell	osteo	bone
cysto	bladder	oto	ear
demi	half	pan	all
derma	skin	para	beside, accessory to
dis	from	path	disease
dorso	back	ped	child, foot
dys	abnormal, difficult	per	by, through
electro	electric	peri	around
en	into, in, within	pharyngo	pharynx
encephal	brain	phlebo	vein
entero	intestine	photo	light
equi	equal	phren	diaphragm, mind
eryth	red	pneumo	air, lungs
ex	out, out of, away from	pod	foot
extra	outside of, in addition to	poly	many, much
ferro	iron	post	after
fibro	fiber	pre	before
fore	before, in front of	proct	rectum
gastro	stomach	pseudo	false
glosso	tongue	psych	mind
glyco	sugar	pyel	pelvis of the kidney
hemi	half	pyo	pus
hemo	blood	pyro	fever, heat
hepa, hepato	liver	quadri	four
histo	tissue	radio	radiation
homo	same	re	back, again
hydro	water	reno	kidney
hygro	moisture	retro	backward
hyper	too much, high	rhin	nose
hypo	under, decreased	sacro	sacrum
hyster	uterus	salpingo	fallopian tube
ileo	ileum	sarco	flesh
in	in, within, into	sclero	hard, hardening
inter	between	semi	half
intra	within	sex	six
intro	in, within, into	skeleto	skeleton
juxta	near, close to	steno	narrowing, constriction
laryngo	larynx	sub	under
latero	side	super	above, excess
lapar	abdomen	supra	above
leuk	white	syn	together
macro	large, big	tachy	fast
mal	bad, poor	thyro	thyroid, gland
mast	breast	trache	trachea
medio	middle	trans	across, over
mega, megalo	large, great	tri	three
meno	menses	ultra	beyond
micro	small, tiny	un	not, back, reversal

Word element	Meaning	Word element	Meaning
uni	one	lithiasis	presence of stones
uretero	ureter	lysis	disintegration
urethro	urethra	megaly	enlargement
uro	urine, urinary organs	meter	instrument that measures
vaso	vessel	oid	likeness, resemblance
		oma	tumor
Suffixes		opathy	disease of
		orrhaphy	surgical repair
able	able to	osis	disease, condition of
algia	pain	ostomy	to form an opening or outlet
cele	tumor, swelling	otomy	to incise
centesis	surgical puncture to remove fluid	pexy	fixation
cide	killing, destructive	phage	ingesting
cule	little	phobia	fear
cyte	cell	plasty	plastic surgery
ectasia	dilating, stretching	plegia	paralysis
ectomy	excision, surgical removal of	rhage	to burst forth
emia	blood	rhea	excessive discharge
esis	action	rhexis	rupture
form	shaped like	scope	lighted instrument for visual examination
genesis, genetric	formation, origin		
gram	tracing, mark	scopy	to examine visually
graph	writing	stomy	to form an opening
ism	condition	tomy	incision into
itis	inflammation	uria	urine
ize	to treat		
lith	stone, calculus		

Appendix B Weight and Volume Equivalents

METRIC EQUIVALENTS

Weights			Volume		
1 picogram	=	10^{-12} gram	1 milliliter	=	1 gram
1 nanogram	=	10^{-9} gram	1 liter	=	1 kilogram = 1000 grams (milliliters)
1 microgram	=	10^{-3} milligram = 10^{-6} gram			
1 milligram	=	1000 micrograms = 10^{-6} gram			
1 centigram	=	10 milligrams = 10^{-1} decigram = 10^{-2} gram			
1 decigram	=	100 milligrams = 10 centigrams = 10^{-1} gram			
1 gram	=	1000 milligrams = 100 centigrams = 10 decigrams			
1 kilogram	=	1000 grams			

APPROXIMATE WEIGHT EQUIVALENTS: METRIC AND APOTHECARIES' SYSTEMS

Metric	Apothecaries'	Metric	Apothecaries'
0.1 mg	1/600 grain	30 mg	1/2 grain
1.12 mg	1/500 grain	40 mg	2/3 grain
0.15 mg	1/400 grain	50 mg	3/4 grain
0.2 mg	1/300 grain	60 mg	1 grain
0.25 mg	1/250 grain	100 mg (0.1 gm)	1-1/2 grains
0.3 mg	1/200 grain	150 mg (0.15 gm)	2-1/2 grains
0.4 mg	1/150 grain	200 mg (0.2 gm)	3 grains
0.5 mg	1/120 grain	300 mg (0.3 gm)	5 grains
0.6 mg	1/100 grain	400 mg (0.4 gm)	6 grains
0.8 mg	1/80 grain	500 mg (0.5 gm)	7-1/2 grains
1 mg	1/60 grain	600 mg (0.6 gm)	10 grains
1.2 mg	1/50 grain	1 gram	15 grains
1.5 mg	1/40 grain	1.5 gm	22 grains
2 mg	1/30 grain	2 gm	30 grains
3 mg	1/20 grain	3 gm	45 grains
4 mg	1/15 grain	4 gm	60 grains (1 dram)
5 mg	1/12 grain	5 gm	75 grains
6 mg	1/10 grain	6 gm	90 grains
8 mg	1/8 grain	7.5 gm	120 grains (2 drams)
10 mg	1/6 grain	10 gm	2-1/2 drams
12 mg	1/5 grain	30 gm	1 ounce (8 drams)
15 mg	1/4 grain	500 gm	1.1 pounds
20 mg	1/3 grain	1000 gm	2.2 pounds (1 kilogram)
25 mg	3/8 grain		

Appendix B Weight and Volume Equivalents

APPROXIMATE VOLUME EQUIVALENTS: METRIC, APOTHECARIES', AND HOUSEHOLD SYSTEMS

Metric	Apothecaries'	Household
0.06 ml	1 minim (m)	1 drop (qt)
0.3 ml	5 minims	
0.6 ml	10 minims	
1 ml	15 minims	15 drops (gtt)
2 ml	30 minims	
3 ml	45 minims	
4 ml	60 minims (1 fluid dram)	60 drops (1 teaspoon [tsp])
8 ml	2 fluid drams	2 teaspoons
15 ml	4 fluid drams	4 teaspoons (1 tablespoon [Tbsp])
30 ml	8 fluid drams (1 fluid ounce)	2 tablespoons
60 ml	2 fluid ounces	
90 ml	3 fluid ounces	
200 ml	6 fluid ounces	1 teacup
250 ml	8 fluid ounces	1 large glass
500 ml	16 fluid ounces (1 pint)	1 pint
750 ml	11/2 pints	
1000 ml (1 liter)	2 pints (1 quart)	1 quart
4000 ml	4 quarts	1 gallon

Glossary

Abdominal (diaphragmatic) breathing Breathing that involves the contraction and relaxation of the diaphragm

Acid-fast bacillus (AFB) A laboratory test to identify the organism *Mycobacterium tuberculosis*

Active–assistive range-of-motion (ROM) exercise The client, with the nurse's assistance, uses a stronger, opposite arm or leg to move each of the joints of a limb incapable of active motion

Active range-of-motion (ROM) exercise Isotonic exercise in which the client moves each joint in the body through its complete range of movement, maximally stretching all muscle groups within each plane, over the joint

Acupressure Compression of blood vessels by means of needles in surrounding tissues

Acute pain Sharp or severe discomfort; sudden onset and short course (as opposed to chronic)

Additive IV setup See Secondary IV setup

Adjuvant Medication or treatment that enhances the effects of other medications or treatments

Adventitious breath sounds Abnormal or acquired breath sounds

Aerobic Requiring oxygen

Aerosolization The production of a colloidal solution dispensed in the form of a mist

Afternoon care Hygienic care offered to the client in late afternoon

Airborne transmission Droplet nuclei or dust particles containing an infectious agent transmitted by air currents to a suitable portal of entry, usually the respiratory tract, of another person

Air-fluidized bed A specialized bed filled with sandlike granules that have air flowing through them to support the client's body

Alginate Derived from kelp, a wound care product that absorbs liquid drainage

Alignment (posture) The proper relationship of body segments to one another

Alopecia The loss of scalp hair (baldness) or body hair

Ambulation The act of walking

Ampule A glass container usually designed to hold a single dose of a drug

Anaerobic Not requiring oxygen to live

Angiocatheter A short intravenous access device (needle) made of plastic or similar material

Anisocoria Unequal pupils

Anorexia Lack of appetite

Anoxemia (hypoxemia) A condition in which the level of oxygen in the blood is below normal

Antiembolism (elastic) stockings Firm elastic hosiery that exerts external pressure to compress the veins of the legs, decrease venous blood from pooling in the extremities, and facilitate the return of venous blood to the heart

Antiseptic An agent that inhibits the growth of some microorganisms

Anuria The failure of the kidneys to produce urine, resulting in a total lack of urination or output of less than 100 mL/day in an adult

Apical pulse A central pulse located at the apex of the heart

Apical–radial pulse Measurement of the apical beat and the radial pulse at the same time

Apnea A complete absence of respirations

Aquathermia To treat with warm water

Arrhythmia (dysrhythmia) A pulse with an abnormal rhythm

Arterial blood pressure The measure of the pressure exerted by the blood as it pulsates through the arteries

Artificial airway Devices inserted to maintain a patent air passage for clients whose airway have become or may become obstructed

Asepsis Freedom from infection or infectious material

As-needed (PRN) care Provision of hygienic care as required by the client

Asphyxia Inadequate intake of oxygen

Astigmatism An uneven curvature of the cornea that prevents horizontal and vertical light rays from focusing on the retina

Asystole Cardiac standstill, absence of heart contractions

Atelectasis A condition that occurs when ventilation is decreased and pooled secretions accumulate in a dependent area of a bronchiole and block it

Atomization Production of large droplets for inhalation

Auscultation The process of listening to sounds produced within the body

Auscultatory gap The temporary disappearance of sounds normally heard over the brachial artery when the sphygmomanometer cuff pressure is high and the sounds reappear at a lower level

Automated external defibrillator (AED) Battery-operated device that senses the cardiac rhythm through two adhesive pads, determines appropriateness of electric shock to convert the rhythm to normal, and can deliver the shock manually or automatically

Axillary crutch Metal or wood pole with padded, crescent-shaped portion at the top for placing in the armpit to aid in walking

Bag bath An adaptation of the towel bath

Balance Stability; steadiness; equilibrium

Bandage A strip of paper or cloth used to wrap a part of the body

Basal metabolic rate (BMR) The rate of energy utilization in the body required to maintain essential activities such as breathing

Basal rate A low continuous infusion delivered by a PCA pump to provide sustained analgesia during times of rest and sleep

Base of support The area on which an object rests

Bevel The slanted part at the tip of a needle

Binder A type of bandage applied to large body areas (abdomen or chest) or for a specific body part (arm sling); used to provide support

Bivalve To cut into two halves such as the top and bottom of a cast

Blanch test Circulation test performed by applying and then quickly releasing pressure to a finger- or toenail and observing the loss and return of color

Bloodborne pathogens Potentially infectious organisms that are carried in and transmitted through blood or materials containing blood

Blood glucose meter A machine that measures capillary blood glucose

Body mechanics The efficient and coordinated use of the body to produce motion and maintain balance during activity

Body substance isolation A system of infection control based on the principles that all people have increased risk for infection from microorganisms placed on their mucous membranes and nonintact skin; all people may have potentially infectious microorganisms in their moist body sites and substances; and an unknown portion of clients and health care workers will always be colonized or infected with potentially infectious microorganisms in their blood and other moist body sites and substances

Bolus intermittent feedings Administration of 300 to 500 mL of enteral formula several times per day

Bradycardia Abnormally slow pulse rate, less than 60 per minute

Bradypnea Abnormally slow respiratory rate, usually less than 10 respirations per minute

Brand name Name of the drug given by the drug manufacturer

Breast self-examination (BSE) A systematic procedure for palpating one's own breast tissues in search of abnormal lumps

Bromhidrosis Foul-smelling perspiration

Bryant's traction A type of skin traction used to stabilize fractured femurs or correct congenital hip dislocation in young children

Buccal Pertaining to the cheek

Buck's extension A type of skin traction used to immobilize fractures of the hip and reduce muscle spasm before surgical repair

Butterfly (wing-tipped) needles Intravenous access needles or catheters with plastic flaps at the proximal end used to stabilize the device

Calorie (C, cal, kcal) A unit of heat energy equivalent to the amount of heat required to raise the temperature of 1 kg of water 1°C

Cane A slender stick held in the hand used for support during walking

Cannula A tube with a lumen (channel) that is inserted into a cavity or duct and is often fitted with a trocar during insertion

Capillary blood glucose (CBG) A measurement of glucose from a capillary blood specimen

Cardiac arrest The cessation of heart function

Cardinal signs See vital signs

Cardiopulmonary resuscitation (CPR) Artificial stimulation of the heart and lungs; also referred to as basic life support (BLS)

Carminative An agent that promotes the passage of flatus from the colon

Cast window A rectangular piece cut from a cast to allow release of pressure and visualization of the skin beneath

Cataract Opacity of the lens or capsule of the eye

Category-specific precautions An infection control system based on the need for strict isolation, contact isolation, respiratory isolation, tuberculosis isolation, enteric precautions, drainage/secretions precautions, or blood/body fluid precautions

Catheter A tube of rubber, plastic, metal, or other material used to remove or inject fluids into a cavity such as the bladder

Center of gravity The point at which the mass (weight) of the body is centered

Central venous line A catheter inserted into a large vein located centrally in the body (e.g., the superior vena cava, right atrium)

Cerumen The waxlike substance secreted by glands in the external ear canal

Chemical name The name by which a chemist knows the drug; describes the constituents of the drug precisely

Chemical restraints Medications used to control socially disruptive behavior

Cheyne–Stokes breathing Rhythmic waxing and waning of respirations from very deep breathing to very shallow breathing with periods of temporary apnea, often associated with cardiac failure, increased intracranial pressure, or brain damage

Chronic obstructive pulmonary disease (COPD) A disease process that decreases the ability of the lungs to perform ventilation

Chronic pain Prolonged pain, usually recurring or persisting over 6 months or longer, which interferes with functioning

Chyme Digested products that leave the stomach through the small intestine and then pass through the ileocecal valve

Clean catch See midstream urine specimen

Cleaning bath A bath given for hygienic purposes

Cleansing enema Introduction of solution into the rectum to stimulate bowel emptying

Clear liquid diet Limited to water, tea, coffee, clear broths, ginger ale or other carbonated beverages, strained and clear juices, and plain gelatin

Closed airway suction system The suction catheter, enclosed in a plastic sheath, attaches to the ventilator tubing, and the client does not need to be disconnected from the ventilator

Closed bed An unoccupied bed with the top covers drawn up to the top of the bed under the pillow

Closed system A system that does not exchange energy, matter, or information with its environment

Closed tracheal suction system The suction catheter, enclosed in a plastic sheath, attaches to the ventilator tubing, and the client does not need to be disconnected from the ventilator

Closed wound drainage system Consists of a drain connected to either an electric suction or a portable drainage suction

Clubbing (of a nail) Elevation of the proximal aspect of the nail and softening of the nailbed

Code blue Term used by an agency such as a hospital to indicate a medical emergency such as cardiac arrest

Colonic irrigation Introduction of a large amount of solution into the colon to flush it out

Colostomy An opening into the colon (large bowel)

Complete bed bath The nurse washes the entire body of a dependent client in bed

Condom A sheath or cover, usually made of rubber or plastic, worn over the penis during coitus to prevent conception or infection; urinary condoms are used to catch urine

Constipation Passage of small, dry, hard stool or passage of no stool for an abnormally long time

Contact precautions An infection control category based on providing barriers to the direct contact route of infectious organism transmission

Continuous feedings Enteral feedings administered over a 24-hour period using an infusion pump that guarantees a constant flow rate

Continuous local anesthetic Continuous subcutaneous administration of long-acting local anesthetics into or near the surgical site

Continuous passive motion (CPM) An electric device used to promote recovery after joint surgery

Continuous suction regulator Device that applies suction continuously; used with double-lumen nasogastric tubes

Continuous sutures A method of suturing; one thread runs in a series of stitches and is tied only at the beginning and at the end of the run

Contracture Permanent shortening of a muscle and subsequent shortening of tendons and ligaments

Contralateral stimulation Stimulating the skin in an area opposite the painful area

Controlled coughing Asking the client to inhale deeply and hold his or her breath for a few seconds and then instructing the client to cough twice while exhaling

Core temperature The temperature of the deep tissues of the body (e.g., thorax, abdominal cavity); relatively constant at 37°C (98.6°F)

Countertraction A force that neutralizes the direct pull of traction

CPR See cardiopulmonary resuscitation

Cross-contamination The transfer or microorganisms from one surface to another

Crutchfield tongs Metal device inserted into each side of the skull to which traction is applied

Cuffed tracheostomy tube Tracheostomy tube that is surrounded by an inflatable cuff that produces an airtight seal between the tube and the trachea

Cutaneous pain Pain that originates in the skin or subcutaneous tissue

Cutaneous stimulation Techniques to distract the client and focus attention on the tactile stimuli, away from the painful sensations, thus reducing pain perception

Cyclic feedings Continuous feedings that are administered in less than 24 hours (e.g., 12 to 16 hours)

Dandruff Dry or greasy, scaly material shed from the scalp

Debridement Removal of infected and necrotic tissue

Decubitus ulcer See pressure ulcer

Deep breathing Taking especially large volumes of inspiration

Deep somatic pain Pain that arises from ligaments, tendons, bones, blood vessels, and nerves

Deep vein thrombosis (DVT) The development of a blood clot in the deep veins of the leg

Defecation Expulsion of feces from the rectum and anus

Delegate To assign responsibility and authority for performing specific tasks to another

Deltoid site Site of the deltoid muscle, which is found on the lateral aspect of the upper arm

Dentifrice A paste or powder used to clean or polish the teeth

Dermatologic preparation A medication applied to the skin

Detrusor muscle The major longitudinal muscle of the urinary bladder

Dialysate The fluid used to remove or deliver electrolytes and other substances when the kidneys are unable to do so properly

Dialysis The movement of solutes and fluid across a semipermeable membrane

Diaphragmatic breathing (abdominal breathing) Breathing that involves the contraction and relaxation of the diaphragm

Diastole The period during which the ventricles relax

Diet as tolerated (DAT) A diet that is ordered when the client's appetite, ability to eat, and tolerance for certain foods may change

Diluent An agent that dilutes the substance or solution to which it is added

Direct transmission Immediate and direct transfer of microorganisms from person to person through touching, biting, kissing, or sexual intercourse

Disease-specific precautions Delineation of the use of private rooms, special ventilation, and use of gowns to care for clients with particular diseases or microorganisms

Disinfectant Agent that destroys all microorganisms

Divided colostomy A colostomy in which both ends of the divided colon are brought to the abdominal surface but at separate locations

DNR (do not resuscitate, no code) A physician's order that requires that no effort be made to resuscitate the client with terminal or irreversible illness in the event of a respiratory or cardiac arrest

Documentation The charting or recording of client data

Dorsal recumbent (back-lying) position A supine position with the head and shoulders slightly elevated

Dorsogluteal site A site that can be used for intramuscular injection for adults and children with well-developed gluteal muscles

Double-barreled colostomy A colostomy in which both ends of the divided colon are brought to the abdominal surface side by side

Drain A substance or appliance that assists in the discharge of serosanguinous fluid and purulent material from a wound and promotes healing of underlying tissues

Dressing A material used to cover and protect a wound

Drip factor (drop factor) The number of drops per milliliter of solution delivered for a particular drip chamber calculating the drip rate

Droplet nuclei Residue of evaporated droplets that may remain in the air for long periods of time

Drug (medication) A chemical compound taken for disease prevention, diagnosis, cure, or relief or to affect the structure or function of the body

Dwell Fluid remaining in place for a specified period of time

Dysphagia Difficulty or inability to swallow

Dysphasia Difficulty speaking

Dyspnea Difficult or labored breathing

Dysuria Painful or difficult voiding

Early morning care Hygienic care offered to clients as they awaken in the morning

Earmold The part of a hearing aid that directs the sound into the ear

Edema The presence of excess interstitial fluid in the body

Effleurage A stroking massage technique

Endotracheal suctioning Removing secretions from an endotracheal tube

Endotracheal tube A tube that is inserted through the mouth or nose into the trachea

Enema A solution introduced into the rectum and sigmoid colon to remove feces and/or flatus

Enteral nutrition (EN) Nutrition that is provided when the client is unable to ingest foods or the upper gastrointestinal tract is impaired and the transport of food to the small intestine is interrupted

Enteral Through the gastrointestinal system

Epidural anesthesia The injection of an anesthetic agent into the epidural space (the area inside the spinal column but outside the dura mater)

Erythema A redness associated with a variety of skin rashes

Eschar Thick necrotic tissue produced by burning, by a corrosive application, or by death of tissue associated with loss of vascular supply, bacterial invasion, and putrefaction

Etiology The causal relationship between a problem and its related or risk factors

Eupnea Normal, quiet breathing

Exhalation (expiration) The movement of gases from the lungs to the atmosphere

Exophthalmos A protrusion of the eyeballs with elevation of the upper eyelids, resulting in a startled or staring expression

Expiration (exhalation) The outflow of air from the lungs to the atmosphere

External catheter A condom applied to the penis to catch urine

Extravasation The escape of blood from a vessel into the body tissues

Exudate Material, such as fluid and cells, that has escaped from blood vessels during the inflammatory process and is deposited in tissue or on tissue surfaces

Face mask A mask covering the client's nose and mouth used to deliver oxygen and/or other gases

Face tent An open-topped device that covers the face used to deliver oxygen

Fasciculation An abnormal contraction or shortening of a bundle of muscle fibers

Febrile Pertaining to a fever; feverish

Fecal impaction A mass or collection of hardened, puttylike feces in the folds of the rectum

Fecal incontinence (bowel incontinence) Loss of voluntary ability to control fecal and gaseous discharges through the anal sphincter

Feces (stool) Body wastes and undigested food eliminated from the rectum

Fenestrated tracheostomy tube A tracheostomy tube that has holes in the outer cannula

Fever Elevated body temperature

Filter needle When using a medication ampule, the filter needle prevents glass particles from being withdrawn with the medication

Flail chest The ballooning out of the chest wall through fractured rib spaces during exhalation

Flange The part of the outer cannula of a tracheostomy tube that rests against the neck and allows the tube to be secured in place with tape or ties

Flatness (of sound) An extremely dull sound produced, during percussion, by very dense tissue, such as muscle or bone

Flow-oriented SMI Flow-oriented sustained maximal inspiration devices

Fomite An inanimate object other than food that can harbor disease-producing microorganisms and transmit an infection

Fowler's position A bed sitting position with the head of the bed raised to 45 degrees

Full liquid diet Contains only liquids or foods that turn to liquid at body temperature such as ice cream

Gastrostomy tube A tube that enters the stomach through a surgical opening in the abdominal wall

Gauge The diameter of the shaft of a needle; the larger the gauge number, the smaller the diameter of the shaft

Generic name (of drug) A drug name not protected by trademark and usually describing the chemical structure of the drug

Gingivitis Red, swollen gingiva (gums)

Glaucoma A disturbance in the circulation of aqueous fluid; causes an increase in intraocular pressure

Glossitis Inflammation of the tongue

Goniometer A device used to measure the angle of a joint in degrees

Guaiac test A test performed for occult (hidden) blood to detect gastrointestinal bleeding not visible to the eye

Guided imagery A relaxation technique using self-chosen positive images to achieve specific health-related goals (i.e., stress reduction, pain control)

Halo-thoracic vest A type of traction in which a circular metal band, secured by two anterior and two posterior pins that penetrate the skull a fraction of an inch, is braced on a chest jacket via metal rods; used to immobilize fractures of cervical or upper thoracic vertebrae

Hand roll A device to prevent flexion contractures of the fingers

Harris flush A return-flow enema, used to expel flatus; alternating flow of fluid into and out of the large intestine stimulates peristalsis

Hearing aid A battery-powered, sound-amplifying device used by hearing-impaired persons

Heave An abnormal lateral movement of the chest related to enlargement of the left ventricle

Heimlich maneuver Subdiaphragmatic abdominal thrusts used to clear an obstructed airway

Hematuria The presence of blood in the urine

Hemiplegia Loss of movement on one side of the body

Hemoptysis The presence of blood in the sputum

Hemothorax A collection of blood in the pleural cavity

Hemovac A portable drainage suction device

Heparin lock (saline lock) The airtight cap covering the end of a client's intravenous or central venous tubing

Hernia A protrusion of an organ or tissue through an opening such as the abdominal or inguinal muscles

High-Fowler's position A bed-sitting position in which the head of the bed is elevated 90 degrees

Hirsutism Abnormal hairiness, particularly in women

Homans' sign Calf pain produced by dorsiflexion of the foot

Hot pack Hot, moist cloth applied to an area of the body

Hour of sleep (hs) care Hygienic care provided to clients before they retire for the night

Hub The part of the needle that fits onto the syringe

Huber needle A noncoring needle used to access implanted ports

Huff coughing After inhaling deeply the client leans forward and exhales sharply with a "huff" sound to keep the airways open while moving secretions up and out of the lungs

Humidifier A device that adds water vapor to inspired air

Hydraulic lift A device used in transferring the client between the bed and a wheelchair, the bed and the bathtub, and the bed and a stretcher

Hydrocolloid dressing Flexible gumlike material such as karaya or gum covered with a water-resistant film

Hydrocolloid A glutinous suspension in which water is the fluid

Hygiene The science of health and its maintenance

Hyperalimentation (total parenteral nutrition, TPN) See total parenteral nutrition

Hypercapnea (hypercarbia) Accumulation of carbon dioxide in the blood

Hyperesthesia Greater-than-normal sensation

Hyperinflation Giving the client breaths that are 1 to 1.5 times the tidal volume set on the ventilator through the ventilator circuit or via a manual resuscitation bag

Hyperopia (farsightedness) Abnormal refraction in which light rays focus behind the retina

Hyperoxygenation Increasing the oxygen flow before suctioning and between suction attempts to avoid suction-related hypoxemia

Hyperpyrexia See Hyperthermia

Hyperresonance An abnormal booming sound produced during percussion of the lungs

Hypertension An abnormally high blood pressure; over 140 mm Hg systolic and/or 90 mm Hg diastolic

Hyperthermia (hyperpyrexia) An extremely high body temperature (e.g., 41°C [105.8°F])

Hyperventilation Very deep, rapid respirations

Hypodermic syringe An instrument used to inject liquids through a hollow needle into subcutaneous tissues

Hypoesthesia (hypesthesia) Less-than-normal sensation

Hypopigmentation Less-than-normal skin color

Hypotension An abnormally low blood pressure; less than 100 mm Hg systolic in an adult

Hypothermia A core body temperature below the lower limit of normal

Hypoventilation Very shallow respirations

Hypoxemia See Anoxemia

Hypoxia Insufficient oxygen anywhere in the body

Ice collar A flexible dressing filled with frozen water or gel that can be molded around the neck

Ileal conduit Urinary diversion in which the ureter is implanted into an isolated section of an ileal pouch, one end of which is closed and the other brought to the abdominal surface to form a stoma

Ileostomy An opening into the ileum (small bowel)

Impaction A condition of being firmly wedged or lodged; in reference to feces, a collection of hardened puttylike feces in the folds of the rectum

Implanted port An intravenous access device placed completely under the skin

Incentive spirometer (sustained maximal inspiration device, SMI) A device that measures the flow of air through a mouthpiece

Incontinence Involuntary urination or defecation

Indirect transmission Vehicle-borne or vector-borne transmission of infectious organisms

Infiltration The diffusion or deposition into tissue of substances that are not normal to it

Infusion controller A device used with intravenous infusions to control the infusion rate by using gravitational force

Infusion pump A device used with intravenous fluids to deliver a desired infusion rate by exerting positive pressure on the tubing or on the fluid

Infusion The introduction of fluid into a vein or part of the body

Inhalation (aerosol) therapy Deliverance of droplets of medication or moisture suspended in a gas, such as oxygen, by inhalation through the nose or mouth

Injection cap A device that may be attached to an existing peripheral intravenous catheter or needle to allow medications to be administered intravenously without requiring a continuous intravenous infusion

In-line suctioning See Closed airway suction system or Closed tracheal suction system

Inner cannula Some tracheostomy tubes have an inner cannula that fits inside the outer cannula and may be removed for periodic cleaning

Insensible fluid loss Fluid loss that is not perceptible to the individual

Inspection Visual examination

Inspiration See inhalation

Instillation Application of a medication into a body cavity or orifice

Insulin syringe An instrument for injecting insulin into subcutaneous tissue

Intermittent feedings Administration of 300 to 500 mL of enteral formula several times per day

Intermittent injection ports Part of IV tubing that allows for intermittent administration of medications intravenously

Intermittent suction regulators Device that applies suction for a set interval (15 to 60 seconds), followed by an interval of no suction; generally used with single-lumen tubes

Interrupted sutures A method of suturing in which each stitch is tied and knotted separately

Intractable pain Pain that is resistant to cure or relief

Intradermal (intracutaneous, ID) Under the epidermis; into the dermis

Intramuscular (IM) Into the muscle

Intraoperative period The phase during surgery; begins when the client is transferred to the operating room and ends when the client is admitted to the recovery room

Intraspinal (intrathecal) into the spinal canal

Intravenous (IV) Within a vein

Intravenous lock See Heparin lock

Intravenous push (IVP, bolus) The direct intravenous administration of a medication that cannot be diluted or that is needed in an emergency

Irrigation (lavage) A flushing or washing-out of a body cavity, organ, or wound with a specified solution

Jacket restraint A cloth vest with straps used to secure a client

Jackson–Pratt A closed wound drainage system

K-pad A device through which warm water circulates to provide heat therapy

Lancet injector A tool that holds a lancet that is used to obtain a blood specimen for a capillary blood glucose reading

Lancet A small, pointed, two-edged surgical knife

Large-bore tube Enteral tube larger than 12 French

Lateral (side-lying) position The person lies on one side of the body

Lavage An irrigation or washing of a body organ, such as the stomach

Lift An abnormal anterior movement of the chest related to enlargement of the right ventricle

Light diet A food plan designed for postoperative and other clients who are not ready for a regular diet; contains foods that are plainly cooked

Line of gravity An imaginary vertical line running through the center of gravity

Lofstrand crutch A type of crutch with supports for the hand and forearm

Logrolling A technique used to turn a client whose body must at all times be kept in straight alignment

Loop colostomy An entire piece of colon is brought through the abdomen and then incised to provide drainage openings

Low air-loss (LAL) bed A specialized bed with air-filled compartments that are constantly exchanging air to reduce pressure on the client's body

Low-Fowler's (semi-Fowler's) position A bed-sitting position in which the head of the bed is elevated between 15 and 45 degrees, with or without knee flexion

Macrodrip The larger size drops delivered by intravenous tubing; can be 10, 12, 15, or 20 drops/mL

Malnutrition A disorder of nutrition; insufficient nourishment of the body cells

Meatus An opening, passage, or channel

Meconium The first fecal material passed by the newborn, normally up to 24 hours after birth

Medical asepsis All practices intended to confine a specific microorganism to a specific area, limiting the number, growth, and spread of microorganisms

Medication (drug) A substance administered for the diagnosis, cure, treatment, mitigation, or prevention of disease

Medication Administration Record (MAR) A form that includes the client's name, room and bed number, drug name and dose, and times and method of administration

Medication history Includes information about the drugs the client is taking currently or has taken recently

Meniscus The crescent-shaped upper surface of a column of fluid

Metered dose inhaler (MDI) A compressed gas delivery system that dispenses a measured amount of medication

Microdrip The smaller size drops delivered by intravenous tubing, 60 drops/mL

Micturition See urination

Midclavicular line (MCL) An imaginary line that runs inferiorly and vertically from the center of the clavicle

Midstream urine specimen A type of urine specimen that is collected when a urine culture is ordered by the physician. Care is taken to ensure that the specimen is as free as possible from contamination by microorganisms around the urinary meatus.

Milk, milking (stripping) a tube The compression and movement of fingers along the length of a tube in order to move its contents toward an opening for removal

Minim The basic unit of measure in the apothecary system, equal to 0.0616 mL

Miosis Constricted pupils

Miter A method of folding the bedclothes at the corners to secure them in place while the bed is occupied

Mitt (hand) restraint A cloth cover for the hand with a strap attached to secure a client's wrist

Mode of transmission In the cycle of infection, the means of the organism reaching another person or host

Moist compress A damp cloth or bandage applied firmly to a body part

Morning care Hygienic care provided after clients have breakfast although it may be provided before breakfast

Multidose vial A small bottle that contains multiple doses of a liquid

Mydriasis Enlarged pupils

Myopia (nearsightedness) Abnormal refraction in which light rays focus in front of the retina

Narcotic A strong analgesic

Nares The nostrils

Naris A single nostril

Nasal cannula (nasal prongs) A device used to administer low-flow oxygen

Nasoenteric tube A tube of soft rubber or plastic that is inserted through a nostril and into the small intestine

Nasogastric (NG) tube A plastic or rubber tube inserted through the nose into the stomach for the purpose of feeding or irrigating the stomach

Nasopharynx The part of the pharynx above the soft palate

Nasopharynx airway A device used to keep the upper air passages open when they may become obstructed by secretions or the tongue

Nasopharyngeal suctioning Removes secretions from the upper respiratory tract

Nebulization The conversion of a fine mist or spray from a liquid

Neuropathic pain The result of a disturbance of the peripheral or central nervous system that results in pain that may or may not be associated with an ongoing tissue-damaging process

No Code Blue Like Do Not Resuscitate, a physician's order that requires that no effort be made to resuscitate the client with terminal or irreversible illness in the event of a respiratory or cardiac arrest

Nonopioids Non-narcotic analgesics; include acetaminophen (Tylenol) and nonsteroidal anti-inflammatory drugs (NSAIDs)

Nonrebreather mask An oxygen delivery device that covers the mouth and nose but allows all exhaled air to exit the system

Nonsteroidal anti-inflammatory drugs (NSAIDs) Drugs that relieve pain by acting on the peripheral nerve endings to inhibit the formation of the prostaglandins that tend to sensitize nerves to painful stimuli; have analgesic, antipyretic, and anti-inflammatory effect; include aspirin and ibuprofen

Normocephalic Normal head size

Nose culture A specimen collected from the mucosa of the nasal passages using a culture swab

Nosocomial Referring to or originating in a hospital or similar institution (e.g., a nosocomial infection)

Nothing by mouth (NPO) Not to orally ingest liquid or solids, *nil per os*

Nutrient An organic and inorganic substance found in food; nutrients are digested and absorbed in the gastrointestinal tract and then used in the body's metabolic processes

Nutrition What a person eats and how the body uses it

Obligatory loss The essential fluid loss required to maintain body functioning

Obstructed airway The blockage of passage of air through the trachea

Obturator A disc or instrument that closes an opening (e.g., the obturator of a tracheostomy set fits inside and closes off the end of the outer tube)

Occult Hidden

Occupied bed A bed currently being used by a client

Official name (of drug) The name under which a drug is listed in one of the official publications (e.g., the *United States Pharmacopeia*)

Oliguria Production of abnormally small amounts of urine by the kidney

Open airway suction system If a client is connected to a ventilator, the nurse disconnects the client from the ventilator, suctions the airway, reconnects the client to the ventilator, and discards the suction catheter

Open bed A bed not presently being used by its occupant, with the top covers folded back

Open system A system in which energy, matter, and information move into and out of the system through the system boundary

Open-tipped catheter A flexible, plastic catheter that has an opening at the end of the catheter and may be more effective for removing thick mucous plugs

Opioids Naturally occurring or synthetic narcotic analgesics

Oral Referring to the mouth

Oropharyngeal airway A device used to keep the upper air passages open when they may become obstructed by secretions or the tongue

Oropharyngeal suctioning Removes secretions from the upper respiratory tract

Orthopneic position A sitting position to relieve respiratory difficulty in which the client leans over and is supported by an overbed table across the lap

Ostomy appliance The equipment used to collect drainage from an ostomy, often a skin barrier, flange or wafer, and pouch

Ostomy pouch A collection bag or reservoir that fits over the stoma

Ostomy A suffix denoting the formation of an opening or outlet such as an opening on the abdominal wall for the elimination of feces or urine

Otoscope An instrument used to examine the ears

Outer cannula The part of the tracheostomy tube that is inserted into the trachea

Ova and parasites One type of stool specimen analysis to confirm the presence of and identify the organism in order to determine appropriate treatment

Overnutrition Obesity—refers to a caloric intake in excess of daily energy requirements resulting in storage of energy in the form of increased adipose tissue

Oximeter A device that measures the arterial blood oxygen saturation

Oxygen concentrator An electrically powered system that manufactures oxygen from room air

Oxygen saturation (SaO$_2$) The amount of hemoglobin fully saturated with oxygen; given as a percent value

Oxygen toxicity Failure of lung ventilation that occurs when very high oxygen concentrations are breathed for extended periods of time

Pain reaction The autonomic nervous system and behavioral responses to pain

Pain threshold (pain sensation) The amount of pain stimulation a person requires before feeling pain

Pain tolerance The maximum amount and duration of pain that an individual is willing to endure

Pallor The absence of underlying red tones in the skin; may be most readily seen in the buccal mucosa

Palpation The examination of the body using the sense of touch

Paradoxical breathing The ballooning out of the chest wall during expiration and depression or sucking inward of the chest wall during inspiration

Paralytic ileus Cessation of intestinal muscle contraction

Parenteral Drug administration occurring outside the alimentary tract; injected into the body through some route other than the alimentary canal (e.g., intramuscularly)

Paresthesia An abnormal sensation of burning or prickling

Parotitis Inflammation of the parotid salivary gland

Partial (abbreviated) bath An abbreviated bath in which only parts of the client's body that might cause discomfort or odor, if neglected, are washed

Partial rebreather mask An oxygen delivery device that covers the mouth and nose but has a reservoir bag that allows the client to rebreathe about the first third of the exhaled air in conjunction with oxygen

Passive range-of-motion (ROM) exercise Exercise in which another person moves each of the client's joints through their complete range of movement, maximally stretching all muscle groups within each plane over each joint

Patient-controlled analgesia (PCA) A pain management technique that allows the client to take an active role in managing pain

Peak expiratory flow rate (PEFR) The maximum amount the client can forcefully expire

Pearson attachment A sling appliance that joins the Thomas splint at the knee level to support the lower leg off the bed and permit the knee to be flexed

Pediculosis Infestation with head lice

Penrose drain A flexible rubber drain

Percussion (clapping, cupping) The forceful striking of the chest with cupped hands to loosen secretions in the lungs

Percussion (in assessment) A method in which the body surface is struck to elicit sounds that can be heard or vibrations that can be felt

Percutaneous endoscopic gastrostomy (PEG) A procedure in which a PEG catheter is inserted into the stomach through the skin and subcutaneous tissues of the abdomen; used as a feeding tube

Percutaneous endoscopic jejunostomy (PEJ) A procedure in which a PEJ catheter is inserted into the jejunum through the skin and subcutaneous tissues of the abdomen; used as a feeding tube

Perineal (peri-) care Cleansing of the perineum

Perioperative period Refers to the three phases of surgery: preoperative, intraoperative, and postoperative

Peripheral parenteral nutrition (PPN) Intravenous nutrition administered through a peripheral (rather than a central) vein

Peripheral pulse A pulse located in the periphery of the body (e.g., foot, wrist)

Peritoneal dialysis The instillation and drainage of a solution (dialysate) from the peritoneal cavity

Peritoneal exchange A complete cycle of instilling, dwelling, and draining dialysate from the abdomen

Personal protective equipment (PPE) Barriers such as gloves, mask, and gown used to protect persons from contact with potentially infective materials

Petalling The application of strips of tape around the edges of a cast

Phantom pain Pain that remains after the perceived location has been removed, such as pain perceived in a foot after the leg has been amputated

Phlebitis Inflammation of the vein

Physical restraints Any manual method or physical or mechanical device, material, or equipment attached to the client's body that restrict the client's movement

Piggy-back IV A secondary IV setup which connects the second IV container to the tubing of the primary IV at the upper port

Pitch The frequency or number of the vibrations heard during auscultation

Pivot A technique in which the body is turned in a way that avoids twisting of the spine

Plaque An invisible soft film consisting of bacteria, molecules of saliva, and remnants of epithelial cells and leukocytes that adheres to the enamel surface of teeth

Plaster of paris A chalk-based material applied to gauze and used to immobilize a body part in a cast

Pleximeter In percussion, the middle finger of the dominant hand placed firmly on the client's skin

Plexor In percussion, the middle finger of the nondominant hand or a percussion hammer used to strike the pleximeter

Pneumatic compression device (PCD) See Sequential compression device

Pneumothorax Accumulation of gas or fluid in the pleural cavity

Point of maximal impulse (PMI) The point where the apex of the heart touches the anterior chest wall

Portal of entry In communicable disease, the opening through which infectious organisms invade the body (e.g., urinary tract, respiratory tract, open wound)

Portal of exit In communicable disease, the location through which infectious organisms leave the body (e.g., respiratory tract, infected wound, skin)

Postanesthesia care unit (PCU) Unit the client is transferred to after surgery

Postanesthesia room (PAR) Unit the client is transferred to after surgery

Postoperative phase Begins with the admission of the client to the postanesthesia area and ends when healing is complete

Postural drainage The drainage,

by gravity, of secretions from various lung segments

Posture The bearing and position of the body; the relative arrangements of the various parts of the body

Preemptive analgesia The administration of analgesics prior to an invasive or operative procedure

Prefilled unit-dose system Injectable medications that are available as prefilled syringes ready for use or as prefilled sterile cartridges and needles that require the attachment of a reusable holder before use

Preoperative phase The period before an operation; begins when the decision for surgery has been made and ends when the client is transferred to the operating room bed

Presbycusis Loss of hearing related to aging

Presbyopia Loss of elasticity of the lens and thus loss of ability to see close objects as a result of the aging process

Prescription The written direction for the preparation and administration of a drug

Pressure ulcer (decubitus ulcers, bedsores) Reddened areas, sores, or ulcers of the skin occurring over bony prominences

Primary port The port on the IV tubing that is furthest from the client

PRN (pro re nata) An order that enables the nurse to give a medication or treatment when, in the nurse's judgment, the client needs it

Progressive relaxation A formalized relaxation technique designed to reduce stress and chronic pain

Prone position Face-lying position, with or without a small pillow

Pruritus Itching

Pulmonary embolus (PE) A blood clot that has moved to the lungs

Pulse deficit The difference between the apical pulse and the radial pulse

Pulse oximeter A noninvasive device that measures the arterial blood oxygen saturation by means of a sensor attached to the finger or other location

Pulse pressure The difference between the systolic and the diastolic blood pressure

Pureed diet A modification of the soft diet wherein food is blended to a semisolid consistency

Purosanguineous Containing pus and blood

Pursed-lip breathing Exhalation of air against resistance after a deep inhalation; performed by clients with chronic obstructive lung disease; carried out by forming a small "O" with the lips and exhaling slowly

Purulent Containing pus

Pus A thick liquid associated with inflammation and composed of cells, liquid, microorganisms, and tissue debris

Pyrexia (hyperthermia) A body temperature above the normal range; fever

Quad cane A stick held in the hand used for support during walking that has a four-pronged base

Radiating pain Pain perceived at the source and in surrounding or nearby tissues

Radiodensity of soft tissues The property that determines the amount of x-ray that passes through

Range of motion (ROM) The degree of movement possible for each joint

Reagent A substance used to produce a chemical reaction to detect, measure other substances

Rebound phenomenon (thermal) The time when the maximum therapeutic effect of a hot or cold application is achieved and the opposite effect begins

Reconstitution The technique of adding a solvent to a powdered drug to prepare it for injection

Recovery room (RR) Unit the client is transferred to after surgery

Rectus femoris site The rectus femoris muscle, situated on the anterior aspect of the thigh, is used only occasionally for intramuscular injections

Referred pain Pain perceived to be in one area but whose source is another area

Refractometer An instrument used to measure the specific gravity of urine

Regular diet A balanced diet that supplies the metabolic requirements

Regulator A device for controlling or adjusting the flow of fluid or gas

Renal failure Inability of the kidneys to perform their vital functions

Reservoir A source of microorganisms

Resonance A low-pitched, hollow sound produced over normal lung tissue when the chest is percussed

Respiration The act of breathing; transport of oxygen from the atmosphere to the body cells and transport of carbon dioxide from the cells to the atmosphere

Respiratory arrest The sudden cessation of breathing

Restraints Protective devices used to limit physical activity of the client or a part of the client's body

Retention enema Solution introduced into the rectum and sigmoid colon and held there to soften the feces or to deliver a medication

Retention sutures (stay sutures) Large sutures used in addition to skin sutures to attach underlying tissues of fat and muscle as well as skin; used to support incisions in obese individuals or when healing may be prolonged

Retraction (mobility) Moving a part of the body backward in same plane parallel to the ground

Return flow enema See Harris flush

Reverse Trendelenburg's position A position with the head of the bed raised and the foot lowered, while the bed foundation remains unbroken

Rh factor An element either present or absent on the surface of erythrocytes; persons without the factor (Rh negative) may have a serious reaction if exposed to blood with the factor (Rh positive)

Rigidity Stiffness or inflexibility of a muscle

Robinson catheter A hollow, straight, flexible tube of rubber or plastic with holes in the distal end

Safety belt A strap used to secure a client

Safety monitoring device An electronic sensor or monitor that triggers an alarm when the client moves beyond preset parameters

Saline lock See Heparin lock

Saliva The clear liquid secreted by the salivary glands in the mouth

Sanguineous Containing blood

Secondary IV setup When more than one IV solution needs to be infused at the same time, secondary setup is used

Secondary port The port on the IV tubing that is closest to the client

Second-voided specimen The client is asked to void and, in 30 minutes, to void again. The second voiding is used for testing as it more accurately reflects the present condition of the body.

Seizure A sudden onset of a convulsion or other paroxysmal motor or sensory activity

Seizure precautions Safety measures taken to protect a client from injury should he or she have a seizure

Self-help bed bath Clients confined to bed are able to bathe themselves with help from the nurse for washing the back and perhaps the feet

Semi-Fowler's (low-Fowler's) position A bed-sitting position in which the head of the bed is elevated 15 to 45 degrees, with or without knee flexion

Sequential compression device (SCD) A device to promote venous return by alternately inflating and deflating plastic sleeves wrapped around the legs

Serial casting The process of applying multiple casts in succession to position an extremity or account for reduction in swelling

Serosanguineous Composed of serum and blood

Serous Of or like serum

Shaft The cannula of a needle

Sharps Any items that can cut or puncture skin

Shower Ambulatory clients use shower facilities for cleansing purposes. Clients in long-term care settings are often given showers with the use of a shower chair.

Sims' (semiprone position) position Side-lying position with lowermost arm behind the body and uppermost leg flexed

Single (end) colostomy Has only one stoma, which arises from the end of the proximal portion of the bowel

Single order An order that is to be carried out one time only at a specified time

Single-dose vial A bottle containing a liquid that is used for only one dose

Skull tongs Devices used to immobilize fractures of the cervical and upper thoracic vertebrae

Sliding board A smooth polyethylene board that is used by a nurse to help transfer a client

Sling A support for an upper extremity, triangular bandage

Small-bore tube A softer, more flexible, and less irritating tube, ranging from 5 to 12 French in diameter

Soft diet A diet that is easily chewed and digested and is often ordered for clients who have difficulty chewing and swallowing

Sordes Accumulation of foul matter (food, microorganisms, and epithelial elements) on the teeth and gums

Spasticity Describing the sudden, prolonged involuntary muscle contractions of clients with damage to the central nervous system

Specific gravity The weight or degree of concentration of a substance compared with that of an equal volume of another, such as distilled water, taken as a standard

Specimen A small sample or part taken to show the nature of the whole, as a small quantity of urine for urinalysis or a small fragment of tissue for microscopic study

Spectrometer A device for measuring the amount of red and infrared light absorbed by oxygenated and deoxygenated hemoglobin in arterial blood, used in pulse oximetry

Sphygmomanometer An instrument used to measure blood pressure

Spica (hip) cast A cast that encircles the lower abdomen and one or both lower extremities

Spica A reverse spiral

Spore A round or oval structure enclosed in a tough capsule

Sputum The mucous secretion from the lungs, bronchi, and trachea

Standard precautions (SP) A set of guidelines outlining steps all health care workers must follow to reduce the chances that bloodborne pathogens and potentially infectious organisms from other body tissues are transmitted from the client to other persons

Standing order A written document about policies, rules, regulations, or orders regarding client care that gives the nurse authority to carry out specific actions under certain circumstances, often when a physician is not available; an order that may be carried out indefinitely until another order is written to cancel it

Staples Wire clips

Stat order Indicates an order that is to be carried out immediately and only once

Status epilepticus A series of grand mal seizures

Steatorrhea Excess fat in the feces due to a malabsorption syndrome or pancreatic enzyme deficiency

Stereognosis The ability to recognize objects by touching and manipulating them

Sterile field A specified area that is considered free from microorganisms

Stockinette Tubular woven material open at both ends

Stoma An artificial opening in the abdominal wall; may be permanent or temporary

Stomatitis Inflammation of the oral mucosa

Stricture A narrowing of a passageway or canal

Stridor A harsh, crowing sound made on inhalation caused by constriction of the upper airway

Stryker wedge frame A bed device consisting of two removable metal frames (anterior and posterior) with canvas stretched across them to hold a person's body and allow it to be turned without bending the spine

Subcutaneous (hypodermic, SC or SQ) Injection beneath the layers of the skin

Sublingual Under the tongue

Suctioning The aspiration of secretions by a catheter connected to a suction machine or wall outlet

Sulcular technique A technique of brushing the teeth under the gingival margins

Suppository A solid, cone-shaped,

medicated substance inserted into the rectum, vagina, or urethra

Suprapubic catheter A tube inserted into the bladder through the abdominal wall above the pubic arch

Surgical asepsis (sterile technique) Practices that keep an area or object free of all microorganisms

Surgical bed (anesthetic, recovery, or postoperative bed) A bed with the top covers fanfolded to one side or to the end of the bed

Sustained maximal inspiration device (SMI) See Incentive spirometer

Sutures (wound) The surgical stitches used to close accidental or surgical wounds; can also refer to the material used to sew the wound

Synthetic cast Artificially prepared cast material such as polyester, fiberglass, and thermoplastics

Syringe pump A method of intermittently administering an IV medication wherein the medication is mixed in a syringe that is connected to the primary IV line via a mini-infuser

Systolic pressure The pressure of the blood against the arterial walls when the ventricles of the heart contract

Systolic The time period during which the ventricles contract

Tandem A secondary IV setup in which a second IV container is attached to the line of the first container at the lower, secondary port

Tartar A visible, hard deposit of plaque and dead bacteria that forms at the gum lines

Therapeutic bath A bath given for physical effects, such as to soothe irritated skin or to treat an area (e.g., the perineum). Medications may be placed in the water.

Thermal Referring to heat

Thomas splint A proximal ring that fits around the upper leg and to which two long, slender steel rods are attached that extend to a smaller ring distal to the foot; used to establish traction on femoral fractures

Throat culture A specimen collected from the mucosa of the oropharynx and tonsillar regions using a culture swab

Tidaling The periodic rise and fall or increase and decrease as in the

level of fluid in a chest tube drainage bottle

Toe pleat A fold made in the top bedclothes to provide additional space for the client's toes and feet

Total enteral nutrition (TEN) See Enteral nutrition

Towel bath A commercially prepared in-bed bath that uses a quick-drying solution containing a disinfectant, a cleaning agent, and a softening agent mixed with water

Tracheostomy A surgical incision in the trachea below the first or second tracheal cartilage

Traction Exertion of a pulling force either manually or by a device in order to stabilize and immobilize

Trademark See Brand name

Transcutaneous electric nerve stimulation (TENS) Noninvasive, nonanalgesic pain control technique that allows the client to assist in the management of acute and chronic pain

Transdermal patch A method of medication administration in which medication is absorbed through the skin

Transfer (walking) belt A belt that has a handle that allows the nurse to control movement of the client during a transfer

Transfusion (blood) The introduction of whole blood or its components into the venous circulation

Transmission-based precautions An infection control system based on the route of movement of microorganisms: airborne, droplet, or contact

Transparent wound barrier A see-through semipermeable membrane dressing

Transtracheal catheter A small plastic cannula inserted between the third and fourth tracheal cartilages; used to deliver oxygen therapy

Tremor An involuntary trembling of a limb or body part

Trendelenburg's position The client is supine on a surface inclined 45 degrees, with the head at the lower end

Trigone A triangular area at the base of the bladder marked by the ureter openings at the posterior corners and the opening of urethra at the anterior corner

Tripod position (a) the proper standing position with crutches; the crutches are 15 cm (6 inches) in front of the feet and 15 cm (6 inches) out laterally; (b) position often assumed by people in respiratory distress in which they sit upright and lean on their arms or elbows

Trochanter roll A rolled towel support placed against the hips to prevent external rotation of the legs

Tub bath Can be used for a cleaning or therapeutic bath

Tuberculin syringe A narrow syringe, calibrated in tenths and hundredths of a milliliter on one scale and in sixteenths of a minim on the other scale

Tuberculosis (TB) An infectious disease caused by the tubercle bacillus *Mycobacterium tuberculosis*

Tympany A musical or drumlike sound produced during percussion over an air-filled stomach and abdomen

Uncuffed tracheostomy tube A plastic or metal tracheostomy tube that allows for air to flow around the tube

Undernutrition Intake of nutrients insufficient to meet daily energy requirements as a result of inadequate food intake or improper digestion and absorption of food

Universal Precautions The original set of guidelines outlining steps all health care workers must follow to reduce the chances that blood-borne pathogens were transmitted from the client to other persons

Unlicensed assistive personnel (UAP) Personnel such as certified nursing assistants, hospital attendants, nurse technicians, and orderlies, who work in health care settings and are responsible for nursing activities requiring less technical skill (e.g., bathing, feeding, specimen collection, hygiene) and that do not require nursing judgment

Unoccupied bed A bed not currently being used by a client

Urgency (of urination) The feeling that one must urinate

Urinary incontinence A temporary or permanent inability of the external sphincter muscles to control the flow of urine from the bladder

Urinary retention The accumulation of urine in the bladder and inability of the bladder to empty itself

Urinary sheath See External catheter

Urination (micturition, voiding) The process of emptying the bladder

Urine pH The measurement of the concentration of hydrogen ions in the urine which indicates its acidity or alkalinity

Urinometer (hydrometer) An instrument used to measure the specific gravity of urine

Vastus lateralis site The middle third of the vastus lateralis muscle is suggested as the site for an intramuscular injection

Vector-borne transmission Microorganisms from an insect or other animal transferred from a reservoir to a host

Vehicle-borne transmission Transport of an infectious agent into a susceptible host via any intermediate substance (e.g., fomites or food)

Venous (vascular) access device Specially designed catheters or ports used to provide a means of entrance to the vascular system for an extended period of time

Ventilation The movement of air in and out of the lungs; the process of inhalation and exhalation

Ventricular fibrillation (VF) The quivering, nonfunctional contraction of individual cardiac ventricle muscle fibers

Ventrogluteal site The preferred site for intramuscular injections

Venturi mask A special mask that delivers a precise concentration of oxygen

Vial A glass medication container with a sealed rubber cap, for single or multiple doses

Visceral pain Results from stimulation of pain receptors in the abdominal cavity, cranium, and thorax

Visual acuity The degree of detail the eye can discern in an image

Visual fields The area an individual can see when looking straight ahead

Vital signs (cardinal signs) Measurements of physiologic functioning, specifically, temperature, pulse, respiration, and blood pressure

Vitiligo Patches of hypopigmented skin, caused by the destruction of melanocytes in the area

Void See Urination

Volume-control infusion set A small fluid container attached below the primary infusion container used to administer intermittent intravenous medications

Volume-oriented sustained maximal inspiration device (SMI) A device that measures the inhalation volume maintained by the client

Walker A metal rectangular frame used as an aid to ambulation

Water-seal A system in which a drainage tube extends into fluid in the bottom of the container and prevents air from entering the tube

Wean To gradually decrease dependence on assisted ventilation until the client is able to breathe spontaneously and independently

Wet-to-damp dressing A wet bandage applied to a wound and allowed to dry until damp before being removed

Wet-to-dry dressing A wet bandage applied to a wound and allowed to dry completely before being removed

Wheal Small raised area like a blister

Wheezing A rasping or whistling sound in breathing caused by constriction in the upper airway

Whistle-tipped catheter Flexible, plastic catheter that has an angle opening at the end of the tip and is less irritating to respiratory tissues

Wound dehiscence Separation of a suture line before the incision heals

Wound evisceration Extrusion of internal organs and tissues through the incision

Wound A break in the continuity of a body tissue

Wrist (ankle) restraint A strap used to secure a client's leg so it cannot be moved

Yankauer suction tube A rigid, plastic tube used for suctioning oral secretions

Z-track technique A technique for intramuscular injection of a substance likely to be irritating, or when deposition of a drug and absorption by muscle tissue is critical

Photo and Art Credits

Chapter 1

1-1, 1-2, 1-3, 1-4: Elena Dorfman/*Fundamentals of nursing: Concepts, process, and practice,* 6th ed., by B. Kozier, G. Erb, A. Berman, & K. Burke, 2000, Upper Saddle River, NJ: Prentice Hall Health. 1-5, 1-6: Alain McLaughlin/*Fundamentals of nursing: Concepts, process, and practice,* 6th ed., by B. Kozier, G. Erb, A. Berman, & K. Burke, 2000, Upper Saddle River, NJ: Prentice Hall Health. 1-7: Precision Graphics/*Fundamentals of nursing: Concepts, process, and practice,* 6th ed., by B. Kozier, G. Erb, A. Berman, & K. Burke, 2000, Upper Saddle River, NJ: Prentice Hall Health. 1-8, 1-9, 1-10: Linda Harris/*Fundamentals of nursing: Concepts, process, and practice,* 6th ed., by B. Kozier, G. Erb, A. Berman, & K. Burke, 2000, Upper Saddle River, NJ: Prentice Hall Health. 1-11: George Draper.

Chapter 2

2-1: Source: E. F. Dubois, *Fever and the regulation of body temperature* (Springfield, IL: Charles C. Thomas, 1948). Courtesy of Charles C. Thomas Publisher, Ltd. 2-4: Nea Hanscomb/*Fundamentals of nursing: Concepts, process, and practice,* 6th ed., by B. Kozier, G. Erb, A. Berman, & K. Burke, 2000, Upper Saddle River, NJ: Prentice Hall Health. 2-2: *Techniques in clinical nursing,* 4th ed., by Barbara Kozier, Glenora Erb, Kathleen Blais, Joyce Young Johnson, & Jean Smith Temple, 1993, Redwood City, CA: Addison-Wesley. 2-3, 2-7, 2-8, 2-15, 2-18, 2-19: Elena Dorfman/*Fundamentals of nursing: Concepts, process, and practice,* 6th ed., by B. Kozier, G. Erb, A. Berman, & K. Burke, 2000, Upper Saddle River, NJ: Prentice Hall Health. 2-5, 2-9, 2-27: Jenny Thomas/*Fundamentals of nursing: Concepts, process, and practice,* 6th ed., by B. Kozier, G. Erb, A. Berman, & K. Burke, 2000, Upper Saddle River, NJ: Prentice Hall Health. 2-14C: Richard Tauber/*Fundamentals of nursing: Concepts, process, and practice,* 6th ed., by B. Kozier, G. Erb, A. Berman, & K. Burke, 2000, Upper Saddle River, NJ: Prentice Hall Health. 2-10, 2-13, 2-24: Anne Erickson, CMI. 2-11, 2-12, 2-26: *Quick reference to pediatric clinical skills,* by R. Bindler & J. Ball, 1999, Upper Saddle River, NJ: Prentice Hall Health. 2-14A, D, E, F, 2-16: *Fundamentals of nursing,* 2nd ed. (vol. 2) (p. 420), by K. J. Berger & M. B. Williams, 1999, Stamford, CT: Appleton & Lange. 2-17, 2-20, 2-21, 2-22: *Fundamentals of nursing: Concepts, process, and practice,* 6th ed., by B. Kozier, G. Erb, A. Berman, & K. Burke, 2000, Upper Saddle River, NJ: Prentice Hall Health. 2-6, 2-14B, 2-14G, 2-25: George Draper. 2-23: Linda Harris/*Fundamentals of nursing: Concepts, process, and practice,* 6th ed., by B. Kozier, G. Erb, A. Berman, & K. Burke, 2000, Upper Saddle River, NJ: Prentice Hall Health. 2-28, 2-29: Courtesy Nonin Medical, Inc.

Chapter 3

3-1, 3-2, 3-3, 3-5, 3-17, 3-18, 3-19, 3-20, 3-21, 3-28, 3-29, 3-30, 3-35, 3-36, 3-37, 3-38, 3-42, 3-43, 3-51, 3-55, 3-65, 3-66, 3-75, 3-76, 3-77, 3-78, 3-79, 3-80, 3-81, 3-82, 3-83, 3-84, 3-91: Richard Tauber/*Fundamentals of nursing: Concepts, process, and practice,* 6th ed., by B. Kozier, G. Erb, A. Berman, & K. Burke, 2000, Upper Saddle River, NJ: Prentice Hall Health. 3-8, 3-10, 3-13, 3-48, 3-50, 3-70: Anne Erickson, CMI. Table photos, 3-4, 3-32, 3-92: Elena Dorfman/*Fundamentals of nursing: Concepts, process, and practice,* 6th ed., by B. Kozier, G. Erb, A. Berman, & K. Burke, 2000, Upper Saddle River, NJ: Prentice Hall Health. 3-6: GTS Graphics/*Fundamentals of nursing: Concepts, process, and practice,* 6th ed., by B. Kozier, G. Erb, A. Berman, & K. Burke, 2000, Upper Saddle River, NJ: Prentice Hall Health. 3-7, 3-74, 3-86, 3-87, 3-88, 3-90: George Draper. 3-9A: SPL/Custom Medical Stock Photo, Inc. 3-9B, 3-89: *Medical surgical nursing: Critical thinking in client care,* 2nd ed., by P. LeMone & K. Burke, 2000, Upper Saddle River, NJ: Prentice Hall Health. 3-11, 3-69, 3-93: *Fundamentals of nursing: Concepts, process, and practice,* 6th ed., by B. Kozier, G. Erb, A. Berman, & K. Burke, 2000, Upper Saddle River, NJ: Prentice Hall Health. 3-12, 3-14, 3-15, 3-16, 3-27, 3-31, 3-34, 3-40, 3-61, 3-71, 3-72: Christopher Burke/*Fundamentals of nursing: Concepts, process, and practice,* 6th ed., by B. Kozier, G. Erb, A. Berman, & K. Burke, 2000, Upper Saddle River, NJ: Prentice Hall Health. 3-22, 3-60: Nea Hanscomb/*Fundamentals of nursing: Concepts, process, and practice,* 6th ed., by B. Kozier, G. Erb, A. Berman, & K. Burke, 2000, Upper Saddle River, NJ: Prentice Hall Health. 3-23: Romaine Lo Prete/Matt Perry/*Fundamentals of nursing: Concepts, process, and practice,* 6th ed., by B. Kozier, G. Erb, A. Berman, & K. Burke, 2000, Upper Saddle River, NJ: Prentice Hall Health. 3-24, 3-44, 3-67B, 3-85: *Health assessment in nursing,* by L. K. Sims, D. D'Amico, J. K. Stiesmeyer, & J. A. Webster, 1995, Redwood City, CA: Addison-Wesley. 3-25, 3-33, 3-62: Matt Perry/*Fundamentals of nursing: Concepts, process, and practice,* 6th ed., by B. Kozier, G. Erb, A. Berman, & K. Burke, 2000, Upper Saddle River, NJ: Prentice Hall Health. 3-26: Dr. Richard Buckingham/*Fundamentals of nursing: Concepts, process, and practice,* 6th ed., by B. Kozier, G. Erb, A. Berman, & K. Burke, 2000, Upper Saddle River, NJ: Prentice Hall Health. 3-39, 3-45, 3-46, 3-52, 3-53, 3-54, 3-59, 3-64, 3-68, 3-73: Romaine Lo Prete/*Fundamentals of nursing: Concepts, process, and practice,* 6th ed., by B. Kozier, G. Erb, A. Berman, & K. Burke, 2000, Upper Saddle River, NJ: Prentice Hall Health. 3-41, 3-47, 3-49, 3-56, 3-57, 3-58, 3-63: Kristin Mount/*Fundamentals of nursing: Concepts, process, and practice,* 6th ed., by B. Kozier, G. Erb, A. Berman, & K. Burke, 2000, Upper Saddle River, NJ: Prentice Hall Health. 3-67A: Precision Graphics/*Fundamentals of nursing: Concepts, process, and practice,* 6th ed., by B. Kozier, G. Erb, A. Berman, & K. Burke, 2000, Upper Saddle River, NJ: Prentice Hall Health. 3-94, 3-95: *Pediatric nursing: Caring for children,* 2nd ed., by J. Ball & R. Bindler, 1999, Stamford, CT: Appleton & Lange. 3-96: Anne Erickson, CMI. Adapted from *Health assessment in nursing,* by L. K. Sims, D. D'Amico, J. K. Stiesmeyer, & J. A. Webster, 1995, Redwood City, CA: Addison-Wesley. Reprinted by permission of Pearson Education, Inc. Upper Saddle River, NJ 07458.

Chapter 4

4-1, 4-10, 4-11: Anne Erickson, CMI. 4-2: GTS Graphics/*Fundamentals of nursing: Concepts, process, and practice,* 6th ed., by B. Kozier, G. Erb, A. Berman, & K. Burke, 2000, Upper Saddle River, NJ: Prentice Hall Health. 4-3: *Quick reference to pediatric clinical skills,* by R. Bindler & J. Ball, 1999, Upper Saddle River, NJ: Prentice Hall Health. 4-4, 4-5, 4-6, 4-7, 4-14: George Draper. 4-8, 4-15, 4-16, 4-17: Elena Dorfman/*Fundamentals of nursing: Concepts, process, and practice,* 6th ed., by B. Kozier, G. Erb, A. Berman, & K. Burke, 2000, Upper Saddle River, NJ: Prentice Hall Health. 4-9: Jenny Thomas/*Fundamentals of nursing: Concepts, process, and practice,* 6th ed., by B. Kozier, G. Erb, A. Berman, & K. Burke, 2000, Upper Saddle River, NJ: Prentice Hall Health. 4-12: Linda Harris/*Fundamentals of nursing: Concepts, process, and practice,* 6th ed., by B. Kozier, G. Erb, A. Berman, & K. Burke, 2000, Upper Saddle River, NJ: Prentice Hall Health. 4-13: Precision Graphics/*Fundamentals of nursing: Concepts, process, and practice,* 6th ed., by B. Kozier, G. Erb, A. Berman, & K. Burke, 2000, Upper Saddle River, NJ: Prentice Hall Health.

Chapter 5

5-1, 5-2, 5-3, 5-8, 5-11, 5-12, 5-13, 5-16, 5-17, unnumbered illustrations: Precision Graphics/*Fundamentals of nursing: Concepts, process, and practice,* 6th ed., by B. Kozier, G. Erb, A. Berman, & K. Burke, 2000, Upper Saddle River, NJ: Prentice Hall Health. 5-4, 5-7: Linda Harris/*Fundamentals of nursing: Concepts, process, and practice,* 6th ed., by B. Kozier, G. Erb, A. Berman, & K. Burke, 2000, Upper Saddle River, NJ: Prentice Hall Health. 5-5, unnumbered photo: George Draper. 5-6: Richard Tauber/*Fundamentals of nursing: Concepts, process, and practice,* 6th ed., by B. Kozier, G. Erb, A. Berman, & K. Burke, 2000, Upper Saddle River, NJ: Prentice Hall Health. 5-9, 5-10, 5-18, unnumbered 5-3: Anne Erickson, CMI. 5-14, 5-15, 5-21, 5-23: Jenny Thomas/*Fundamentals of nursing: Concepts, process, and practice,* 6th ed., by B. Kozier, G. Erb, A. Berman, & K. Burke, 2000, Upper Saddle River, NJ: Prentice Hall Health. 5-19, 5-20, 5-22: Elena Dorfman/*Fundamentals of nursing: Concepts, process, and practice,* 6th ed., by B. Kozier, G. Erb, A. Berman, & K. Burke, 2000, Upper Saddle River, NJ: Prentice Hall Health.

Chapter 6

6-1, 6-3: 2000 Hill Rom Services, Inc. Reprinted with Permission—All Rights Reserved. 6-2: Courtesy Kinetic Concepts. 6-4, 6-5, 6-6, 6-7, 6-8: Courtesy Stryker Medical. 6-9, 6-16, 6-18C, 6-19A, 6-24, 6-25: George Draper. 6-10, 6-11, 6-12, 6-13, 6-15A: Elena Dorfman/*Fundamentals of nursing: Concepts, process, and practice,* 6th ed., by B. Kozier, G. Erb, A. Berman, & K. Burke, 2000, Upper Saddle River, NJ: Prentice Hall Health. 6-14: Jenny Thomas/*Fundamentals of nursing: Concepts, process, and practice,* 6th ed., by B. Kozier, G. Erb, A. Berman, & K. Burke, 2000, Upper Saddle River, NJ: Prentice Hall Health. 6-15B: *Fundamentals of nursing,* 2nd ed. (vol. 3) (p. 1216), by K. J. Berger & M. B. Williams, 1999, Stamford, CT: Appleton & Lange. 6-17: Precision Graphics. 6-18A & B, 6-19B, 6-20, 6-21, 6-22, 6-23: Anne Erickson, CMI. 6-26, 6-27, 6-28: Richard Tauber/*Fundamentals of nursing: Concepts, process, and practice,* 6th ed., by B. Kozier, G. Erb, A. Berman, & K. Burke, 2000, Upper Saddle River, NJ: Prentice Hall Health.

Chapter 7

7-1: Courtesy AlertCare, Mill Valley, California: 7-9, 7-10A: George Draper. 7-2: Courtesy of J. T. Posey Company. *Fundamentals of nursing: Concepts, process, and practice,* 6th ed., by B. Kozier, G. Erb, A. Berman, & K. Burke, 2000, Upper Saddle River, NJ: Prentice Hall Health. 7-5: Linda Harris/*Fundamentals of nursing: Concepts, process, and practice,* 6th ed., by B. Kozier, G. Erb, A. Berman, & K. Burke, 2000, Upper Saddle River, NJ: Prentice Hall Health. 7-3, 7-4: Nea Hanscomb/*Fundamentals of nursing: Concepts, process, and practice,* 6th ed., by B. Kozier, G. Erb, A. Berman, & K. Burke, 2000, Upper Saddle River, NJ: Prentice Hall Health. 7-6: Jenny Thomas/*Fundamentals of nursing: Concepts, process, and practice,* 6th ed., by B. Kozier, G. Erb, A. Berman, & K. Burke, 2000, Upper Saddle River, NJ: Prentice Hall Health. 7-7: Precision Graphics/*Fundamentals of nursing: Concepts, process, and practice,* 6th ed., by B. Kozier, G. Erb, A. Berman, & K. Burke, 2000, Upper Saddle River, NJ: Prentice Hall Health. 7-8: Precision Graphics/Matt Perry/*Fundamentals of nursing: Concepts, process, and practice,* 6th ed., by B. Kozier, G. Erb, A. Berman, & K. Burke, 2000, Upper Saddle River, NJ: Prentice Hall Health. 7-10B: *Quick reference to pediatric clinical skills,* by R. Bindler & J. Ball, 1999, Upper Saddle River, NJ: Prentice Hall Health.

Chapter 8

Unnumbered photo, 8-3, 8-6, 8-10, 8-11, 8-20, 8-21, 8-22, 8-23, 8-25, 8-26, 8-29, 8-30, 8-32, 8-33, 8-34, 8-35, 8-36, 8-37: George Draper. Unnumbered illustration, 8-1, 8-2, 8-4, 8-5, 8-7, 8-8, 8-9, 8-12, 8-13, 8-14, 8-15, 8-16, 8-17, 8-18, 8-19, 8-24, 8-27, 8-28: Precision Graphics/*Fundamentals of nursing: Concepts, process, and practice,* 6th ed., by B. Kozier, G. Erb, A. Berman, & K. Burke, 2000, Upper Saddle River, NJ: Prentice Hall Health. 8-31: Anne Erickson, CMI.

Chapter 9

9-1A–D: *Medical surgical nursing: Critical thinking in client care,* 2nd ed., by P. LeMone & K. Burke, 2000, Upper Saddle River, NJ: Prentice Hall Health. 9-1E: *Pediatric nursing: Caring for children,* 2nd ed., by J. Ball & R. Bindler, 1999, Stamford, CT: Appleton & Lange.

Chapter 10

Unnumbered photos, 10-3, 10-17: Jenny Thomas/*Fundamentals of nursing: Concepts, process, and practice,* 6th ed., by B. Kozier, G. Erb, A. Berman, & K. Burke, 2000, Upper Saddle River, NJ: Prentice Hall Health. Unnumbered illustrations: Linda Harris and Nea Hanscomb/*Fundamentals of nursing: Concepts, process, and practice,* 6th ed., by B. Kozier, G. Erb, A. Berman, & K. Burke, 2000, Upper Saddle River, NJ: Prentice Hall Health. 10-1: George Draper. 10-2, 10-11, 10-12, 10-13: Linda Harris/*Fundamentals of nursing: Concepts, process, and practice,* 6th ed., by B. Kozier, G. Erb, A. Berman, & K. Burke, 2000, Upper Saddle River, NJ: Prentice Hall Health. 10-4: Precision Graphics/Matt Perry/*Fundamentals of nursing: Concepts, process, and practice,* 6th ed., by B. Kozier, G. Erb, A. Berman, & K. Burke, 2000, Upper Saddle River, NJ: Prentice Hall Health. 10-5, 10-6: Christopher Burke/*Fundamentals of nursing: Concepts, process, and practice,* 6th ed., by B. Kozier, G. Erb, A. Berman, & K. Burke, 2000, Upper Saddle River, NJ: Prentice Hall Health. 10-7: Anne Erickson, CMI. 10-8, 10-9, 10-10, 10-14, 10-15: Precision Graphics/*Fundamentals of nursing: Concepts, process, and practice,* 6th ed., by B. Kozier, G. Erb, A. Berman, & K. Burke, 2000, Upper Saddle River, NJ: Prentice Hall Health. 10-16, 10-18: Elena Dorfman/*Fundamentals of nursing: Concepts, process, and practice,* 6th ed., by B. Kozier, G. Erb, A. Berman, & K. Burke, 2000, Upper Saddle River, NJ: Prentice Hall Health.

Chapter 11

11-1, 11-2, 11-3, 11-4: Nea Hanscomb/*Fundamentals of nursing: Concepts, process, and practice,* 6th ed., by B. Kozier, G. Erb, A. Berman, & K. Burke, 2000, Upper Saddle River, NJ: Prentice Hall Health. 11-5, 11-8: Alain McLaughlin/*Fundamentals of nursing: Concepts, process, and practice,* 6th ed., by B. Kozier, G. Erb, A. Berman, & K. Burke, 2000, Upper Saddle River, NJ: Prentice Hall Health. 11-6, 11-7: George Draper. Table art: *Fundamentals of nursing: Concepts, process, and practice,* 6th ed., by B. Kozier, G. Erb, A. Berman, & K. Burke, 2000, Upper Saddle River, NJ: Prentice Hall Health.

Chapter 12

12-1: Nea Hanscomb/*Fundamentals of nursing: Concepts, process, and practice,* 6th ed., by B. Kozier, G. Erb, A. Berman, & K. Burke, 2000, Upper Saddle River, NJ: Prentice Hall Health. 12-2, 12-3, 12-4, 12-5, 12-13, 12-14, 12-15, 12-16, 12-17, 12-18, 12-19: Linda Harris/*Fundamentals of nursing: Concepts, process, and practice,* 6th ed., by B. Kozier, G. Erb, A. Berman, & K. Burke, 2000, Upper Saddle River, NJ: Prentice Hall Health. 12-6, 12-7: Elena Dorfman/*Fundamentals of nursing: Concepts, process, and practice,* 6th ed., by B. Kozier, G. Erb, A. Berman, & K. Burke, 2000, Upper Saddle River, NJ: Prentice Hall Health. 12-8, 12-9: Alain McLaughlin/*Fundamentals of nursing: Concepts, process, and practice,* 6th ed., by B. Kozier, G. Erb, A. Berman, & K. Burke, 2000, Upper Saddle River, NJ: Prentice Hall Health. 12-10, 12-11, 12-12: George Draper.

Chapter 13

13-1, 13-2: Richard Tauber/*Fundamentals of nursing: Concepts, process, and practice,* 6th ed., by B. Kozier, G. Erb, A. Berman, & K. Burke, 2000, Upper Saddle River, NJ: Prentice Hall Health.

Chapter 14

14-1: Precision Graphics/*Fundamentals of nursing: Concepts, process, and practice,* 6th ed., by B. Kozier, G. Erb, A. Berman, & K. Burke, 2000, Upper Saddle River, NJ: Prentice Hall Health. 14-2: Matt Perry/*Fundamentals of nursing: Concepts, process, and practice,* 6th ed., by B. Kozier, G. Erb, A. Berman, & K. Burke, 2000, Upper Saddle River, NJ: Prentice Hall Health. 14-3: Source: *Wong's essentials of pediatric nursing,* 6/e, by D. L. Wong, M. Hockenberry-Eaton, D. Wison, M. L. Winkelstein, & P. Schwartz, 2001, p. 1301, St. Louis: Copyrighted by Mosby, Inc. Reprinted with permission. 14-4: Courtesy of Aprille Ciavarella, RN, and Lori Townsend, RN, at Sunrise Hospital and Medical Center and Sunrise Children's Hospital, Las Vegas, Nevada. 14-5: Jenny Thomas/ *Fundamentals of nursing: Concepts, process, and practice,* 6th ed., by B. Kozier, G. Erb, A. Berman, & K. Burke, 2000, Upper Saddle River, NJ: Prentice Hall Health.

Chapter 15

15-1, 15-15: George Draper. 15-2, 15-3: *Fundamentals of nursing,* 2nd ed. (vol. 3) (pp. 912–913), by K. J. Berger & M. B. Williams, 1999, Stamford, CT: Appleton & Lange. 15-4: Nea Hanscomb/*Fundamentals of nursing: Concepts, process, and practice,* 6th ed., by B. Kozier, G. Erb, A. Berman, & K. Burke, 2000, Upper Saddle River, NJ: Prentice Hall Health. 15-6, 15-8B, 15-9: Anne Erickson, CMI. 15-10, 15-13: Elena Dorfman/*Fundamentals of nursing: Concepts, process, and practice,* 6th ed., by B. Kozier, G. Erb, A. Berman, & K. Burke, 2000, Upper Saddle River, NJ: Prentice Hall Health. 15-5, 15-7, 15-8A: Courtesy of Ross Products Division of Abbott Laboratories, Columbus, Ohio. 15-11: Christopher Burke/ *Fundamentals of nursing: Concepts, process, and practice,* 6th ed., by B. Kozier, G. Erb, A. Berman, & K. Burke, 2000, Upper Saddle River, NJ: Prentice Hall Health. 15-12, 15-14: Precision Graphics/*Fundamentals of nursing: Concepts, process, and practice,* 6th ed., by B. Kozier, G. Erb, A. Berman, & K. Burke, 2000, Upper Saddle River, NJ: Prentice Hall Health.

Chapter 16

16-1: Jenny Thomas/*Fundamentals of nursing: Concepts, process, and practice,* 6th ed., by B. Kozier, G. Erb, A. Berman, & K. Burke, 2000, Upper Saddle River, NJ: Prentice Hall Health. 16-2, 16-6: Elena Dorfman/*Fundamentals of nursing: Concepts, process, and practice,* 6th ed., by B. Kozier, G. Erb, A. Berman, & K. Burke, 2000, Upper Saddle River, NJ: Prentice Hall Health. 16-3, 16-22, 16-23: George Draper. 16-5: Christopher Burke/*Fundamentals of nursing: Concepts, process, and practice,* 6th ed., by B. Kozier, G. Erb, A. Berman, & K. Burke, 2000, Upper Saddle River, NJ: Prentice Hall Health. 16-7, 16-24: Anne Erickson, CMI. 16-9, 16-11, 16-12, 16-13, 16-14: Matt Perry/*Fundamentals of nursing: Concepts, process, and practice,* 6th ed., by B. Kozier, G. Erb, A. Berman, & K. Burke, 2000, Upper Saddle River, NJ: Prentice Hall Health. 16-4, 16-8, 16-10, 16-21: Linda Harris/*Fundamentals of nursing: Concepts, process, and practice,* 6th ed., by B. Kozier, G. Erb, A. Berman, & K. Burke, 2000, Upper Saddle River, NJ: Prentice Hall Health. 16-15: Courtesy Cymed Ostomy Co., Princeton, New Jersey. 16-16, 16-17, 16-18: Cory Patrick. 16-19, 16-20, 16-25: Courtesy Convatec, A Bristol-Myers Squibb Company. 16-26: *Techniques in clinical nursing,* 4th ed., by Barbara Kozier, Glenora Erb, Kathleen Blais, Joyce Young Johnson, & Jean Smith Temple, 1993, Redwood City, CA: Addison-Wesley.

Chapter 17

17-1, 17-2, 17-16, 17-20, 17-24: Christopher Burke/*Fundamentals of nursing: Concepts, process, and practice,* 6th ed., by B. Kozier, G. Erb, A. Berman, & K. Burke, 2000, Upper Saddle River, NJ: Prentice Hall Health. 17-3: Anne Erickson, CMI. 17-4: Jenny Thomas/*Fundamentals of nursing: Concepts, process, and practice,* 6th ed., by B. Kozier, G. Erb, A. Berman, & K. Burke, 2000, Upper Saddle River, NJ: Prentice Hall Health. 17-5: Courtesy Viscot Industries, Inc., East Hanover, New Jersey. 17-19, 17-21: *Fundamentals of nursing,* 2nd ed. (vol. 3) (p. 988), by K. J. Berger & M. B. Williams, 1999, Stamford, CT: Appleton & Lange. 17-7: George Draper. 17-6, 17-8, 17-9, 17-10, 17-11, 17-12, 17-13, 17-22: Courtesy Bard Medical Division, Covington, California. 17-14, 17-15, 17-17, 17-18: Precision Graphics/*Fundamentals of nursing: Concepts, process, and practice,* 6th ed., by B. Kozier, G. Erb, A. Berman, & K. Burke, 2000, Upper Saddle River, NJ: Prentice Hall Health. 17-23: Kristin Mount/*Fundamentals of nursing: Concepts, process, and practice,* 6th ed., by B. Kozier, G. Erb, A. Berman, & K. Burke, 2000, Upper Saddle River, NJ: Prentice Hall Health. 17-25: Courtesy Cymed Ostomy Co., Princeton, New Jersey.

Chapter 18

18-1: Anne Erickson, CMI. 18-2: Courtesy HealthCare Specialties, LLC/Fresenius, San Diego, California.

Chapter 19

19-1, 19-2: Elena Dorfman/*Fundamentals of nursing: Concepts, process, and practice,* 6th ed., by B. Kozier, G. Erb, A. Berman, & K. Burke, 2000, Upper Saddle River, NJ: Prentice Hall Health. 19-3: *Fundamentals of nursing,* 2nd ed. (vol. 3) (p. 1078), by K. J. Berger & M. B. Williams, 1999, Stamford, CT: Appleton & Lange. 19-4: Jenny Thomas/*Fundamentals of nursing: Concepts, process, and practice,* 6th ed., by B. Kozier, G. Erb, A. Berman, & K. Burke, 2000, Upper Saddle River, NJ: Prentice Hall Health.

Chapter 20

20-1, 20-2: *Fundamentals of nursing,* 2nd ed., (vol. 3) (pp. 1015, 1043), by K. J. Berger & M. B. Williams, 1999, Stamford, CT: Appleton & Lange. 20-3, 20-4: George Draper.

Chapter 21

21-1, 21-11, 21-12: *Fundamentals of nursing,* 2nd ed. (vol. 3) (pp. 1067, 1069), by K. J. Berger & M. B. Williams, 1999, Stamford, CT: Appleton & Lange. 21-2, 21-13, 21-14: George Draper. 21-3: *Emergency care,* 9th ed., by D. Limmer, M. F. O'Keefe, H. D. Grant, R. H. Murray, Jr., & J. D. Bergeron, 2001, Upper Saddle River, NJ: Brady/Prentice Hall Health. 21-4, 21-6, 21-8: Jenny Thomas/*Fundamentals of nursing: Concepts, process, and practice,* 6th ed., by B. Kozier, G. Erb, A. Berman, & K. Burke, 2000, Upper Saddle River, NJ: Prentice Hall Health. 21-5, 21-7: Elena Dorfman/*Fundamentals of nursing: Concepts, process, and practice,* 6th ed., by B. Kozier, G. Erb, A. Berman, & K. Burke, 2000, Upper Saddle River, NJ: Prentice Hall Health. 21-9: Christopher Burke/*Fundamentals of nursing: Concepts, process, and practice,* 6th ed., by B. Kozier, G. Erb, A. Berman, & K. Burke, 2000, Upper Saddle River, NJ: Prentice Hall Health. 21-10: *Quick reference to pediatric clinical skills,* by R. Bindler & J. Ball, 1999, Upper Saddle River, NJ: Prentice Hall Health.

Chapter 22

22-1, 22-2, 22-3, 22-4: Precision Graphics/*Fundamentals of nursing: Concepts, process, and practice,* 6th ed., by B. Kozier, G. Erb, A. Berman, & K. Burke, 2000, Upper Saddle River, NJ: Prentice Hall Health. 22-5: Nea Hanscomb/*Fundamentals of nursing: Concepts, process, and practice,* 6th ed., by B. Kozier, G. Erb, A. Berman, & K. Burke, 2000, Upper Saddle River, NJ: Prentice Hall Health. 22-6, 22-10, 22-13: George Draper. 22-7, 22-11, 22-12: Jenny Thomas/*Fundamentals of nursing: Concepts, process, and practice,* 6th ed., by B. Kozier, G. Erb, A. Berman, & K. Burke, 2000, Upper Saddle River, NJ: Prentice Hall Health. 22-8, 22-9: Linda Harris/*Fundamentals of nursing: Concepts, process, and practice,* 6th ed., by B. Kozier, G. Erb, A. Berman, & K. Burke, 2000, Upper Saddle River, NJ: Prentice Hall Health.

Chapter 23

23-1: Nea Hanscomb/*Fundamentals of nursing: Concepts, process, and practice,* 6th ed., by B. Kozier, G. Erb, A. Berman, & K. Burke, 2000, Upper Saddle River, NJ: Prentice Hall Health. 23-2, 23-5: Elena Dorfman/*Fundamentals of nursing: Concepts, process, and practice,* 6th ed., by B. Kozier, G. Erb, A. Berman, & K. Burke, 2000, Upper Saddle River, NJ: Prentice Hall Health. 23-3: Courtesy Bivona Medical Technologies, Gary, Indiana. 23-4, 23-10: Courtesy Passy-Muir, Inc., Irvine, California. 23-6, 23-8: Jenny Thomas/*Fundamentals of nursing: Concepts, process, and practice,* 6th ed., by B. Kozier, G. Erb, A. Berman, & K. Burke, 2000, Upper Saddle River, NJ: Prentice Hall Health. 23-7: Linda Harris/*Fundamentals of nursing: Concepts, process, and practice,* 6th ed., by B. Kozier, G. Erb, A. Berman, & K. Burke, 2000, Upper Saddle River, NJ: Prentice Hall Health. 23-9: George Draper.

Chapter 24

24-1: Anne Erickson, CMI. 24-2: *Medical surgical nursing: Critical thinking in client care,* 2nd ed., by P. LeMone & K. Burke, 2000, Upper Saddle River, NJ: Prentice Hall Health. 24-3: Elena Dorfman/*Fundamentals of nursing: Concepts, process, and practice,* 6th ed., by B. Kozier, G. Erb, A. Berman, & K. Burke, 2000, Upper Saddle River, NJ: Prentice Hall Health. 24-4, 24-5, 24-6, 24-7, 24-8, 24-9, 24-10: George Draper.

Chapter 25

25-1, 25-2: Anne Erickson. 25-3, 25-9C, 25-25, 25-28, 25-29, 25-30: George Draper. 25-4, 25-9A, 25-11, 25-12, 25-14, 25-16: *First responder,* 5th ed., by J. D. Bergeron & G. Bizjak, 1999, Upper Saddle River, NJ: Prentice Hall. 25-5, 25-6: *Emergency care,* 9th ed., by D. Limmer, M. F. O'Keefe, H. D. Grant, R. H. Murray, Jr., & J. D. Bergeron, 2001, Upper Saddle River, NJ: Brady/Prentice Hall Health. 25-7, 25-8, 25-17, 25-18, 25-19, 25-20, 25-21, 25-22, 25-26, 25-27: *Quick reference to pediatric clinical skills,* by R. Bindler & J. Ball, 1999, Upper Saddle River, NJ: Prentice Hall Health. 25-9B, 25-15: *Prehospital emergency care,* 6th ed., by J. J. Mistovich, B. Q. Hafen, & K. J. Karren, 2000, Upper Saddle River, NJ: Prentice Hall Health. 25-10: Supplement to accompany *Fundamentals of nursing: Concepts, process, and practice,* 6th ed., by B. Kozier, G. Erb, A. Berman, & K. Burke, 2000, Upper Saddle River, NJ: Prentice Hall Health. 25-13: *First responder,* 5th ed., by J. D. Bergeron & G. Bizjak, 1999, Upper Saddle River, NJ: Prentice Hall. 25-23: *Health assessment in nursing,* by L. K. Sims, D. D'Amico, J. K. Stiesmeyer, & J. A. Webster, 1995, Redwood City, CA: Addison-Wesley. 25-24: *Medical surgical nursing: Critical thinking in client care,* 2nd ed., by P. LeMone & K. Burke, 2000, Upper Saddle River, NJ: Prentice Hall Health.

Chapter 26

26-1, 26-5, 26-7, 26-8, 26-9, 26-10: George Draper. 26-2, 26-3: Precision Graphics/*Fundamentals of nursing: Concepts, process, and practice,* 6th ed., by B. Kozier, G. Erb, A. Berman, & K. Burke, 2000, Upper Saddle River, NJ: Prentice Hall Health. 26-4: GTS Graphics/*Fundamentals of nursing: Concepts, process, and practice,* 6th ed., by B. Kozier, G. Erb, A. Berman, & K. Burke, 2000, Upper Saddle River, NJ: Prentice Hall Health. 26-6, 26-11: Elena Dorfman/*Fundamentals of nursing: Concepts, process, and practice,* 6th ed., by B. Kozier, G. Erb, A. Berman, & K. Burke, 2000, Upper Saddle River, NJ: Prentice Hall Health. 26-12: Linda Harris/*Fundamentals of nursing: Concepts, process, and practice,* 6th ed., by B. Kozier, G. Erb, A. Berman, & K. Burke, 2000, Upper Saddle River, NJ: Prentice Hall Health. 26-13: Nea Hanscomb/*Fundamentals of nursing: Concepts, process, and practice,* 6th ed., by B. Kozier, G. Erb, A. Berman, & K. Burke, 2000, Upper Saddle River, NJ: Prentice Hall Health.

Chapter 27

27-1: George Draper. 27-2, 27-3, 27-15: Jenny Thomas/*Fundamentals of nursing: Concepts, process, and practice,* 6th ed., by B. Kozier, G. Erb, A. Berman, & K. Burke, 2000, Upper Saddle River, NJ: Prentice Hall Health. 27-4, 27-7, 27-8: *Quick reference to pediatric clinical skills,* by R. Bindler & J. Ball, 1999, Upper Saddle River, NJ: Prentice Hall Health. 27-5, 27-9, 27-10, 27-11, 27-12, 27-16: Christopher Burke/*Fundamentals of nursing: Concepts, process, and practice,* 6th ed., by B. Kozier, G. Erb, A. Berman, & K. Burke, 2000, Upper Saddle River, NJ: Prentice Hall Health. 27-6: Elena Dorfman/*Fundamentals of nursing: Concepts, process, and practice,* 6th ed., by B. Kozier, G. Erb, A. Berman, & K. Burke, 2000, Upper Saddle River, NJ: Prentice Hall Health. 27-13: Courtesy MABIS Healthcare, Inc., Lake Forest, Illinois. 27-14: *Prehospital emergency care,* 6th ed., by J. J. Mistovich, B. Q. Hafen, & K. J. Karren, 2000, Upper Saddle River, NJ: Prentice Hall Health. 27-17: Anne Erickson, CMI. 27-18: Courtesy Trudell Medical International.

Chapter 28

28-1, 28-2, 28-5, 28-15, 28-34: Nea Hanscomb/*Fundamentals of nursing: Concepts, process, and practice,* 6th ed., by B. Kozier, G. Erb, A. Berman, & K. Burke, 2000, Upper Saddle River, NJ: Prentice Hall Health. 28-3, 28-4, 28-12, 28-13, 28-14, 28-20, 28-30, 28-31, 28-32, unnumbered photos: Elena Dorfman/*Fundamentals of nursing: Concepts, process, and practice,* 6th ed., by B. Kozier, G. Erb, A. Berman, & K. Burke, 2000, Upper Saddle River, NJ: Prentice Hall Health. 28-6, 28-7: Anne Erickson, CMI. 28-16, 28-17, 28-18: Precision Graphics/*Fundamentals of nursing: Concepts, process, and practice,* 6th ed., by B. Kozier, G. Erb, A. Berman, & K. Burke, 2000, Upper Saddle River, NJ: Prentice Hall Health. 28-19, 28-21, 28-22, 28-23, 28-24, 28-25, 28-26, 28-27, 28-28, unnumbered illustration: Christopher Burke/*Fundamentals of nursing: Concepts, process, and practice,* 6th ed., by B. Kozier, G. Erb, A. Berman, & K. Burke, 2000, Upper Saddle River, NJ: Prentice Hall Health. 28-9: Richard Tauber/*Fundamentals of nursing: Concepts, process, and practice,* 6th ed., by B. Kozier, G. Erb, A. Berman, & K. Burke, 2000, Upper Saddle River, NJ: Prentice Hall Health. 28-10, 28-11, 28-29, 28-39, 28-40, 28-41: Jenny Thomas/*Fundamentals of nursing: Concepts, process, and practice,* 6th ed., by B. Kozier, G. Erb, A. Berman, & K. Burke, 2000, Upper Saddle River, NJ: Prentice Hall Health. 28-8, 28-33, 28-37, 28-42: George Draper. 28-35, 28-36C, 28-38: *Fundamentals of nursing,* 2nd ed. (vol. 3) (pp. 1312, 1313), by K. J. Berger & M. B. Williams, 1999, Stamford, CT: Appleton & Lange. 28-36A & B: *Fundamentals of nursing: Concepts, process, and practice,* 6th ed., by B. Kozier, G. Erb, A. Berman, & K. Burke, 2000, Upper Saddle River, NJ: Prentice Hall Health. 28-43: *Techniques in clinical nursing,* 4th ed., by Barbara Kozier, Glenora Erb, Kathleen Blais, Joyce Young Johnson, & Jean Smith Temple, 1993, Redwood City, CA: Addison-Wesley. 28-44: *Medical surgical nursing: Critical thinking in client care,* 2nd ed., by P. LeMone & K. Burke, 2000, Upper Saddle River, NJ: Prentice Hall Health.

Chapter 29

29-1, 29-11: Linda Harris/*Fundamentals of nursing: Concepts, process, and practice,* 6th ed., by B. Kozier, G. Erb, A. Berman, & K. Burke, 2000, Upper Saddle River, NJ: Prentice Hall Health. 29-2: Precision Graphics/*Fundamentals of nursing: Concepts, process, and practice,* 6th ed., by B. Kozier, G. Erb, A. Berman, & K. Burke, 2000, Upper Saddle River, NJ: Prentice Hall Health. 29-3, 29-16, 29-27, 29-32, 29-34: *Quick reference to pediatric clinical skills,* by R. Bindler & J. Ball, 1999, Upper Saddle River, NJ: Prentice Hall Health. 29-4, 29-17, 29-18, 29-19A, 29-20A: Elena Dorfman/*Fundamentals of nursing: Concepts, process, and practice,* 6th ed., by B. Kozier, G. Erb, A. Berman, & K. Burke, 2000, Upper Saddle River, NJ: Prentice Hall Health. 29-5: Matt Perry/*Fundamentals of nursing: Concepts, process, and practice,* 6th ed., by B. Kozier, G. Erb, A. Berman, & K. Burke, 2000, Upper Saddle River, NJ: Prentice Hall Health. 29-6A, 29-13, 29-14, 29-25, 29-26, 29-28: *Fundamentals of nursing,* 2nd ed. (vol. 3) (pp. 1309, 1312, 1313, 1318, 1321, 1327), by K. J. Berger & M. B. Williams, 1999, Stamford, CT: Appleton & Lange. 29-6B, 29-10, 29-15, 29-19B, 29-20B, 29-22, 29-23, 29-30, 29-35: George Draper. 29-7: Courtesy of Becton Dickinson. 29-8, 29-33: Nea Hanscomb/*Fundamentals of nursing: Concepts, process, and practice,* 6th ed., by B. Kozier, G. Erb, A. Berman, & K. Burke, 2000, Upper Saddle River, NJ: Prentice Hall Health. 29-9, 29-29: *Fundamentals of nursing: Concepts, process, and practice,* 6th ed., by B. Kozier, G. Erb, A. Berman, & K. Burke, 2000, Upper Saddle River, NJ: Prentice Hall Health. 29-12: Richard Tauber/*Fundamentals of nursing: Concepts, process, and practice,* 6th ed., by B. Kozier, G. Erb, A. Berman, & K. Burke, 2000, Upper Saddle River, NJ: Prentice Hall Health. 29-21: Courtesy of ALARIS Medical Systems, Inc., San Diego, California. 29-24: Courtesy Alta Bates/Summit Medical Center, Oakland, California. 29-31: Anne Erickson, CMI.

Chapter 30

30-1 Photos: Caliendo/Custom Medical Stock Photos, Inc. 30-2, 30-15, 30-16: Anne Erickson, CMI. 30-3, 30-12, 30-13: Elena Dorfman/*Fundamentals of nursing: Concepts, process, and practice,* 6th ed., by B. Kozier, G. Erb, A. Berman, & K. Burke, 2000, Upper Saddle River, NJ: Prentice Hall Health. 30-4: *Techniques in clinical nursing,* 4th ed., by Barbara Kozier, Glenora Erb, Kathleen Blais, Joyce Young Johnson, & Jean Smith Temple, 1993, Redwood City, CA: Addison-Wesley. 30-5: *Fundamentals of nursing,* 2nd ed. (vol. 3) (p. 851), by K. J. Berger & M. B. Williams, 1999, Stamford, CT: Appleton & Lange. 30-6, 30-7, 30-18: Precision Graphics/*Fundamentals of nursing: Concepts, process, and practice,* 6th ed., by B. Kozier, G. Erb, A. Berman, & K. Burke, 2000, Upper Saddle River, NJ: Prentice Hall Health. 30-8: Jenny Thomas/*Fundamentals of nursing: Concepts, process, and practice,* 6th ed., by B. Kozier, G. Erb, A. Berman, & K. Burke, 2000, Upper Saddle River, NJ: Prentice Hall Health. 30-9: Courtesy Convatec, A Bristol-Myers Squibb Company, Princeton, New Jersey. 30-10, 30-11: George Draper. 30-14, 30-17, 30-19, 30-20: Linda Harris/*Fundamentals of nursing: Concepts, process, and practice,* 6th ed., by B. Kozier, G. Erb, A. Berman, & K. Burke, 2000, Upper Saddle River, NJ: Prentice Hall Health.

Chapter 31

31-1, 31-3, 31-4: George Draper. 31-2B, C, D: *Medical surgical nursing: Critical thinking in client care,* 2nd ed., by P. LeMone & K. Burke, 2000, Upper Saddle River, NJ: Prentice Hall Health. 31-2A, E, F: Anne Erickson, CMI.

Chapter 32

32-1: Christopher Burke/*Fundamentals of nursing: Concepts, process, and practice,* 6th ed., by B. Kozier, G. Erb, A. Berman, & K. Burke, 2000, Upper Saddle River, NJ: Prentice Hall Health. 32-2, 32-3, 32-10, 32-11: Linda Harris/*Fundamentals of nursing: Concepts, process, and practice,* 6th ed., by B. Kozier, G. Erb, A. Berman, & K. Burke, 2000, Upper Saddle River, NJ: Prentice Hall Health. 32-4: *Medical surgical nursing: Critical thinking in client care,* 2nd ed., by P. LeMone & K. Burke, 2000, Upper Saddle River, NJ: Prentice Hall Health. 32-5, 32-12, 32-16, 32-20: *Fundamentals of nursing: Concepts, process, and practice,* 6th ed., by B. Kozier, G. Erb, A. Berman, & K. Burke, 2000, Upper Saddle River, NJ: Prentice Hall Health. 32-15: Anne Erickson, CMI. 32-6, 32-7, 32-9, 32-13, 32-14: *Fundamentals of nursing,* 2nd ed. (vol. 3) (pp. 678, 679, 852, 853), by K. J. Berger & M. B. Williams, 1999, Stamford, CT: Appleton & Lange. 32-8, 32-19: George Draper. 32-17: Jenny Thomas/*Fundamentals of nursing: Concepts, process, and practice,* 6th ed., by B. Kozier, G. Erb, A. Berman, & K. Burke, 2000, Upper Saddle River, NJ: Prentice Hall Health. 32-18: Richard Tauber/*Fundamentals*

Index